国家出版基金项目
NATIONAL PUBLICATION FOUNDATION

National Key Book Publishing Planning Project of the 13th Five-Year Plan

"十三五"国家重点图书出版规划项目

International Clinical Medicine Series Based on the Belt and Road Initiative

"一带一路"背景下国际化临床医学丛书

Traditional Chinese Medicine

中医学

Chief Editor　Huang Yong　Zhu Lifang

主编　黄　泳　　朱荔芳

U0339678

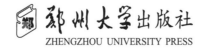

郑州大学出版社

ZHENGZHOU UNIVERSITY PRESS

图书在版编目(CIP)数据

中医学 = Traditional Chinese Medicine：英文／黄泳，朱荔芳主编. — 郑州：郑州大学出版社，2020. 12

("一带一路"背景下国际化临床医学丛书)

ISBN 978-7-5645-6557-2

Ⅰ. ①中… Ⅱ. ①黄…②朱… Ⅲ. ①中医学 – 临床医学 – 英文 Ⅳ. ①R24

中国版本图书馆 CIP 数据核字(2019)第 217861 号

中医学 = Traditional Chinese Medicine：英文

项目负责人	孙保营　杨秦予	策 划 编 辑	李龙传	
责 任 编 辑	刘宇洋	装 帧 设 计	苏永生	
责 任 校 对	张彦勤	责 任 监 制	凌　青　李瑞卿	

出版发行	郑州大学出版社有限公司	地　　址	郑州市大学路 40 号(450052)	
出 版 人	孙保营	网　　址	http://www.zzup.cn	
经　　销	全国新华书店	发行电话	0371-66966070	
印　　刷	河南文华印务有限公司			
开　　本	850 mm×1 168 mm　1 / 16			
印　　张	34.75	字　　数	1 340 千字	
版　　次	2020 年 12 月第 1 版	印　　次	2020 年 12 月第 1 次印刷	

书　　号	ISBN 978-7-5645-6557-2	定　　价	159.00 元	

Staff of Expert Steering Committee

Chairmen

Zhong Shizhen   Li Sijin   Lü Chuanzhu

Vice Chairmen

Bai Yuting	Chen Xu	Cui Wen	Huang Gang	Huang Yuanhua
Jiang Zhisheng	Li Yumin	Liu Zhangsuo	Luo Baojun	Lü Yi
Tang Shiying				

Committee Member

An Dongping	Bai Xiaochun	Cao Shanying	Chen Jun	Chen Yijiu
Chen Zhesheng	Chen Zhihong	Chen Zhiqiao	Ding Yueming	Du Hua
Duan Zhongping	Guan Chengnong	Huang Xufeng	Jian Jie	Jiang Yaochuan
Jiao Xiaomin	Li Cairui	Li Guoxin	Li Guoming	Li Jiabin
Li Ling	Li Zhijie	Liu Hongmin	Liu Huifan	Liu Kangdong
Song Weiqun	Tang Chunzhi	Wang Huamin	Wang Huixin	Wang Jiahong
Wang Jiangang	Wang Wenjun	Wang Yuan	Wei Jia	Wen Xiaojun
Wu Jun	Wu Weidong	Wu Xuedong	Xie Xieju	Xue Qing
Yan Wenhai	Yan Xinming	Yang Donghua	Yu Feng	Yu Xiyong
Zhang Lirong	Zhang Mao	Zhang Ming	Zhang Yu'an	Zhang Junjian
Zhao Song	Zhao Yumin	Zheng Weiyang	Zhu Lin	

专家指导委员会

主 任 委 员

钟世镇　李思进　吕传柱

副主任委员（以姓氏汉语拼音为序）

白育庭　陈　旭　崔　文　黄　钢　黄元华　姜志胜

李玉民　刘章锁　雒保军　吕　毅　唐世英

委　　　员（以姓氏汉语拼音为序）

安东平　白晓春　曹山鹰　陈　君　陈忆九　陈哲生

陈志宏　陈志桥　丁跃明　杜　华　段钟平　官成浓

黄旭枫　简　洁　蒋尧传　焦小民　李才锐　李国新

李果明　李家斌　李　玲　李志杰　刘宏民　刘会范

刘康栋　宋为群　唐纯志　王华民　王慧欣　王家宏

王建刚　王文军　王　渊　韦　嘉　温小军　吴　军

吴卫东　吴学东　谢协驹　薛　青　鄢文海　闫新明

杨冬华　余　峰　余细勇　张莉蓉　张　茂　张　明

张玉安　章军建　赵　松　赵玉敏　郑维扬　朱　林

Staff of Editor Steering Committee

Chairmen

Cao Xuetao   Liang Guiyou   Wu Jiliang

Vice Chairmen

Chen Pingyan   Chen Yuguo   Huang Wenhua   Li Yaming   Wang Heng

Xu Zuojun   Yao Ke   Yao Libo   Yu Xuezhong   Zhao Xiaodong

Committee Member

Cao Hong   Chen Guangjie   Chen Kuisheng   Chen Xiaolan   Dong Hongmei

Du Jian   Du Ying   Fei Xiaowen   Gao Jianbo   Gao Yu

Guan Ying   Guo Xiuhua   Han Liping   Han Xingmin   He Fanggang

He Wei   Huang Yan   Huang Yong   Jiang Haishan   Jin Chengyun

Jin Qing   Jin Runming   Li Lin   Li Ling   Li Mincai

Li Naichang   Li Qiuming   Li Wei   Li Xiaodan   Li Youhui

Liang Li   Lin Jun   Liu Fen   Liu Hong   Liu Hui

Lu Jing   Lü Bin   Lü Quanjun   Ma Qingyong   Ma Wang

Mei Wuxuan   Nie Dongfeng   Peng Biwen   Peng Hongjuan   Qiu Xinguang

Song Chuanjun   Tan Dongfeng   Tu Jiancheng   Wang Lin   Wang Huijun

Wang Peng   Wang Rongfu   Wang Shusen   Wang Chongjian   Xia Chaoming

Xiao Zheman   Xie Xiaodong   Xu Falin   Xu Xia   Xu Jitian

Xue Fuzhong   Yang Aimin   Yang Xuesong   Yi Lan   Yin Kai

Yu Zujiang   Yu Hong   Yue Baohong   Zeng Qingbing   Zhang Hui

Zhang Lin   Zhang Lu   Zhang Yanru   Zhao Dong   Zhao Hongshan

Zhao Wen   Zheng Yanfang   Zhou Huaiyu   Zhu Changju   Zhu Lifang

编审委员会

Editorial Staff

Wang Xiaoyan	Shandong University of Traditional Chinese Medicine
Xiong Ying	Nanjing University of Chinese Medicine
Yang Yang	Hebei University of Chinese Medicine
Yang Zhonghua	Guangzhou University of Chinese Medicine
Yang Zongbao	Xiamen University
Yao Zengyu	Southern Medical University
Yu Bin	Jining Medical University
Yuan Xiaoxia	Xinjiang Medical University
Zhai Fengting	Shandong University of Traditional Chinese Medicine
Zhang Jiping	Southern Medical University
Zhang Zhinan	Southern Medical University
Zhu Mingmin	Jinan University

Illustrator

Pan Boqun

作者名单

主　审
　　唐纯志　　广州中医药大学
主　编
　　黄　泳　　南方医科大学
　　朱荔芳　　济宁医学院
副主编
　　郑桂芝　　济宁医学院
　　王欣君　　南京中医药大学
　　王　颖　　浙江中医药大学
　　张　梁　　广州中医药大学
编　委（以姓氏汉语拼音为序）
　　别明珂　　湖南中医药大学
　　蔡晓雯　　南方医科大学
　　崔瑞琴　　宁夏医科大学
　　何玲玲　　福建中医药大学
　　黄焕琳　　新西兰中医针灸学校
　　李　琳　　山东中医药大学
　　李乃奇　　南方医科大学
　　刘彦玲　　遵义医科大学
　　罗华丽　　重庆医科大学
　　曲姗姗　　南方医科大学
　　宋观礼　　中国中医科学院广安门医院
　　隋　华　　大连医科大学
　　孙　闵　　济宁医学院
　　唐利龙　　宁夏医科大学
　　屠文展　　温州医科大学
　　王　蕊　　河北中医学院
　　王蔚琳　　广州医科大学
　　王晓燕　　山东中医药大学
　　熊　英　　南京中医药大学

杨　阳　　河北中医学院
杨忠华　　广州中医药大学
杨宗保　　厦门大学
姚锃钰　　南方医科大学
于　斌　　济宁医学院
袁晓霞　　新疆医科大学
翟凤婷　　山东中医药大学
张继苹　　南方医科大学
张治楠　　南方医科大学
朱明敏　　暨南大学

绘图者
　　潘伯群

Preface

At the Second Belt and Road Summit Forum on International Cooperation in 2019 and the Seventy-third World Health Assembly in 2020, General Secretary Xi Jinping stated the importance for promoting the construction of the "Belt and Road" and jointly build a community for human health. Countries and regions along the "Belt and Road" have a large number of overseas Chinese communities, and shared close geographic proximity, similarities in culture, disease profiles and medical habits. They also shared a profound mass base with ample space for cooperation and exchange in Clinical Medicine. The publication of the International Clinical Medicine series for clinical researchers, medical teachers and students in countries along the "Belt and Road" is a concrete measure to promote the exchange of Chinese and foreign medical science and technology with mutual appreciation and reciprocity.

Zhengzhou University Press coordinated more than 600 medical experts from over 160 renowned medical research institutes, medical schools and clinical hospitals across China. It produced this set of medical tools in English to serve the needs for the construction of the "Belt and Road". It comprehensively coversaspects in the theoretical framework and clinical practicesin Clinical Medicine, including basic science, multiple clinical specialities and social medicine. It reflects the latest academic and technological developments, and the international frontiers of academic advancements in Clinical Medicine. It shared with the world China's latest diagnosis and therapeutic approaches, clinical techniques, and experiences in prescription and medication. It has an important role in disseminating contemporary Chinese medical science and technology innovations, demonstrating the achievements of modern China's economic and social development, and promoting the unique charm of Chinese culture to the world.

The series is the first set of medical tools written in English by Chinese medical experts to serve the needs of the "Belt and Road" construction. It systematically and comprehensively reflects the Chinese characteristics in Clinical Medicine. Also, it presents a landmark achievement in the implementation of the "Belt and Road" initiative in promoting exchanges in medical science and technology. This series is theoretical in nature, with each volume built on the mainlines in traditional disciplines but at the same time introducing contemporary theories that guide clinical practices, diagnosis and treatment methods, echoing the latest research findings in Clinical Medicine.

As the disciplines in Clinical Medicine rapidly advances, different views on knowledge, inclusiveness, and medical ethics may arise. We hope this work will facilitate the exchange of ideas, build common ground while allowing differences, and contribute to the building of a community for human health in a broad spectrum of disciplines and research focuses.

Nick Lemoine

Foreign Academician of the Chinese Academy of Engineering
Dean, Academy of Medical Sciences of Zhengzhou University
Director, Barts Cancer Institute, London, UK
6th August, 2020

Foreword

The Belt and Road Development Plan of *TCM* (2016–2020) was put forward to implement *Vision and Action on Jointly Building Silk Road Economic Belt and the* 21*st Century Maritime Silk Road* (the Belt and Road, B&R), issued by the National Development and Reform Commission, Ministry of Foreign Affairs, and Ministry of Commerce of the People's Republic of China, with State Council authorization in March 2015. We aim to enhance communication and strengthen cooperation with foreign countries, and create a new pattern of all-facet opening up in TCM field. Nowadays, TCM has been spread to 183 countries and regions. As an important part of the international medical system, TCM is playing an active role in protecting human health.

In order to introduce TCM with its unique advantages to the world and make contribution to human health cause, Zhengzhou University Press organized the compilation of this book to promote and spread TCM culture.

TCM is a comprehensive discipline, including fundamental theories of TCM, diagnostics of TCM, Chinese materia medica, prescription, acupuncture and moxibustion, traditional Chinese tuina and clinical discipline such as internal medicine, surgery, gynecology, and pediatric of TCM etc. All these essential parts of TCM are included in this textbook. We cover all the contents from theoretical basis to clinical practice comprehensively, which are under the guideline of classic inheritance and the essence of TCM. The clinical practical parts are also emphsized to enable students to turn knowledge into useful skills. Different topics are designed detailedly or briefly under a systematical framework, while practical clinical skills and information are highlighted comparatively.

This is a TCM book in English compiled by 37 teachers and experts in universities, colleges and hospitals with experiences of teaching in English to ensure the accuracy of TCM theory and language expression. During the compilation, drafts were modified, revised and collated with the help of a great number of professors.

In this book, philosophical foundation, physiology and pathology, etiology, differentiation and diagnostics, and health-preservation of TCM, Chinese materia medica and prescription, acupuncture and moxibustion, characteristic therapies, and common clinical disease are systematically arranged. From Chapter 1–4, a clear picture of the philosophical foundation of TCM from yin-yang, five-element, qi, blood, body fluids and zang-fu viscera theory is presented. From Chapter 5–7 include etiology, pathogenesis, diagnostic and differentiation of syndromes. Chapter 8 is one of the most popular chapters with a topic of health-preservation. Chapter 9 and Chapter 10 are about Chinese materia medica and prescription, presenting the tropism of natures, flavors and meridians, as well as commonly used prescription. Acupuncture and moxibustion therapy is the topic of Chapter 11, meridians and acupoints and acupuncture techniques are explained systematically and thoroughly. Chapter 12 is about some particular therapies such as massage, dietary therapy, qigong and Tai Chi. Chapter 13 mainly presents clinical TCM therapies of common diseases. And the last is appendix which provides supplementary materials as references.

Prof. Tang Chunzhi, dean of Clinical Medical College of Acupuncture, Moxibustion and Rehabilitation, Guangzhou University of TCM, is the chief reviser of the compilation board. Prof. Huang Yong, director of Acupuncture and Moxibustion Department, School of TCM, Southern Medical University, and Prof. Zhu Li-fang, vice director of International Exchanges & Cooperation Deparment, Jining Medical University, are chief editors in charge of the compilation. All the editorial board members worked hard with clear division and efficient cooperation of work in compiling this book.

It is a great challenge to compile an English book of TCM. If you find any errors or mistakes that might exist in the book, please do not hesitate to let us know. We are always open to suggestions and comments, and strive to improve it for a new edition.

Authors

Contents

Chapter 1

Introduction

1.1　General introduction to Traditional Chinese Medicine

Traditional Chinese Medicine(TCM) which is an alternative therapy, originated in China and has evolved over thousands of years. TCM practitioners use herbal medicines, acupuncture and moxibustion, traditional Chinese tuina, dietary therapy and tai chi, etc. , for diseases prevention and treatment.

The formation and the development of TCM were through the daily life of ancient Chinese people and in the process of their fight against diseases over thousands of years. In ancient times, people found that eating some specific food, using grinding stones or heat stimulating on special parts of body could relieve pains. These usages gradually resulted in herbal therapy, acupuncture and moxibustion therapy, and traditional Chinese tuina therapy.

During the Spring and Autumn Period(770B. C. −476B. C.), the Warring States Period(475B. C. − 221B. C.) and the Han Dynasty(202B. C. −220A. D.), the rapid development of the science and the culture made a foundation for TCM theoretical system.

From the Han Dynasty(202B. C.) to the Qing Dynasty(1912A. D.), lots of physicians practiced TCM and continuously promoted its development. During that time, many famous doctors appeared and they published a lot of books about their theories.

Since the founding of the People's Republic of China in 1949, Chinese government has set great store by TCM and rendered vigorous support to its development. In 1950, Chairman Mao Zedong made a speech in support of TCM stating the combination of Chinese traditional medicine and Western medicine can better protect people from diseases and improve public health.

TCM represents a combination of natural sciences and humanities, and profoundly embraces the philosophy of the Chinese nation. Applying such principles as "harmony of nature and human", "balance of yin and yang", and "treatment should aim to the essence", TCM embodies the core value of Chinese civilization. It is also advocated that "the environment, the individual constitution, and the conditions of climate and season should be fully considered during the syndrome differentiation practicing and therapeutic determination". Ideas such as "reinforcing the fundamental, cultivating the vital energy, and strengthening tendons and bones", and "mastership of medicine lying in proficient medical skills and lofty medical ethics", provide an enlightened base on which the world is studied. This is a major means to help Chinese people to maintain health, cure diseases, and live a long life.

There are four conditions for the formation of TCM theoretical system.

Firstly, the social changes and the contention among the hundred schools of thought created a social condition for the TCM theoretical system. The idea "harmony of nature and human" at that time was a great influence on TCM, emphasizing the relationship between nature and human beings.

Secondly, natural science in the Qin and Han Dynasty (221B. C. – 220A. D.) had outstanding achievements in astronomy, geography, meteorology, science of calendar, phenology, agriculture, botany, mineralogy, smelting technology and zymotechnique, and it was also an inner power for TCM theoretical system development.

Thirdly, Chinese ancient doctors accumulated and summarized lots of medicine knowledge in long-term medical practice. For example, in Shang Dynasty (1600B. C. – 1046B. C.), ancient doctors used herbal medicines to treat diseases; in Western Zhou Dynasty (1046B. C. – 771B. C.), ancient doctors established the name of the diseases and advanced herbal therapy theory; in Spring and Autumn Period (770B. C. – 476B. C.), a doctor called Yi He advanced the first etiology theory; and in the Warring States Period, professional doctors appeared such as Bian Que and Cang Gong, who established the diagnostic methodology.

And fourthly, ancient Chinese philosophy provided for TCM the method of thinking. The theory of qi, or monism of qi, which was one of the representative theories of the developmental traditional Chinese philosophy in the pre-Qin Period (before 221B. C.), then the theory of yin and yang, and the theory of five elements are the three most basic ideas of traditional Chinese philosophy, forming the unique thinking mode and cultural concept of Chinese nations. Ancient Chinese people would use philosophic concepts and terms to illustrate their ideas.

To enrich treatment methods, TCM also absorbed the essence of other civilizations. Chinese people discovered the frankincense and myrrh could be used for therapeutic disease. Meanwhile, with its development, TCM was gradually spread throughout the world. As early as in Qin and Han Dynasties (221B. C. – 220A. D.), TCM was popular in many neighboring countries and influenced their traditional medicines at the same time. The technique of smallpox vaccination in TCM was spread outside China during the Ming and Qing Dynasties (1368A. D. – 1912A. D.). The *Bencao Gangmu* (*Compendium of Materia Medica*) was translated into various languages, and was hailed as "ancient Chinese encyclopedia" by Charles Darwin, the British biologist. The acupuncture and moxibustion has won the popularity throughout the world for the remarkable effects. The discovery of Qinghaosu (artemisinin, an anti-malaria drug) has saved millions of lives, especially in developing countries.

In recent years, TCM has got more and more domestic and international recognition. Many countries cover the acupuncture and Chinese herbs in hospitalization insurance systems. An increasing number of foreigners come to China to study TCM, and many countries such as America, England, Germany, Japan, Malaysia and Singapore, etc. , have set up educational bases to train TCM talents. All these improvements have aroused more interest in TCM study and application.

1.2 Brief history of TCM

1.2.1 The beginning of TCM

In the primitive society, our ancestors spontaneously formed the perceptual treatment knowledge for surviving in the fight with nature and beasts. During the process of gathering foods, Chinese ancestors came to realize the harms and the benefits of plants, minerals and the different parts of animals, and then consciously made use of them. Acupuncture appeared after Neolithic Age. Firstly, people begun to grasp the technology of forging, controlling and grinding, then they made more types of stones(also the Stone for medicine), and over time the acupuncture techniques were developed. When people lit fire for heating, they found it could help to relieve pain. They wrapped hot stones or sand with animal skins or tree bark and attached them to a part of body to relieve pain. This is the beginning of heat ironing. This period was before the Spring and Autumn(770B. C. –476B. C.) and was the beginning of TCM, and manifested the initial tools, techniques and the fundamental thought.

1.2.2   Marks of formation of TCM

During the Qin Period(221B. C. –207B. C.) and the Han Period(202B. C. –220A. D.), the publishment of *Huangdi Neijing*(*Internal Classic*), *Nanjing* (*Classic of Difficult Issues*), *Shanghan Zabing Lun* (*Treatise on Cold Damage and Miscellaneous Diseases*) and *Shennong Bencao Jing*(*Shennong's Classic of the Materia Medica*) marked the establishment of the TCM theoretical system.

Internal Classic was divided into *Suwen*(*Plain Questions*) and *Lingshu*(*Miraculous Pivot*), and was written in the Spring and Autumn Period(770B. C. –476B. C.) to Qin and Han Periods(221B. C. –220A. D.). It was the summary of medical achievements from the pre-Qin Period(before 221B. C.) to Western Han Dynasty(202B. C. –9A. D.), including medical experience and theoretical accumulation. The book systematically expounded the contents of yin and yang, five elements, visceral manifestations, meridians and collaterals, etiology, pathogenesis, disease and syndrome, diagnostic methods, principles of treatment, acupuncture and moxibustion, and herbology. It was the earliest medical anthology in China, establishing the principal theories and laying the theoretical basis of TCM.

Classic of Difficult Issues is believed to be written in the Western Han Dynasty(202B. C. –9A. D.) by Qin Yueren(Bian Que). It took the form of "questions and answers" to discuss the zang-fu viscera, meridians and collaterals, pulse taking, acupoints and techniques of acupuncture, and is regarded as a classic medical book comparable to *Internal Classic*. Both of *Classic of Difficult Issues* and *Internal Classic* are the foundation of the TCM theoretical system and the clinical practice.

Treatise on Cold Damage and Miscellaneous Diseases was written by Zhang Zhongjing at the end of the Eastern Han Dynasty(25A. D. –220A. D.). It was the first monograph of TCM in which treating diseases was based on syndrome differentiation. The book was divided into *Shanghanlun*(*Treatise on Cold Damage Diseases*) and *Jingui YaoLue*(*Synopsis of Golden Chamber*). *Treatise on Cold Damage Diseases* advanced a new theory called syndrome differentiation of six meridians, and made a comprehensive and systematic analysis for the contents of the exogenous contraction diseases such as etiology, clinical features, diagnostics, treatments and prognosis. *Synopsis of Golden Chamber* suggested that the miscellaneous diseases should be dealt with through the syndrome differentiation of zang-fu viscera, and recorded the etiology, pathogenesis, diagnostics and treatment for nearly forty kinds of diseases. The book intergrated basic theory of TCM and clinical practice tightly together, and established the guidelines of treatments based on syndrome differentiation relevant to diagnostic treatments. Many prescriptions in this book are even in use now, so it is known as "the ancestor of prescriptions".

Shennong's Classic of the Materia Medica was written approximately in the Han Dynasty(202B. C. –220A. D.). It was the earliest monograph of herbal medicines in China. The book summarized the achievement about the pharmacology before the Han Dynasty(202B. C. –220A. D.). There are 365 herbs recorded in this book, which were divided into upper, middle and lower grades according to the effectiveness, toxicity and different applications. It recorded the performance and indications of each herb, and additionally discussed the theory of medicinal properties of four natures and five flavors, establishing the principle of medication and the theory of compatibility of medicines, and provided the basis of pharmacology for TCM theoretical system. It combined the pharmacology and the pathology together, and enriched the TCM theoretical system.

Above all, with the help of these medical works, the past achievements were summarized respectively as basic theory, clinical medicine and medicinal knowledge. The scattered medical knowledge and experience were assembled into a systematic theory. The ancient Chinese doctors in this period were good at combining theory and practice, formed and constantly improved the unique theoretical system of TCM, including treating principle and prescription. This system laid the foundation for the later development of TCM(Table 1–1).

Table 1–1   **Representative works in Spring and Autumn States, Warring States, Qin and Han Dynasties**

Dynasty	Name of work	Author	Achievement and contribution
The Spring and Autumn States (770B.C.–476B.C.)	*Internal Classic*	Numerous experts	Summarizing medical achievements including experiences and theories from the pre-Qin period to Western Han Dynasty. As the earliest medical anthology in China, it represented the highest level of Chinese medical theory
The Warring States (475B.C.–221B.C.)	*Yinyang Shiyimai Jiujing* (11 *Yin and Yang Meridians for Moxibustion*) and *Zu Bi Shi Yi Mai Jiu Jing* (11 *Hand and Foot Meridians for Moxibustion*)	Anonymous	One of the origins of acupuncture and moxibustion
	Daoyintu (*Guided Maps*)	Anonymous	The earliest monograph of medical exercises in China
The Western Han Dynasty (202B.C.–9A.D.)	*Classic of Difficult Issues*	Bian Que	Another classic of TCM, the supplementation of *Internal Classic*, laying the foundation of the theoretical system of TCM
	52 *Bingfang* (*Formulas for Fifty-two Diseases*)	Anonymous	The earliest monograph of prescriptions in China
The Eastern Han Dynasty (25A.D.–220A.D.)	*Shennong's Classic of the Materia Medica*	Numerous experts	The earliest monograph of material medica recorded in China
The end of Eastern-Han Dynasty (184A.D.–220A.D.)	*Treatise on Cold Damage and Miscellaneous Diseases*	Zhang Zhongjing	The first clinical medical monograph of TCM treating diseases based on syndrome differentiation

1.2.3 Development of TCM

1.2.3.1   Period of Wei, Jin, Sui and Tang Dynasties(220A. D. –960A. D.)

As a link between the pre-accumulation and post-development, the construction of clinical medicine during this period well prepared for the development of the theoretical system of TCM. In this period, numbers of the TCM branch subjects emerged and became more mature. With the development of the politics, economics and culture, the level of the medical theory and clinical skills were improved. Meanwhile, social stability and economic prosperity promoted the communication between Chinese and foreign medicine. For instance, TCM spread to Japan, Korea and Southeast Asian countries, while Indian and Persian medicine enriched TCM with Buddhism introduced into China. Many famous doctors and medical works appeared in this period.

Maijing (*Pulse Classic*) was written in Jin Dynasty(265A. D. –420A. D.) by Wang Shuhe. It is the first monograph of sphygmology in China, promoting the application of pulse taking method. The book comprehensively and systematically expounded upon pulse diagnostics, described and explained 24 kinds of morbid pulse conditions, and advanced the method to identify eight groups of similar pulses.

Zhenjiu Jiayijing (*A–B Classic of Acupuncture and Moxibustion*) was written by Huangfu Mi in the Jin Dynasty(265A. D. –420A. D.). It is the earliest existing acupuncture monograph in China, summarizing acupuncture achievements before the Wei and Jin Dynasties, containing pathogenesis, diagnostics, zang-fu viscera, meridians, acupoints, manipulations, indications and contraindications of acupuncture and moxibustion. It confirmed the location, indication and operation of 349 acupoints in human body, including 49 single and 300 double acupoints. This book made a great contribution to the development of the acupuncture and moxibustion.

Zhubing Yuanhoulun (*Treatise on the Origins and Manifestations of Various Diseases*) was written by Chao Yuanfang in the Sui Dynasty(581A. D. –618A. D.). It is the first monograph for etiology, pathogenesis and symptomatology. It discussed the pathogenic factors, pathogenesis and symptoms of diseases in various clinical subjects such as internal medicine, surgery, gynecology, pediatric, ophthalmology, otorhinolaryngology, and dermatology and so on. This book promoted the development of diagnostics and treatment based on syndrome differentiation.

Beiji Qianjin Yaofang (*Essential Prescriptions Worth a Thousand Gold for Emergencies*) and *Qianjin Yifang* (*Supplement to the Essential Prescriptions Worth a Thousand Gold*) were written by Sun Simiao in the Tang Dynasty(618A. D. –907A. D.). These two books are the earliest medical encyclopedias in China, containing the differentiation of pulse syndrome, diagnostic method, treating principles, prescription, acupuncture method and dietary supplements which were used before Tang Dynasty(618A. D. –907A. D.). These two books represented the level of medical development at that time. Moreover, the author as a physician, put forward the standards of medical ethics that "an excellent doctor should have perfect skill and absolute sincerity", which became the essence of the medical ethics in China.

This was the period for massive development of clinical medicine. In China the first monographs of pediatrics, gynecology, orthopedics and surgery all emerged in this period(Table 1–2).

Table 1-2   **Representative works in Wei,Jin,Sui and Tang Dynasties**

Dynasty	Name of work	Author	Achievement
The Jin Dynasty (266A. D. –420A. D.)	Zhouhou Beijifang (Handbook of Prescriptions for Emergency)	Ge Hong	The first emergency manual in China
	Pulse Classic	Wang Shuhe	The first sphygmology monograph in China
	A – B Classic of Acupuncture and Moxibustion	Huangfu Mi	The first monograph for acupuncture and moxibustion in China
The Northern and Southern Dynasties (420A. D. –589A. D.)	Bencao Jingjizhu (Collective Commentaries on the Classic of Materia Medica)	Tao Hongjing	Putting forward the classification method of medicines
	Leigong Paozhilun (Master Lei's Discourse on Medicinal Processing)	Lei Xiao	The first monograph for herbs processing in China
	Liujuanzi Guiyifang (Liu Juanzi's Ghost-Bequeathed Formulas)	Gong Qingxuan	The first monograph for surgery in China
The Sui Dynasty (581A. D. –618A. D.)	Treatise on the Origins and Manifestations of Various Diseases	Chao Yuanfang	The first monograph for etiology,pathogenesis and symptomatology in China
The Tang Dynasty (618A. D. –907A. D.)	Xinxiu Bencao (Newly Revised Materia Medica)	Su Jing(chief editor)	The first pharmacopoeia enacted by the government and the world's earliest pharmacopeia
	Luxinjing (Cranial Fontanelle Classic)	Shi Wu	The first monograph for pediatrics in China
	Jingxiao Chanbao (Tested Treasures in Obstetrics)	Zan Yin	The first monograph for gynecology in China
	Xianshou Lishangxu Duanmifang (Surgical Care of the Injuring)	Lin Daoren	The first monograph for orthopedics in China
	Essential Prescriptions Worth a Thousand Gold for Emergencies and Supplement to the Essential Prescriptions Worth a Thousand Gold	Sun Simiao	The first medical encyclopedia in China
	Waitai Miyao (Arcane Essentials from the Imperial Library)	Wang Tao	Comprehensive medical work compiled with literature

1.2.3.2　Period of Song,Jin,and Yuan Dynasties(960A. D. –1368A. D.)

In this period,TCM theoretical system and various clinical subjects developed rapidly,and new schools of thoughts came into formation. A large number of Chinese medical works began to be compiled in some other countries and published at that time,and the authorities also began to normalize the prescription,meridians and acupoints.

Sanyinji Yibingzheng Fanglun(*Treatise on Diseases*,*Patterns*,*and Formulas Related to the Unification of the Three Etiologes*) was written by Chen Wuze in the Song Dynasty(1127A. D. –1279A. D.). The book combined the etiology and the syndromes,and put forward and expounded the classification of etiology as three aspects:exogenous,endogenous and non-endo-exogenous cause. It was a great influence on the development of etiology.

In the Jin and Yuan Dynasties(1115A. D. –1368A. D.),the most celebrated representatives were the "four great physicians of Jin and Yuan Dynasties",namely Liu Wansu, Zhang Congzheng,Li Gao and Zhu Zhenheng(Table 1–3).

Table 1–3　**Four great physicians of Jin and Yuan Dynasties**

Name	School	Academic view	Therapy characteristics	Medical works
Liu Wansu	School of cold and cool	Six climatic factors transformed into fire and extremely hyperactivity of five emotions can all lead to fire	Mainly cooling and purging fire	*Su Wen Xuan Ji Yuan Bing Shi* (*Explanation of Mysterious Pathogeneses and Etiologies Based on the Plain Questions*) ,*Su Wen Xuan Ming Lun Fang* (*Formulas from the Discussion Illuminating the Plain Questions*)
Zhang Congzheng	School of eliminating pathogen	Eliminating pathogen is the key for treating disease and tonic shouldn't be used too frequently	Mainly inducing sweating,emesis and purgation	*Ru Men Shi Qin*(*Confucians' Duties to Their Parents*)
Li Gao	School of strengthening the earth (spleen)	The occurrence of disease is mostly related to the endogenous injury of spleen and stomach	Mainly nourishing spleen and stomach	*Pi Wei Lun*(*Treatise on the Spleen and Stomach*)
Zhu Zhenheng	School of nourishing yin	Yang is always excessive while yin is always in deficiency	Mainly nourishing yin and reducing fire	*Ge Zhi Yu Lun*(*Further Discourses on the Acquisition of Knowledge through Profound Study*)

The advocating theories and clinical practice of the "four great physicians of Jin and Yuan Dynasties" are breakthrough innovations in the theory and practice of TCM and also the milestone in the development of TCM(Table 1–4).

Table 1-4   Representative works of TCM in Song, Jin and Yuan Dynasties

Dynasty	Name of work	Author	Achievement
The Song Dynasty (960A. D. – 1279A. D.)	*Taiping Huimin Hejiju Fang* (*Benedicial Formulas from the Taiping Imperial Pharmacy*)	The Imperial Medical Bureau (set up by Song government)	The first monograph of patent medicine preparation enacted by government
	Bencao Tujing (*Illustrated Classic of Materia Medica*)	Su Song	The first engraved block printing of illustrations for medicinal herbs
	Furen Daquan Liangfang (*The Complete Compendium of Fine Formulas for Women*)	Chen Ziming	Comprehensive monograph of gynecology and obstetrics
	Sanyinji Yibingzheng Fanglun (*Treatise on Diseases, Patterns, and Formulas Related to the Unification of the Three Etiologies*)	Chen Wuze	Putting forward the classification of etiology as three aspects: exogenous, endogenous and non-endo-exogenous causes
	Xiyuanji Lu (*Records for Vindication*)	Song Ci	The first Chinese monograph of forensic medicine that has great effects both domestically and internationally
The Yuan Dynasty (1271A. D. – 1368A. D.)	*Aoshi Shanghan Jinjing Lu* (*Ao's Golden Mirror Records for Cold Pathogenic Diseases*)	Du Qingbi	The first monograph of tongue diagnostics

1. 2. 3. 3   Period of Ming and Qing Dynasties(1368A. D. –1911A. D.)

In the Ming and Qing Dynasties, TCM theoretical system further developed. In this period, the significant achievement was the development of life gate doctrine and the innovation of the theory of epidemic febrile diseases. Moreover, a large number of integrated medical encyclopedia, series, and works enriched and developed the TCM theoretical system, including *Zhengzhi Zhunsheng* (*Standards for Diagnostics and Treatment*) , *Jingyue Quanshu* (*The Complete Works of Zhang Jingyue*) , and *Yizong Jinjian* (*Golden Mirror of Medicine*) , etc.

New contents were added to the zang-fu viscera theory of TCM by the development of the life gate doctrine. Many doctors like Zhang Jingyue and Zhao Xianke, attached importance to the life gate doctrine, and innovated the concept and the function of the life gate doctrine. The life gate doctrine greatly influenced the development of TCM theory and clinical practice, with important guiding significance up to now.

Epidemic febrile disease is a collective name for various acute febrile diseases, which are mostly infectious and epidemic. The epidemic febrile disease doctrine originated from *Internal Classic*, *Classic of Difficult Issues* and *Treatise on Cold Damage and Miscellaneous Diseases*. The theory of epidemic febrile disease gradually became more mature and more independent in the late Ming Dynasty and the early Qing Dynasty.

Wenyilun (*Treatise on Epidemic Febrile Diseases*) was written by Wu Youxing. In this work, he put forward the theory of "epidemic pathogen (pestilential qi)", holding that the epidemic febrile diseases were caused by pestilential qi rather than the six exogenous pathogenic factors. And such pestilential qi that is often infectious invades body from nose and mouth and can cause regional pandemics, with similar symptoms and course.

Wang Qingren is the author of *Yilin Gaicuo* (*Correction of Errors in Medical Works*). The book corrected some errors in human anatomy in ancient medical books and developed the theory of blood stasis. It also established many effective formulas to treat the symptoms of blood stasis. The book made certain contributions to the development of qi and blood theory.

In this period, theories and experiences in early ages were coordinated and a large number of monographs were established. For example, *Compendium of Materia Medica* was a great monograph of herbal medicine written by Li Shizhen in the Ming Dynasty (1368A. D. – 1644A. D.). It covered 1892 kinds of Chinese medicinal herbs with more than 1000 pictures and 11 096 prescriptions. Herbal medicines are classified into 16 classes and 62 topics by the most advanced and scientific classification. After publication, the book was translated into Korean, Japanese, Latin, English, French, German, and Russian and was spread internationally with a great influence in the world. *Gujin Yitong Daquan* (*Ancient and Modern Medical Complete Book*) was a famous medical encyclopedia written by Xu Chunfu in the Ming Dynasty (1368A. D. – 1644A. D.). *Standards for Diagnostics and Treatment* was a famous clinical medical series of TCM written by Wang Kentang in the Ming Dynasty (1368A. D. –1644A. D.) (Table 1–5).

Table 1–5   **Representative works of TCM in the Ming and Qing Dynasties**

Dynasty	Name of work	Author	Achievement
The Ming Dynasty (1368A. D. –1644A. D.)	*Compendium of Materia Medica*	Li Shizhen	Chinese medical herbs cyclopedia in the ancient China, regarded as the great pharmacopoeia in the orient
	Pujifang (Formulas for Universal Relief)	Teng Shuo, Liu Chun	The maximal prescription work in Ancient China, including 61 739 prescriptions
	The Complete Works of Zhang Jingyue	Zhang Jingyue	The summarization of TCM theory and experience of the Ming Dynasty and before
	Yiguan (*Key Link of Medicine*)	Zhao Xianke	Putting forth the theory of Mingmen doctrine
	Waike Zhengzong (*Orthodox Lineage of External Medicine*)	Chen Shigong	The first monograph of surgery that recorded and discussed tumor

Continue to Table 1-5

Dynasty	Name of work	Author	Achievement	
The Qing Dynasty (1644A. D. –1912A. D.)	*Treatise on Epidemic Febrile Diseases*	Wu Youxing	Putting forward the theory of "epidemic pathogen(pestilential qi)"	Formation and development of warm febrile disease
	Wenrelun (Treatise on Warm-Heat Diseases)	Ye Gui	Putting forward syndrome differentiation of defense-qi-nutrient-blood	
	Shire Tiaobian (Systematic Differentiation of Damp-Heat Diseases)	Xue Xue	The monograph of dampness-heat diseases	
	Wenbing Tiaobian (Systematic Differentiation of Epidemic Febrile Diseases)	Wu Tang	Putting forward syndrome differentiation of *sanjiao*	
	Wenre Jingwei (Warp and Woof of Warm-Heat diseases)	Wang Mengying	Focus on latent-qi warm febrile disease	
	Yifang Jijie (Medical Formulas Collected and Analyzed)	Wang Ang	Useful clinical prescription book classified according to functions and indications	
	Correction of Errors in Medical Works	Wang Qingren	Focus on anatomy and develop the theory of blood stasis as a cause of disease	
	Fuqing Zhu Nvke (Fu Qingzhu's Obstetrics and Gynecology)	Fu Shan	The monograph of gynecology	
	Youyou Jichen (The Grand Compendium of Pediatrics)	Chen Fuzheng	The monograph of pediatrics	
	Shenshi Yaohan (Precious Book of Ophthalmology)	Fu Renyu	The monograph of ophthalmology, particular discussion of cataractopiesis with acupuncture therapy	
	Chonglou Yuyao(Jade Key to the Secluded Chamber)	Zheng Meijian	The monograph of laryngology	
	Golden Mirror of Medicine	Wu Qian as the chief editor	Medical textbook edited by the government and collected into *Si Ku Quan Shu(Library in Four Divisions)*	
	Wuyi Huijiang (Compiled Medical Discourses of the Southern China)	Tang Dalie as the chief editor	The earliest magazine of Chinese medicine	

1.2.3.4   Modern times(After 1912A. D.)

At the end of Qing Dynasty, Western medicine was introduced to China. After the controversy in modern times(1912A. D. –1949A. D.), the Chinese medicine practitioners took in and combined the theories of Western medicine gradually. The development of TCM theory shows the trend of the coexistence of the old and the new.

On the one hand, people continued to organize and summarize the achievements of the predecessors. For instance, Cao Bingzhang edited *Zhongguo Yixue Dacheng*(*Compendium of Chinese Medicine*) in 1930's. On the other hand, the school of combination of TCM and Western medicine expound that they should inherit the advantages of TCM, but they also have to learn the advantages of Western medicine.

The book *Zhongxi Huitong Yijing Jingyi*(*The Gist in the Medical Classic of Combination of Chinese and Western Medicine*) was written by Tang Zonghai and the book *Yixue Zhongzhong Canxilu*(*Integrating Chinese and Western Medicine*) by Zhang Xichun, and both were the magnum opus of the school of combination of Chinese and Westen medicine.

After the foundation of the People's Republic of China(1949), the government recognized that it was very important to support and promote the development of TCM. Chairman Mao Zedong emphasized the importance of inheriting and expanding TCM, and pointed out that "TCM is a great treasure which ought to be studied more and improved further". At that time, TCM adhered to the principle of people-oriented and prevention-oriented. But in the inheritance of TCM, traditional Chinese doctors should fully use the modern scientific technology to meet the requirements of the times and the growing needs of people for health care. The national health conference in 1996 also emphasized that equal attention should be paid to Chinese and Western medicine, which greatly promoted the development of TCM. With the expanding popularity and influence of TCM in the world and the development of studies, major breakthrough will be made in TCM theory, promoting the development of life science. Medical treatment, education, scientific research and products of traditional Chinese medicine earn more internationalization. Government promotes the development of TCM based on the principle of "pay equal attention to inheritance and innovation, coordinate the developmental Chinese medicine and Chinese herbs, promote the modernization and internationalization of TCM, and advocate multidisciplinary integration".

1. 3   The essential charactcristics of TCM theoretical system

The holism concept and syndrome differentiation are two especially outstanding basic characteristics of TCM theoretical system.

1.3.1   Concept of holism

The concept of holism is the guiding ideology of the theoretical system of TCM. Holism means unity, integrity and interconnection. This unique concept originated from the ancient Chinese materialism and dialectic ideology. It is an academic idea of TCM for knowing the human body itself and the interconnection among the zang-fu viscera and the integrity between the human body and the external environment. It also provides a way to understand the close relationship between things and phenomena. It is based on the monism of qi, theory of yin and yang, and theory of five elements. When we observe and analyze life by the holistic view, we will focus on the integrality of human body and the unity of human and nature. So, holism is one of the most essential characteristics of TCM, manifested throughout the theory system, including physiology, pathology, diagnostics, syndrome differentiation and treatment. It offers important guidance to clinical work.

1.3.1.1   The human body is an organic whole

In TCM theoretical system, the human body is composed of viscera, meridians and the basic substance of life(essence, qi, blood and body fluids). Each part of the human body is inseparable in structure, mutually connected and restricted in physiology, and mutually affected in pathology. The human body consists of five zang viscera(liver, heart, spleen, lung, and kidney), six fu viscera (gallbladder, small intestine, stomach, large intestine, bladder, and triple energizer), tissues(tendons, veins, muscles, skin, and bones), and the five sense orifices(eyes, tongue, mouth, nose, ears, external genitalia and anus). And as the centered system the five zang viscera are connected to the six fu viscera, the sense orifices and all other tissues, with the help of the meridian system. They are closely related and form a unified whole to perform functional activities by the circulation of essence, qi, blood and body fluids. With such a unity of body structures and interdependent mutual restriction of the function of each organ, the body can maintain its normal life activities. Above all, no organ is isolated, and the human body is an interrelated organic whole.

The essence, the qi, and the spirit are very important to human body. Among them, the essence is the most basic substance of the human body. It is stored in all viscera, especially in kidney, and is under the control of the spirit and the qi. Qi is the origin of the human body and maintains the life activity, also the basic material of the spirit. The formation and operation of qi are controlled by the spirit. Spirit also means the consciousness and thought, and is the manager of the life activity.

The pathological changes in a certain part of the human body are often related to the condition of the viscera, qi, blood, and yin and yang. When we diagnose a disease, we can speculate the pathological changes of viscera through the observation and analysis of the external pathological feature.

1.3.1.2   The unity of human and nature

The natural living of human and various changes in the natural environment can directly or indirectly affect human life activities. Therefore, there are balanced and integrated relationships between the body's physiological and pathological activities and the natural environment, which is the TCM's point—holism of human and nature. The natural environment includes the climatic and the geographical environment providing human with basic conditions for survival and reproduction. Holism of human beings and nature holds that nature will change according to yin and yang and five elements, while the human body has its own inner movement of yin and yang, qi and viscera accordingly. As a result of this kind of close relationship, in order to survive better, humans should comply with nature, adapt to nature, and not go against the laws of nature.

The human body reacts according to the change of seasonal climate. For example, the pulse changes with the seasons, wiry in spring and slippery in late summer. And in summer, there is profuse sweating, in cold winter, there is frequent urination and scanty sweating. All these conditions are caused by yang qi which moves in human body according to the change of seasonal climate in the nature. This shows that human body changes with the climatic seasons.

There are some different effects on human physiology across day and night. During the day, yang qi in human body goes outward to the body surface in order to drive the functional activities of the tissues and viscera, and hides interior the body at night. This phenomenon reflects the self-regulation of human body to adapt the yin and yang changes of the nature.

The differences of geography and living habits, also affect the body physiology and constitution to some extent. Human being can adapt to nature while diseases occur if the adaptation is hindered for various reasons.

Human beings correspond to nature through a positive and active way. People should actively adapt to nature and keep in harmony with nature in order to keep health and prevent diseases. TCM emphasizes the harmony between the functions of the various viscera, the moderate status of the emotion, and adaption to different environments. The most vital essence is the dynamic balance between yin and yang. The fundamental cause of disease is the internal or external dynamic balance disturbed. Therefore, maintaining health actually means conserving the dynamic balance, and curing diseases means restoring the state of coordination and harmony.

1.3.1.3   The unity of human and social environment

Everyone is the member of the society with social attributes, and must be influenced by social environment. Therefore, human and social environment are unified and connected with each other. Different social environments like politics, economy, culture, law, religion, relationships are bound to affect the physiological and psychological activities and pathological changes. And people also maintain the stability of the life activities orderly and harmonious balance in the exchange of social environment.

Different social environment and background can make the differences to physical and mental function and physical constitution of individuals. Generally speaking, a good social environment and harmonious relationship can make people energetic, enterprising and healthy, while unstable social environment and tangled relationships can make people depressed, nervous and anxious. The social status and economic conditions often change according to social environment. Such sudden changes in the social environment as family disputes, neighborhood disagreements, interpersonal tension may greatly impact the physiological and psychological functions of the human body, even can cause death.

The environmental changes mainly affect the mental activities, the viscera function and the operation of qi and blood. So, the prevention and treatment of disease must fully consider the influence of social factors such as the favorable social environment, strong social support and the ability to adapt social environment on the human body and mind.

To sum up, the holistic view of Chinese medicine adheres to "people-oriented", not only considers human as life organics, but also focuses on the integrity of the whole. Moreover, it believes that human beings belong to nature and society, emphasizing the unity of human and nature and social environment. Through physiology, pathology, diagnostics, treatment and health prevention, the essential thinking mode of TCM is of especially important guiding significance in diagnosing and treating physical or mental diseases, and in maintaining the balance between human and nature.

1.3.2   Treatment determination based on syndrome differentiation

Syndrome differentiation is the basic principle of diagnosing and treating diseases.

Syndrome differentiation means collecting the data including the specific symptoms and physical signs through inspection, auscultation, olfaction, inquiry and palpation for analyzing and diagnosing a certain syndrome. Treatment determination means to define the treating approach by corresponding therapeutic principle according to the syndrome differentiation. TCM therapies focus on the person who is sick rather than the disease that the patient contracts, i. e. , aiming to restore the harmonious state of body functions that is disrupted by pathogenic factors.

The pivotal issue to syndrome differentiation is "differentiation", meaning screening and identification. And syndrome, means the pathological summaries of the body in a certain stage of disease course. It includes the causes of disease(such as wind or blood stasis), the infected viscera(such as lung or kidney), and the characters of disease(such as cold or heat), situations of disease(such as mild, serve, chronic and acute), relationship between the pathogenic factors and the healthy qi(such as deficiency or excess)(Table 1-6).

Table 1-6　**Differences and connections between disease, symptom and syndrome**

Concept	Meaning	Significance	Mutual relationship
Disease	A complete morbid process including specific cause, mode of onset, typical clinical presentation, developing law and outcome	Reflect the basic law of occurrence, development and prognosis of whole process of a disease	A series of syndrome and symptoms. In different stages of the process, different syndromes, relevant to different climate, environment and individuality
Symptom	Subjective uncomfortable feelings or objective abnormal changes of the body, such as headache and fever	Reflect one aspect on part of the nature of a disease	The basic element of syndrome and disease to manifest extremely. The main evidence for syndrome differentiation and diagnostics of a disease
Syndrome	A pathological summary of the body in a certain stage of disease course	Reveal the nature of a disease at a certain stage. Reflect the body's adaptability and its connection with environment. Provide the evidence and direction for treatment	The sum of connected symptoms. Combining symptom patterns with diseases, revealing the connection of the two

As shown in the table, there are differences and connections among the syndrome, symptom and disease. "Syndrome" reveals the pathological changes in a certain stage of the disease, and gives more comprehensive and precise information than "symptom" or "disease". It demands practitioners to do analysis by synthesis, to sort out the most important information and then to summarize the correct syndrome. Therefore, the process of syndrome differentiation is to analyze the patient's condition to make correct, reasonable judgment for diagnosis.

Based on syndrome differentiation, treatment is performed by selecting and establishing a suitable treating principle and process, which corresponds to the result of syndrome differentiation. That means syndrome differentiation is the premise and basis to determine treatment, and disease therapy and the examining. Correctness of syndrome differentiation leads to correct ways and methods of treatment. The two are closely linked and inseparable.

In clinical practice, a guiding principle is that treatment is based on syndrome differentiation, in order to recognize the relationship among disease, symptom and syndrome, and to realize that one disease presents a different "syndrome" during its course, while different diseases can appear a similar "syndrome" at some stages in the process development. Therefore, "different treatments for the same disease", and "the same treatment for different diseases" can be applied to clinical treatment according to the result of syndrome differentiation. In conclusion, syndrome differentiation is the process of understanding and treating disease and is the clinical application of all treatment methods, formulas and pharmaceutical selection in TCM. Only with a correct syndrome differentiation, doctors can treat correctly and effectively.

In TCM, individual difference has to be noticed and highly emphasized, combining syndrome differentiation with disease differentiation, focusing on both the whole and part, and stressing the relationship between the macro and micro. With these guidelines, one needs to choose the most suitable treatment according to different conditions in the process of disease and takes into account the climate, environment, and individuality. These are the essences of treatment determination based on syndrome differentiation.

1.3.3   Other characteristics of TCM

Preventative treatment is a core belief of TCM. It lays great emphasis on preventing before a disease arises, guarding against pathological changes when falling sick, and protecting the recovering patients from relapse. TCM believes that lifestyle is closely related to health, so it advocates health should be maintained in daily life. TCM believes that a person's health can be improved through the emotional adjustment, the balance between labor and rest, the sensible diet and a regular life. By these all means, people can cultivate vital energy to protect themselves from harm and keep healthy.

In addition to medication, TCM has many alternative approaches such as acupuncture and moxibustion, traditional Chinese tuina, cupping and guasha(scraping). There is no need for complex equipment in TCM therapy. TCM tools, for example, the small splints used in Chinese osteopathy, the spoons used in guasha, or the cups used in cupping therapy, can draw from materials in our daily life, so that such treatments can spread easily.

To sum up, during its course of development spanning a couple of millennia, TCM keeps drawing and assimilating the advanced elements of natural science and humanities. Its theoretical base through many innovations is covered more scope, and its remedies expand to against various diseases and are displayed unique characteristics.

Huang Yong, Yao Zengyu

Chapter 2

Philosophical Bases of TCM

TCM is built on the foundation of ancient Chinese philosophy, containing the unity of qi, yin and yang, and the five-element theory. These philosophical ideas are the further abstraction and purification of long terms of observation of human life phenomena in combination with the understanding and reasoning of natural phenomena, and become the simple materialism and dialectics that support TCM in establishing its theoretical system and promoting its development. This chapter focuses on the basic viewpoints and methods of Chinese philosophy and their applications in Chinese medicine, and summarizes the main characteristics of TCM thinking method.

2.1 Unity of qi

The unity of qi, also called "qi monism", is the most fundamental thought in ancient Chinese philosophy. Its core idea is that primordial qi is the origin of the universe, and every phenomenon reveals different form and statement of primordial qi. This thought is applied in TCM to understand natural phenomena and life activities, and becomes the fundamental worldview and methodology of TCM.

2.1.1 Basic concept of qi

Qi initially refers to the floating clouds in the sky. The ancients noticed that clouds are blowing, moving, gathering and dispersing under the flow of wind, and can cause various changes in nature, such as wind brings up clouds, clouds condensed into rain, and gentle rain nourishes everything while storms may bring disasters. These phenomena include the invisible, shapeless and capricious things, like wind and clouds, create the nature and cause countless changes. Gradually, an important concept came up as "tangibility born from intangibility". Such intangible things are eventually named "qi" and all physical and tangible things in nature are transformed by this kind of invisible qi.

Qi is a very complicated and important category in ancient Chinese philosophy. The basic concept of qi mainly refers to the invisible and constantly moving substance that exists in the universe, which forms into every visible object in the universe. And the movements and changes of qi drive the development and changes of the universe. It is the medium of the interaction of everything. In the course of development, there are names like "qi", "primordial qi" and "essence qi".

2.1.2　Main contents of the unity of qi

2.1.2.1　Qi is the origin of all things

Before the heaven and earth were formed, the whole universe was thought to be in a state of chaos, filled with clouds of qi under uncertain forms. Yet constantly moving and changing of qi caused the deviation of yin and yang, two opposite but closely connecting matters, making qi the contradictory unity of yin qi and yang qi. Yang qi in the universe rise and dispersed as the intangible heaven, while yin qi descended and condensed into tangible earth. The rising, descending and mutual interaction between yin and yang forms numerous things and phenomena in the universe. Therefore, under the action of qi, the world appeared and everything happened. Thus, it is believed that qi is the origin of all things and is the prime matter of the universe. And human, as a special outcome of the nature, is formed by the condensation of qi, and maintains life activities by the moving and changing of qi.

Qi is neither illusory nor supersensible. The premier form of qi is intangible, which consists in every space of the universe with a state of dispersion and constant motion. In certain conditions, it can be changed and formed into another tangible type of qi that has concrete, visible shape, which is in a cohesive and relatively stable state. Usually the diffuse state of intangible qi is named "qi", and the physical entity formed by qi is called "shape". The invisible qi condenses into the form of a shape, while the visible matter collapses and return to the invisible qi. Thus, there is a constant transformation between "intangible" and "tangible".

2.1.2.2　Qi is the material with unceasing movements that produces all kinds of changes in the universe

Qi has the characteristic of moving, and is often in the state of moving and changing. All the processes and changes that take place in the universe, such as growing and reproduction of plants and animals, as well as accumulation and dispersion of lives, are the results of the movement of qi. Movement of qi depends on the interaction between yin and yang within, and the contradictions and the unity of yin and yang is the root of the movements and changes of qi and the basic law of the universe.

2.1.2.3　Qi is the medium of the interaction of all things in the universe

All things in the universe are formed by qi, interconnected and interacted with each other through the moving and changing of invisible qi filled within the universe. Qi, therefore, is an intermediary between all things in the universe. By means of this, qi keeps the interconnection between the universes, making them into a whole. And this idea holds the primary understanding of holism in TCM, that human, as a part of the universe, are closely connected with the nature through the interaction of qi.

Qi can also maintain the mutual induction of all things in the universe, helping them interact with each other and react accordingly. For example, music instruments resonate, tides are induced by the waxing and waning of the moon, and the physiological and pathological changes of human body are influenced by the changing of days and nights. The mutual inductance between all things is not affected by the distance of space, and is not obstruct by physical objects. It is because the universe is made up of qi and the qi that filled within the universe is the intermediary of all things.

2.1.3　Application of the unity of qi in TCM

Qi monism, as a physiological concept, is theorized into the "unity of qi" of TCM after applied in medicine, and became the methodology of TCM, to help elaborating the basic problems of life, explaining physiological and pathological changes of the body, and guiding clinical diagnosis, treatment and health care, etc.

On one hand, since it is stated that qi is the origin of all things, including human body, the interaction of qi inside the body and between the body and the environment will have great influence on the normal life activities. On the other hand, qi, as the basic substance of human body, not only forms various tissues and viscera, but also diffuses intangibly between them, making the various components of human body closely connected to each other to form a unified whole. Therefore, it will be possible to have local lesions spread to the whole, and overall lesions be reflected at the local. Also lesions of viscera can spread to each other, and functions of internal viscera can also be reflected as the external changes. These perfected the concepts of holism of TCM.

For the human body, the life of a person begins with a breathing of qi and ends with the dissipation of qi. Qi runs through the whole body, providing the original source of energy, and maintaining the function of viscera of the body. The whole process of material metabolism, various life activities, including emotional activities of a person are all regarded as the result of qi movement, and the deficiency and abnormal movements of qi will also be reflected as corresponding symptoms. Thus, clinically, through the analyzing of qi's statement and abnormal movements, the person's health situation and pathological changes can be studied.

Furtherly, the key to prevent the pathogenic qi from attacking the body and to maintain health is to sustain the abundance and coordination of qi. Therefore, regulating qi is one of the important principles of health preserving in TCM, including adaptation to the seasons, regulating emotions, and keeping regular resting and diet. Such laws help to promote the health of the body and prolong life.

2.2 Yin-yang theory

The yin-yang theory is a plain dialectical thought founded on the basis of qi monism. Through the observation of natural phenomena, it is realized that there are two aspects within everything of the universe, that have mutually contradictory and unified relationship, and the moving and changes of the two aspects promote the occurrence and development of all phenomena. These two aspects are named yin and yang, and such understanding gradually formed the theory of yin-yang, holding that the world is material, yet not static. Proposed by *Yi Jing*(*The Book of Changes*), alternating between yin and yang is called "Tao". "Tao" means regulation and principle. *Plain Question* also stated that "yin-yang is the way of heaven and earth, the guiding principle of everything, the parents of change, the root and source of life and death, and the house of spirit".

The yin-yang theory of TCM is formed by the integration of the yin-yang theory of ancient Chinese philosophy and became the philosophical basis and important component of TCM theory. It helps to explain the various phenomena and changes of nature, as well as the physiological functions, pathological changes of the human body, and the basic law of diagnosis, treatment and prevention.

2.2.1 Basic concept of yin and yang

Yin and yang are the general terms for two opposing aspects of a thing, or of interrelating things and phenomena in the universe. The original concepts of yin and yang simply refer to the orientation toward or opposite to the sunlight. The side facing the sun is yang and the opposite side is yin. Since the yang side is always warm, bright and exuberant while the yin side is always cold, dim and depressed, the meaning of yin and yang is gradually extended. Based on this, it is observed and realized that all relatively connected things and phenomena contain two opposite aspects whose interactions promoted the development and changes of the universe. Then, with further extended understanding, yin and yang turned into a pair of philosophical categories used to explain two opposite and interrelated material powers in universe, and the characteristics and interactions between them deduce the law of developing and changing.

The best interpretations of the features of yin and yang are water and fire. Water is cold, moist, quiet, settling and tangible, so it belongs to yin. Fire is warm, dry, moving, rising and intangible, so it belongs to yang. Thus, the basic characteristics of water and fire can represent the basic characteristics of all things' attributes of yin and yang. In general, all those with properties of being dynamic, outward, rising, warm, hot, bright, active, enterprising, strong and intangible, functionally hyperactive attribute to yang, while those with properties of being static, inward, falling, cold, dark, negative, weak, retreating, soft and tangible, functionally hypoactive attribute to yin. According to these characteristics, all things and phenomena in nature can be classified into the categories of yin and yang.

After introduced into the medical field, the theory of yin-yang became an important methodology in studying the human body. It classifies those things that have the effect of moving, warming and exciting the body into yang. Things that have the effect of accumulating, moistening and storing are classified into yin. For example, qi belongs to yang and blood belongs to yin; the six fu viscera of the body belong to yang and the five zang viscera belong to yin.

The properties of yin and yang are conditional. Firstly, there is correlation between yin and yang. Yin-yang theory can only be used to explain the property of two interconnected things or two connected but opposite aspects of one thing, such as day and night, sky and earth. If the two things, such as night and earth, are not mutually related, or are not the opposite sides of a unity, they cannot be distinguished by yin-yang theory to analyze their relative properties and relationships.

Secondly, there is the relativity of yin and yang. Yin-yang properties of things or phenomena are not absolute, but relative. Under certain conditions, yin and yang can be transformed into the opposite. Yin can be converted to yang, and yang can also be converted to yin. And there is infinite divisibility of yin and yang. With the changes of the dividing scope and conditions of two sides, each side of yin and yang can be further divided into yin and yang. For example, the daytime is yang, while the night is yin, if the daytime is further divided into yin and yang, then the morning is yang within yang; the afternoon is yin within yang. Likewise, the night can be further divided.

The formation of the Tai Chi diagram illustrates the formation, characteristics and interrelations of yin and yang(Figure 2-1).

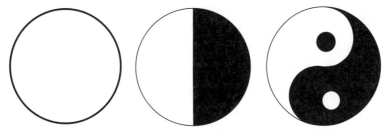

Figure 2-1　**Diagram of Tai Chi**

2.2.2　Basic contents of yin-yang theory

The basic contents of yin-yang theory mainly encompass the opposition and restriction of yin and yang, mutual rooting and interaction of yin and yang, the equilibrium and waxing and waning of yin and yang, and the conversion of yin and yang. They are used to study and understand the inner law and connection of the happening, developing and changing of all things and phenomena.

2.2.2.1　Opposition and restriction between yin and yang

All related things or phenomena in the universe would have two opposites within, such as sky and earth, up and down, outside and inside, active and stable, rising and falling, day and night, bright and dark, hot and cold, etc. Such a relationship between the two opposites is called the opposition of yin and yang.

And restriction of yin and yang refers to the two opposites of yin and yang always represent the relationship of mutual restraint. For example, the changes of climate from one season to another are the results of mutual restriction of yin qi and yang qi of the nature. In spring and summer, yang qi rises and restricts yin qi, leading to warm and hot weather; while in autumn and winter, yang qi falls and yin qi restricts yang qi in term, leading to a cool and cold weather.

For the human body, the contradictory and restricted relationship between yin and yang constitutes the dynamic balance of the body. Once the balance is broken, there will be disharmony of yin and yang within the body, which might cause diseases to occur. And during the onset, development, transformation and recovery of a disease, the restriction of yin and yang can also be manifested as the mutual resistance and predominance between the healthy qi and the pathogenic qi. And any excessive or insufficiency of yin and yang will cause the weakening or hyperactivity of the other.

2.2.2.2　Mutual rooting and interaction between yin and yang

Mutual rooting and interaction of yin and yang represents the relationship of mutual dependence and interaction between contradictory things or phenomena. Yin and yang, as the opposite aspects of a unity, depend on each other and take the existence of each other as a prerequisite for existence. Neither side can be separated from the other and exists alone. For example, brightness belongs to yang and dimness belongs to yin, without brightness, there would be no dimness.

And based on the dependence of each other, yin and yang interact and promote with each other. As for the relationship between qi and blood of the body, qi belongs to yang, and blood belongs to yin. As the commander of blood, qi can generate blood, promote blood circulation and control the circulation of blood, so the normal functioning of qi is helpful for the generation and circulation of blood; as the mother of qi, blood can carry qi and nourish qi, and hence the sufficiency of blood can make full use of the function of qi.

If the relationship of mutual rooting and interaction of yin and yang are damaged, one side of yin or yang will be weakened and cannot support the other, which gradually results in the deficiency of the other side, and causing the pathological changes; what is more, as one side tends to vanish, it would cause the loss of the existing premise of the other, resulting as the separation of yin and yang, essential qi will be exhausted, and this signifies the end of life.

2.2.2.3　Waxing and waning and equilibrium of yin and yang

The two opposite sides of related things or phenomena are always in a constant changing of reducing or increasing, which keeps a relative dynamic balance of things in a certain range. Such characteristics are called the waxing and waning and equilibrium of yin and yang. The waxing and waning is the driving force of the development of all things, and equilibrium is the indispensable condition to maintain a normal state.

The key reason for waxing and waning of yin and yang is the existence of opposition and restriction, as well as mutual rooting and interaction between them. For some situations, the relations of yin and yang are dominated by opposition and restriction, and for others, the relations are dominated by mutual rooting and interaction. Therefore, the changes of waxing and waning of yin and yang are also in various forms.

Based on the relations of opposition and restriction, the waxing and waning of yin and yang are shown as alternate waxing and waning. The increase of one side of yin and yang will lead to the decrease of the other side, and vice versa, stated as "yang waxing and yin waning" or "yang waning and yin waxing". Take the climate of four seasons as an example, from spring to summer, climate changes gradually from warm to hot, which is the process of yang waxing and yin waning; from autumn to winter, climate changes gradually from cool to cold, which is the process of yang waning and yin waxing.

Based on the relations of mutual rooting and interaction, the waxing and waning between yin and yang will present as simultaneous waxing and waning. The increase of one side of yin and yang will also lead to the increase of the other side, and vice versa. Taking qi and blood as an example, qi is yang, and blood is yin. Qi generates blood and blood carries qi. If qi deficiency persists for a long time without recovery, the function of generating blood will decline, which will lead to deficiency of both qi and blood. And in the case of a sudden loss of a large amount of blood, qi will also be lost together with blood, leading to deficiency of both qi and blood. In terms of treatment, tonifying qi can generate blood, and nourishing blood can replenish qi. Such examples represent the statements of "both yin and yang are waxing" and "both yin and yang are waning".

Equilibrium of yin and yang refers to waxing and waning of yin and yang being stable within a certain range, therefore, the human body and the environment can maintain a normal state of balance. If the waxing and waning changes between yin and yang go beyond a certain limit, the balancing condition of yin and yang will be broken, causing disasters in the natural world and diseases in the human body.

2.2.2.4 Mutual conversion of yin and yang

Mutual conversion of yin and yang refers to that the opposite side of yin and yang can transform into the other side under certain conditions. Only when things develop into a certain degree or onto a certain stage, will the property of yin and yang be transformed, such as "extreme yin turns into yang, and extreme yang turns into yin". Here, "extreme" is the required condition for the conversion of yin and yang. Take the climate of four seasons as an example again, from summer to autumn, yang waxing reaches a limit of its range, reaching the condition for transformation, and it converses into yin, leading to cooler weather; from winter to spring, yin waxing reaches a limit of its range, and converses into yang, leading to warmer weather. Therefore, in the development process of things, if waxing and waning of yin and yang is a process of quantitative change, then the conversion of yin and yang is a qualitative change on the basis of quantitative change.

2.2.3 Application of yin-yang theory in TCM

Yin-yang theory has permeated into every aspect of TCM, thereby constructing the basic frame of the TCM theoretical system, and guiding the medical thinking and clinical practice of TCM.

2.2.3.1 Explaining tissues and structures of human body

The human body is an integrated whole, and according to the contents of yin-yang theory, every tissue or structure of the human body has its property of yin or yang. In terms of parts of human body, the upper part is yang and the lower part is yin; the exterior is yang and the interior is yin; the back is yang and the abdomen is yin. As for the four limbs, the lateral sides are yang and the medial sides are yin. In terms of viscera, the six fu viscera are yang and the five zang viscera are yin. Furthermore, each of the zang-fu viscera can be divided into yin and yang, such as heart yin and heart yang; kidney yin and kidney yang, etc.

2.2.3.2　Explaining physiological functions of human body

TCM states that the normal physiological activities of the human body are the result of keeping the unity and opposite relationship of yin and yang inside the body and maintaining a dynamic balance.

The basic laws of human physiological activities can be summarized as the movement of yin essence (substance) and yang qi(function). Life substances belong to yin, while the functional activities belong to yang. Functional activities must be based on the life substances, and functional activities are the driving force of life substances. If yin and yang are imbalanced, it implies the occurrence of diseases; if yin and yang are separated from each other, the movement between yin-essence and yang qi will disappear and life will come to an end. As *Plain Questions* says, "The equilibrium of yin and yang makes vitality well-conserved; the separation of yin and yang makes essential qi exhausted."

2.2.3.3　Explaining pathological changes of human body

Based on the yin-yang theory, the occurrence of diseases is due to pathogenic factors acting on the body, resulting in the imbalance of yin and yang, leading to abnormal exuberance or decline of yin and yang. The occurrence and development of diseases are related to the two aspects of healthy qi and pathogenic qi. Healthy qi is the general concept for all the normal body tissues and structures, physiological functions, and the body's resistance and tolerance ability to repair the injury. Pathogenic qi refers to a variety of pathogenic factors. Both healthy qi and pathogenic qi can be divided into two aspects, yin and yang, namely, yin essence and yang qi, yin pathogens and yang pathogens. The course of diseases is the process of healthy qi struggling with pathogenic qi that leads to the imbalance of yin and yang in the human body. Common forms of imbalance between yin and yang are as follows.

(1) Abnormal exuberance of yin or yang

It refers to the pathological state caused by either yin or yang being higher than a normal level, which causes an excess syndrome of cold(superiority of yin resulting in cold) or heat(superiority of yang resulting in heat).

(2) Abnormal decline of yin or yang

It refers to the pathological state caused by either yin or yang being lower than the normal range, which causes a deficiency syndrome of cold(deficiency of yang leading to cold) or heat(deficiency of yin leading to heat).

(3) Mutual affection of yin and yang

It refers to the eventual pathological changes of dual deficiency of yin and yang caused by yin or yang deficiency that inevitably affects each other.

(4) Yin-yang conversion

It refers to the change of yin and yang properties under certain conditions in which the exuberance of yin or yang reaches its extreme. For instance, patients with acute heat syndrome manifested with high fever, red complexion, irritability, rapid and powerful pulse, if the disease further develops, with heat severely damaging healthy qi in the body, the patient will experience a sudden drop in body temperature, pale complexion, cold limbs, listlessness, feeble and impalpable pulse, etc. This kind of changing belongs to the conversion of yang heat(excess) syndrome into yin cold(deficiency) syndrome.

2.2.3.4　Guiding diagnosis of diseases

The fundamental mechanism of the occurrence and development of diseases is the disharmony of yin and yang. No matter what complicated manifestations a disease shows, it can be summarized and explained by yin and yang.

In the process of four diagnostic methods, the property of yin and yang of the disease can be distinguished through identifying the property of yin and yang of colors, sound, and pulse, etc. For example, bright and lustrous color belongs to yang, while dark and dull color belongs to yin; loud and sonorous voice, talkativeness and restlessness belong to yang; while low and feeble voice, reticence and quiet belong to yin. Rapid and surging pulse belongs to yang, while slow and thready pulse belongs to yin.

After the symptoms are collected, distinguishing the yin-yang property of the syndrome is the key to the diagnosis of diseases in TCM. Take the eight-principle syndrome differentiation for example, among the eight principles, yin and yang are the most general and fundamental principles. Then, exterior, heat and excess belong to yang, while the interior, cold and deficiency belong to yin. Only by distinguishing yin and yang first and foremost, can doctors identify the nature of the diseases and effectively guide the clinical syndrome differentiation.

2.2.3.5　Guiding prevention and treatment of diseases

Under the guidance of holism, TCM holds that people can maintain health and avoid diseases by conforming all life activities to the waxing and waning and conversion laws of yin and yang in the nature. For example, in spring and summer when there is more yang qi in the natural world and most living things are growing and developing, people should pay attention to cultivate yang qi, which is good for the active life activities of the body; while in autumn and winter, since there is more yin qi in the natural world and most living things are storing food or hibernating, people should also pay attention to cultivate yin qi, which is helpful for energy storing in the body. This is a fundamental rule for diseases prevention and health maintenance.

For the treatment of diseases, the application of yin-yang theory mainly represents in the aspects of the determination of therapeutic principles and the summarization of the properties of Chinese medicinal.

(1) Determining therapeutic principles

The disharmony of yin and yang is one of the fundamental causes of the occurrence and development of diseases. Therefore, it is one of the basic principles to treat the diseases by regulating yin and yang, reinforcing the deficiency, purging the excess, and restoring the relative balance of yin and yang. Specifically, excess heat syndrome caused by abnormal exuberance of yang should be treated with cold medicinal to reduce the excessive yang and to purge the heat, namely, "treating heat with cold". Excess cold syndrome caused by abnormal exuberance of yin should be treated with warm medicinal to reduce the excessive yin and to dissipate the cold, namely, "treating cold with heat".

For deficiency syndrome, deficiency cold syndrome caused by abnormal debilitation of yang should be treated by warming yang to reinforce the deficiency of yang. Deficiency heat syndrome caused by abnormal debilitation of yin should be treated with the therapeutic principle of nourishing yin to reinforce the deficiency of yin.

According to the principle of mutual rooting of yin and yang, the therapeutic approach of "treating yin for yang", "treating yang for yin" may also be adopted in the treatment of abnormal debilitation of yin and yang. That is to say, when using warming yang medicinal, nourishing yin medicinal should be used concurrently; and when using nourishing yin medicinal, warming yang medicinal should be added in order to maintain a harmonious interaction between yin and yang.

(2) Summarizing properties and actions of Chinese medicinal

Yin-yang theory can be used to summarize the properties, flavors, and acting tendency of Chinese medicinal.

Chinese medicinal has four properties: cold, hot, warm and cool. Among them, cold and cool natures belong to yin, and can reduce or disperse heat syndrome; while hot and warm natures belong to yang, and can reduce or eliminate cold syndrome. Chinese medicinal also have five flavors, namely, acrid, sweet (bland), sour(astringent), bitter, and salty. Among these flavors, acrid, sweet, and bland belong to yang, while sour, bitter, and salty belong to yin. Different flavors pertain to different effects. And for the actions of medicinal on the body, there are ascending, descending, floating and sinking. Medicinal with the action of ascending and outward properties belong to yang; while descending and inward properties belong to yin.

2.3 Five-element theory

The five-element theory is an ancient philosophic thought which states that the material world is composed of five basic matters of wood, fire, earth, metal and water. Within these elements, there are relations of generation, restriction and transformation, which promote and maintain the development and changing of the world. As is said in *Shang Shu* (*Book of History*), "water and fire are concerned with people's food, wood and metal are concerned with people's working, and the earth gestates everything. "With such fundamental understanding, the five elements are gradually used to conclude all the things and phenomena in the universe according to their properties and characteristics. Thus, the five-element theory becomes the methodology of understanding the universe, and applied in TCM, this theory is used to elaborate the viscera relations among partial, partial and the whole of human body, as well as the unity of human body and the external environment. It played an enormous role in the formation of the unique theoretical system of TCM and primary methodology for TCM to further understand human life activities.

2.3.1 Basic concepts of five elements

In Chinese terms, five elements are named "Wu Xing", "Wu" means the basic material elements of wood, fire, earth, metal and water, and "Xing" means rank, order and movement. "Wu Xing" emphasizes the concept of holism, and represents the characteristics, relations and moving forms of things and phenomena.

2.3.2 Basic contents of five-element theory

2.3.2.1 Characteristics of five elements

Through observation over a long time, the ancients found that wood, fire, earth, metal and water each have their respective characteristics. Through abstract analogy, deduction, analysis and induction, the reasonable and abstract recognition about the characteristics of the five elements are formed.

● Characteristics of wood are "bending and straightening", which show the straight growing and outward extending attitude of trees. Things and phenomena with characteristics of growing, rising, extending and flourishing belong to the category of "wood".

● Characteristic of fire is "flaring up", which means that fire has the attitude of warming, rising and upward going. Things and phenomena with these characteristics belong to the category of "fire".

● Characteristics of earth are "sowing and reaping", which mean the earth is used for human to sow and harvest crops. By extension, things and phenomena with the characteristics of generating, transforming, receiving and bearing belong to the category of "earth".

● Characteristic of metal is "changing", which means metal has the ability to conform to external forces, and it is extended to the ability of descending, restraining, killing and clearing. Things and phenomena with these characteristics belong to the category of "metal".

● Characteristics of water are "moistening and descending", which refer to the nature of water to moisten and to flow downward. Things and phenomena with properties of cooling, moistening, downward going and concealing belong to the category of "water".

2.3.2.2　Classifications of things and phenomena by five elements

Based on the characteristics of the five elements, the properties, characteristics and functions of things and phenomena are compared and classified, things and phenomena with the similar characteristics are classified into the corresponding element's category, forming into the category of five elements(Table 2-1).

Table 2-1   Classification of things by five elements

Five time intervals	Nature							Human Body						
	Five flavors	Five colors	Five changes	Five qi	Five orientations	Five seasons	Five elements	Five zang viscera	Five fu viscera	Five sense viscera	Five body constituents	Five outward manifestations	Five minds	Five fluids
Daybreak	Sour	Blue	Generation	Wind	East	Spring	Wood	Liver	Gallbladder	Eye	Tendon	Nail	Anger	Tear
Midday	Bitter	Red	Growth	Summer heat	South	Summer	Fire	Heart	Small intestine	Tongue	Vessel	Face	Joy	Sweat
Down of sun	Sweet	Yellow	Transformation	Dampness	Middle	Late summer	Earth	Spleen	Stomach	Mouth	Muscle	Lip	Thinking	Saliva
Sunset	Spicy	White	Contraction	Dryness	West	Autumn	Metal	Lung	Large intestine	Nose	Skin	Gland and pores	Anxiety	Nasal discharge
Midnight	Salty	Black	Storage	Cold	North	Winter	Water	Kidney	Bladder	Ear	Bone	Hair	Fear	Spittle

There are two kinds of classification methods, direct classification and indirect deduction. Direct classification is also called analogy, one of the basic concepts of logic, which means to find the individual correlations that have common characteristics from the figure of things(i. e. nature, function and shapes). For example, the sun rises from the east, which is similar to the ascending and dispersing characteristics of wood, so east belongs to wood; liver has the function of governing rise and dispersion, which is also similar to the characteristics of wood, so liver also belongs to wood. Indirect deduction is used for those that cannot be fit into the five elements by direct classification. For example, liver belongs to wood, it governs tendons, opens to eyes, and is exteriorly-interiorly related to gallbladder, so gallbladder, tendons and eyes, etc. , are attributed to wood. From the above, it can be seen that the category of five elements is actually a general summarization of functional characteristics of various things and phenomena.

2.3.2.3   Relations of generation, restriction, over-restriction and counter-restriction among five elements

Apart from classifying and deducing all things and phenomena in the nature, five-element theory explores and explains the inter-connections and self-regulation mechanism among various things or phenomena, using the relations of generation and restriction. This is the essence of five-element theory.

(1)Generation among five elements

Generation among five elements refers to the orderly generative and promoting relations among wood, fire, earth, metal and water. Just as the corresponding seasons appeared in turn, changes of life and phenomena in the universe embody the relations of generation. Based on these generative and promoting rules, the universe has flourishing prospects, and the life process is expansive. The orders of the generation cycle of five elements are as follows: wood generates fire, fire generates earth, earth generates metal, metal generates water, and water generates wood(Figure 2-2).

Among the relationships of generation, each element has two aspects of "being generated" and "generating", and they are called the "mother-child" relation. The element that generates is called the "mother" while the element that is generated is called the "child". Take wood for instance, wood generates fire and is generated by water, so wood is the mother of fire and is the child of water.

(2)Restriction among five elements

Restriction among five elements refers to the restrictive relationships among wood, fire, earth, metal and water. Since it is noticed that one thing is often inhibited and restrained by another, the restriction of the five elements was then induced. Based on this restricting rule, things and phenomena could be prosperous but not hyperactive. The orders of the restriction cycle of five elements are as follows: wood restricted earth, earth restricted water, water restricted fire, fire restricted metal, and metal restricted wood(Figure 2-2).

Among the relations of the restriction, each element has two aspects of "being restricted" and "restricting". The restricting element is the "suppressor" and the restricted element is the "suppressed". Take wood for instance again, wood restricted earth and is restricted by metal, so wood is the suppressor of earth and is the suppressed of metal.

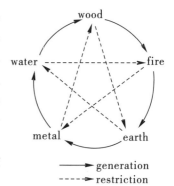

Figure 2 - 2   **Generation and restriction of the five elements**

(3)Mutual restriction and generation among five elements

Mutual restriction and generation among the five elements refer to the coordinating relations of restriction within generation and generation within restriction. Without generation, there are no growth and development of things; without restriction, things cannot be developed and changed in a normal range. For instance, water generates wood, wood generates fire, and water restricts fire. Such mutual relations make it possible to maintain the coordinate balance among the three elements. Through these, it is illustrated that everything is controlled and regulated by the entirety while affecting the entirety itself. It prevents the hyperactivity or hypoactivity of things so as to maintain a dynamic balance. Once the balance is broken, there will be abnormal phenomena in nature and pathological changes in the human body.

(4) Over-restriction and counter-restriction among five elements

Over-restriction and counter-restriction among the five elements are actually the restrictive changes under abnormal conditions, causing abnormal development and changes of things and phenomena.

1) Over-restriction

Over-restriction refers to the abnormal changes of restriction among the five elements, and its order is the same with that of restriction, i. e. wood over-restricts earth, earth over-restricts water, water over-restricts fire, fire over-restricts metal, and metal over-restricts wood (Figure 2-3). It means that there is restriction beyond normal limit, which may lead to an imbalance among the five elements.

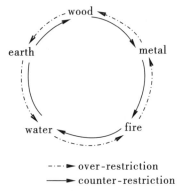

--→ over-restriction
——→ counter-restriction

Figure 2 - 3   **Over-restriction and counter-restriction of the five elements**

There are three reasons for the over-restriction: firstly, the restricted element is deficient, which leads to the restricting element relatively excessive; secondly, the hyperactivity of a certain element that leads to the suppressed element overly restricted; thirdly, both deficiency of the restricted element and hyperactivity of the restricting element exist. Take wood restricting earth as an example, earth itself is deficient, or wood is overly excessive, or they happen simultaneously, can cause wood over-restricts earth.

2) Counter-restriction

Counter-restriction refers to the abnormal adverse restriction among the five elements. Its order is opposite to that of restriction or over-restriction, i. e. wood counter-restricts metal, metal counter-restricts fire, fire counter-restricts water, water counter-restricts earth, and earth counter-restricts wood (Figure 2-3).

There are three reasons for counter-restriction: firstly, the restricted element is overly excessive, which leads to the restricting element relatively deficient and being suppressed by the restricted one; secondly, the restricting element is overly deficient, which causes the restricted element to be relatively excessive and suppresses the restricting element adversely; thirdly, both deficiency of the restricting element and excessive of the restricted element exist. From these above, it can be seen that counter-restriction of the five elements is the abnormal and adverse restriction phenomena when the balance among them is broken. Take metal restricting wood as an example, metal itself is deficient, or wood is overly excessive, or they happen simultaneously, can cause wood counter-restricts metal.

It should be noted that generation and restriction are normal relations in the nature and the human body, while both over-restriction and counter-restriction are abnormal phenomena in the nature and pathological condition in the human body. The order of over-restriction is opposite to that of the counter-restriction, but they can appear simultaneously for a certain element. The orders of restriction and over-restriction are same, but restriction is the normal relation, while over-restriction is abnormal case.

2.3.3   Application of five-element theory in TCM

Five-element theory plays a very important role in the formation of TCM's theoretical system. On one hand, it helps to analyze and conclude the characteristics and properties of tissues and viscera, as well as to illustrate the physiological functions of the zang-fu viscera. On the other hand, it helps to analyze and study the mutual relations among the physiological functions of the zang-fu viscera by the relations of generation, restriction and mutual generation and restriction among the five elements; what's more, by the relations of generation, restriction, over-restriction and counter-restriction among the five elements, it can elaborate the mutual effects of zang-fu viscera under pathological conditions. Therefore, five-element theory is not only used for theoretical elaboration, but also for the guidance of diagnosis and treatment of clinical diseases.

2.3.3.1　Explaining physiological functions and mutual relations among zang-fu viscera

TCM classified the internal viscera of the human body into five zang systems by the five-element theory (Table 2-1). The generation, restriction and mutual restraint among the five-zang systems maintain the internal dynamic balance, and they can help to illustrate the physiological functions and their mutual relations of the internal viscera.

(1) Illustrating physiological functions of five zang viscera

Five-element theory attributes the zang viscera to the five elements respectively, and helps to illustrate the physiological characteristics of each. Liver belongs to wood and governs the free flow of qi. Heart belongs to fire and governs blood and vessels. Spleen belongs to earth and governs transportation and transformation. Lung belongs to metal, governs qi, controls breathing, and links with all vessels, governing management and regulation as well as the water passage. Kidney belongs to water, stores essence and is in charge of urination and defecation.

(2) Illustrating mutual relations of five zang viscera

The functions of five zang viscera are not isolated, but mutually related.

Liver storing blood is helpful for the supply of heart blood, which is called liver generates heart, or wood generates fire. Heart yang is helpful for the transportation and transformation of spleen, and it is called heart generating spleen, or fire generating earth. The normal transportation and transformation of spleen can nourish lung qi, and it is named spleen generating lung, or earth generating metal. The descending and clearing function of lung qi is helpful for kidney to receive qi, and it is called lung generating kidney, or metal generating water. The essence stored in kidney can nourish liver blood, and it is called kidney generating liver, or water generates wood. These are the mutual generations among the five zang viscera.

Liver governing the free flow of qi can smooth spleen qi, keeping it from becoming obstructed. This is liver restricting spleen, which is also called wood restricting earth. Normal function of spleen in transportation and transformation can control kidney water to prevent from overflowing, which is called spleen restricting kidney or earth restricting water. Kidney water can suppress heart yang, so as to avoid the hyperactivity of heart fire, calling kidney restricting heart or water restricting fire. Heart yang can restrain the over purification of lung, calling heart restricting lung or fire restricting metal. The purification and descent of lung can inhibit the excessive ascent and dispersion of liver, calling lung restricting liver or metal restricting wood. These are the mutual restrictions among the five zang viscera.

2.3.3.2　Explaining pathological effects among zang-fu viscera

Five-element theory can help illustrating the mutual effects among zang-fu viscera under pathological conditions. The disease of one zang-fu viscera can transmit to another, and vice versa. The mutual and pathological effects among the zang-fu viscera are called transmission and change in TCM.

(1) Transmission and change based on generation among five elements

It means the order of transmission and change goes along or against the sequence of the generation among five elements. The premier one is named the disorder of mother-viscera affecting child-viscera, and the latter one is named disorder of child-viscera affecting mother-viscera.

Transmission from the mother-viscera to the child-viscera is also called sequential transmission. For example, kidney belongs to water and liver belongs to wood. Water generates wood, so kidney is the mother of liver. If kidney disease affects liver, it is called "disorder of mother-viscera affecting child-viscera". Clinically, deficiency of kidney yin will lead to deficiency of liver blood, and then the syndrome of both liver and kidney deficiency may occur.

Transmitting from the child-viscera to the mother-viscera is also called reverse transmission. Ether hyperactivity or deficient of the child-viscera can lead to the disorder of the mother-viscera, causing both child and mother organs to become hyperactive or deficient, or hyperactivity of the child and deficiency of the mother. For example, liver belongs to wood and heart belongs to fire. Wood generates fire, so hyperactivity of heart fire may lead to hyperactivity of liver fire, causing "blazing of heart-liver fire".

(2) Transmission and change based on restriction among five elements

This refers to the transmission follow or against the order of restriction among the five elements. The premier one is named over-restriction, and the latter one is named counter-restriction.

In the relation of restriction, ether hyperactivity of the suppressor or deficiency of the suppressed can lead to over-restriction. Take liver and spleen as an example, normally liver should restrain spleen, but if the liver qi is too strong(hyperactivity), it may affect spleen and stomach, causing a series of diseases, which is called liver wood over-restricting earth. If the over-restriction of liver to spleen is caused by spleen qi deficiency, the clinical manifestations may be different, and it is called disharmony between liver and spleen.

In another situation, if the suppressed is hyperactive or the suppressor is deficient, it may cause a pathological transmission of counter-restriction. Take the relation between lung and liver as an example, normally lung can restrain liver. However, under some pathological conditions, lung deficiency or liver hyperactivity, it may lead to pathological transmission of liver wood counter-restricting lung, which is also called "wood fire tormenting metal".

In conclusion, the key point for TCM to recognize the mutual transmission of zang-fu diseases is that the diseases of all the viscera can affect and involve one another. However, it also should be noted that the transmission of disease is not absolute based on the generation, restriction, over-restriction and counter-restriction of the five elements. It is not advised to automatically apply it to every disease presentation in clinic.

2.3.3.3   Guiding diagnosis and treatment of diseases

(1) Guiding diagnosis of diseases

Human body is an organic whole, and the diseases of internal organs can be manifested to the complexion, voice, taste and pulse, etc. of the exterior, which become the basis of diagnosing diseases. The five zang viscera have some certain relations with the five colors, five flavors and the changes of relative pulses, so the attribution to the five elements can be used to deduce the location and condition of diseases. For example, bluish complexion, preferring to sour food and wiry pulse may indicate liver diseases.

(2) Guiding control of diseases' transmission and change

Based on the relations among five elements, the occurrence and transmission tendency of diseases is closely related with the generation, restriction, over-restriction and counter-restriction of zang-fu viscera, so besides the treatment of the affected zang-fu viscera, it is also needed to control its transmission and achieve the aim of holistic treatment. For example, in the case of liver diseases, the hyperactivity of wood may over-restrict earth, so replenishing spleen and protecting stomach is the priority in the treatment in order to block the progression and transmission of disease.

(3) Determining therapeutic principles and methods

1) Therapeutic principles and methods based on generation rules

"Reinforcing the mother-viscera to treat deficiency of the child-viscera" and "purging the pathogen of the child-viscera to treat the excess syndrome of the mother-viscera" come from *Classic of Difficult Issues*, which are two therapeutic principles based on generation of the five elements. For deficiency syndrome of a certain zang-fu viscera, reinforcing its mother-viscera can be a good method, and for excess syndrome, reducing its child-viscera can be applied. Such principles are mainly used for the deficiency or excess syndrome of both the mother and child organs, which emphasize that reinforcing or purging should not only focus on the certain organ itself, but also on the connected organ.

The following are the therapeutic methods that formulated by the premier principles.

Nourishing water to moisten wood, also called nourishing liver and kidney, means to nourish kidney yin to promote liver yin deficiency.

Strengthening earth to generate metal, also called nourishing spleen and lung, refers to the method of replenishing lung qi by reinforcing spleen qi.

Replenishing fire to nourish earth, also called warming yang and strengthening spleen, which means to nourish spleen and stomach by warming kidney yang.

Reducing heart to treat hyperactivity of liver, refers to the method of dealing with hyperactivity of liver fire by reducing heart fire.

2) Therapeutic principles and methods based on restriction rules

According to the restriction rules of the five elements, once the pathological changes of abnormal restriction occur, the main manifestations include over restriction, insufficient restriction and counter restriction. The restricting side is hyperactive, while the restricted side is deficient. Therefore, the key point is to restrain the excess and reinforce the deficiency, namely inhibiting excessiveness and supporting weakness.

The following are the therapeutic methods that formulated by the premier principles.

Inhibiting wood and promoting earth, also called smoothing liver and reinforcing spleen, pacifying liver and harmonizing stomach, or regulating liver and spleen, means to treat hyperactivity of liver and deficiency of spleen by smoothing and pacifying liver to strengthen spleen.

Strengthening earth to control water, also called warming kidney yang and reinforcing spleen, means to deal with the retention of water and dampness by warming and activating spleen yang, or warming kidney yang and reinforcing spleen. It is suitable for the edema and fullness due to spleen deficiency and overflow of water and dampness.

Purging south to nourish north, also called purging fire and nourishing water, which means to treat kidney yin deficiency, hyperactivity of heart fire, and disharmony between heart and kidney by purging heart fire and nourishing kidney water.

In conclusion, the application of five element theory in clinical is helpful to ensure the therapeutic principles and methods and help deciding the essential of treatment. Besides, the generation and restriction rules of five elements are also applied to guide the prescription and acupoints selection, as well as the regulation of spiritual and emotional diseases, etc. However, there are some limitations of five-element theory, so it should be applied flexibly based on the specific conditions, syndrome differentiation and treatment.

Wang Weilin

Chapter 3

Visceral Manifestation

Basic concept of visceral manifestation is based on the different physiological functions or morphological characters, and zang-fu viscera can be classified into five zang viscera, six fu viscera and extraordinary viscera according to their physiological function and anatomical structure. The five zang viscera include heart, liver, spleen, lung and kidney. Gallbladder, stomach, small intestine, large intestine, urinary bladder and triple energizer are known as six fu viscera. In addition, there are extraordinary fu viscera which contain the brain, medulla, bone, blood vessel, gallbladder and uterus with its appendages.

The visceral manifestation theory involves not only the observation and understanding of the external manifestations, but also the relationships among viscera and sensitive organs, emotions, body fluids, and even human nature.

3.1 Viscera manifestation

3.1.1 Basic content of visceral manifestation theory

This theory gradually evolved into a relatively complete theoretical system with the guidance of the philosophy of dialectical materialism from ancient China, and further developed into a core system which uniquely understood the functions of human body by the following factors as ancient anatomical knowledge, a long term observation of physiological and pathological phenomena and the summation of life experience and clinical practice.

Anatomical observations have been done on the human body by the ancestors since the ancient China. The book *Internal Classic* contains numerous records concerning the dissection of bones, stomach and the intestines of the human body especially the blood circulation system. During the Qing Dynasty, Wang Qingren verified existing anatomical records through the examination of cadavers and wrote the *Correction of Errors in Medical Works* with more than 20 picture illustrations. It is praiseworthy to the perfection of TCM. Owing to the limitation of the traditional habits, historical conditions as well as the restricted development of science, ancient medical practitioners acquired the anatomy knowledge roughly and superficially.

Even though limited to the adverse factors such as naked eye observation, ancient medical practitioners took cognizance of external manifestations of the physiological and pathological phenomena of the human body for such a long time. Gradually the principles of the physiology and pathology of the body organs were summarized. For example, being angry often leads to congestive eyes, poor appetite, distention of hypochondrium and ribs region, insomnia, etc. The predecessors correlate the phenomena to connect anger, emotional problems, to the free flow of liver qi. Thus, the viewpoints of anger as liver emotion and rage injuring liver were formed.

During the long period of fighting against the nature and diseases, the observations show that certain pathological changes are related to the dysfunction of internal viscera. One example is that lung trouble often manifests itself through a rhinocnesmus, nasal discharge and stuffed nose which can be cured with some special and certain acupoints. As the other example, certain herbs reinforcing spleen can treat some bleeding diseases such as uterine bleeding, purpura, gingival hemorrhage, etc. Eventually' ancient doctors concluded it as spleen dominating blood control. These recognitions had been tested, verified and repeated through daily life and clinical practice, furthermore, been analyzed and composed into the visceral manifestation theory gradually.

3.1.2 The characteristics of zang-fu viscera according to visceral manifestation theory

The five zang viscera are abundant in tissues and have the functions of producing and storing essential qi. Most of them do not open to the exterior directly. They should keep the state of fullness all the time because they house essential qi without leaking freely.

On the contrary, six fu viscera have cavities with the functions of receiving, digesting, transmitting and excreting water and food. Most of them open directly to the exterior and do not have the functions of storing the refined materials but rather merely the passages for food and water. They receive and decompose water and food, absorb the nutrient substances and discharge the waste and unwanted water. It is a continuous process, alternating between emptiness and fullness. Therefore, they take descending and unobstructed as their normal state.

Similar to six fu viscera morphologically, extraordinary fu viscera have the cavities but not the pathways for the water and food. Like the five zang viscera functionally, they also store essential qi. That is so-called extraordinary fu viscera. With the exception of gallbladder, extraordinary fu viscera have no exterior-interior relationships. The bile stored in gallbladder is clear and clean, differing from the turbid contents of stomach, the intestines and the urinary bladder. Therefore, gallbladder belongs to six fu viscera as well as to the extraordinary fu viscera.

3.1.3 The different concepts of internal organs between TCM and Western medicine

The formation of visceral manifestation theory was based on the observations focused on the external symptoms and signs of physiological functions and pathological changes of living bodies rather than morphology of the tissues. Therefore, TCM places much emphasis on the importance of the synthetic functional manifestations of the internal organs.

Although the name of zang-fu viscera in TCM is identical with those used in Western medicine, their concepts are different yet. The physiological function of a viscus may contain part of the functions of the organs with the same name in Western medicine as well as including certain functions of other related organs. And the viscera of TCM are characterized by multi-functions. Generally speaking, zang-fu viscera in TCM is considered not only anatomical units, but also conceptually are parts of physiology and pathology, and the latter is more important. For example, spleen in TCM refers to not only some of the functions of blood coagulation and body fluid metabolism, but also the functions of digestive system in Western medicine. The functions of reproductive system in modern medicine are closely related to that several viscera in TCM, those being kidney, uterus with its appendages and liver.

TCM pays a great deal of more attention to the wholeness of the human body. On the view of holistic concepts, it forms inseparable, harmonious and interactive relationships between zang-fu viscera in both physiology and pathology. Furthermore, it stresses the relationship between human beings and the external environment, including the social and the natural environment. Guided by these concepts, changes in climatic variations, daily living conditions, even economic or political conditions will affect the human body directly or indirectly.

Moreover, TCM places much more emphasis upon the role of zang viscera as the center organs. With them as the center, the five sense organs, the body orifices, the six fu viscera and the tissues are all interconnected through meridians and collaterals to form the functional activities of systems, including heart system, lung system, spleen system, liver system and kidney system. The functional activities of systems manifest the inter-promoting and inter-restraining actions between each other. The viscera in the system can be divided into yin aspect and yang aspect, which keep the balance and interaction. In sum, the visceral manifestation theory is practically developed from the yin and yang and five element theories and goes beyond them. It expounds upon the physiological functions and pathological changes of the zang-fu viscera and extraordinary fu viscera, concentrating on the five zang viscera than about others.

3.2 Five zang viscera

3.2.1 Heart

Heart lies in the chest, above the diaphragm, takes a position left of the center, and is around with the pericardium. Heart corresponds to fire in the five-element theory. It is the most important organ of the human body in TCM because it controls the life process and governs all functions of all the viscera. So it is termed as the monarch of all the organs. In the light of the yin and yang, heart can also be divided into two aspects: heart yin and heart yang, the former refers to the material structures, including blood of heart, the later means the functional activities or heat, including qi. The main physiological function of heart is dominating blood and vessels and housing mind. Heart manifests in complexion and dominates tongue. Joy is as heart emotion. Heart dominates perspiration. Heart connects with small intestine to form a close interior and exterior relationship through heart meridian of hand shaoyin and small intestine meridian of hand taiyang.

3.2.1.1 Main physiological functions of heart

(1) Heart dominating blood and vessels

In TCM, doctors believe that the original blood is a complex substance of body liquid and nourishing qi transformed by spleen and stomach from the diet, which further mixed and transformed into red blood by heart qi. So it is called as heart-blood, and provides the material energy for keeping the physiological activities of the human body. According to the yin and yang theory, heart qi pertains to yang while heart blood to yin. That is the theoretical basis of terms heart yang and heart yin.

Heart dominates both blood and blood vessels, and they form a close blood circulating system. The blood circulates within the vessels via heartbeat. Heart qi is the motive force for blood circulation, propelling the blood flow through the vessels to nourish the whole body and maintain all functional activities with the orderly, regular rhythm.

As it is known, the normal blood circulation is based on the following three factors: sufficient blood, smooth vessels and vigorous driving force of heart qi. If heart blood and heart qi are insufficient or weakened, many symptoms and signs such as palpitation, chest distress, stabbing pain in the precordial region, etc., will occur. Stagnation of the blood and the vessels characterized by purple tongue and lips, rough or intermittent pulse and stuffed chest may result from the obstruction directly or the deficiency indirectly.

Whether or not heart's function in dominating the blood and vessels is normal will guide clinical practice. In TCM, the pulse-taking is referred to the pulsation of an artery. Owing to relating to heartbeat, the pulse's strength may reflect the functional state of heart. For instance, the sufficient heart blood and vigorous heart qi may maintain a harmonic, rhythmic and forceful pulse beat at a frequency of 4–5 beats per breath. On the contrary, an insufficient heart qi will lead to an uneven, weak and thin pulse caused by obstructive blood circulation.

Besides the pulse, color of tongue and complexion and the feelings of chest are attributable to the condition of heart. A ruddy tongue, high color and radiant complexion and comfortable feelings in the chest indicate sufficient heart blood, while pale tongue and wan complexion can suggest the vitality less heart qi and insufficient heart blood accompanied by the clinical symptoms of severe palpitation, short breath, forgetfulness, dream-disturbed sleep, stuffed sensation in the chest, etc.

(2)Heart housing the mind

That heart controls mental activity is the same meaning as heart housing the mind. Traditional Chinese Medicine considers the term mind as an abstract concept. In its narrow sense, it means the mental activities as vitality, consciousness and thinking, etc. However, in its broad meaning, the mind refers to the outward manifestations of the whole life activities including the vitality of the body, eyesight, appearance, complexion, response, speech, etc. Western medicine theory is of the opinion that all the mental activities are attributed to the physiological function of the brain. However, on the view of holism, TCM believes that even heart houses the mind, but these mental activities are ascribed to the physiological functions of the internal organs separately. Furthermore, they are classified into five aspects which correspond to the five zang viscera respectively. The book *Plain Questions* says that heart stores the vitality, lung houses corporeal soul, liver is concerned with housing soul, spleen houses thought, and kidney is housing the will. Even though the five zang viscera are involved in the mental activities, but TCM places much emphasis on the importance of the physiological functions of heart. Heart controls all the activities of the body, including the mental activities.

It should be pointed out that the physiological functions of both heart dominating blood and vessels and heart housing mind are complementary to each other. The former function is controlled by the later one. For example, when an athlete is ready to run, but hasn't really started yet, heart beat and blood flow rate will increase significantly. This is the obvious evidence of heart housing mind influences heart dominating blood and vessels. On the other hand, heart blood is the material basis of mental activities. Only when heart blood is abundant to nourish the mind, can mental activities keep normal. If heart qi and heart blood are insufficient, the mind may be affected, and the manifestations of restlessness, poor memory, excessive dreaming will be found. Moreover, if heart-fire flames up to disturb the mind, there will be delirium, unconsciousness, even coma. If phlegm-fire clouds the mind, it will appear as derangement of the mind, such as dysphoria, aggressive and violent behavior.

3.2.1.2 The relationship of heart with body, aperture, emotional activity and fluid

(1)Heart corresponding to vessels and manifesting in face

According to holistic view of TCM, the state of essential qi of the internal viscera can manifest in the sense organs of the exterior body. This theory has been formed in the long term medical practice. Whether or not the physiological function of heart qi or heart blood is normal, its condition will be reflected in the complexion. The face has abundant small vessels and tender skin, and always is exposed to the external world. So it is as the mirror of heart. Observe the face, therefore, the prosperity or decline of the qi and blood of heart can be deduced. The flourish heart qi and heart blood will lead to lustrous and moist face. Pathologically, deficient qi and blood of heart may bring about pale and dull complexion, stagnated heart blood, purplish or congestive complexion.

(2) Heart dominating tongue

Here, dominating refers to opening or aperture in original intention. Guided by the theory of TCM, tongue is as the specific body opening of heart attributed to the interconnection between the internal organs and the external sense organs in the head and face. It exists a close and influential relationship between them, which not only manifests in physiology, but also in pathology. The tongue is connected with heart via heart meridian so that the qi and blood of heart can go up to arrive at the tongue through the meridian and its collaterals, maintaining the normal functions of tongue such as taste and expressing the speech. If heart works well, the tongue will be red, moist, sensitive, soft and flexible, and coherent to speech. In the pathological process, the changes of heart will be reflected on the tongue. Observation of the shape and color of the tongue can be used for deducing the pathological changes of heart. For instance, flaming up of heart-fire may cause crimson and erosional tongue; obstructive heart blood may cause a purple or blue tongue, or purple spots in the tongue. In the extreme stage of heart fire invading the pericardium or combined with phlegm covering heart-orifice may cause a swollen, stiff tongue, further stuttering even aphasia. In brief, heart is very closely related to the tongue physiologically and pathologically.

(3) Heart related to sweat

As we mentioned above, blood circulation is controlled by heart. Sweat comes from body fluid which is the most important component part of the blood. Simultaneously, heart controls all the activities of the whole body, including the mental activities. TCM believes that sweating caused by stress is directly related to heart. What's more, too much sweat tends to consume heart qi, and causes to perspire spontaneously.

(4) Heart corresponding to joy in the emotions

The concept of heart corresponding to joy in the emotions mean that the physiological function of heart is concerned with joy of the mind. Moderate joy is beneficial and advantageous for the mind, but excessive joy tends to impair heart.

Pericardium is called as xinbao in TCM. It refers to the envelope outside heart, with the small vessels attached, having the function to protect heart and as a substitute for heart to resist external pathogenic factors. The pericardium meridian connects with the triple-energizer meridian of hand shaoyang. In physiology, it has the functions of protecting heart and promoting the circulation of qi and blood. In pathology, TCM considers that the evil invading heart may firstly affect the pericardium. When the heat-evil invades pericardium, the symptoms of mental derangement such as coma and delirium occur. All the disorders pertain to those of heart. In view of this reason, the pericardium is apt to be considered as an attached organ rather than an independent organ of heart.

3.2.2 Lung

Lung is situated in the thorax, connected with the trachea and open to the outside world through the nose, including the two lobes, one on the left and right separately. In theory of five elements, lung corresponds to metal. The main physiological functions of lung is dominating the qi, linking with all the vessels, dominating management and regulation, dominating regulation of water passage.

Lung dominates skin and hair and manifests in hair. Grief is as lung emotion. Lung dominates snivel. Lung connects with large intestine to form a close interior and exterior relationship through lung meridian of hand taiyin and large intestine meridian of hand yangming.

Lung occupies the uppermost position among all the internal viscera and is termed canopy. Lung is the main organ controlling respiration. It is also called delicate viscus owing to lung is delicate and tender, and is directly exposed to external environment and predisposed to attack from every kind of external pathogenic factor.

In TCM theory, lung is generally divided into two aspects: lung yin, namely the material structures of lung and lung yang, namely the physiological functions of lung. While the terms lung yang and lung blood are rarely used. Most of time, they are generally replaced by lung qi and lung yin.

The movement of lung qi mainly manifests two ways, exhaling and inhaling.

3.2.2.1   Main physiological function of lung

(1) Lung dominating qi

Lung dominating qi means that lung has the functions of taking charge of respiration and controlling the qi of the whole body.

The respiratory function is one of the most important physiological functions of the human body because people cannot stop breathing even several minutes. The life activities must consume a lot of fresh air inhaled by lung. In other words, lung is not only the key role in respiratory movement, but also the place at which gas exchange between the interior and exterior of the body occurs. The cognition is similar to Western medicine. But in TCM, performing this function well should depend on the dispersing, purgation and descending functions of lung qi and nourishing of lung yin. If lung is diseased, the respiratory system will be affected with the symptoms and signs such as cough, asthma, dyspnea, etc.

Such the function of lung controlling the qi of the whole body refers to the following aspects:

One is that lung participates in the formation of pectoral qi. The pectoral qi distributing in the chest is a complex of fresh air inhaled by lung and essential qi is transformed from diet by spleen and stomach. It can promote the respiratory activities, warm and protect the internal organs, and maintain the normal physiological functions of them. The second is that lung operates on dominating the qi of the whole body with the forms of ascending, descending, entering and exiting. In addition, lung qi may help heart to propel the blood circulating in the blood vessels as mentioned in Western medicine.

In summary, the function of lung controlling respiration is related to the exhaling and inhaling movement of lung qi. Furthermore, the movement is identical to that of ascending, descending, entering and exiting of the qi of the whole body.

Therefore, if the function of lung dominating qi is in the physiological state, the respiration will be normal and smooth. When lung is diseased, it will lead to disorders of respiration as well as the dysfunction of the qi of the whole body. For instance, deficient lung qi may cause weak respiration, prolonged cough and shortness of breath. Disturbance of lung qi may lead to cough, asthma, stuffy in the chest. If the pectoral qi is affected by the dysfunction of lung, it will manifest short, low voice, spontaneous sweating, lassitude, and so on.

(2) Lung linking with all vessels

All the vessels of the human body meet in lung. In the physiological course of blood circulation and respiration, the blood of the whole body converges through the blood vessels to lung to exchange gases through respiration, then redistributing oxygenated blood back to the whole body via the vessels, which depends on the normal functions of dispersion and ascent, purification and descent of lung. This process will assist heart to control and regulate normal circulation of qi and blood.

(3) Lung dominating water movement

Lung dominating water movement here means maintaining normal body fluid metabolism. The food essence and water transformed and absorbed by spleen and stomach may be transmitted upward to lung. Then they are distributed to all over the body by the function of dispersing and ascending, flourishing and warming the viscera and tissues. After that, they are transformed into sweat to be excreted through the pores. Meanwhile, amount of water is discharged via the respiration. Because of the highest location among all the viscera, lung is apt to keep lung qi descend as its normal state. The spent water may be descent downwards into the urinary bladder to form urine by means of descending. Synchronously, part of water is reabsorbed by large intestine and discharged as defection. This is so-called lung is the upper source of water. Under appropriate physiological states, the dispersing and descending of lung ensures the suitable amount of sweating and urination so as to regulate water metabolism. Pathologically, lung fails to regulate water metabolism due to abnormal purgation and descending functions, then distribution and excretion of water will be affected, and symptoms and signs such as edema, enuresis, and difficult urination will occur.

(4) Lung dominating management and regulation

In TCM theory, heart is considered as the monarch of the whole body. Thus it was said lung is the prime minister who is responsible for managing and regulating functions in *Plain Questions*. Here, lung is ranked as prime minister to assist the monarch in governing their kingdom; to coordinate with heart in managing and regulating the whole body. Although TCM acts heart as the chief of all the internal viscera in maintaining the coordinated and harmonious relationships, it is depended on assistance of lung. Only when lung plays the perfect role of coordination with heart can the internal organs maintain normal functions physiologically.

All in all, the function of lung dominating management and regulation mainly manifests in the following aspects. One is that lung assists heart in promoting and regulating blood circulation. The second is that lung controls the qi of the whole body via controlling the respiration with the exhaling and inhaling movement. The third is that it regulates the formation and distribution of pectoral qi so as to regulate the physiological functions of the viscera. The last one is, as mentioned above, lung regulates the water movement by its functions of dispersing, descending, purifying and ascending. Actually, this function derives from its total physiological functions. If this function is abnormal, the formation and distribution of pectoral qi should be affected, the pathological changes such as tiredness, shortness of breath, feeble voice will be found. Lung qi and blood circulation will be disturbed also with the symptoms of cough, asthmatic breath, stuff and tingling in the chest may appear.

3.2.2.2 The relationship of lung with body, aperture, emotional activity and fluid

(1) Lung dominating skin and hair and manifesting in hair

TCM believes that the exterior skin of the body is a protective fence against exogenous evils and has the function of excreting sweat, adjusting the temperature. All the functions of skin should depend on the normal states of lung. Based on the function of dispersing, descending, purifying and ascending, lung qi may distribute, warm and nourish the skin and body hair. And the opening and closing of sweat pores are dominated by the vigorous lung qi and normal respiration. Synchronously, the skin and hair help lung to regulate the respiration and modulate the water metabolism. Resulting the inter-coordinating relationship, lung impacts upon the skin mutually. For instance, when the exogenous pathogens attack the human body, the skin and hair will be invaded firstly. When serious impairments occur in lung, it will result symptoms such as aversion to cold, high fever, bad cough and stuffy nose. The failure of dispersing of lung qi always leads to the fading skin and withered hair attributed to the insufficient nourishment. Furthermore, the seriously deficient lung qi manifests spontaneous perspiration and being susceptible to cold. The obstructed lung qi may affect the normal opening and closing of the sweat pores, resulting in anhidrosis or cough, etc.

(2) Lung dominating nose

The nose, throat, trachea and bronchus are the pathway through which the fresh air inhaled and exhaled. All of them are classified into lung system and connect with each other with lung meridian. The nose is the portal of lung with the function of ventilating and smelling. Only when lung qi is in functional, can the nose breathe and smell actively. Pathologically, they often influence each other whoever falls ill. For example, if lung is attacked by the exogenous pathogens and fails to perform its dispersing function, the nose would be involved and resulting stuff nose, running nose, sneeze and anosmia, etc. In the clinic, allergic rhinitis is often cured by reinforcing lung qi. It is the clear and unquestionable evidence of this theory.

(3) Lung dominating snivel

Lung dominating snivel is associated with lung dominating nose. Nose is the window of lung, and snivel is the mucus secreted by the nasal mucosa and has the function of moistening the nasal cavity. The condition of snivel can reflect the function of lung. If lung is affected by the cold pathogen, the running nose will be found; the heat pathogen, turbid and yellow snivels; dryness pathogen, dry sensation in the nose and dried snot.

(4) Grief is as lung emotion

The concept of grief is as lung emotion means that the physiological function of lung is concerned with grief of the mind. When lung is diseased, the tolerance to the external world will be reduced and it is easy to call up grief to impair lung qi.

3.2.3　Liver

Liver lies in the upper part of the abdomen on the right side, under the diaphragm, slightly to the right hypochondriac region. Its meridians are distributed throughout the right and left ribs. On the view of theory of five elements, liver corresponds to wood. Liver meridian of foot jueyin connects gallbladder meridian of foot shaoyang to form an exterior and interior relation. Its physiological functions are dominating free flow and rise of qi, storing the blood, promoting the function of digestion, regulating the normal circulation of qi, blood and water. The specific body opening is eyes. Liver dominates design of strategy, and controls tendon and manifests in nail. Here, liver yin refers to the material structures, and liver yang, functions of heat. Liver qi simply means its functions.

The concept of anger is as liver emotion means that the physiological function of liver is concerned with anger of the mind. When liver is diseased and fails to dominate free flow and rise of qi functionally, and anger will be called up easily.

3.2.4　Spleen

Spleen is located in the middle energizer underneath the diaphragm. According to the five-element theory, spleen corresponds to earth. On the view of yin-yang theory, spleen yin refers to material structures while spleen yang, including spleen qi, pertains to functions.

The function of spleen in TCM is similar to the digestive system function in Western medicine. Spleen is associated with stomach with meridians and collaterals to form a pair.

3.2.4.1 Main physiological function of spleen

(1)Spleen dominating transportation and transformation

The main physiological function of spleen is dominating transportation and transformation. Transportation means conveying and distributing the essential substance all over the body, but the form of essential substance will not be changed. Transformation implies changes, digestion and absorption. During the process of transformation, water and food will be digested and assimilated into essence. Here, water and food are implied to all kinds of diet. The function of spleen dominating transportation and transformation denotes that spleen digests the water and food and assimilates the essence.

TCM considers that the digestive function is related to spleen, stomach and small intestine. Together with stomach and small intestine, spleen is responsible for the main digestive process. The diet taken in stomach is primarily composed and digested by both spleen and stomach, then sent downward into small intestine. Then small intestine undergoes separating the clear part from the turbid. The clarity is named essence, it refers to qi and blood, which is conveyed all over the body so as to nourish the internal viscera, organs and tissues. Next step, essence is transported upward to heart and lung by spleen, then conveyed throughout the whole body to support the life activities. TCM holds that spleen is a major organ of the digestive system either the physiological functions or the pathological changes.

The dysfunction of spleen leads to pathological changes of digestion, the symptoms and signs such as abdominal distention, diarrhea and lassitude will occur. Because spleen cannot produce sufficient qi and blood, heart and brain wouldn't have enough material basis to afford their normal functions, insomnia, anemia, and even memory loss will appear.

The other function of spleen is promoting water metabolism and maintaining the balance of water metabolism. At the same time of transporting and transforming the qi and blood, spleen has the function of absorbing, distributing and excreting water-dampness which refers to excess water in the body.

On the one hand, the water taken into the body is transported and transformed into body fluid by spleen. Then the body can be nourished and moistened by the body fluid.

On the other hand, spleen transmits unusable water from the metabolism to the related organs, such as lung, kidney, urinary bladder and skin. Then the unusable water is eventually changed into sweat or urine to be excreted out of the body. From the above, it can be concluded that spleen plays an important role in circulation and excretion of water. The process of water metabolism mainly depends on spleen qi. Only when it acts well, can spleen be able to digest and assimilate the nutrients effectively, transport and distribute the essence appropriately, and transmit and excrete water-fluid normally. It maintains the relative balance of the body fluid metabolism. For these reasons, spleen is termed source of phlegm, while lung as container of phlegm.

Dysfunction of spleen causes disorders of water metabolism also. If excessive water retention occurs in the body, edema, diarrhea, obesity will appear. If the dampness is stagnated in the four limbs, numbness and swollen joints will occur. If the dampness retains in lung, abundant phlegm and bad cough will be found.

After birth, food and drinks provide a major source of the nutrients required by the human body, to support the life activities as the material basis.

As spleen is so important in the process of producing qi and blood, it is based on the foundation of postnatal life and the source of qi and blood. In Jin Dynasty, there was a famous doctor named Li Dongyuan who created the school of invigorating the earth. He considered various diseases are attributing to the internal impairment of spleen. Being of the acquired foundation, spleen and stomach act on the health care and preservation of health obviously. So more attention must be paid not only to diet nutrition, but also to the protection of spleen and stomach in the daily life, and protect spleen and stomach with proper herbs, acupuncture and moxibustion treatments, or exercises under clinical guidance.

(2) In charge of sending up

Sending up means rising, ascending and leading up. The clarity transformed by spleen, stomach and small intestine from the food and water, is then sent up to the upper energizer by spleen, and is distributed throughout the whole body. The direction of this process is rising and ascending. If it is abnormal, the upper part of the body cannot obtain enough nutrients and function well. So dizziness, vertigo, memory loss and blurred vision may occur.

The other meaning is leading up. It means that spleen can fix the internal organs at their original locations. This function is attributed to the strong spleen qi. If spleen qi is deficient to ascend, that is to say, spleen qi is weak. It may result in ptosis of stomach, kidney and uterus, and prolapse of rectum.

(3) Spleen commanding the blood

Spleen commanding the blood means that spleen controls the blood in its circulation within the vessels to prevent it from extravasation. This function relies on the strength of spleen qi also. If spleen qi is declined, the blood will often escape from the vessels, resulting in various types of hemorrhage, such as blood in the stool, gum bleeding, hematuria, uterine bleeding and purpura, etc.

3.2.4.2   The relationship of spleen with body, aperture, emotional activity and fluid

(1) Spleen dominating limbs and muscles

TCM considers that spleen dominates the limbs and muscles. It is a direct reflection of the domination of spleen in transportation and transformation. The muscles and the limbs depend on the nourishment of essence derived from water and food transformed and distributed by spleen. Abundant essential substance ensures adequate energy for muscular movement. If spleen function is normal, the muscles will be reinforced and develop well and be strong and endurable, so as the four limbs move powerfully and limberly. In contrast, a lack of essence due to the poor spleen qi functions, can result in lassitude, weakness or atrophy. In clinical practice, emaciation and feebleness due to some certain chronic diseases can be treated by the method of invigorating spleen to reinforce qi, in accordance with the theory of spleen dominating muscles and limbs.

(2) Spleen manifesting in lips and mouth as window of spleen

Spleen dominates the muscles including the lips which are components of the muscles, and spleen is the source of growth and development of qi and blood. It indicates that the brilliance of spleen appears externally on the lips. When spleen functions well and produces sufficient qi and blood, the lips will manifest as ruddy and lustrous for being nourished adequately.

The mouth is the uppermost opening of the digestive system. A hearty appetite and good taste depend on the normal spleen qi in both transportation and transformation. Only when spleen functions well can the mouth enjoy the five kinds of flavor. Conversely, if the dampness or other pathogens affect spleen, it may result in an impairment of digestive system such as sticky, sweetish sensation in the mouth, poor appetite, tastelessness, etc.

(3) Spleen producing sputum

The sticky part of the saliva is called sputum. It has the function of moisturizing oral cavity and protecting oral mucosa. The increase of salivary secretion during the intake of food contributes to the swallowing and digestion of food. If spleen functions well, the sputum will be secreted normally to assist the digestive function of spleen and stomach, but not outflow from the mouth. Conversely, if spleen and stomach work disharmoniously, it will lead to the overflow of salivary secretion and spilling out of the mouth.

（4）Overthinking as spleen emotion

There are certain relationships between spleen and emotional activities. Under normal conditions, thinking problems have no harmful effects on the physical activities of the human body. But overthinking may disturb the functions of spleen, resulting in symptoms and signs such as anorexia, abdominal distension, etc. TCM considers that spleen as the pivotal point of ascending and descending qi due to its location being in the middle energizer. When overthinking happens, qi stagnation will occur, and spleen is always first to be affected.

It should be pointed out that the theory of spleen in TCM is concerned with most of the functions of the digestive system that Western medicine deals with, but is also related to blood coagulation and body fluid metabolism.

3.2.5 Kidney

Kidney is situated in the lumbar zone, one on either side of the spinal column. Since kidney stores the congenital essence, which is the foundation of all the viscera and life activities as the primary driving force, it is ranked foundation of prenatal life.

According to the theory of five elements, kidney corresponds to water.

Based on the theory of yin and yang, kidney yin refers to the material structures, including its essence of life, and kidney yang refers to the functions and heat. Meanwhile, kidney qi is produced by kidney's essence of life which is the driving force on the human body's growth development and reproduction.

Its physiological functions are storing the essence of life, regulating the water metabolism, controlling and promoting inspiration. The specific body opening is ears and urinogenital orifice and the anus. Kidney determines the condition of the bone and marrow. The brilliance of kidney appears externally on the hair of the head. Kidney corresponds to fear in the emotions. Saliva is as the fluid of kidney.

In addition, kidney and urinary bladder make a pair of zang-fu. Kidney meridian connects with the urinary bladder to form an exterior-interior relationship.

3.2.5.1 Main physiological function of kidney

（1）Storing the essence of life

The essence refers to one of the kinds of the most important and valuable materials of the human body. It can be classified into two aspects as congenital essence of life and postnatal essence.

Congenital essence of life is inherited from the parents. Both the quality and quantity of congenital essence is determined by the parents before birth. It is the material basis in the development of the embryo and reproduction. It determines the body shape, character even life-span. Only on the sufficient basis of the congenital essence, can the embryo develop, and can the life come into being.

The second part means postnatal essence, also known as acquired essence. After birth, postnatal essence is produced by spleen and stomach constantly to support the life activities such as growth, development and other physiological activities. It is the basic material constituting a human body, which forms the viscera, tissues, bone, tendons and muscles, skin and hair of the human body. Only when the postnatal essence is abundant, can the physique be strong and smart, can the life activities keep normal, and can the rest part be stored in kidney to nourish and reinforce the congenital essence and be in preparation for future needs.

After birth, the congenital essence is enriched and strengthened by postnatal essence. The transformation of postnatal essence relies on the replenishment of vitality from the congenital essence. Although the resources are different, both of them are mixed and stored in kidney and are inseparable. In brief, the prosperity or decline of kidney essence places much emphasis on the importance of the postnatal essence than the other. Thus, kidney is considered as the foundation of prenatal life.

TCM believes that kidney essence will be transformed into the vital energy under certain conditions, called kidney qi. It should be pointed out that, they are actually the different states of the same substance just like the water and steam. Kidney qi is responsible to promote the growth, development and reproduction of the body.

From the childhood, with the promotion of kidney qi, the rapid growth of permanent teeth and fast growth of hair appear. Subsequently, the further enrichment of kidney essence promotes genital development and maturation of the sexual instinct for maintaining the animated reproductive function. When human reaches the age of puberty, the tian gui was produced by the richest kidney qi for promoting a process of maturity of the reproductive function. It can promote the development of sperm in boys and the menarche in girls. When it develops a certain level, the reproductive functions for both male and female are fully matured. With the increase of age, kidney essence may be from prosperity to decline. Similarly, tian gui gradually attenuates to exhaustion.

Since the growth, development and reproductive function are closely related to prosperity or decline of kidney essential qi. pathologically, an insufficient kidney essence will lead to hypogenesis of bone and intelligence and developmental retardations such as metopism, runtishness, amentia, or five kinds of retardation (retardation of standing, walking, hair-growing, teeth eruption and delayed speech) and five kinds of softness(softness of four limbs, head, nape, muscles and mastication) in children. In adults, frailty and premature senility may result from excessive consumption of kidney essence characterized by hair loss, baldness, looseness of teeth, memory loss, tinnitus and dizziness, sexual dysfunction, etc. The method of reinforcing and tonifying kidney is often used to treat these diseases in clinic.

As mentioned before, kidney essence which is stored in kidney transforms into kidney qi mutually, is called essential qi. On the view of yin-yang theory, the essence pertains to material, being yin, while qi to function, being yang. These two are termed as the primordial yin and primordial yang.

Kidney yin is the foundation of the yin-fluid of the whole body which moistens and nourishes the internal organs and tissues. Kidney yang is the foundation of the yang qi of the body. It functions in warming and promoting the whole body as the primal driving force of the life. Similar to the relationship of yin and yang, under normal conditions, both of kidney yin and kidney yang restrict, depend and interact mutually in a dynamic state in order to keep balance of yin and yang. If it fails to maintain the balance, many pathological changes will occur. The deficiency of kidney yin leads to endogenous heat and causes yin deficiency of other organs, brings on symptoms of heat sensation in palms and soles, night sweat, vertigo, tinnitus, soreness and weakness of waist and knees, spermatorrhoea, etc.

The deficiency of kidney yang will lack in functions of warming and promoting, brings on symptoms of external cold, cold and pain in the lumbar zone, infertility, frequent urination at night, etc. Concurrently, deficiency of kidney yang will fail to warm and promote the other viscera manifesting other disorders. For instance, if heart is short of warm from kidney yang, it will manifest in the syndrome of deficiency of heart yang such as palpitation, edema, cyanosis, etc. On the contrary, the prolonged diseases will result in the deficiency of yin or yang in the corresponding viscera and may involve kidney finally.

(2)Dominating the water metabolism

Kidney dominating the water metabolism indicates that kidney plays a key role in regulating and managing the water metabolism of the human body although lung, spleen, liver and triple energizer are involved in. Kidney disseminates body fluid derived from food essence to nutritive and nourish all over the body.

Then the body fluid is used and consumed by the viscera and bowels, after that, kidney discharges the waste produced by this process. The normal function of kidney dominating the water metabolism depends on kidney qi and kidney yang.

As mentioned before, the body fluid is classified into the clear and turbid parts during the water metabolism. The clear part refers to the nutrients while the turbid means the metabolic spend and waste. The clear is transformed and transported from the food and water by spleen and stomach, and consequently conveyed to lung and heart upward. Part of water is excreted through the respiration and sweat pores due to the purgation function of lung. The turbid water may descent downwards into kidney by the function of descending of lung. Here this fluid still has some nutrient composition, and is further absorbed by the functions of evaporation and fractional distillation of kidney yang. The turbid then flows down to the urinary bladder to form the urine. The whole process relies on kidney qi and kidney yang.

Even the urinary bladder stores and discharges urine, the opening and closing of it should be reliant upon the transformative function and retentive ability of kidney qi. During the whole process of water metabolism, kidney plays a positive and irreplaceable role in promoting the functions of lung, spleen, liver and triple energizer, etc. It is only by the warming and evaporating function of kidney yang that lung can regulate water metabolism, spleen transporting and transforming water and dampness, liver promoteing water metabolism, the triple energizer smoothing the passages of water, and the urinary bladder controling the opening and closing normally.

If the function of kidney is abnormal, the water metabolism will be disturbed and symptoms such as oliguria, edema, polyuria, anuria and frequent urination arise.

(3) Controlling and promoting inspiration

TCM considers that although lung controls the respiration, it needs the assistance of kidney to receive and absorb gases from lung, to aid in inhaling the air downwards.

The clear qi inhaled by lung should descend to kidney, termed received and absorbed by kidney. Here kidney qi may maintain the inhalation depth and prevent hypopnea. Otherwise, more exhalation and less inhalation, pulmonary emphysema, pulmonary-cardiac disease, dyspnea and hypopnea will be found.

3.2.5.2　The relationships of kidney with body, aperture, emotional activity and fluid

(1) Dominating bones and teeth, generating marrow to fill up the brain

Domination of bones and generation of marrow to fill up the brain depends on the function of kidney storing essential qi and dominating growth and development. Essence is the basic substance of different forms of structures including bones and teeth, marrow and brain.

Sufficient essence generates abundant marrow to nourish the bones to be solid and hard. Teeth are a part of bones, so it is called that teeth are the surplus of the bones.

Furthermore, bone marrow, spinal cord and brain form a closed system which is inter connected. The prosperity or decline of kidney essence has a great effect on not only bones and teeth, but also the condition of marrow. TCM terms the brain as the sea of marrow.

Only when kidney essence is sufficient, can the marrow be full, and the brain function well. Pathologically, insufficient kidney essence will lead to mal-development of bones, scanty marrow and hypogenesis of the brain manifesting loosening tooth, easily fractured bones, fragile bone, low intelligence, memory loss, blurred vision, tinnitus, etc.

(2) The brilliance of kidney manifesting in hair

Here, the hair refers to the hair on the head. TCM holds that hair is the surplus of the blood. Kidney stores the essence, and liver stores the blood. Liver blood depends on nourishment from the essence of kidney, while the essence of life stored in kidney relies on the replenishment from liver blood. Both the blood and essence have the same resource that is the qi and blood transformed and transported by spleen and stomach, and they can transform mutually when necessary. Hair is the mirror of kidney. It can reflect the condition of kidney essence.

(3) Opening into ears and urinogenital orifice and anus

Different from the other four viscera, kidney have upper and lower specific body openings, the upper means the ears and the lower refers to urinogenital orifice and the anus.

Actually, the audition, the function of ears depends on the prosperity or decline of kidney essential qi. So the hearing may response the condition of kidney essential qi.

The urinogenital orifice and the anus are closely related with kidney due to the function of controlling water metabolism.

(4) Saliva as the fluid of kidney

Saliva refers in particular to the clear and rarefied foam in the mouth. Kidney yin is sent upward through kidney meridian of foot shaoyin, reaches under the tongue, and secreted into the mouth to moisten it.

(5) Fear as kidney emotion

Fear is concerned with kidney. Intense fear may affect the distribution of kidney qi, causing urinary incontinence. The pathologic changes of kidney may result in symptoms of fear and uneasiness.

3.3 Six fu viscera

3.3.1 Gallbladder

Gallbladder is one of the six fu viscera, but also belongs to the extraordinary fu viscera. Gallbladder is a small pouch that sits just under liver. Gallbladder and liver are in an interior and exterior relationship to each other by the connection of gallbladder meridian of foot shaoyang and liver meridian of foot jueyin. The main physiological function of gallbladder is to store and excrete bile and dominate decision.

3.3.1.1 Storing and excreting bile

Gallbladder stores bile produced by liver. The bile is produced by gallbladder qi and stored in gallbladder. The bile is yellow in color and bitter in taste, and excretes into small intestine to participate in the process of digestion and absorption of food and promotes small intestine to separate the lucid from the turbid. Since the bile plays an important role in assisting the absorption of food, it is called the essential juice or the lucid juice and gallbladder is called the fu-viscera of essential juice or the fu-viscera of lucid juice in TCM.

Whether the excretion of the bile is normal or not is concerned with the dredging and dispersing functions of liver on the one hand and the unobstructed condition of gallbladder on the other. Failure of liver to dredge and disperse the obstruction of gallbladder itself will affect the excretion of the bile and disturb digestion and absorption, frequently leading to anorexia, abdominal distension, vomiting, hypochondriac pain or even jaundice if the bile is extravasated in the muscles and skin.

3.3.1.2 Dominating decision

The dominating decision means that to make judgment and make a decision. And this function is related to the strength of gallbladder qi. If gallbladder qi was very strong, the decision is made very quickly and decisively. If gallbladder qi was very weak, one could not make decision very quickly and be hesitant to do everything. Deliberation comes from liver and decision dominating from gallbladder, so liver and gallbladder control our strategy and decision together. If gallbladder qi and liver qi were sufficient, some mental disorders or emotional symptoms such as fear and palpitation, insomnia, dream-disturbed sleep, etc. , will be occurred.

3.3.2 Stomach

Stomach is located in the upper-left area of the abdomen below liver and next to spleen. Stomach cavity is usually divided into three parts, namely shangwan(the upper part of stomach and cardia), zhongwan(the middle part of stomach) and xiawan(the lower part of stomach and pylorus). Its main function is to store and breakdown foods and liquids that we consume before those contents travel to other organs to be further digested. Stomach and spleen are in an interior-exterior relationship to each other by the connection of stomach meridian of foot yangming and spleen meridian of foot taiyin.

The main physiological function of stomach is dominating reception and decomposition.

3.3.2.1 Stomach dominating reception

The physiological function of stomach is to receive and digest food. The dominating reception function means that stomach has the function of receiving and holding the food and water of the diet. Since stomach is big and can contain large amount of food, and the food received and digested by stomach is the main substance for producing qi and blood, stomach is called the sea of food and water in *Internal Classic*. While the food essence can be changed into body essence and produced under the function of stomach, stomach is also known as the reservoir of five zang viscera and six fu viscera.

3.3.2.2 Stomach dominating decomposition

The dominating decomposition function means that the food will be transformed into chyme in stomach. Food is digested here, and then sent downward to small intestine, where the essential substances are transformed and transported by spleen to the whole body.

Stomach depends on stomach qi to perform its function. Stomach qi is the basic motive power for transmitting food and water in stomach downwards. The canal connecting stomach and small intestine must be kept unobstructed so that the chyme can smoothly be transmitted from stomach to small intestine. That is why the physiological function of stomach is often described as stomach functions to descend and the unobstructed condition is prerequisite to the normal function of stomach in TCM, usually abbreviated as stomach governing descent. Dysfunction of stomach will lead to distending stomachache and poor appetite due to disharmony of stomach qi, or belching, vomiting, nausea and hiccup due to failure of stomach qi to descend or upward flow of stomach qi.

3.3.3 Small intestine

Small intestine is located in the middle of the abdomen, and connected to stomach on the top end and to large intestine(colon) on the bottom end. Small intestine and heart are in an interior-exterior relationship to each other by the connection of small intestine meridian of hand taiyang and heart meridian of hand shaoyin. The main physiological functions of small intestine are dominating reception and digestion, and separation of the refined from residue.

3.3.3.1 Dominating reception and digestion

The function of stomach in receiving and digesting food and water should coordinate with the transportation and transformation effect of spleen, so that the food and water are able to be changed into subtle substance. The digestive function of spleen and stomach is crucial to the life and health of human beings. If the dominating reception and digestion function is weak, the patient will be abdominal pain, diarrhea and stool.

3.3.3.2　Separation of the refined from residue

The physiological function of small intestine is to receive the chyle and separate the lucid from the turbid. The lucid refers to refined nutritious substances and fluid, which is absorbed by small intestine and transported to the whole body by the function of spleen. The turbid means the food residue and a part of water, which is transported to large intestine by the function of stomach and small intestine. Spleen transports the clean essential substances to all parts of the body, and part of the water contained in food to the urinary bladder. Small intestine transfers the turbid residues to large intestine. Therefore, if diseased, small intestine will not only affect the function of digestion and absorption, but also lead to urinary problems.

3.3.4　Large intestine

The upper end of large intestine is connected to small intestine by the ileocecum, and its lower end connects to the anus. Large intestine and lung are in an interior-exterior relationship to each other by the connection of large intestine meridian of hand yangming and lung meridian of hand taiyin. Its main physiological function is to receive the wastes from small intestine and, in the process of transporting it to the anus, absorbing a part of its fluid, and converting it into feces to be excreted from the body.

Large intestine can receive the residue of food from small intestine, absorb some fluid, transport the waste down, and expel the stool from the anus. Dysfunction of large intestine produces the symptoms of borborygmus and diarrhea, if the fluid is further exhausted, the symptoms will be constipation and so on.

3.3.5　Bladder

The urinary bladder, or bladder, is a hollow organ in the pelvis. Most of it lies behind the pubic bone of the pelvis, but when full of urine, it can extend up into the lower part of the abdomen. Bladder and kidney are in an interior-exterior relationship to each other by the connection of bladder meridian of foot taiyang and kidney meridian of foot shaoyin. The main physiological function of bladder is dominating fluid storage.

Bladder is known as the minister of the reservoir and is responsible for storing and excreting the urine or waste fluid from kidney. The turbid fluid is formed after the water metabolism, and is transported downwards to kidney, where it turns into urine under the function of kidney qi transformation. Bladder function of transforming fluids depends on kidney yang. If kidney yang is deficient, bladder will lack qi and heat to transform fluids and symptoms will include profuse, clear urine, frequent urination or even incontinence.

3.3.6　Triple energizer

Triple energizer is a special fu viscera, serving to generalize certain functional systems of the body. The concept of triple energizer has two meaning. First, it is one of the six fu viscera, and has a function of passing through original qi and passing through water. Second, it represents the partition of human body, including the upper energizer, middle energizer and lower energizer.

3.3.6.1　Triple energizer of six fu viscera

As one of six fu viscera, triple energizer is located in the abdomen. Triple energizer and pericardium are in an interior-exterior relationship to each other by the connection of triple energizer meridian of hand shaoyang and pericardium meridian of hand jueyin. The main physiological function of triple energizer is passing through original qi and water.

(1) Passing through original qi

The original qi, also known as the root source of qi, is the primary motivation of life activity. The original qi is derived from kidney and distributed to all parts of human body through the transportation and transformation function of triple energizer so as to activate and promote the physiological function of other viscera and tissues. Once the original qi is deficient and the transportation of triple energizer is not smooth, qi deficiency in certain areas in the body will occur.

(2) Passing through water

All of our body fluids(blood, sweat, tears, saliva, urine, etc.) originate from the food and drink we consume. Food and drink are transformed and separated by spleen into clean and dirty parts. Clean fluids are directed to lung and skin, while kidney and small intestine process dirty fluids to be excreted as urine. According to Chinese Medicine, this process is a simplified version of how our body metabolizes fluids. The triple energizer is responsible for the generation, transportation and removal of all body fluids. Although the distribution and excretion of body fluids inside the body are accomplished by the synergistic function of many organs, including lung, spleen and kidney, etc., the normal circulation of body fluid must be based on the meridian function of triple energizer.

3.3.6.2 Physiological function of triple energizer according to its position

As a region, triple energizer can be divided into three parts, for example, the upper energizer, middle energizer and lower energizer. The upper energizer includes the thorax, heart and lung, the middle energizer includes the upper abdomen, spleen, stomach, liver, gallbladder and small intestine, the lower energizer includes the lower abdomen, kidney, bladder and large intestine.

(1) Upper energizer

The main physiological function of upper energizer is dispersing the defense qi, distributing the food essence and fluid to nourish and moisten the whole body. The main physiological process of the upper energizer is distributing the body's fluids via the action of lung. Often referred to as a mist, the upper burner is responsible for transforming the body's energy into a vapor that maintains the lubrication necessary for healthful respiration. This vapor also assures the skin's moisture, a necessary immunity guard to prohibit pathogens from invading the body. Our physical shield against viruses and bacteria, skin is our first line of defense against airborne illnesses.

When the misting function of the upper energizer is impaired, it typically leads to a breakdown of our defenses. This can result in a cold, with symptoms such as sneezing, running nose, temperature, sore throat, body aches, etc.

(2) Middle energizer

The main physiological processes in the middle energizer relate to digestion. In the process of digestion, the middle burner's spleen and stomach break down food and drink by separating what is to be absorbed from what is to be excreted. Referred to as the maceration chamber, the middle energizer is where nourishment is garnered and transported throughout the body.

When the macerating function of the middle energizer is impaired, there is an imbalance in the digestive process. Most typical of a triple energizer imbalance are food retention issues, such as bloating, nausea, heartburn and excessive belching.

(3) Lower energizer

The main physiological process in the lower energizer is the separation of fluids for excretion in the form of urine. Referred to as the drainage ditch, the lower energizer incorporates the functions of small intestine, kidney and urinary bladder.

When the drainage ditch is not functioning properly, there are problems with water retention and urination. Imbalances involving the triple energizer can include lower leg edema, burning urination, urinary retention, loss of bladder control and frequent urination.

3.4　Extraordinary fu viscera

3.4.1　Brain

The brain is located in the skull and is composed of marrow. That is why the brain is called the sea of marrow in *Internal Classic*. The physiological functions of the brain include the following aspects.

3.4.1.1　Governing vital activities and vitalitys

The brain plays a very important role in life activities. It governs the five zang viscera and six fu viscera and regulates life activities. Impairment of the brain will threaten life. That is why it is said in *Internal Classic* that stabbing the brain will cause immediate death. The brain is an organ responsible for cognition and thinking. All the mental activities result from the reflection of things in the objective world. Though theory of viscera manifestation attributes the mental activities to heart, it never neglects the role of the brain. Li Shizhen, a great doctor in the Ming Dynasty, pointed out that the brain is the place where the primordial vitality is kept. When the brain is normal in function, people will be full of vigor, clear in thinking, fluent in speaking and strong in memory. If the brain is abnormal in function, it will lead to devitalization, retard thinking, dizziness, poor memory or mental disorder.

3.4.1.2　Governing sense and movement

There are various sensory organs in the body, such as the eyes, ears, nose, tongue and skin that respectively receive sound, light and flavor as well as the stimulation of pain, cold and heat. The brain receives such stimulation through the meridians. The brain also governs the limbs. The brain transmits the order to move through the meridians to the limbs. The brain also constantly regulates the movement of the limbs. That is why the movement of the limbs is rhythmical and accurate. If the brain is abnormal in governing and regulating the limbs, it will cause bradyesthesia and dyskinesia.

The theory of viscera manifestation emphasizes the importance of the five zang viscera, so the functions of the brain are attributed to the five zang viscera respectively. For example, the mental activities are divided into shen(vitality), po(inferior spirit), hun(inferior soul), yi(idea) and zhi(will) which are attributed to the five zang viscera respectively, for example, heart storing vitality, lung storing inferior spirit, liver storing inferior soul, spleen storing memory and kidney storing conception. Clinically mental activities are most closely related to heart, liver and kidney. Because heart governs the mind and all mental activities; liver governs dredging and dispersing and regulates mental activities; and kidney stores yin essence in order to produce marrow to enrich the brain. That is why mental diseases are clinically treated from heart, liver and kidney.

3.4.2　Marrow

Marrow is controlled and produced by kidney, and is equivalent to the brain and spinal cord. Marrow includes brain marrow, spinal marrow, and bone marrow. The main physiological function of marrow is to nourish the brain and spinal cord through essence and transformed into blood.

3.4.2.1　Nourish the brain and spinal cord through essence

Marrow is controlled and produced from kidney essence. Kidney essence can be transported to brain and nourish the brain so as to maintain the function of brain. If the sea of marrow is abundant, vitality is good, the body feels light and agile, and the span of life will be long, which is expounded in *Internal Classic*. If it is deficient there will be dizziness, tinnitus, blurred vision, fatigue, and a great desire to lie down as the brain and spinal cord are not adequately nourished and become deficient.

3.4.2.2　Transformed into blood

Since kidney essence can be transformed into marrow, and marrow can be transformed into blood, the marrow can transform into blood. In clinic, the method of nourishing kidney essence and marrow is sometimes used to treat the blood deficient syndrome.

3.4.3　Uterus

The uterus is located in the lower abdomen. The physiological function of the uterus is to produce menses and conceive fetus.

3.4.3.1　Produce menses

The uterus usually maturates at the age of fourteen and begins to produce menses, a periodic phenomenon of uterine bleeding. In adult women, blood is periodically accumulated in the uterus for conceiving and nourishing fetus. If pregnancy does not take place, the accumulated blood will be excreted out of the body. Such an excretion of blood from the uterus is known as menstruation. After excretion of the accumulated blood, the uterus begins to accumulate blood again for another periodic menstruation. Menstruation takes place once a month regularly like morning and evening tides. That is why menstruation is also called monthly tide in Chinese Medicine.

3.4.3.2　Conceive fetus

After pregnancy, the uterus is the place to nourish the fetus. There is no menstruation during pregnancy. But great quantity of blood is constantly transported to the uterus to nourish the fetus. The uterus becomes larger and larger with the development of the fetus. After delivery there is still no menses because blood is transported upwards and transformed into milk. After weaning, milk gradually stops secreting. Then blood is transported downwards into the uterus and menses begin to occur again.

The function of the uterus to produce menses and to conceive fetus is a complicated process and depends on the nourishment and coordination of other viscera.

When essence, yin and yang stored in kidney develop to a certain level, tian gui (reproductive substance) occurs. Tian gui can promote the development and maturation of the genitals, including the uterus. When the uterus becomes maturated, it is ready to produce menses and conceive fetus. When a woman becomes old, essence, yin and yang stored in kidney are gradually reduced, and so is tian gui. Eventually menstruation stops and the uterus can no longer conceive fetus.

Liver plays a very important role in the physiological functions of the uterus. On the one hand, liver governs dredging and dispersing activities and regulates the movement of qi. With the assistance of liver, the uterus functions normally, producing menses and conceiving fetus. On the other hand, liver stores blood and regulates the volume of blood. Such a function of liver is closely related to the quantity of menses and nourishment of the fetus. Since the function of the uterus is closely related to liver qi and liver-blood, there is an old saying that liver is the congenital base of life for women.

The thoroughfare and conception vessels start from the uterus. The thoroughfare vessel is the sea of blood and regulates qi and blood in the twelve regular meridians. The conception vessel governs the uterus and pregnancy. If these two vessels function well, blood will be transported smoothly into the uterus to ensure regular menses and conception of fetus. The functions of these two vessels are assisted and regulated by kidney and liver. In fact, kidney, liver, the thoroughfare and conception vessels physiologically coordinate with each other to influence the uterus.

Besides, heart, lung and spleen also influence the functions of the uterus. Because heart governs blood and propels the circulation of blood; lung governs qi and directs the flow of blood; and spleen commands blood, governs transportation and transformation and serves as the source of qi and blood.

Luo huali, Yu bin, Bie Mingke

Chapter 4

Qi, Blood, Essence and Body Fluids

Qi, blood, body fluids, and essence are the basic substances for life activities of human body. Qi refers to a refined material in the body which is energetic, invisible and continuously moving. It is an important component for human body as well as a motivation for life activities. The blood refers to the red liquid moving inside the vessels. Essence refers to various essential substances in the body. Body fluids are a generic term for normal fluid in the body. Qi, blood, body fluids, and essence are the products of physiological activities of zang-fu viscera, meridians and collaterals, meanwhile, they are the substantial basis to maintain physiological functions of zang-fu viscera, meridians and collaterals.

4.1　Qi

The concept of qi has occupied Chinese philosophers throughout history, from the beginning of Chinese civilization to our modern times. Qi refers to asubtle or formless entity that is in continual and perpetual motion. It is at the basis of all phenomena in the universe and provides continuity between coarse material forms and tenuous, rarefied, non-material energies.

Ancient philosophers and doctors then had applied the idea of qi to understand human beings and consequently to explain phenomena in medicine. Just as qi is the material substratum of the universe, it is also the material and mental-spiritual substratum of human life. As *Plain Questions* explains: "A human being results from the qi of Heaven and Earth...The union of the qi of Heaven and Earth is called human being."

4.1.1　The concept of qi

In TCM books, qi is always mentioned along with blood, essence and body fluids, for they all are fundamental substances constituting the human body and maintaining its life activities. However, among them qi is particularly important for the human body.

In concern of the concept of qi in medicine, two aspects of qi are especially relevant to medicine:

Qi is in a constant state of flux and in varying states of aggregation. When qi condenses, energy transforms and accumulates into physical shape; when qi is dispersed, it gives rise to more subtle forms of matter.

Qi is an energy that manifests simultaneously on the physical and mental-spiritual level.

Philosophers and doctors also perceived the existence and influence of qi in the human body by observing the phenomena of human life such as the qi of breathing, hot air over the body during exercise, and so on.

Qi is scalable and defines both health and pathological developments in the body. All of the physiological activities, changes or movements in the body are explained by qi. The endless motion of qi promotes and regulates human metabolism through the body. Just as *Classic of Difficult Issue* says: "Qi is the roof of human being", so when the movement of qi stopped, human life comes to an end.

4.1.2   The origination of qi

Qi in the body comes from two main sources. The first source of qi is the transformation of the innate essence called the "innate vital substance", which forms the material basis for functional activity. The second source is derivation from essential substances in nature such as food, water, herbs and other food supplements, as well as air. Both the inherited and the acquired vital energies are further processed and transformed by the viscera. Kidney first sends the innate vital substance upwards where it combines with food essence derived from spleen. It further mixes with the fresh air from lungs where it finally forms into qi of the body.

Yuan qi(primordial qi) originates from kidney. This qi is closely related to essence. Actually, primordial qi is nothing but essence in the form of qi. Kidney stores innate essence, and is supported by acquired essence. Kidney essence is mainly composed of innate essence, where a person's qi is fundamentally composed of original qi that is transformed from innate essence. Therefore, only when the function of the kidney in storing essence is normal, it can produce enough qi.

The gu qi (food qi) originates from spleen and stomach. The spleen and stomach function together to complete the digestion and absorption of water and grain. In the middle energizer, food essence rise to chest heading first to the lung and then to the heart with the help of the ascending function of spleen qi, where it is then transformed into blood and fluids. Then three scurces, innate essence, acquired food essence and air, are used to genarate qi. The spleen and stomach transform food and water into refined essences, and then into qi for distribution to zang-fu viscera and the rest of the body.

The zong qi(pectoral qi) originates from lung. Lung governs qi and is in charge of the generation of pectoral qi. On the one hand, lung governs respiratory qi by inhaling fresh qi into the body and exhaling turbid qi outside. On the other hand, lung combines the inhaled air with pectoral qi as transformed by spleen. Pectoral qi accumulates inside chest and penetrates into the heart vessels in order to move qi and blood. It then flows upward into the respiratory tract to promote breathing and also downward to an area below the navel called the Dantian(cinnabar field) in order to supplement primordial qi.

By understanding the formation of qi, TCM has identified two important factors for maintaining health healthy diet and breathing fresh air. Following these simple principles are the first steps towards creating a healthy balance in the body.

4.1.3   The movement of qi

Qi, as a refined substance, flows in every point of the body actively and constantly, to drive and maintain various physiological activities of human body.

Qi moves in four irection: ascending, descending, exiting and en-tering. Upward movement of qi means ascending while downward movement of qi means descending. Though ascending and descending are opposite, they can be transformed into each other. When qi ascends to the supreme point, it begins to descend.

Such a transformation is known as "extreme ascending changes into ascending". These are the upward and downward movement of qi under normal conditions. Entering and existing, two opposite moving styles of qi, take place alternately. When qi disperses existing to a certain degree, it begins to restrain itself entering to a certain degree, it begins to disperse existing. These are the external and internal movement of qi under normal conditions.

Ascending descending, exiting and entering of qi are very important to life. The movements of qi can regulate physiological function so as to attain the relative equilibrium. The concrete performance consists in two aspects: On the one hand, viscera, meridians, body, sense organs and orifices are harmonious and sequential in physiological function through the movement of qi. Essence, blood and body fluid have to depend upon the movement of qi to constantly circulate, so as to nourish and moisten viscera, tissues, body constituents, sense organs and orifices. On the other hand, the exchange of qi between outside and inside of the body, or absorbing essential qi from the nature and expelling the turbid qi and terminal metabolic products renews human qi and supples continuously so as to maintain life activity and regulate physiological balance. If the movements of qi are broken down, it will result in pathological changes due to imbalance among viscera, tissues, body, sense organs and orifices.

The state of coordinative balance without obstruction among ascending, descending, exiting and entering of qi is known as "free flow of qi". On the contrary, if the movements of qi in ascending, descending, exiting and entering are obstructed, or fails to maintain harmony, the "disorder of qi dynamic" arises.

Therefore, there are also four kinds of pathology qi movements called "disorder of qi dynamic". Qi pathology can manifest in four different ways as follows.

4.1.3.1 Qi deficiency

Qi deficiency has various causes most commonly, overwork and dietary irregularity. The qi of stomach, spleen, lungs or kidneys are especially prone to being deficient.

4.1.3.2 Qi sinking

If qi is deficient, it is likely to sink, causing prolapsing of the organs. This applies mostly to spleen qi and kidney qi.

4.1.3.3 Qi stagnation

Qi can fail in its movement and stagnate. This applies mostly to liver qi, but also, to a lesser extent to other organs such as intestines and lungs.

4.1.3.4 Qi counterflow

Qi can flow in the wrong direction: this is called "rebellious qi". Examples are stomach qi failing to descend and flowing upwards, causing nausea or vomiting; spleen qi failing to ascend and flowing downwards, causing diarrhea.

4.1.4 The functions of qi

Qi of human body is the essential substance that makes up the body and maintains basic activities. Generally, the function of qi exerting in the life activity can be summarized as six aspects.

4.1.4.1 Propelling function

Qi is the refined substance with very strong activity. The propelling function of qi can stimulate and maintain the physiological function of the viscera and other organs. When qi within body is abundant, the physiological functions are sound and normal, life is full of vitality. Weakness of qi in promotion will lead to the hypofunction of the viscera as well as metabolite disorders of essence, blood, body fluid, even retarded growth and development, marked by various pathological states with hypofunction.

4.1.4.2   Warming function

Qi warms body as the source of heat energy in the body. Warming is an essential function of qi, as all physiological processes depend on "warmth". This is especially crucial with fluids as they are yin in nature and therefore need yang to promote their transformation, transportation and excretion.

The source of yang and warmth in the body is primarily kidney yang and the minister fire. Spleen yang also warms body but it, derives its warmth primarily from kidney yang.

The warming function of qi means qi can produce thermal energy and make body warm and remove the cold.

4.1.4.3   Defending function

The defending function of qi also called "protecting function", it means qi can guard the body invasion of exogenous pathogens or drive the pathogens out. As to pathogenic factors, qi that protects the body is called "healthy qi" or "genuine qi".

When human body is invaded by exogenous pathogens, qi has the function of fighting against the pathogens and expelling them out. When exogenous pathogens invade the body through a part, qi will gather in the affected place and exert its defending function to fight against the pathogens. When the defending function of qi is normal, human body will be hardly invaded by pathogens; or invaded by pathogens, hardly get diseased; it suffering from disease, recover easily. If the defending function of qi is weak, the resistant ability will fall down gradually, and exogenous pathogens will take advantage of the insufficiency to invade and make body contracted.

4.1.4.4   Controlling function

The controlling function of qi means qi(yang in nature) holds fluids and blood(yin in nature) in their proper places. This is essential so that fluids or blood do not leak out.

Examples of the holding by qi are: spleen qi holds blood in blood vessels and fluids in proper spaces. Both spleen qi and kidney qi hold blood in uterus vessels. Kidney qi and bladder qi hold urine, and lung qi holds sweat.

4.1.4.5   Nourishing function

The nourishing function of qi mainly manifests in three aspects.

(1) To nourish the body surface through the defensive qi flowing the muscular striae.

(2) To transport nutrients so as to moisten and nourish the tissues and organs through the meridian qi.

(3) To nourish the whole body through the nutritive qi transforming into blood.

4.1.4.6   Qi transforming function

Qi(yang in nature) is essential for the transformation of food and fluids(yin in nature) into clear (yang) and turbid(yin) parts. This process of transformation is another aspect of the change in the state of aggregation/dispersion of qi mentioned above. Material, dense forms of matter such as food and fluids need the power of qi to be transformed into more subtle forms of matter. For example, food is transformed into food qi, which is, in turn, transformed into genuine qi.

Examples of transformation of various substances by qi are: spleen qi transforms food into food qi, stomach qi digest food, kidney qi transforms fluids, bladder qi transforms body fluids into urine, heart qi transforms food qi into blood, and lung qi transforms air into genuine qi.

4.1.5   The types of qi and their movements

Qi of the human body, according to its production, distribution and functional characteristics, is classified into four different kinds, yuan qi(primordial qi) , zong qi(pectoral qi) , ying qi(nutritive qi) and wei qi (defensive qi).

4.1.5.1 Primordial qi

The primordial qi refers to the most fundamental and important qi of the human body and is the motivating power of life activity. So, primordial qi is also called "the innate qi", or "genuine qi".

Production and distribution of the primordial qi: primordial qi comes mainly from innate essence stored in kidney, being continuously supplemented and nourished by acquired essence produced by the spleen-stomach. Therefore, the rise and falls of primordial qi have direct relation with natural endowment. In addition, food condition, physical exercises and marital adjustment can influence primordial qi. Insufficient primordial qi due to inadequate natural endowment can usually be cultivated after birth. Primordial qi is stored in the kidney and distributed to all parts of the body through triple energizer. It goes everywhere inward to the five zang viscera and the six fu viscera and outward to the body constituents, sense organs and orifices.

4.1.5.2 Pectoral qi

The pectoral qi accumulate in thorax and it is an acquired essential qi. Because thorax is the part where pectoral qi gathers, it is called "the sea of qi".

The formation and distribution of pectoral qi: pectoral qi is the combination of the natural fresh air inhaled by the lung and the food essential qi transformed by spleen-stomach. Accumulating in thorax, pectoral qi goes up along the upper respiratory tract, permeates heart and lung, and distributes to the whole body by continuously going downward through triple energizer. On the one hand, the pectoral qi goes up out of lung and flows along the respiratory tract to throat to promote respiration. On the other hand, it permeates heart and vessels to propel blood circulation. Triple energizer is the passage for all qi to circulate. Through triple energizer the pectoral qi continues to go downward and to be stored in the elixir field so as to supply primordial qi and permeates the stomach meridian of foot yangming via acupoint Qijie(ST 30).

4.1.5.3 Nutritive qi

Nutritive qi refers to a kind of qi circulating within vessels and having nutritive action. It is an important component of the blood. It can be different but cannot be separated from blood, hence named "nutritive-blood". Compared with the defensive qi, nutritive qi pertains to yin, so it is also called "nutritive-yin".

Production and distribution of nutritive qi: the nutritive qi comes from the most refined and nutritive part of foodstuff essence. Nutritive qi flows inside the vessels to circulate throughout the body, interiorly into viscera and exteriorly onto limbs and joints, repeatedly in the cycle without an end.

4.1.5.4 Defensive qi

Defensive qi means the qi circulating outside the vessels and having protective function to the body. Compared with nutritive qi, the defensive qi comes from of "defensive yang", the fierce and swifts part of the foodstuff essence. Because of quick activity and strong vitality, defensive qi does not be limited by vessels and goes outward over skin and muscular striae, inward to thorax and abdomen, spreading the whole body.

Although nutritive qi and defensive qi come from foodstuff essence, they have different property, distribution and physiological function. Nutritive qi comes from "the most essential part" of foodstuff essence, flowing inside vessels, producing blood and nourishing the whole body, so it belongs to yin. Defensive qi comes from "the most active and powerful part" of foodstuff essence, flowing outside vessels, defending the body surface and warming the body, so it belongs to yang. Only when these two qi coordinate with each other, can they exert their own physiological function respectively.

Besides there are "visceral qi" and "meridian qi". They all derive from primordial qi, which is distributed to a viscus or meridian and combined with foodstuff essence or fresh air so as to become qi of a viscus or meridian. In clinical, the rise and fall of visceral qi and meridian qi can be determined according to their functional conditions.

4.2 Blood

Blood is generated from food essence and kidney essence through the processes of qi transformation by spleen, stomach, heart, lung and kidney.

The meaning of "blood" is different in Chinese and Western medicine. In Chinese medicine, blood is a form of very dense and material qi. Moreover, blood is inseparable from qi, as qi infuses vitality into blood; without qi, blood is inert.

4.2.1 The concept of blood and its origination

Blood is a red liquid material circulating within vessels and possessing strong nourishing and moistening functions.

The basic substance of blood production is essence including congenital essence, as known as kidney essence, and acquired essence, food nutrients.

Essence is transformed into blood durig its production, which gives blood vitality. The essence and blood are the same kind, being of inter-promotion and inter-transformation. Essence is the beginning of life, and blood is a special form of essence. Original essence is stored kidney. Sufficient kidney essence can provide necessary nourishment for liver. Liver stores blood, as the essence enters the liver and transfarmed into blood. The mutual supporting and conversion of essence and blood outstandingly reflect the close relationship of the liver and the kidney in their physiological functions. If the function of liver or kidney is weakened, particularly deficiency of kidney essence or kidney yin. The formation of blood lead to syndrome of blood deficiency will be affected.

Food assimilate into body are converted into foodstuff essence through the decomposition by the stomach and transformation and transportation by spleen. The pure and refined part of which is transformed into the nutritive qi. The nutritive qi permeates the vessels and combines with body fluid to become blood. The nutritive qi comes from the most pure and refined part of the foodstuffs. It insures that the blood has extremely abundant nourishing composition. The body fluid is also are important part of blood, and has the functions of maintaining and regulating blood volume, diluting blood and lubricating the vessels, thus guaranteeing ample blood and its enduring circulation. Nutritive qi and body fluid are the main material basis of blood production. Balanced diet and robust spleen-stomach function are important assurance for blood production.

4.2.2 The circulation of blood

Blood circulates endlessly within the vessels and meridians, like a circle without an end, thus to nourish the whole body to support the life activity. Basically, the propelling and controlling function of qi, the integrity and smoothness of vessels, the quality and temperature of blood maintain normal blood circulation. Heart, lung, spleen and liver play important roles in maintenance of normal blood circulation. Heart governs blood circulation, lung connects with many large vessels, spleen controls blood and liver stores blood.

Blood is propelled by heart to circulate in the vessels. Apart from heart, other internal organs are also involved in the circulation of blood, including lung, spleen and liver. Structurally lung is connected with all the vessels in the body. Depending on the association with vessels, lung distributes nutrient substances, like pectoral qi, to the whole body and accumulates qi and blood from the whole body to assist the heart to propel blood circulation. Spleen commands blood, making the vessels compact, directing blood to circulate normally in vessels and preventing it from flowing out of vessels. The liver stores blood and regulates the volume of blood. Besides, liver also governs dredging and dispersing, thus smoothing the activity of qi to promote blood circulation.

The factor that directly acts on blood circulation is qi. Other factors that may affect blood circulation are the state of vessels and the changes of cold and heat, such as phlegm, dampness, blood stasis, swelling and nodules.

4.2.3   The functions of blood

The blood is life material with abundant nourishment and yin liquid. Its functions include nourishing and moistening body, material basis for mental activities and transport the turbid qi.

It should be noted that blood is also an important material base for mental activities. If blood is sufficient, there will be sufficient vitality; if blood is deficient, there will be dispiritedness; if blood is in disturbance, there will be mental disorder. Since blood contains fluid, it can moisten viscera and body. When the fluid flows out of vessel, it moistens orifice and lubricate joint.

Besides, blood also transports turbid qi. When turbid air is transported to lung, it is excreted from respiration. When it is transported to kidney, it is discharged from urination. When it is transported to superficies, it is excreted from sweating.

In addition, blood is also material basis for generation of the sperm, menstrual blood, and milk.

4.3   Essence

In ancient Chinese philosophy, essence is an invisible and ever-moving foundational substance that constitutes the entire universe. In Chinese medicine, essence is more specifically related to human life, and is generally thought of as being fluid-like in that it flows between the organs in which it is stored.

Essence in Chinese medicine has a variety of meanings, in the narrow sense, in the broad sense and in the general sense. Essence is initially defined as reproductive essence with function of producing offspring, which is called essence in the narrow sense, and is also the initial concept of essence in Chinese medicine. From this point of view of liquid essence, blood, fluids, innate essence, foodstuff essence, reproductive essence, and visceral essence all belong to the scope of the broad sense of essence. However, in terms of formation and function of a specific substance, there is a difference between essence and blood or fluids in concept. In general, the concept of essence is limited to the innate essence, foodstuff essence, reproductive essence and visceral essence, not including blood and fluids. Essence in Chinese medicine usually refers to the general sense.

4.3.1   The concept of essence

Essence is a type of refined nutritious substances in the body. In a broader sense, it refers to the refined nutritious substances transformed by qi and constituting the human body and maintaining its life activity,including qi,blood,body fluids,foodstuff essence,marrow,etc. In a narrow sense,it means the reproductive essence having function of producing offspring and stored in kidney,acting as basic substance promoting growth,development and reproductive function of human body.

4.3.2　The origination and types of essence

Essence of human body is originally endowed from parents and is constantly replenished and nourished after birth. Based on the original differenee,there are innate and acquired essences.

Innate essence includes kidney essence,inherited from parents,and the original substance constitutes embryo. Life material endowed from parents is essence coming from birth,which is the innate essence. Through the observation and experience of the multiplying process of mankind,the ancients recognized that the combination of reproductive essence of parents can produce a new individual life. From embryo's formation to the fetur's maturity,which all depends on nutrition of qi-blood in uterus. Therefore,innate essence is an original substance of life,mainly stored in kidney.

Acquired essence comes from foodstuffs,and is called "foodstuff essence". After birth,human body depends on spleen-stomach to digest and absorb foodstuff,converting it into foodstuff essence so as to nourish every viscera,thus maintaining its normal life activity. Because this part comes from acquirement,it is called the acquired essence.

4.3.3　The functions of essence

The essence has functions of producing offspring,promoting growth and developing,transforming itself into marrow and blood,producing qi and spirit.

4.3.3.1　Producing offspring

Reproductive essence is the congenital material of basic life. Combining the reproductive essence of couple can produce a new individual life. It has the function of reproduction,It comes from combination of the innate and acquired essence and stores in kidney,constituting essential qi of kidney. With its abundance that is marked by full development of body,to the period of youth,"tiangui" (reproduction-stimulating essence) is generated,granting function of producing offspring. Therefore,essential qi of kidney can not only contain the reproductive essence but also transform into kidney qi to promote reproduction.

4.3.3.2　Promoting growth and development

Essential qi of kidney has the function of promoting growth and development. After birth,the body constantly grows and develops till matures as the it gradually becomes abundant;then body gradually gets senile along with continual decline of it. If kidney essence is abundant,growth and development of the body will be normal;if kidney essence gets deficient,it will result in pathological changes marked by hypoevolutism,five kinds of flaccidity and developmental delay.

4.3.3.3　Moistening and nourishing viscera

The essence can moisten and nourish viscera,tissues,sense organs and orifices. As the essence is sufficient,human body can get necessary nourishment to perform its normal physical function. If kidney essence is deficient due to inadequate natural endowment or disturbed production of acquired essence,the essence of five zang viscera will decline,and viscera,tissues,sense organs and orifices fail to get the nourishment and supplement,wich cause their physical functions will be insufficient or even fail.

4.3.3.4　Transforming itself into marrow and blood

Kidney stores essence which can transform itself into the marrow including brain marrow and bone marrow. Brain marrow can nourish the brain. Its sufficiency provides alert mind, agile thinking and clear speech. Bone depends on the nourishment of marrow. As kidney essence is sufficient, the bone marrow will be abundant, and then skeleton will be firm and flexible. Teeth are the extension of the bones which are nourished by marrow transformed from kidney essence. As kidney essence is abundant, teeth are firm and lustrous, If kidney essence is deficient which affects production of marrow, and then skeleton loses its nourishment for teeth, leading to looseness, even loss of teeth. If brain marrow is deficient, it will result in symptoms such as dizziness, vertigo, mental weakness, amnesia and retarded intelligence.

Essence produces marrow, which is one of the sources for blood production. Sufficient essence in kidney provides necessary nourishment for liver, which replenishs blood. Therefore, essence and blood promote each other, so there is a saying "essence and blood have the same origin".

4.3.3.5 Producing qi and spirit

Innate essence can generate innate qi(primordial qi). Transformed from the foodstuff essence the foodstuff qi which is combines with fresh air inhaled by the lung to form acquired qi. Qi constantly drives and regulates metabolism of human body, maintaining life activity. Essence can produce both qi and spirit. It is the substantial basis for mental activity. Only when the essence is enough, can spirit be sound, which is the basic assurance for life existence.

4.4 Body fluids

Body fluids refer to the different kinds of physiological fluids in the body, including fluid existing in zang-fu viscera and tissues, and secretions and excretion of human body. Like qi and blood body fluids are also the essential substance constituting the human body. The flowing mainly makes an introduction of the origination, distribution, excretion and function of body fluid.

4.4.1 The concept of body fluids

Body fluids are general terms for all normal physiological fluids in the body, including internal fluids that act to moisten various organs and tissues, and also their secretions and excretions in the body such as tears, saliva, sweat, nasal discharge, gastric juice, intestinal juice, urine and so on. Just like qi and blood, Body fluids are also ones of the essential substances constituting the human body and maintaining its life activities.

Body fluids can be divided into two parts: jin(fluid) and ye(liquid). Jin is clear and thin and flows easily. It follows along with the circulation of defensive qi and blood, in fact assisting their smooth flow, spreading throughout skin, muscles and orifices, coming out as sweat, tears, saliva and mucus. Furthermore, it permeates blood vessels to keep them moistened and becomes a component part of blood. Ye, on the contrary, is thick and viscous, moving relatively slowly and circulating with nutritive qi under the control of spleen and kidney as well as middle and lower burner. It is distributed in bones, joints, brain, marrow and internal organs to nourish the related parts of the body, lubricating orifices of sense organs of eyes ears nose and mouth. Jin and ye both come from food and water transformed by the spleen and stomach, functionally permeate, supply and transform into each other. These two fluids are closely related. For this reason, they are jointly referred to as "jinye"(body fluids)(Table 4–1).

Table 4–1　**Differentiation of jin and ye**

Jin	Ye
Yang	Yin
Thin,clear and watery	Thick,sticky
Found superficially under skin, perfuses and warmsthe tissues	Found in zang-fu viscera
Flow with qi and blood	Not flowing with qi and blood
Functioning as sweats,saliva and urine	Functioning as moistening lubricant,found in bone marrow,joints and deep yin areas of the body

4.4.2　The origination,distribution and excretion of body fluids

According to TCM theory,body fluids originate from food and water. The formation,distribution and excretion of body fluid are a complex physiological process in which they are accomplished by the joint action of many organs. As is stated in *Plain Questions*,"After food and drink enter into the stomach,they are decomposed into food essence and then,transported to spleen,which disperses essence upward to lung and lung regulates water pathways downward to urinary bladder. By doing so,body fluids are finally disseminated throughout the body along meridians and collaterals. "

Body fluids mainly come from foodstuff and it is produced by digesting and absorbing function of stomach,spleen and small intestine. The metabolism of body fluids come through a series of physiological activities,including "receiving and digesting" of stomach; "transporting, transforming and transmitting" of spleen,"transmitting and changing" of large intestine and "separating the clear from turbid" of small intestine(Figure 4–1). As different viscera may exert different effect on thes whole process,the spleen transports body fluids to heart and lung by governing transportation and transformation;lung distributes body fluids to the whole body and down into kidney by governing the regulation of water passage;kidney transports body fluids that are steamed during the formation of urine upward into heart and lung. So the distribution of body fluids mainly depends on the action of lung,spleen and kidney(Figure 4–2). After the body fluids are utilized by human body,the rest of them should be excreted out of body. Also the excretion involves several organs coordination. Lung disseminates body fluids transformed into sweat outwardly to the surface of the body;the terminal metabolic product urine is excreted out of body through the qi transformation of kidney and urinary bladder;parts of body fluids are carried out through defecation and respiration by large intestine and lung. In addition,smoothness of water passage of triple energizer and free flow of liver qi can also help the distribution and excretion of body fluids(Figure 4–3).

In brief,the production of body fluids mainly depends on the transformation and transportation of spleen and stomach;their distribution depends on the spleen and the lung;their excretion depends on the lung and the kidney. So the dysfunction of these organs will certainly cause disturbance of the distribution and excretion of body fluids,giving rise to phlegm,edema or urine disorders.

Appendix:five zang viscera transforming five kinds of liquids

Five kinds of liquids include sweat,snivel,tear,saliva and drool. TCM believes that these liquids are transformed by five zang viscera.

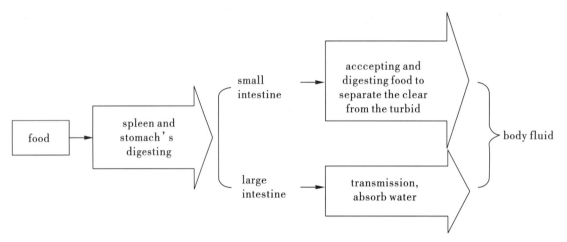

Figure 4-1   **Thegeneration of body fluid**

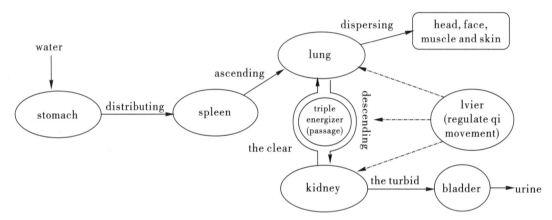

Figure 4-2   **The distribution of body fluid**

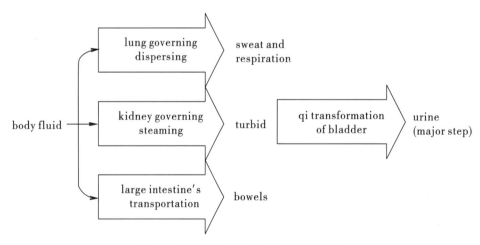

Figure 4-3   **The excretion of body fluid**

The relationships between five zang viscera and five kinds of liquids are described this way: sweat is the liquid of heart, snivel is the liquid of lung, tear is liquid of liver, saliva is the liquid of spleen and drool is the liquid of kidney.

(1) Sweat comes from body fluids and is excreted out of the body through sweat pores under the steam-

ing of yang qi. Heart pertains to fire in the five elements. Heart fire transforms into yang qi to steam body fluids which comes out of the skin and becomes sweat. Thus sweat is regarded as the fluid of heart. Insufficiency of heart yang results in oligohidrosis while superabundance of heart fire brings on polyhidrosis.

(2) Snivel refers to the nasal mucus that can moisten nostrils. Since nose is the orifice of lung, so snivel is the liquid of the lung. If lung qi fails to disperse, nose will become stuffy and running; if lung-heat impairs body fluids, nose will be dry with scanty snivel.

(3) Tear comes from the eyes and can moisten eyes. Since eyes are the orifices of the liver, tear is the liquid of liver. If there is wind-heat in liver, eyes will become tearing; if livery in is insufficient, the eyes will become dry because of scanty tear.

(4) Saliva refers to the thin part of the fluid in mouth. It can promote the intake of food. Since mouth is the orifice of spleen, saliva is liquid of spleen. If spleen is weak, there will be profuse of saliva running out of mouth; if spleen yin is insufficient, mouth will be dry because of scanty saliva in mouth.

(5) Drool refers to the thick part of the fluid in mouth. It nourishes kidney essence by not only wetting and dissowling food for smooth swallowing but also keeping and health.

4.4.3　The functions of body fluids

4.4.3.1　Moistening and nourishing

Body fluids are mainly responsible for providing moisture and nourishment to tissues. When distributed to the surface of the body, body fluids moisten skin and hair and maintain smooth and elastic texture of skin. Body fluids also moisten, nourish and protect different orifices in the body. For example, body fluids allow eyes to blink smoothly, the nasal cavity to maintain an open airway without blockage and lips and mouth to remain moist without becoming dry. Internal body fluids also penetrate different organs, tissues and even bone marrow to provide moisture and nourishment. The spinal cord and brain are examples of organs surrounded by body fluids that protecting and nourishing them.

4.4.3.2　Transporting

Body fluids can hold various turbid qi and waste materials produced by qi transformation and transport them to the involved organs to be excreted out of the body by urinating, sweating and respiration. The liquid waste materials are directly excreted in the form of fluid through urination and sweating. But the turbid qi excreted through respiration is transported to the lung first by body fluid and then exhaled out of the body. If body fluids are insufficient, the turbid qi cannot be quickly excreted out of the body, seriously affecting qi transformation and causing various pathological changes.

When body fluids metabolize, they can also produce the waste after metabolism in the body, and transmit the poisonous substances to go outside of the body by sweating and urination, thus maintaining the cleanliness of the body itself and ensuring the normal physiological functions of the viscera, bowels, meridian and collaterals, tissues and other organs.

4.4.3.3　Transforming into blood

Body fluids seep into blood vessels through the wall of blood vessels, performing nourishing and lubricating function and becoming a component of blood. When the body is short of water, the fluid in blood will seep out of vessels to supplement the body fluids and rectify dehydration. Through the process of permeating into and out of vessels, human body can maintain the effective blood volume and ensure normal blood circulation.

Disharmony of body fluids is manifested in two ways. When body fluids can no longer nourish and provide moisture to the body, symptoms such as dry skin, flaccid muscles, brittle hair, dry eyes, parched lips and a dry nose or throat occur. When there is dysfunction of distribution or excretion of body fluids, symptoms can present as swollen eyelids, edema(retention of fluid in the tissues), obesity or other conditions.

Wang Ying, Li lin

Chapter 5

Etiologies and Pathogenesis

According to Traditional Chinese Medicine, the human body is an organic whole. There is a relatively dynamic balance between the viscera, tissues and the external environment, so as to maintain the normal life activities of the body. If this balance is broken and cannot recover in timely manner, the body catches disease. There is a close relationship among etiology, pathogenesis and symptoms. Etiology and pathogenesis mainly discuss the causes of the destruction of this balance and the mechanism of disease's occurrence, development and evolution.

Etiology and pathogenesis of TCM elaborate upon the causes of disease, including the theory, knowledge and disciplines of its occurrence, development and variation. Etiology is classified into four classes, exogenous pathogenic factors, endogenic pathogenic factors, pathological products and the others. Pathogenesis theory explains the mechanism of disease onset, progression and prognosis, and mainly elaborates upon the basic pathogenesis and disease transmission variations and outcomes.

5.1　Etiology

The cause of the disease, which can destroy the relative balance of the human body, is called the pathogenic factor. Also known as "disease evil", "pathogenic" and so on. Identifying the cause of the patient's disharmony is an important part of Chinese medical practice. By doing that, we can advise the patient how to avoid it, minimize it or prevent disease. Any kind of factors that can influence the relative balance of the physiological state of the human body is called "cause of disease". The causes of diseases can be divided into three types, which are external pathogenic factors, internal pathogenic factors, and the pathogenic factors belonging to neither external nor internal.

Therefore, except the traumatology, TCM divides diseases into exogenous diseases and internal damages. Accordingly, this section is divided into two categories for discussion.

5.1.1　Exogenous factors

Exogenous diseases originate from the natural world, such as six climatic influences and pestilent qi which invade human body mainly through skin, nose or mouth. The onset of exogenous diseases is associated with seasons. It is more urgent, and the pathogenic factors may transmit from the exterior to the interior. If mixed with pestilent qi, it has the epidemic and infectious characters.

5.1.1.1   Six excesses

Under normal circumstances, wind, cold, summer heat, dampness, dryness and fire are called six qi. They are six different factors in nature, which are the normal condition of nature and are harmless to human body. When abnormal climate occurs, for example, excessive or deficient climate (e. g. , too hot in summer or too cold in winter), and rapid climate changes (e. g. , intense bursts of cold or heat), the body cannot adapt and disease occurs. On the other hand, when the people have low resistance and cannot adapt even to normal climatic changes, the six qi will also become pathogenic factors that attack and cause disease. Under these circumstances, the six qi are called six climatic influences. The characteristics of six climatic influences are as follows.

Six excesses invade through skin, or from the nose and mouth, or both at the same time.

They have a close relationship with seasonal changes. For example, in spring there may be more wind diseases, summer more heat diseases, late summer more dampness diseases, autumn more dry diseases, and winter more cold diseases.

They have a relationship with dwelling place. Residing in a wet place causes more dampness diseases and living in a hot climate causes more heatstroke or summer heat syndrome.

Six pathogenic factors can invade the body respectively and simultaneously. For example, common cold due to wind-cold, diarrhea due to dampness-heat, and arthralgia due to wind-cold-dampness.

In the disease process the six pathogenic factors not only influence each other, but also can be mutually transformed into each other under certain conditions, for example, inward attack of cold changing into heat, long stagnation of summer heat-dampness turning into dryness, which may further impair yin, etc.

In addition, there are some clinical pathologic changes that are not caused by the six climatic influences, but because of the dysfunction of zang-fu viscera, or qi, blood and fluid, which may lead to wind, cold, dampness, dryness, heat and fire. Though the clinical features correspond with the exogenous six climatic influences, they are endogenous, so they are referred to as the internal five pathogens, namely internal wind, internal cold, internal dampness, internal dryness and internal fire (heat).

(1) Wind

Wind is the dominant weather in spring, yet existing in all seasons. So diseases caused by wind are not limited in spring, but also in other seasons. According to TCM, wind is an extremely important exogenous pathogenic factor of disease. Wind qi attacks through skin and pores to produce wind diseases. Wind is characterized by the following features.

Wind belongs to yang pathogen. It tends to float, move and attack the upper part, the back or the surface of the body. The wind in the nature has no shape. Its major characteristic is upward and outward movement. As head and skin is always attacked first, the typical symptoms to appear are headache, running nose, sweating and aversion to wind. When pathogenic wind attacks the lung, nasal congestion, throat itching and cough will occur as consequences.

Wind tends to be mobile and causes diseases with no fixed place. Sometimes it is light and soft, sometimes it is mad. So diseases caused by wind are characterized by constant movement, and the location of disease is not fixed, for example, syndrome of wind-prevailing migratory arthralgia. On the other hand, wind diseases are unpredictable and attack quickly, such as urticaria, which is not only itchy, but also moves around the body as one hive resolves and another rises.

Wind tends to cause vibration. In the nature, wind is easy to make objects rocking, so diseases caused by pathogenic wind have the same characteristics. Clinically, there may appear dizziness and convulsion. For example, invasion by pathogenic wind after some external injuries may lead to symptoms like limb convulsion. Wind often causes common symptoms like tremor, vertigo, convulsions, stiff neck, opisthotonos and so on.

Wind is the primary pathogen that tends to be complicated by other pathogenic factors. Because pathogenic wind is the mainfactor among the exterior pathogenic factors, the six climatic influences often attack the body in combination with the wind. For example, wind-cold, wind-heat, wind-dampness, etc. So pathogenic wind is also called the head of six climatic influences. Cold, dampness, dryness and fire tend to be attached to wind when attacking the human body, causing syndromes like wind-cold, wind-heat, wind-dampness, etc. Wind attacks in any season, and the ancient doctors regarded it as the lead of the exogenous pathogenic factors.

(2) Cold

Cold pathogen refers to excess cold that causes coagulation and involuntary muscular contraction. Cold is the normal climatic factor in winter, but it can also be seen in other seasons or the time when temperature rapidly decreases. For example, being caught in rain or wading in water, being exposed to wind while sweating and indulgence in exposure to cold or sleeping in the open air or drinking too much cold drink, all the aforementioned factors can cause the invasion of pathogenic cold.

The cold weather in the nature mainly manifest itself through cold air, storage of everything, water being difficult to evaporate, things that are not easily erosive and animals that roll up and sleep quietly with skin and hair contracted, etc.

The diseases caused by pathogenic cold can be divided into two kinds, the exogenous cold disease and the endogenous cold disease. Cold disease due to invasion of exogenous pathogenic is different from those caused by endogenous pathogenic cold, which mainly resulting from deficiency of yang qi within the body. But the two kinds of cold diseases could be internally related—yang deficient body tends to suffer from the attack of external pathogenic cold, while external cold retaining in the body may impair the body yang and leads to endogenous cold disease.

In exogenous cold disease, there are differences of cold-attack and cold-stroke according to the invading location. The condition that pathogenic cold injures skin surface, which depresses the wei yang. This is called "cold attack", marked by chills, fever, etc. The condition that pathogenic cold directly invade the interior of the body and injure yang qi of the zang-fu viscera is called "cold stroke", shown as epigastralgia, vomiting, diarrhea, etc.

Cold, as a kind of yin pathogen, tends to damage yang qi. Pathogenic cold and pathogenic heat are opposite. In nature, pathogenic cold pertains to yin while pathogenic heat pertains to yang. Normally, yang qi of the human body may restrain pathogen cold. But excessive cold attacking the surface of the body will impair yang qi and lead to symptoms including aversion to cold, fever, headache, lacking of sweat, running nose and body pain. If cold attacks the zang-fu viscera directly, visceral yang will be impaired and lead to symptoms including aversion to cold, abdominal cold pain, diarrhea, cold limbs, clear abundant urine, etc.

Cold can easily lead to stagnation in the body, such as stagnant qi, blood, and body fluid, blocking meridians and causing pain. It is said that cold is characterized by pain. Continuous and smooth circulation of qi and blood fully rely on the warming and promoting function of yang qi. Whenever yin pathogen invades the body, yang qi is affected. Therefore, qi and blood of the human body will lose the warmth of yang qi. When qi and blood in the channels are condensed and obstructed, circulation of qi and blood will become slow, unsmooth or even stagnant, which leads to various pains. For example, if pathogenic cold attacks the taiyang meridian, pain in the whole body will occur. If pathogenic cold invades the middle and lower energizer, there will appear cold-pain in the abdomen, even acute pain. The pain can be relieved by warmth and aggravated by coldness.

Cold has the characteristics of constriction and traction which tend to astringe the qi movement, leading to the contraction of striae, meridians and tendons. For cold attacking the exterior, there may be aversion to cold, and fever without sweating. When cold attacks meridians and joints, the symptoms include difficulty in joint flexion and extension, spasm and pain.

Cold has the characteristic of limpidity. If one's excretion is clear, for example clear nasal discharge or white clear sputum, it is likely to be attacked by cold.

(3) Summer heat

Summer heat is the dominant qi in summer. If summer heat (the natural weather) makes one ill, it is called pathogenic summer heat. The diseases caused by summer heat are mostly seasonal. That is to say, summer heat only flourishes in summer, chiefly after the summer solstice, and before the beginning of autumn. *Plain questions* said, the one first lasting to the summer solstice is disease warmth while that later, disease summer heat. However, summer heat is purely external pathogen and there is no internal summer heat. It is developed from heat, and has characteristics as follows.

Summer heat is a kind of yang pathogen that has the characteristic of being torrid. Pathogenic cold belongs to yin whereas summer heat pertains to yang. So when pathogenic summer heat invades the body, yang qi of the body is relatively excessive, usually appearing a series of obvious yang (heat) symptoms clinically, such as high fever, profuse sweating, thirst with desire to drink, red complexion, and surging pulse. Moreover, the summer heat forces the fluids to leak out and pathogenic heat consumes and scorches the yin fluids inside, resulting in damage of yin in the body. So diseases caused by pathogenic summer heat often manifest in combination with symptoms of fluids deficiency, sud as thirst, indulgence in drink, dry lips and tongue, scanty red urine, dry stools, etc.

Summer heat ascends and disperses, and is likely to disturb the mind, attack the head and offend pericardium directly. It opens the pores and causes excessive sweating which will lead to qi consumption. So symptoms caused by pathogenic summer heat usually occur in the upper portion of the body, such as flushed face, dry mouth, etc. And sweating is the main way for the human body to dissipate heat. So invasion of pathogenic summer heat may make the striae of the skin and muscles open, resulting in profuse sweating, which consumes fluids, causing scanty and dark urine, and disorders of qi, blood, body fluid, etc. While a lot of sweat is excreted, qi consumption will occur in consequence, because qi is excreted together with excretion of fluids. So, symptoms of deficiency of qi may appear, such as shortness of breath, fatigue, weakness, etc.

Summer heat is usually accompanied with dampness when invading the body. Besides being very hot, the summer is often full of rain and dampness, so dampness and heat intermingle and mix to fill with air. That is why summer heat often mixes with the dampness when it invades human body. Clinically, there are symptoms manifest both summer heat syndrome and dampness stagnation syndrome, such as fever and thirst with fidgets, heavy limbs, stuffy chest, sticky thin and sloppy stool, greasy tongue coating, soggy pulse, etc.

(4) Dampness

Dampness is the dominant qi in late summer, a period of time between summer and autumn. During this time summer heat has not disappeared, and rain comes more frequently, resulting in fullness of moisture in the air. It is the dampest period of the year. Thus damp disease often occurs in late summer.

But in other seasons, if living or working in damp conditions, or being exposed to rain and wading in water, sweating to make clothes damp. one may also be ill due to external affection of pathogenic dampness.

So disease caused by pathogenic dampness may occur in four seasons, not limited in late summer. The diseases caused by external dampness are different from internal dampness diseases which results from spleen deficiency. But the two factors often influence each other during the occurrence of a disease. Pathogenic dampness may disturb the function of the spleen in transportation and transformation, leading to generation of internal dampness. On the contrary, if the spleen fails to transport and transform water-dampness due to the deficiency, internal dampness disease will occur and the patient is vulnerable to the invasion of external dampness.

Dampness has the character of stickiness, turbidity and descending tendency. It is a yin pathogen, therefore tending to damage yang qi, and it can also obstruct the function of qi. Its nature is similar to that of water, so dampness pertains to yin. A famous physician once said "when dampness is strong enough, yang qi will become weaker". Pathogenic dampness injures the human body, retains the zang-fu viscera and meridians. It most incidentally blocks qi movement. For example pathogenic damp accumulating on the chest leads to chest oppression due to its disturbance of qi movement pathogenic damp blocking the spleen and stomach leads to descending and stagnation of the flow of qi there will appear epigastric fullness, abdominal distension and sloppy diarrhea; it staying in the lower energizer impedes the qi movement in the lower energizer, marked by scanty urine.

Dampness is yin pathogen excess yin would cause illness of yang. So the invasion of pathogenic dampness may damage yang qi of the human body. The spleen like the dryness has aversion to dampness. Hence when pathogenic damp invades the body, it will disturb the spleen first, then lead to restrain of the spleen yang, and the spleen yang fails to transport and transform, resulting in retention of water-dampness. Therefore, there may appear poor appetite, epigastric fullness, abdominal distension and sloppy diarrhea, scanty urine, edema and ascites.

Dampness is characterized by heavy and turbid. Among six climatic influences, dampness is the heavy and turbid pathogen. Heaviness implies that the feature of diseases caused by pathogenic damp is heavy. For example, if dampness invades the body, the symptoms can be characterized by heavy head with the feeling of being swathed, heavy body, and sluggish or heavy limbs. If pathogenic dampness stays in the channel and joints, there will be pain and numbness in the joint, therefore, arthralgia caused by pathogenic damp is called damp or heavy arthralgia.

Turbidity means that diseases caused by pathogenic dampness are represented by filthy and foul discharge or secretion. For example, if pathogenic dampness stays in upper part of the body, dirty complexion and excessive secretion from the eyes will occur. When pathogenic damp stagnates in the large intestine, sloppy diarrhea or dysentery appears. If dampness goes downward, turbid urine and leukorrhagia for women occur.

Dampness is viscous and lingering, refering to that the diseases caused by pathogenic dampness are characterized by the sticky and stagnant. These characteristics mainly manifest in the two aspects. One is sticky symptom. For example, when dampness accumulates in the large intestine, the flow of bowl-qi will be unsmooth, which is marked by mucopurulent stools. The other is in the course of disease. Besides the long duration, it is refractory in healing and easily relapses. This is because of the stickiness of dampness which makes it prone to block the circulation of qi. For example, the courses of eczema, damp-arthralgia and cold caused by pathogenic wind-damp, are long.

Dampness tends to move downward. Dampness is similar to water in nature. Water is descending, heavy and turbid in nature. So, pathogenic damp has the descending tendency and easily to injure the yin position of the human body. So the diseases caused by pathogenic damp usually start from the lower position, or the symptoms in the lower position are predominant. For example, edema caused by pathogenic water-dampness mainly occurs in the lower limbs, and so does stranguria with turbid urine, diarrhea and dysentery, leucorrhea or ulcer caused by pathogenic damp.

(5) Dryness

Dryness is the dominant climate in autumn, and the climate in autumn is dry. So in this season, things always lack moisture, and everything is withered and splitting in the nature. External pathogen in the nature of dryness descends and is called pathogenic dryness. Diseases caused by pathogenic dryness are called external dry diseases. Pathogenic dryness often invades the lung and damages defensive qi through the mouth and nose to cause diseases.

Pathogenic dryness can be divided into warm dryness and cold dryness. In early autumn, it is sunny, rainless and hot. Dryness and heat associate with each other to attack people during this period of time, and cause warm dryness syndrome. In late autumn near winter, it is cold. Dryness invades human body in company with cold, and cause cold dryness syndrome.

It is characterized by dryness and tends to consume body fluid. Pathogenic dryness is the dry and pucker pathogen. So, dryness is most likely to consume and injure fluids of the human body, which leads to various dry and pucker symptoms. The clinical manifestations of such symptoms usually concentrate on orifices of skin and hair of the head and face, defecation and micturition, resulting in dry mouth and lips, dry nose and pharynx, dry and rough skin, even chapped skin, dry and unlustrous hair, scanty urine and constipation.

Another character is impairment of lung. Lung, a "fragile organ", is delicate, and likes to be moistened and dislikes dryness. It controls respiration, governs skin and hair externally, opens at the nose. Pathogenic dryness often damages the fluids through the mouth and nose. So it is prone to damage the lung, causing symptoms such as dry cough, scanty and sticky sputum, chest pain, difficult breath, etc. If lung collateral vessels are damaged, bleeding will appear in the sputum. The lung is exteriorly-interiorly related to the large intestine, so pathogenic dryness in the lung may influence the large intestine, resulting in dry stools.

(6) Fire(heat)

Fire(heat) is the predominant factor in summer. Fire(heat) is the climate with excess yang qi in the natural field, characterized by of being warm and hot. Fire(heat) weather rages in hot summer. But it has no obvious seasonal nature like pathogenic summer heat. Because in other seasons, there may also appear hot climate, or when working under the high temperature, people can easily be affected by Fire(heat) pathogen. Hence, Fire(heat) pathogen has no specific seasonal nature.

In TCM, the nature of warm and pathogenic fire is similar to pathogenic heat. Generally, warmness is the lesser of the heat while fire is the greater of the heat. Therefore, they are collectively called warm(heat) and fire(heat) pathogen in general. Generally, pathogenic warm and heat belongs to external pathogen, such as wind(heat), summer(heat) and dampness(heat), but dysfunction of zang-fu viscera like liver or heart can also generate fire, produced by excess of yang qi of the body, which is called endogenous fire or internal fire.

As a yang pathogen, it has an ascending tendency. Pathogenic fire (heat) is produced by excessive yang in the nature, which is scorching moving, elevating and flaring in nature. So the diseases caused by pathogenic fire usually occur in the upper portion of the human body, particularly predominancing in fire (heat) symptoms on the head and face. For example, scorching heat is the nature of fire presenting with high fever, flushed face, red eyes, red tongue, headache, rapid pulse, erosion of mucous membrane in the mouth, swelling and aching of gingiva, etc.

Fire disturbs the mind. The heart corresponds to heat in five elements. So when being invaded by pathogenic fire(heat), heart spirit tends to be harassed, which results in dysphoria, insomnia, mania, unconsciousness, delirium, etc.

Fire is likely to consume qi and body fluid. Fire is yang pathogen, scorching and steaming in nature. So if pathogenic fire(heat) invades the body, there appears a series of heat symptoms. At the same time, it consumes the body fluids and drives the fluids out, causing sweating and yin deficiency. So in addition to high fever, diseases caused by pathogenic fire are usually accompanied with symptoms of fluids insufficiency, such as thirsty with a desire for cold drink, dry mouth and tongue, scanty and dark urine, difficult and painful urination, constipation, red tongue with yellow coating, etc. Moreover, as fire(heat) forces fluids excrete outside, and causes profuse sweating, qi might be consumed together with the loss of fluids. Since the fluids and qi are injured, there may appear symptoms of deficiency of qi, such as shortness of breath, fatigue, or even qi collapses in severe cases.

Fire is prone to produce bleeding and internal wind. Blood congeals when getting cold, circulates when getting warmth. So, pathogenic heat makes the vessel expanded and circulation of blood accelerated. In severe cases, pathogenic heat burns and injures the vessels, resulting in different kind of bleeding, such as hematemesis, epistaxis, skin rash, hypermenorrhea, metrorrhagia, ecchymosis, bloody stool and hematuria. When pathogenic fire(heat) invades the body, excessive heat in the liver channel results in hyperactivity of the liver yang, and consumes liver yin, so muscles and tendons cannot be nourished and moistened. Liver wind stirring up internally is manifested as headache, painful stiff nape, high fever, coma, convulsions of the limbs, upward squint of the eyes, opisthotonus, etc.

Fire is likely to cause sores and carbuncles. When pathogenic fire invades blood aspect, it is likely to be accumulated locally and cause qi and blood stagnation, which is the reason of erosion of muscles in local position, such as abscess, furuncle, ulceration and carbuncle, presenting with redness, swelling, heat and pain.

5.1.1.2 Pestilent qi

Pestilent qi is a kind of exogenous pathogenic factor with strong pathogenicity and infectivity. In TCM literature, it is also called epidemic toxin, plague, unusual evil, etc. Pestilent qi spreads through air, nose and mouth invasion, animal bites, diet, skin contact, etc. It includes a wide range of epidemic diseases such as mumps, facial erysipelas, scarlatina, chickenpox, etc.

(1)Three unique features are quite prominent when compared with the six climatic influences, urgent and dangerous, infectious and epidemic, and each pestilent qi only causes one disease but with similar symptoms.

1)Strong contagiosity and being epidemic

Pestilent qi can be spread in many ways, so they have strong contagiosity and are epidemic. It can attack people in all ages and both sex in the epidemic area. And the patient with infection of the same pestilent qi may have similar manifestations and symptoms.

2)Rapid onset and being dangerous

In general, the onset of the diseases caused by six climatic influences is more acute than that of the diseases caused by internal injury, but pestilent qi is more rapid and dangerous when compared with the onset caused by the six climatic influences. So diseases caused by epidemic qi are characterized by being acute on the onset, violent in occurrence, fatal in disease condition. The characteristic of varied in change and quick in transforming to cause disease is similar to fire(heat) evil in six climatic influences. But pestilent qi is stronger than pathogenic fire in toxicity. For example, high fever, harassing heart spirit, bleeding, and stirring wind often occur during the course of the disease. So in terms of causing diseases, it is stronger, more dangerous, and with higher rate of death.

3) One pestilent qi causing one kind of disease

There are many kinds of epidemic qi. One kind of the pestilent pathogen causes one kind of pestilent disease. Different people have the same clinical manifestations if they are invaded by same pestilent qi. For example, no matter a man or a woman, the mumps patients all appear swelling cheeks under the ears.

(2) Climate factors, environmental factors, special factors and preventive measures all affect the eruption of the epidemic.

The formation of pestilent qi and its causing disease has a certain condition. In general, it is related to the following factors.

1) Abnormal climate or abnormal change of natural climate, e. g. prolonged drought, heat, damp fog, malaria, etc.

2) Polluted environment and unclean diets, e. g. polluted air, source of water or food.

3) Having not done preventive and separating work in time.

Social factors, e. g. , incessant war, unstable society, bad working environment, extremely poor life, pestilence continuously occurs and epidemic. If a country is safe and stable and pays attention to health and pestilence work by adopting a series of active and effective anti-pestilence and therapeutic measures, the infectious diseases can be effectively controlled.

5.1.2   Internal factors

The "internal cause" of disease refers to the pathogenic factors related with emotional strain, overstrain, over ease, etc. Traditionally, internal, emotional causes of disease injure the internal viscera directly; while the external, climatic causes of disease affect the exterior of the body first. Internal factors include seven emotions, improper diet, overstrain and over ease and chronic disease caused deficiency syndrome.

5.1.2.1   Seven emotions

Seven emotions refer to the seven kinds of human mental activities, namely joy, anger, anxiety, thought, sorrow, fear and fright. They are the different emotional reactions to the various objective things and outside phenomena. In normal condition, the seven emotions are the external manifestations of the functional activities of the zang-fu viscera, and cannot cause any disease. When sudden, strong or prolonged emotional stimuli go beyond the body's adaptability and endurance, the emotional stimuli will become pathogenic factors, which cause dysfunction of healthy qi, blood and zang-fu viscera, and imbalance between yin and yang, hence lead to diseases. This is known as "internal damages" caused by seven emotions.

Seven emotions have the following common characteristics.

(1) Directly damaging internal organs

Different from the six climatic influences, the seven emotions directly affect the corresponding zang viscera and result in diseases, because a certain zang viscera is closely related to a certain emotional activity. The basic rules are as follows. The heart governs joy and excessive joy damages heart. The liver governs anger and excessive anger damages liver. The spleen governs thought and excessive thought damages spleen. The lung governs sorrow and anxiety, so excessive sorrow or anxiety damages lung. The kidney governs fear and fright, and excessive fear and fright damages kidney. All these show that the changes in five zang viscera would cause the emotional reactions accordingly. Meanwhile, excessive emotional changes damage the five zang viscera respectively. The theory that seven emotions are rooted in five zang viscera opposed to influencing functions of the organs has a vital significance on diagnosis and treatment. The diseases caused by seven emotions are usually marked by abnormal emotional symptoms such as melancholia, hysteria, insomnia, fright palpitations and mania. On the contrary, abnormal changes of qi-blood and the zang-fu viscera can also influence emotions.

Seven emotions originate from the heart. The heart is the governor of living activities of the human body. It not only governs physiological activities of the human body, but also governs psychological activities.

(2) Disordered activity of qi

When the seven emotions damage the internal organs, they mainly affect the activity of visceral qi, leading to disorder of qi and blood circulation. Generally speaking, joy can harmonize qi and blood, ease the mind, but over-joy causes qi to slacken, leading to inability to concentrate and even mania. Anger can drive liver qi upward, so rage causes qi to rise, leading to dizziness, headache, red eyes, and even sudden syncope. Excessive anxiety causes qi inhibition, leading to chest oppression, hypochondriac distension and fullness or pain. Excessive thought causes qi stagnation, leading to abdominal distension and fullness, anorexia and loose stool. Sorrow causes qi consumption, leading to lassitude and dispiritedness. Fear leads qi to sink, resulting in incontinence of urine and feces. Fright causes qi disturbance, leading to palpitation and bewilderment. Details are as follows.

1) Rage causes qi adversely rising

The liver governs the rise and dispersion of the qi and blood. So, furious anger can lead to dysfunction of the liver. As the liver qi rises adversely and blood follows qi, it will result in symptoms of irritability, headache, dizziness, flushed face, even sudden fainting.

2) Over joy causes qi to slacken

In normal condition, joy can relax tension, making the mind eased. Over joy injures the heart, slacken qi movement and the spirit cannot get rest, which is the reason of absent-mindedness, insomnia, and even mental confusion.

3) Sorrow causes qi consumption

It means that over worry and sorrow would lead to pathologic changes which injure lung qi, resulting in shortness of breath, listlessness and lassitude.

4) Fear causes qi sinking

Great fear would lead to the kidney qi unconsolidated and sinking. Clinically, there may appear symptoms as incontinence of urine and stools, and spermatorrhea.

5) Fright causes disorder of qi

Over fright would injure heart qi, leading to disharmony between qi and blood, and abnormal mind. There appear symptoms of palpitation, panic, or mental confusion.

6) Pensiveness causes qi stagnation

Excess over thinking, long-term thinking injure the spleen, leading to depression and stagnation of spleen qi of the middle energizer, and even damage to the transporting and transforming function of the spleen, resulting poor appetite, epigastric fullness, abdominal distension, loose stools.

7) Excessive anxiety causes qi stagnation

Excessive anxiety may cause damage to lung, frequently manifest as qi stagnation, which is the reason for oppression in the chest, signing, and abdominal distension.

8) Mostly cause mental diseases

Seven emotions damage the related zang viscera, especially influence the heart which stores the spirit, so seven emotions mostly lead to mental diseases.

(3) Affecting state of illness

Good and optimistic emotions are in favor of the recovery of diseases. Whereas emotional stimulation may make diseases aggravated or rapidly exacerbated. In the course of many diseases, the state of illness often deteriorates as the result of severe fluctuation of the patients' moods.

Above all, the seven emotions, causing disturbances of qi activity under abnormal conditions, play an important role in etiology of TCM. Studying the principles of the seven emotions will be beneficial for health care and recovery. As emotional factors inducing diseases, TCM emphasizes keeping peaceful and empty, observing the spirit of the field of life cultivation and health preservation. For example, many heart diseases can be aggravated by the seven emotions. In clinic, epigastria pain and diarrhea due to liver qi disorder caused by the internal injury of the seven emotions may usually be aggravated by emotional stimulations.

5.1.2.2　Improper diet

Diets are the source of nutrients, and the material to maintain vital activities of the body. Food is transformed into food essence, which can be transformed into qi and blood to maintain living activities. Improper diet can also be a pathogenic factor. It is composed of three aspects, uncontrolled diet, contaminated food and food predilection. Improper diet causes damage to the function of spleen and stomach, leading to internal dampness, phlegm, and other internal diseases.

(1) Uncontrolled diet

People need to eat a certain amount of food at a timed interval in the day. Starvation refers to the insufficient intake of food or drink, which will induce insufficiency of vital energy and blood. It may cause insufficient qi and blood, the ability of body resistance decreases, so the invasion of external pathogenic factors is more likely to occur. The following symptoms often appear, like lusterless complexion, palpitations, shortness of breath and exhaustion. Because of weakness of healthy qi, people become vulnerable to other diseases. On the other hand, overeating refers to excess intake of foods. It will damage the transformation and transportation ability of the spleen and stomach, and lead to food accumulation. It leads to food stagnation in the gastrointestinal tract, causing abdominal fullness and distension, anorexia, vomiting, diarrhea, etc. Another important factor is the fixed time for meal. Eating regularly can facilitate activities of the digestion and absorption. As the function of the spleen and stomach of children is weak and they do not know proper time and proper volume of food intake, food accumulation often occurs among children.

(2) Contaminated food

Contaminated food refers to the intake of unclean, unhygienic, erosive or toxic foods. It may cause stomach and intestine diseases, parasitic disease or even food poisoning. Contaminated food may give rise to symptoms such as abdominal pain, vomiting, diarrhea, etc. In severe cases mental confusion and coma may appear, and even lead to death.

(3) Food predilection

In order to meet the demand of the body for various nutrients, various kinds of food should be taken. As an etiological factor, it refers to being addicting to a special tropism taste of food. Indulgence in taking certain foods may cause excess or deficiency of some nutrient composition in the body, which results in the imbalance between yin and yang and leads to certain kinds of diseases. Food predilection may be divided into three respects: addiction to cold/hot foods, addiction to five tastes foods, and addiction to alcohol.

1) Addiction to cold/hot foods

In general, diets require moderate warmth. If cold-nature foods are overeaten, pathogenic cold will directly attack the spleen-stomach, injure yang qi of the spleen and the stomach, leading to internal generalization of cold-dampness, resulting in abdominal pain and diarrhea. If pungent, dry and hot foods are eaten frequently, the stomach and intestine may have accumulating heat, resulting in thirst, constipation, even hemorrhoid, etc.

2) Addiction to five-taste foods

Diets of five tastes have different nutritional actions. The tastes and five zang viscera have their affinity for each other. The five tastes respectively enter the five zang viscera, i. e. the sour flavor enters the liver, the bitter flavor enters the heart, etc. Indulgence in eating five-taste food may not only result in dysfunction of correspondence between zang viscera, but also disorder the balance between the five zang viscera, which may cause other pathologic changes.

3) Addiction to alcohol

Drink proper alcohol may promote the circulation of qi and blood of the human body, but drinking alcohol without control may cause diseases. The alcohol is hot and damp in nature. Indulgence in drinking may injure the spleen and stomach, produce internal damp-heat, and cause a series of diseases. Epigastria distention, poor appetite, bitter and sticky mouth, greasy tongue fur, etc. These are frequently seen in clinic.

5.1.2.3 Overstrain and lack of exercise

Reasonable arrangement of labor and rest is a necessary requirement of people's health. Adequate labor and physical exercise help blood circulation and enhance physical fitness. On the other hand, enough rest can eliminate fatigue, restore physical and mental energy.

Overstrain refers to overwork, excess use of mental resources or excess sexual activity. Excessive physical labor will cause consumption of qi and muscle, joints and bones damages while excessive thought and preoccupation will cause the consumption of blood, impairment of spleen and heart, leading to symptoms like palpitations, forgetfulness, insomnia, dreaminess or indigestion, abdominal distension and loose stool, exhaustion. Sexual indulgence will directly lead to deficiency of kidney essence, and the common signs are lumbar debility, dizziness, tinnitus, depression, spermatorrhea, decreased sexual function and impotence.

On the other hand, the body needs proper daily activities to make the circulation of qi and blood fluent and smooth. Without working or exercise, the poor circulation of qi and blood will also bring about diseases.

5.1.3 Pathological products

Besides the cause of external and internal pathogenic factors, the pathogenic products formed during the course of disease can also become pathogenic factor. It mainly includes phlegm and fluid retention, blood stasis, calculus. They act on the human body, leading to new pathologic changes and forming various diseases.

5.1.3.1 Phlegm and fluid retention

(1) Formation of phlegm-fluid retention

Phlegm and fluid retention are the pathologic product formed by the water metabolic disturbance of the body, which can be a new pathogenic factor to block the channels and collaterals, obstruct the movement of qi and blood, and damage the activity of zang-fu viscera. Phlegm and fluid can be caused by six climatic influences, seven emotions, improper diet, or overstrain and over rest. When the qi transformation of lung, spleen, liver, kidney, and triple energizer are disturbed because of the reasons above, the circulation of body fluid tends to be stagnant, causing visible or invisible phlegm. The latter usually manifests as clinical symptoms and pathological changes that cannot easily be perceived and understood.

Generally speaking, phlegm is thick and turbid, while fluid retention is thin and clear. In the narrow sense, phlegm is pathologic secretions of the respiratory tract, also called sputum; in a broader sense, phlegm has no form, it is a viscous turbid pathological product coming from the disorder of water metabolism, which can be accumulated anywhere in the body, and cause a variety of diseases. Fluid retention is movable, which may be retained and accumulated in the inter-place of the zang viscera and tissues of the human body with loose location.

(2) Characteristics of causing diseases by phlegm-fluid retention

1) Block the movement of qi and blood

Phlegm-fluid retention is a shaped pathologic product. When it is formed, the movement of qi and blood will be obstructed. Also the phlegm-fluid may flow into the channel to retard circulation of qi and blood. The accumulated phlegm-fluid causes phlegm plum scrofula, etc. If it stays in the lung, and the lung fails in dispersing and descending, then oppression in the chest, dyspnea, cough, spitting sputum will occur. If they block the spleen and stomach, there will appear intestine nausea, vomiting, abdominal distention and poor appetite.

2) Causing a wide range of and changeable diseases

Phlegm-fluid retention flows together with qi, so it can accumulate anywhere: upward to the head, downward to the foot, inward to the zang viscera, and outward to skin. In clinic, the diseases formed by phlegm-fluid retention have changeable symptoms. So there is a saying "hundreds of diseases are caused by phlegm". For example, epilepsy does not have symptoms in the ordinary, but when some factors induce its onset, there will appear sudden faint, convulsion, trismus and frothy salivation. So it is caused by phlegm.

3) Disease tending to be lingering and long in the course

Disease caused by phlegm and excess fluid is manifested as lingering of disease tendency of long course. For example, cough caused by phlegm-fluid retention often occurs again and again, and cannot be cured completely. Especially, the course of some disorders resulting from stubborn phlegm or latent stagnant fluid is longer.

4) Tending to disturb the spirit

Phlegm-fluid's retention is turbidity, while the heart spirit is clear and clean. If phlegm-fluid adversely ascends with qi, the seven orifices and the pericardium would be likely to be clouded. Patients will suffer from dizziness with sensation of heaviness of the head, listlessness, irritability, and even mania.

5) Frequently seen in slippery and greasy coating of tongue

A slippery and greasy coating is one of the characteristics of causing disease by phlegm and excess fluid.

5.1.3.2 Static blood

Static blood is a pathological product, formed when blood stops circulating properly, which belongs to the category of secondary pathogenic factors. Normal circulation of blood depends on the internal organs coordinating function, the driving and the consolidation of qi, unobstructed vessels, and other internal and external environmental factors. Thus, deficiency of qi, stagnation of qi, cold, heat, and trauma can all lead to the formation of blood stasis.

(1) Formation of static blood

Any factors that can inhibit the blood circulation or cause the blood out of the vessel can produce static blood. Generally speaking, there are five ways to form static blood.

1) Stasis caused by trauma

Various trauma, such as falls, knife injury, trauma due to surgical operation, can make the vessel break causing the blood to spill from the channels. It can also be the reason of blood stasis.

2) Stasis due to qi stagnation

Qi movement would make blood move, and qi stagnation would make blood stasis. When emotional depression, dampness, water, and phlegm-fluid accumulate in the body, block collaterals, and influence zang viscera and qi movement, blood circulation would be unsmooth. It can also be the reason of blood stasis.

3) Stasis due to qi deficiency

Normal circulation of blood depends on qi promoting and controlling. If qi and blood are sufficient, the circulation of blood would move normally. If qi is deficient, it gives rise to slow movement of blood or fails to control blood, and the blood stasis would appear in or out of the blood vessels.

4) Stasis caused by blood cold

Blood moves when it is heated, blood coagulates when it is cold. If external cold pathogen enters into blood, or internal cold originated from yang deficiency influences the blood, and blood could not be warmed or maintain normal circulation. Blood will be stagnant and move not freely, leading to stasis of blood in certain part of the body.

5) Stasis due to blood heat

When the pathogenic fire(heat) enters the blood, or internal fire(heat) is transformed internally, fluids in blood would be scorched, which makes blood mucoid and greasy and move slowly. Or when heat scorches blood vessel, force blood moves out of the vessel, the blood will stagnate at certain parts of the body, and blood stasis occurs.

(2) Characteristics of causing disease by static blood

When the blood is stagnated, its function of nourishing would be influenced and generation of new diseases might take place.

1) Tending to block qi movement

Qi promotes blood circulation. They are supplemented, and cooperating in function. When blood stagnates, qi movement would be influenced in the vessel. Further stagnated blood can aggravate qi stagnation.

2) Influence the blood circulation

Static blood is the pathologic product of the abnormal movement of blood. But after the formation of stagnant blood, no matter in or out of the vessels, the function of the heart and liver may be influenced, which leads to local or whole abnormal movement of blood.

3) Influence the generation of fresh blood

Static blood is the pathologic product, which has lost the nourishing function. If static blood blocks for a long period of time, the movement of qi and blood would be influenced, and cause malfunction of zang-fu viscera, affecting the formation of new blood. Hence, there is the saying that "if stagnant blood does not go away, new blood cannot generate".

(3) Clinical characteristic of the diseases caused by static blood

As the locations being blocked by static blood are different, the reasons of stagnant blood formation are numerous, the accompanied pathogens are different, and the change of the diseases is complex. Hence its pathologic manifestations vary. The common characteristics of clinical manifestations include pain(fixed, aggravated by pressing, severer at night), masses or swelling(fixed, dark-green swelling and distention), hemorrhage(dark purplish blood mixed with masses), cyanosis, dark-purplish tongue proper and retarded or irregularly intermittent pulse.

In addition, in clinic there may always appear amnesia, thirst but no desire to drink, incrusted skin, etc. The above-mentioned clinical manifestations should be mastered by the doctors. So when the patient had the history of trauma, hemorrhage and giving birth before the onset or during the course of disease, the possibility of blood stasis should be considered.

5.1.3.3　Calculus

The pathological product like sand and stone caused by prolonged accumulation of pathogenic dampness-heat in the body is called "calculus". The commonly seen ones are gastric stones, gallbladder stones, kidney stones, etc. Calculus is the pathologic product formed in the course of disease, which can also become pathogenic factor of certain diseases.

(1) Formation of calculus

Factors forming stones are comparatively complex, the commonly seen ones include difference of water quality(hard water), improper diets(fatty and oily diet, overeating persimmons or date in an empty stomach), prolonged taking of medicinal calcium and magnesium, individual difference and internal injury of emotion.

(2) Characteristics of causing diseases by calculus

1) Frequently occurring in liver, gallbladder, kidney, etc.

2) Long course of disease and changeable symptoms. Calculus is formed by prolonged blockage of damp-heat and qi-blood. Clinically, there are different symptoms according to the size and position of calculus. Generally speaking, if the calculus is small, the illness will be mild, or no symptoms appear. On the contrary, if the calculus is big, the illness will be severe, and there may appear obvious and complex symptoms.

3) Easy to cause pain. In mild cases, the blocking calculus may cause distention and pain. In severe cases, colic pain occurs.

4) Easy to block qi movement and damage channels. As calculus stays in the zang-fu viscera, movement of qi, circulation of blood and fluids will be blocked, the bile will not be excreted smoothly in the liver and gallbladder, and water fluid cannot be moved to kidney and bladder.

5.1.4　Other factors

5.1.4.1　Traumatic injury

Trauma usually refers to the injury in the tissues, organs or qi-blood of zang-fu viscera due to external power, or burns, freezing, insect bite, etc. External injuries are wide in scale, including injury of fall, injury due to heavy loading, injuries of press, guns, operation, burns, frost, insect bite, etc. There is usually an obvious history of external injuries for diseases caused by external wounds. In mild cases, traumata of skin, tendons and bones; in severe cases, it may affect the zang viscera, and even more dangerous. Hence, the nature and degree of trauma should be specially differentiated.

(1) Burns and scalds

Burns mainly refers to the scorching of the human body by objects of high temperature, e. g. , boiling water, hot oil, steam, fire, thunder electricity attack, etc. The wound of burns is mainly due to fire toxic. In mild cases, the skin would be scorched, and the injured location is red and swelling, painful, or blisters. In severe cases, muscles and tendons would be injured, and the injured location is like the leather or wax-white, yellow or carbonizing-like change. If the wound is a large-scale burn, not only the local part is severely scorched, but also the zang-fu viscera and body fluids would also be involved due to excessive heat toxic. When fluids are exuded, life would be threatened.

(2) Frostbite

Frostbite refers to the whole or local injury of the body caused by the invasion of pathogenic cold under the low temperature. The degree of frostbite depends on the temperature of the frostbite and the length of the frost time. The lower the temperature, the longer the time of frost, the severe damage would be. In general, local frostbite occurs on the hand, foot, nose, cheek, and other exposed locations. At the early stage, the local skin is pale, numbness with cold, then swelling, dark and purplish, pain with itching, scorching, and later, ulcer would occur. General frostbite is usually due to excess of yin cold of external affection, leading to severe impairment of yang qi in the body, loses the warming function; resulting in chills, decrease of body temperature, purplish lips, tongue and finger nails, numbness, retarded reaction, or weak breath, slow and thready pulse, etc. If no treatment is given in time, yang collapse may lead to death.

5.1.4.2　Drug pathogens

Drug pathogens refer to a pathogenic factor leading to the occurrence of disease due to improper process and use of drugs. As practitioners of Chinese medicine, we should be aware of the side-effects and adverse reactions of medicines in order to diagnose the condition properly, so we should be able to separate which symptoms are caused by the drugs and which are not.

Some drugs influence changing pattern of pulse and tongue. For example, beta blockers affect the pulse deeply by making it slow and rather deep. In such cases, the pulse cannot be used for diagnosis. Antibiotics clearly affect the tongue by making it peeled in patches, that is, with patches without coating, when such kind of tongue appears, the patient should be asked whether he or she is using antibiotics up to 3 weeks before the consultation. Oral steroids also change the tongue, tending to make it swollen and red.

5.1.4.3　Wrong treatment

In TCM, wrong treatment means wrong herbal treatment. An example of wrong treatment is tonifying yang when nourishing yin. Wrong treatment would lead to aggravation of the disease conditions.

5.1.4.4　Congenital factors

Every person is born with a certain constitution, which is dependent on the parent's health in general, their health at the time of conception specifically, and the mother's health during pregnancy. Many dysplasia and malformation of the fetus are due to insufficiency or abnormalities of essence and blood inherited from parents.

5.2　Pathogenesis

Pathogenesis, or mechanism of disease, is the basic law for the clinical manifestations, development and prognosis of disease, as well as for diagnosis and treatment. The theory of pathogenesis based on the theory of yin and yang, five-elements, blood and fluids, etc. The occurrence, development and change of disease are closely related to the patients' healthy qi, pathogenic properties, degree of disease, location of disease, etc.

Pathogenesis reveals the characteristics and basic laws in which diseases emerge, develop and change. It also provides the intrinsic basis and theoretical foundation one can follow when analyzing clinical manifestation, syndrome differentiation, prevention and treatment of the disease. Diseases are numerous with complex clinical signs and various prognoses. Each disease or syndrome has its own pathogenesis, but the general rules are struggle between healthy qi and pathogenic qi, imbalance between yin and yang, disorder of qi and blood, body fluids disorders.

Chinese medicine does not analyze the pathogenic factors in a detailed, microscopic fashion, but is concerned only with the broad picture. In TCM, it is believed that the occurrence, development and changes of the disease are closely related to the state of physical constitution of the affected body and the nature of the pathogenic factors. When a pathogenic factor invades a human body, the right qi fights against the pathogenic qi, during the battle the dynamic balance of yin and yang may be broken, causing disorders of physiological functions of zang-fu viscera, meridians, collaterals, qi or blood, etc., resulting in diseases either locally or of the whole body.

The occurrence of a disease is mainly related to two kinds of power, healthy qi and pathogenic qi, and the struggle between them sets the basic ground where a disease occurs and develops.

Healthy qi is the comprehensive ability of the body to maintain normal functional activitiessuch as disease resistance, eliminating pathogen, and adjustment and repairment of body. Pathogenic qi refers all kinds of pathogenic factors, including all sorts of pathogenic factors existing outside or inside the body, such as the six climatic influences, pestilent qi, seven emotions, phlegm-dampness, static blood, etc.

5.2.1   Occurrence of disease

Deficiency of healthy qi is the internal basis of disease occurrence. Only when the body's healthy qi is deficient, causing low disease resistance and difficulty in eliminating pathogenic qi, the pathogenic qi will invade the body and cause diseases. This is called "pathogenic qi prevails over healthy qi". Weakness of healthy qi may attract pathogens. Meanwhile, healthy qi deficiency may also cause diseases by generating "deficient pathogen". In addition, the intensity of the healthy qi determines the nature of the onset syndrome.

The healthy qi plays a predominant role in the occurrence of the disease. Invasion of pathogen and the struggle with healthy qi are the essential factors in the process of disease occurrence and development. Pathogenic qi can induce disorder of physiological function, causing imbalance between yin and yang, dysfunction of qi, blood, meridians and viscera; morphological damage to viscera and tissues can occur, such as damaging the skin, bones, muscles and organs, consuming essential qi, blood and body fluid. The occurrence of a disease and its pathological changes mainly depend on the nature of the pathogenic qi, its location and to what extent it influences the body.

Under certain conditions, the pathogenic qi may even play a leading role, for example, in insect and animal bites, gunshot injuries, food poisonings, etc. Therefore, it is necessary to emphasize "firmly maintain the healthy qi to fend off pathogenic qi". Meanwhile, the doctor needs to keep perspective of intensity of invasion of pathogens.

The occurrence and development of illness is shaped by the outcome of the struggle between healthy qi and pathogenic qi. Healthy qi, pathogenic qi and the struggle between them are affected by various internal and external factors of the body.

5.2.2   Predomination and decline of pathogenic qi and healthy qi

It refers to the waxing and waning of healthy qi and pathogenic factors during the course of a disease and it determines the prognosis of the disease.

Heathy qi is a collective designation for all normal functions of the human body and the abilities to maintain health, including the abilities of self-regulation, adaptation to the environment, resistance against pathogens and self-recovery from illness, the same as normal qi or genuine qi. Essence, qi, blood and fluids are the material basis for the formation of heathy qi. When they are sufficient the physiological functions of zang-fu viscera, channels and collaterals are abnormal, and then the heathy qi of the body is exuberant. Pathogenic qi is an agent causing disease, also called pathogenic factor or pathogen. Pathogenic qi mainly refers to six external pathogens, seven emotion damages, improper diet, pathological products, traumatic injure, parasites, etc.

When a pathogenic factor tries to invade the human body, there is a struggle taking place between the pathogen and the heathy qi, which is related to its occurrence, development and prognosis, at the same time, influencing the variation between deficiency and excess, either of the following conditions would happen.

If heathy qi is strong enough, then the body is strong to resist disease and difficult for pathogens to invade; even the disease does occur in the body at all, and the patient is easily to recover. If heathy qi is deficient, pathogenic factor would invade the body, and cause diseases. Then it can damage organs, essential qi, blood, and fluids, bring about functional disorders of zang-fu viscera, meridians and collaterals, even change individual constitutions. *Plain Question* states that "exuberance of pathogen causing excess syndrome, lack of essential qi causing deficiency syndrome". That is the basic rule of deficiency and excess. One thing that should be mentioned is that the deficiency and excess are relative but not absolute concepts.

5.2.2.1   Deficiency and excess syndromes

In the case that the pathogenic qi has overwhelming privilege and the healthy qi is still enough for the struggle, it mainly reflects as syndrome of excess. Such a syndrome with relatively severe reaction of the body is often seen at the early and medium stages of diseases caused by six climatic influences, phlegm, blood stasis, etc. On the other hand, lack of healthy qi and mild struggle against the pathogenic qi show a series of pathological manifestations with insufficient anti-pathogenic energy, which is called deficiency syndrome, often seen at the advanced stage of exogenous diseases.

5.2.2.2   Further pathological statement of deficiency and excess

During the course of disease, the exuberance and debilitation of pathogenic qi or healthy qi may lead to either simple deficiency syndrome and excess syndrome, or complexity of the both. Under certain conditions, excess and deficiency may transform into each other. Sometimes the manifestation and the real syndrome are not the same, or are even on the contrary that needs to be analyzed comprehensively.

5.2.2.3   Effect on prognosis of disease

Domination of healthy qi and decline of pathogenic qi are the necessary conditions for improvement and cure of disease. If healthy qi is sufficient for the resistance of pathogenic qi, or with timely and proper treatment, pathogenic qi is gradually eliminated and functions of organs are improved. On the contrary, domination of pathogenic qi and decline of healthy qi are the basic causes of aggravation of disease or death. Furthermore, in the course of the exuberance and debilitation of pathogenic qi or healthy qi, if healthy qi is not strong enough to eliminate pathogenic qi, and pathogenic qi is not strong enough to further develop, it will bring on such a condition in which both qi are at a stalemate, or healthy qi is deficient and pathogenic qi is still lingering, making the disease change from acute into chronic condition or causing certain sequelae.

5.2.3   Yin-yang disharmony

Normally, yin and yang in the body maintain a dynamic balance. If such balance is impaired by pathogenic factors, the normal relationships among zang-fu viscera, meridians, qi and blood will be affected, leading to various complicated pathological changes, and these changes can be seen through the nature of the disease such as cold or heat, deficiency or excess. The disharmony between yin and yang is not only the internal essential cause of the occurrence, development and change of disease, but also the key to recovery or deterioration. Details of disharmony between yin and yang are discussed in Table 4-1.

Disorders of qi and blood are pathological states that occur during the process of a disease because of either struggle between the healthy qi and the pathogenic qi, or disturbance of visceral functions, including deficiency, disturbance in circulation or physiological function of qi and blood. The pathological changes are always reflected through the abnormal physiological function of zang-fu viscera.

5.2.4   Disorders of body fluids

The normal metabolism of body fluids is a relatively constant condition that maintains the formation, distribution and excretion of fluid. The normal generation of fluid depends upon the qi movement; distribution and excretion rely on the transportation of spleen, ascent and descent of lung, free flow of liver qi, qi transformation of kidney and triple energizer. When the relating functions of zang-fu viscera are abnormal, pathological changes like deficiency or abnormal distribution and excretion of body fluid will occur.

5.2.4.1　Deficiency of body fluids

Deficiency of body fluids implies a pathological state that manifests a series of dry and deficiency symptoms which affect the zang-fu viscera, sense organs and orifices not being sufficiently moistened and nourished due to shortage of body fluid. There are three main contributing factors. One is excessive heat causing impairment of fluid, such as exogenous heat pathogen or internal heat due to yin deficiency or qi stagnation. The second is over consumption, for example, serious vomiting, diarrhea or extensive bums. The third one is chronic disease that makes people weak with insufficient production of body fluid.

5.2.4.2　Disorder of distribution and excretion of body fluids

The distribution of body fluids refers to the transportation, dispersion and circulation of fluid, which is the process of its metabolism. And the excretion of body fluids means after metabolism the fluids discharges in forms like sweat, urine and vapor. If the circulation of fluid is slow or stagnated, the internal dampness generates and results in phlegm and fluids retention or even leads to edema. The disorder of distribution and excretion of body fluids have different manifestations but share mutual effects, which cause pathologic changes like accumulated phlegm and retained fluid.

Zheng Guizhi, Zhang Zhinan, Zhu Lifang

Chapter 6

The Four Examinations

Diagnostics of traditional Chinese medicine is related to treatment based on syndrome differentiation as it provides the diagnostic tools to syndrome differentiation, and it is the basic method to collect message from the patients. Diagnostics of TCM is based on the fundamental principle that signs and symptoms reflect the condition of the zang-fu viscera. There are three fundamental principles of diagnostics of TCM: "inspect the exterior to examine the interior", "a part reflects the whole", and "find the abnormal obey the normal". Diagnostics of TCM includes four methods: inspection, auscultation and olfaction, inquiring, and pulse diagnosis. Inspection is to observe the patient's mental activity, complexion, appearance, movement, body shape and secretion, discharge, etc. Auscultation and olfaction is to distinguish whether there is something abnormal in patient's speaking, breath, cough, voice and odor of secretion and discharge by means of doctor's auditognosis and osphresis. Inquiring is disease data collecting course that doctor questions patient about the patient's symptoms, the cause or predisposing factors of disease, the process of clinical development and treatment. Pulse diagnosis means to feel certain parts of pulse beating on the body surface or to press-touch some parts of the body. All the four examinations should be applied simultaneously to diagnosis to ensure the correct diagnosis.

6.1 Inspection

Inspection is a method by which doctors use vision to observe the patient's systemic and local manifestations, tongue images, excretions, and so on, in order to collect information on the patient's condition.

6.1.1 Inspection of vitality, complexion, figure, posture

6.1.1.1 Inspection of vitality

Vitality is the generalization of all the physiological activities of human body. It can reflect the normal or abnormal life activities. Vitality can be distinguished in broad sense and narrow sense. Vitality in broad sense means the total external manifestations of the life activities of human body which are the reflection of visceral functions. Vitality in narrow sense means the mental activities including consciousness and thinking of human being. Inspection of vitality includes observing the vitality state in the two senses.

Inspection of vitality plays an important role in diagnosis. By means of vitality inspection, we can know the patient's conditions such as the state of qi and blood, the state of zang-fu viscera and the seriousness of disease.

Four conditions should be distinguished in the vitality observation: full vitality, lack of vitality, loss of vitality and false vitality.

(1) Full vitality

Full vitality is also called "having vitality". It is the normal manifestation of sufficient essence and qi and exuberant vitality. Even if suffering from certain illness, it means the stomach qi has not been injured and the vitality has not been weakened. What we can know is that the illness is not serious. Full vitality is manifested by the lustrous complexion, alert and lustrous eyes, natural express, clear speech, normal mentality, well rhythmic breath, plump muscles, free movement of limbs and agile reaction. Among them, those reflecting the sufficiency of heart qi are the lustrous complexion, natural expression, clear speech, normal mentality and agile reaction. That reflecting the sufficiency of lung qi is well rhythmic breath. Those reflecting the sufficiency of spleen qi are the plump muscles and free movement of limbs. Those reflecting the sufficiency of liver and kidney qi are the alert and lustrous eyes. The sufficiency of the five zang visceral essence and qi means health or favorable prognosis, though suffering from illness.

(2) Lack of vitality

It is condition of no enough vitality, which seems to be the most common one in clinic cases. It is manifested by less lustrous complexion, less lustrous eyes, shortness of breath, indolence of speaking, retarded reaction and sleeplessness. Lack of vitality is due to the insufficiency of blood and qi of the five zang viscera and is commonly seen in deficient syndromes.

(3) Loss of vitality

Loss of vitality is the reflection of essence insufficiency, declined vitality and serious damage of the vital qi. It marks the failure of visceral functions and means critical condition and unfavorable prognosis.

Loss of vitality is manifested by the dim complexion, dull and gloomy eyes, indifferent expression, sag mentality, sluggish reaction, feeble or intermittent breath, lean muscles, difficulty in acting, even coma with murmuring, sudden fall with unconsciousness, close eyes with opened mouth, paralyzed hands, urinary and fecal incontinence. Among them, that reflecting the failure of heart is sluggish reactions. That reflecting the failure of lung essence and qi is the feeble or intermittent breath. Those reflecting the failure of spleen and stomach essence and qi are lean muscles and difficulty in acting. Those reflecting the failure of liver and kidney essence and qi are dull and gloomy eyes. As for the coma with murmuring, opened mouth with paralyzed hands, urinary and fecal incontinence, they reflect the crisis due to the pathogen sinking into the pericardium or prostration of the essence and qi.

(4) False vitality

False vitality means a kind of pseudo-phenomenon of temporary improvement. As a result of patient's essence and qi deficiency caused by chronic disease or serious disease, false vitality appears suddenly at the crisis stage. The false vitality marks the essence and qi will be exhausted and means the exacerbation of disease condition. The yin and yang will be divorced because of the failure of yin in astringing yang which results in the outward escape of deficient yang.

6.1.1.2   Inspection of complexion

Inspection of complexion is to inspect the face color and luster of skin in order to understand the conditions of disease.

Observation of the face color is an extremely important part of visual diagnosis. The face color reflects the state of qi and blood and is closely related to the condition of the vitality. We are supposed to know the rise and fall of stomach qi through changes of luster.

Various pathological colors are usually described, but before analysis the particular color itself, one has to distinguish a clear, shining type of color from a dull, dry type of color. If the color is clear and has a rather moist appearance, it indicates that stomach qi is still intact. This is a positive indication, even if the color itself is pathological. If the color has a rather dry and lifeless look, it indicates that stomach qi is exhausted, which is always a negative indication and points to poor prognosis.

(1) Normal complexion

It refers to color and luster of the complexion in healthy people and it differs according to races. For Chinese people, the normal complexion seems to be light yellow, ruddy and lustrous.

(2) Abnormal complexion

Abnormal complexion means changes of color on faces and body skin caused by disease, including five unfavorable complexions. The five abnormal complexions are described as follows.

1) Green

A green color of the face indicates any of the following conditions: liver syndrome, interior cold, pain or interior wind. Pain is often the result of blockage and obstruction of meridians, so there is green color. The stagnated blood in vessels is often shown by green color. In cases of liver disease, since the functional activity of qi fails to disperse, which leads to stagnation, there will also be green color.

2) Red

Red is the color of blood. Heat accelerates blood flow and makes the vessels fill up, so the skin presents red color. Red indicates heat. This can be excessive or deficiency heat. In excessive heat, the whole face is red, while in deficiency heat only the cheekbones are red. If the chronic disease or serious disease results in exhaustion of essence and qi, so that yin fails to astringe yang and the deficient yang floats upwards, there will be reddish complexion like being made-up, or wandering reddish color on the zygomatic region. This is called the floating yang syndrome.

3) Yellow

Yellow suggests spleen deficiency or dampness, or both. The spleen dominates transportation and transformation. It is the source of the regeneration of qi and blood. If the spleen fails in transporting, the food essence cannot be transformed into qi and blood, then the skin will be yellow complexion without well nourishment. If the water and dampness accumulate inside because the deficient spleen fails to transport them, there will be yellow complexion, too.

The luster yellowness on glabella and nose tip predicts the decline of disease, while the lusterless marks the disease is difficult to be cured.

4) White

White suggests cold syndrome or deficiency syndrome (loss of blood or qi). It is the manifestation of insufficient qi and blood failing to nourish the body. The declined yang qi fails to promote the flow of qi and blood, so that qi and blood cannot nourish the face and skin. It can also be the result of loss of qi and blood which could not fill up vessels.

5) Black

It suggests kidney deficiency, water or fluid retention, blood stasis, pain syndrome and cold syndrome. Black is related to yin cold and water.

The dim bluish complexion is due to insufficiency of kidney yang regardless whether it is a new manifestation or protracted disease. Black complexion with dried face is usually due to the chronic consumption of kidney essence and the essence failing to nourish the face. Blackness surrounding the orbits is usually seen in administrator which is due to the insufficiency of kidney yang that leads to interior retention of water-dampness or pours down of cold-dampness. The blood stasis is manifested by the black complexion with squamous and dry skin. The butterfly-like black spots on female's face are due to kidney deficiency and blood stasis.

(3)The facial portions corresponding to the zang-fu viscera

The zang-fu viscera have their certain corresponding portions on the face. Combining it with the color observation will be contributory to making better diagnosis.

With the method to divide the facial portions proposed in *Internal Classic* we can establish relationship between facial portions and zang-fu viscera. The throat portion is above the glabella. The lung portion is between the glabella. Below the glabella is heart portion and below the heart portion is liver portion. Lateral to liver portion is gallbladder portion and below liver portion is the spleen. The stomach portion is on the wing of nose. The large intestine portion is on the cheek. On lateral side of large intestine portion is the portion kidney. Below kidney portion is the portion of umbilicus. Above cheek is the portion of small intestine. The portion of urinary bladder and uterine is between the nose and lip.

6.1.1.3　Inspection of figure

The figure inspection is to observe the robustness or weakness and corpulence or emaciation of the patients' body, and the condition of different parts of the body and the constitution, etc., so as to understand the internal changes of disease of the human body. The five zang viscera pair with the five elements respectively in the interior, while the figure pair with the five zang viscera in the exterior. The robustness or weakness of the body's outer figure is related to the exuberance or declination of the functions of five zang viscera. In virtue of observing the patient's figure, it is possible to speculate the solidness or fragileness of zang-fu viscera, the exuberance or declination of qi and blood, the wax or wane of the genuine qi and pathogen qi.

(1)Robustness, weakness, corpulence and emaciation

Robustness refers to a strong physique. It is shown by bulky skeleton, wide and thick chest, plump muscle and luster skin. It is regarded as a favorable sign even though suffering from disease.

Weakness refers to a feeble physique. It is reflected by the thin skeleton, narrow chest, lean muscle and lusterless skin. The prognosis is seemed to be unfavorable if suffering disease.

Corpulence with a good appetite is thought as exuberant figure, while corpulence with poor appetite as exuberant figure with qi deficiency. The former means sturdiness and latter means insufficiency of yang qi and infirmity.

Emaciation with polydipsia(too much food intake) pertains to the fire-flaming in the middle energizer, however, emaciation with small food intake refers to the deficiency of spleen and stomach.

(2)Five body constituents and five houses

The five body constituents, namely skin, muscle, tendon, bone and vessel, match with the five zang viscera. The five zang visceral functions are the roots of the five body constituents which can reflect the exuberance or declination of the five zang viscera. The so-called five houses refer to the head, back, lumbar, knee and bone. It is likely to speculate the disease location of zang-fu viscera and the severity of the disease by observing the five houses.

(3)Constitution

There are certain relations between the body type and constitution. The relationship among body type, constitution and disease is always emphasized in TCM. So the different constitutions are susceptible to different disease.

6.1.1.4　Posture

The kinetic and static postures of patients are closely related to disease. Different diseases show different mobile postures, so the different posture of patients can speculate the nature of disease and its prognosis.

Patient's sitting and lying position and activity can lead to a useful diagnosis of disease.

Supine position pertains to yang while prone position to yin. Sitting with raised head and asthma with plenty of expectoration pertain to the lung excess. The condition of sitting with droopy head and shortness of breath with less talk pertains to the lung deficiency. Stiffness of neck and back is due to the pathogen in bladder meridian of foot taiyang. Shiver is the phenomenon of struggling between genuine qi and the pathogen, which can be seen in exopathic disease, or tetanus, or in the condition of inward sinking of purulent poison in surgical case.

6.1.2　Location inspection

6.1.2.1　Inspection of head, neck and five sensory organs

Inspection of head, neck and five sensory organs belong to local inspection, and the local inspection plays an important role in the inspection.

（1）Inspection of head

The head is known as the confluence of all yang meridians and the residence of intelligence. At the same time, the brain is called the house of original mentality and as sea of marrow and the hair is surplus of blood. Because the kidney produces bone marrow, so the state of head is related in the disorders of brain and kidney and to the exuberance or declination of qi and blood.

The key contents of the inspection of head are the conditions of the size, shape, fontanel, action, color and distribution of hair.

The size of the head can be measured by the head circumference, and the change of it in the development stage is: the newborn is about 34 cm, 1 year old is about 46 cm, 2 years old is about 48 cm, 5 years old is about 50 cm, and reaching adult at 15 years old is about 54-58 cm.

1）The shape of the head

The abnormal shapes of head can be often found in infant, mainly macrocrania, microcephalia, caput quadratum.

● Macrocrania: The forehead, parietal bone, ossa temporale and occipital are projecting, inflated and round; in contrast, the face is very small. At the same time the eyes are downcast and the sclera expose. Macrocrania is mostly due to insufficiency of congenital essence, kidney essence insufficiency and stagnation of fluid.

● Microcephalia: The head is small, accompanying with round head tip, craniosynostosis, and mental retardation. Microcephalia is mostly due to kidney essence insufficiency and poor development of the skull.

● Caput quadratum: It refers that the forehead protruds and the top of the head is flat and square. It is due to kidney essence insufficiency, spleen-stomach weakness or the dysplasia of the skull, and is more common in children's rickets or congenital syphilis.

2）Fontanelle

Fontanelle is a kind of spatium interosseum formed by the untight joint of the skull in infants. Fontanelle can be divided into anterior and posterior fontanelle. Anterior fontanelle closure time is in 12-18 months after born of, and the posterior fontanelle closure in 2-4 months after born of. Fontanelle is one of the main parts to observe the growth and nutritional status.

● Bulging fontanel: It mostly is an excess syndrome. It is due to the fire pathogen attacking upward, or the brain lesions, or intracranial stagnation of fluid.

● Sunken fontanel: It mostly is a deficiency syndrome. And it is due to the depletion of body fluid caused by vomiting and/or diarrhea, deficiency of both qi and blood, or the insufficiency of the brain marrow.

● Infantile metopism: It is due to the kidney qi deficiency or hypogenesis, and it is common in children's rickets.

3) Movement

Whether it is an adult or a child, the uncontrollable shaking head is usually the presymptom of the internal stirring of liver wind. If this occurs in the elderly, it may be due to the deficiency of both qi and blood.

4) Hair

Thick black hair is a sign of the exuberant kidney qi and the adequate essence and blood. Therefore, the observation of hair color and density can understand the rise and fall of kidney qi and the situation of the essence and blood.

● Color and lustre: If the hair is yellow and dry, sparse and easy to fall, it may mean the asthenia of essence and blood, and can be seen in chronic deficiency patients or long time disease. Adolescent white hair, accompanied by lumbar acid, tinnitus and other diseases, it is mostly due to kidney deficiency; with insomnia and absent-mindedness, it is due to the blood deficiency. Children's hair is thin and yellow and soft, growth retarded, or even the slow growth of hair, which is mostly due to insufficiency of congenital essence or poor feeding, insufficiency of qi and blood.

● Lipsotrichia: Sudden flaky hair loss, revealing or elliptical bright scalp without conscious symptoms, is called "alopecia areata", which is due to the blood deficiency and be attacked by wind meanwhile, or the injury by seven emotional factors like the long-term mental tension, consuming the essence and blood, failure of blood to nourish hair. If the head is bald, hair removal and often exhausted, it is mostly caused by mental exhaustion, consuming the essence and blood or is due to congenital inheritance. That the hair is sparse and easy to fall in the young and middle-aged, accompanied by vertigo, forgetfulness, lumbar knee acid, is due to kidney deficiency; with the scalp itching, much dandruff and oil, it's mostly blood heat.

5) Face

Heart manifests in complexion, and the face is nourished by the essential qi of zang-fu viscera. So inspection of the face can know the condition of the zang-fu viscera and qi and blood.

● Swollen face: The swelling of the face is often seen in the edema disease. It is due to the spleen, kidney and lung dysfunction, and stagnation of fluid-dampness. If the skin is scorching redness, swollen and sore, and the red will discolor because of pressure, called "head fire cinnabar", which is due to the wind-heat and fire toxin attacking upward.

● Swelling of the gills: Cheek swells around the lobe, and the edge is not clear, skin color is not red, companying with pain or haphalgesia, that is called "mumps", which is due to externally-contracted warm toxin.

● Emaciated face: The facial muscles are thin with sunken eye socket and cheeks, and the whole body is thin. This is due to the extreme lack of qi and blood of the zang-fu viscera and common in the critical stage of chronic disease.

● Deviation of the mouth and eyes: The condition that only one side of the mouth and eyes are wry, which is characterized by flabby facial muscles, disappearance of frontal wrinkle, unclosed eyes, flat nasolabial groove, and ptosis of labial angle, without half body paralysis, usually can be seen in facial paralysis. If deviation of the mouth and eyes accompanying with half body paralysis, it is often seen in wind stroke.

　● Unusual facies: The panic face can be usually seen in infantile convulsion, lupomania or goiter. lumps on forehead or around eyes, loss of brows and hair and leontiasis (the face looks like a lion's face) is usually seen in leprosy. Sardonic feature is a special appearance of the mimetic convulsion and could be seen in neonatal tetanus, lockjaw and other diseases.

(2) Inspection of neck

The neck is the connecting part of the head and trunk, with the passage of the trachea, the esophagus, the spinal cord and the meridians. The front part of the neck is called "collum" and the back part is called "nape". The normal person's neck is upright, both sides are symmetrical andcan move with ease. The male's laryngeal prominence is prominent. The pulsation of the lateral carotid artery is not easy to see when people are quiet.

The raised head shows the disease pertains to yang while the droopy head to yin. Stiffness of neck means excess of pathogen and the suspended head leaning on something means deficiency of the vital qi. Soft neck indicates the kidney qi deficiency.

(3) Inspection of five sensory organs

1) Eyes

Eyes, as window of liver, have a close relationship to zang-fu viscera. The *Miraculous Pivot* says: "All the essential qi of the five zang viscera and six fu viscera pours upward into the eyes." So inspection of the eyes is an extremely important part of diagnosis.

Five orbiculi theory of the traditional Chinese medicine believes the different parts of eyes corresponding to the five zang viscera respectively. The upper and lower eyelid parts correspond to the spleen (flesh orbiculus); the blood vessels of the two canthi region correspond to the heart (blood orbiculus); the conjunctiva and sclera correspond to the lung (qi orbiculus); the location of the cornea correspond to the liver (wind orbiculus) and the location of the pupil correspond to the kidney (water orbiculus).

Therefore, observing the eyes is not only the important part of the inspection of vitality, but also the diagnosis of ophthalmology or medical diseases.

　● Vitality: If the eyes are clear and flashy, that means, that the vitality and the essence are in a good condition.

If one has good eyesight, obvious distinguishable black and white of the eyeball, lustrous eye-light, with little tears and eye secretion, it indicates the disease pertains to yang syndrome and is easily to be cured. While one has blurred vision, the cloudy white of the eye, blurred color in the black of eye, gloomy eye-light, without tears and eye secretion, it means the disease pertains to yin syndrome and is difficult to be cured.

　● Color: The normal human eyelid conjunctiva and two canthi are ruddy, the sclera is white, the cornea is colorless and transparent, and the iris is brown.

There are several kinds of abnormal changes.

Swollen eyes: Most of them belong to the excess heat syndrome. If red appears in the corners of the eye, it may indicates heart fire; and a red color in the sclera means lung heat. If the reddish color appears in canthus, it represents the heart fire flaming. If the whole eye is red, painful and swollen, it indicates an exterior invasion of wind-heat in liver meridian. The reddish and blear eyelid indicates the spleen fire.

White eyes yellowed: This is the main manifestation of jaundice, caused by the overflowing bile due to the steaming dampness-heat or the cold-dampness.

Two canthi pale white:This phenomenon belongs to the blood deficiency. The deficiency of blood cannot nourish eyes.

Eyelid black and gloomy:It mostly belongs to the kidney deficiency,which is due to kidney essence insufficiency or kidney yang deficiency.

● Shape:Puffy swelling of eyelids:This is usually a sign and a common manifestation of edema. If it accompanies with redness,heat,pain and other symptoms,it is mostly due to wind-heat attacking upward. Slow swelling of eyelids with flabbiness is mostly because of the spleen deficiency failing to transport water-dampness while a swelling under the eyes indicates kidney deficiency.

Depressed eye socket:A slight depression is mostly due to the depletion of body fluid caused by vomiting and/or diarrhea or deficiency of both qi and blood. Deep sunken eye socket with lose the sight means the exhaustion of visceral essential qi,and critical illness.

Exophthalmos:Protruding eyeballs with hyperpnoea,fullness sensation in chest,usually belong to lung distention. If the eyes protrusion with diffuse swollen next laryngeal prominence in front of the throat,moving up and down accompanied by swallowing movement,mostly belong to gall disease. And the single protruding eyeball mostly indicates the intracranial tumor.

Stye and eyelid cellulitis:The edge of the eyelid is swollen like wheat. If the redness and swelling is slight,it is usually called "stye". While the redness and swollen is severe red,swollen and hard,it is usually called "eyelid cellulitis". All of them are due to the wind-heat or the spleen-stomach amassing heat and the heat attacks the eyes.

● Normal state:The pupils of the normal are rounding,bilateral and large. The diameter of the pupils is 3–4 mm in the natural light. The pupillary light reflex is sensitive,and the movement of the eyeball is flexible.

The main abnormal changes have the following points.

Myosis:This is mostly due to poisoning,such as radix aconite,wild aconite,poisonous mushroom,organophosphorus pesticide or the reaction of morphine and other drugs. This can also be seen in eye diseases.

Mydriasis:It usually can be seen in eye diseases like green glaucoma and so on. This can also be affected by trauma and certain medications. Bilateral mydriasis with pupillary light reflex disappears indicates kidney essence insufficiency,which is a dying crisis.

Froward-staring eyes:It refers to looking straight ahead forwardly with clouded vitality,which is due to the exhaustion of visceral essential qi.

Upcast eyes:It means the patient keeps looking up and the eyeballs could not turn. Most of this is due to internal stirring of liver wind or the exhaustion of visceral essential qi,which is in danger.

The eye tending to one side is called "strabismus",which is mostly caused by trauma or congenital.

Eyes closure obstacle:Both of the eyes closure obstacle usually means goiter. Exposure of the eyeballs in children's sleeping is caused by the spleen deficiency. This symptom can usually be seen in the depletion of body fluid caused by vomiting and/or diarrhea,infantile spleen-stomach weakness or chronic infantile spleen wind.

Ptosis:It is also known as "invalid eyelid". The double blepharoptosis is mostly due to the congenital deficiency or spleen-kidney deficiency. One sided blepharoptosis is mostly due to the spleen qi deficiency or trauma.

Others:Photophobia with tears can usually be due to the acute contagious conjunctivitis or the fulminant exogenous wind-heat. Eyelid twitching is mostly due to the attack of wind-heat or deficiency of qi and blood.

2) Ears

Ears are windows of kidney. Shaoyang meridians are encircling and entering the ear. And ears are also the syncretistical organs of various meridians. There are reaction points about zang-fu viscera and body parts on the auricle. So the inspection of ears is of great significance for the diagnosis of general disease.

The main contents of the inspection of ears are to observe the ears' color, shape, and the changes of theauditory canal.

- Color: Normal ears have a rosy color, and it is the expression of ample qi and blood. A pale color of the helices mostly indicates deficiency of both qi and blood. Red and swollen helices means dampness-heat in liver and gallbladder or fire toxin attack upward. A bluish or black color indicates yin cold excess or throe. Kraurotic and ustal helices indicates essence prostration and the condition is dangerous. Rosy papules on the back of ears and hairline of infant is usually the premonitory symptoms of measles.

- Shape: A normal person's ears are thick and big and have symmetry of shape, which means ample kidney qi. A thin ear indicates congenital deficiency and kidney qi deficiency. A squamous and dry skin of the ears means blood stasis for a long time.

- Auditory canal: Local redness and swelling pain of auditory canal indicate furuncle of auditory canal, which is due to the pathogen and heat entanglement. Efflux of the auditory canal with pus is called "purulent ear", which mostly is due to the dampness-heat in liver and gallbladder.

3) Nose

Nose, as the window of lung, relates to zang-fu viscera.

The main contents of the inspection of nose are to observe the color, shape, and changes in nasal cavity.

- Color: The color of a healthy person's nose is ruddy and lustrous, meaning that the stomach qi is adequate. And the slightly moist and shiny nose indicates that any disease might be is not serious. The white tip of the nose indicates the deficiency of both qi and blood or blood collapse. The red color of tip indicates heat in lung and spleen. The green or blue color of tip indicates abdominal pain caused by yin cold. The black color of tip indicates kidney deficiency and water retention. If the tip of the nose is dim and desiccated, it indicates deficiency of stomach qi and disease severity.

- Shape: Swelling of nose indicates the exorbitance of the pathogen while the sunken nose mostly indicates deficiency of vital qi. Flaring of the nostrils means the lung fails to govern diffusion and purification resulting in breathing difficulties, which is mostly due to phlegm-heat accumulated in lung and can be seen in asthma, etc.

- Changes in nasal cavity: Black and dry nostril shows the exorbitant heat injuring yin, and the black, cool and slippery nostril indicates the extremity of yin. A clear snivel indicates affection of exogenous wind-cold or yang deficiency. a thick nasal discharge indicates affection of exogenous wind-heat or the heat accumulating in lung and stomach. Epistaxis is usually due to heat injuring the lung and stomach. Fishy purulent nasal discharge for long time is called "sinusitis" and is mostly due to wind-heat in lung meridian or dampness-heat in liver and gallbladder. Neoplasm in the nostril is called "nasal polyp" and indicates the dampness-heat hiding in the nasal cavity.

4) Mouth

Mouth is the window of spleen and spleen manifests in lips. Both the stomach meridian of foot yangming and large intestine meridian of hand yangming travel around lips. So the abnormal changes of mouth and lip could show the disorders of spleen and stomach, as well as large intestine.

The main contents of the inspection of mouth and lips are to observe the color and abnormal shape.

● Color: A normal person's lips are ruddy, moist and shiny, indicating that the stomach qi is adequate and coordination between qi and blood. Pale lips mean blood deficiency or the blood loss. Cherry lips are usually seen in carbon monooxide poisoning. Red lips indicate excess heat. if the lips are dark red and dry, it is usually due to the heat injures the body fluids. The purple or bluish lips indicate stasis of blood which is common in patients with severe dyspnea or heart yang deficiency. The black lips may indicate excess yin or excruciating pain, and it is mostly caused by the cold congealing in the blood vessel, excruciating pain.

● Shape: Hare lip is due to congenital malformations. Drooling form the corner of the mouth seen in children belongs to spleen qi deficiency, while in adults it belongs to wind striking the meridians and collaterals or the sequela of wind stroke. Anabrotic lips indicate the spleen-stomach amassing heat. Whitish vesicles on the lip of the mouth with redness and pain after festering is called "mouth sore", which is mostly due to the spleen-stomach amassing heat. If children's mouth and tongue are covered with white scale and look like the mouth of the goose, it is usually due to the deficiency of vital qi. If the small, hoar spots surrounded by a flush, appear in the children's buccal mucosa which is near the molar teeth, it is known as "koplik spots" and is the omen of measles.

● Movement: The abnormal state of lips is summed up as "six abnormalities of the mouth".

Opening of the mouth: If the mouth is always open, it is a sign of deficiency syndrome. If the mouth is always open like fish and the breath is only out of the way, it indicates the lung qi will soon lose and the patient is in danger.

Clenched jaw: Mouth is closed and difficult to open with teeth clenched, which is a sign of deficiency syndrome and due to the internal stirring of liver wind. It can be seen in wind stroke, epilepsy, fright wind, lockjaw, etc.

Deviated mouth: The corner of the mouth is skewed to one side, which is usually due to the wind striking collateral or stroke syndrome of wind-phlegm blocking collateral.

Pursed lips: The upper and lower lips are tightly clustered together which can be seen in the neonatal tetanus or tetanus patients.

Mouth vibration: Shivery jaw and quivery lips indicate yang deficiency, exuberant yin or struggle between vital qi and pathogen.

Mouth movement: If mouth frequently opens and closes and cannot control, it may indicate stomach qi deficiency. The corner of the mouth twitched is a sign of wind symptom.

5) Teeth

The teeth are known as "surplus of bone" and kidney governs bones. The stomach meridian of foot yangming and large intestine meridian of hand yangming run in the gums, the stomach meridian of foot yangming runs around the superior gum while the large intestine meridian of hand yangming inferior. It is especially important to observe the changes of teeth and gum to know the changes of stomach, kidney and fluid and liquid.

The main contents of the inspection of teeth and gums are to observe the color, wet or dry, and movement.

● Teeth: If the teeth are white, moist and firm, it is the performance of the kidney qi excess and enough body fluid. Dry teeth indicate the excess heat injuring stomach fluid. The bright and dry teeth like a stone indicate heat in the bright yang and the serious injury of body fluid. Dry teeth like dead-bone indicate the deficiency heat due to kidney yin deficiency. Gnathospasmus indicates the liver wind stirring up internally. The gnashing of teeth in the sleep is the sign of stomach heat or malnutrition which is due to the parasitic infestation.

　● Gums：Normal gums are ruddy, and it means that the stomach qi is adequate and coordination between qi and blood. Pale gum means blood deficiency or deficiency of both qi and blood. The swollen and painful gums indicate blazing of stomach fire. Loss of teeth with exposed root of teeth is called "gaping gums" and is usually due to flaring fire of the kidney yin deficiency. If the gums are bleeding, it is called "gum bleeding". If the gums are red swollen and pain, it indicates blazing of stomach fire, while the gums are slightly swollen, it means the failure of spleen to control blood or flaring fire due to deficiency of kidney yin.

6.1.2.2　Inspection of idiosoma

（1）Inspection of chest

When observing the chest, we should pay attention to the changes of chest shape and breathing.

The chest of normal people is symmetrical on both sides, in an elliptical shape. The anteroposterior diameter of the adult is shorter than the left-right diameter, and the proportion is 1 : 1.5. Both sides of the clavicle are symmetrical.

　● Chicken breast：The chicken-breast-like chest in child is named chicken breast, which is usually due to insufficiency of congenital essence, acquired dystrophy, spleen-kidney deficiency and is common in children's rickets.

　● Flat chest：The thoracic cavity is flat, and anteroposterior diameter is obviously shorter than left-right diameter. It can be seen in a slender person, the people of deficiency of both qi and yin, or the man of yin deficiency of lung and kidney, deficiency of qi and blood.

　● Barrel chest：The anteroposterior diameter of the chest is almost equal to the left-right diameter. It can be seen in the lung distention diseases.

（2）Inspection of abdomen

The abdomen of thenormal is flat and symmetrical, and can be slightly raised when standing upright, approximately equal to the chest level. The abnormal shape of abdomen mainly includes abdominal distention, abdominal retraction and protruding umbilicus.

1）Abdominal distention

The anterior abdominal wall in the supine is obviously higher than the line of the sternum to midpoint of the pubic symphysis. If the abdominal distention with obviously engorged vessels, it is difficult to be cured, but the one without the vessel exposure is curable.

Abdominal mass can also lead to abdominal distention. The unmovable abdominal lump is mostly known as "abdominal mass" while the movable one is called as "abdominal gathering". The upper and down movement of lump is usually due to parasitic infestation.

2）Abdominal retraction

The anterior abdominal wall in the supine is obviously lower than the line of the sternum to midpoint of the pubic symphysis. The abdominal retraction with emaciation may be due to extreme spleen-stomach weakness in chronic disease, deficiency of both qi and yin or over use of emetic or purgative in newly occurred disease.

3）Protruding umbilicus

Protruding umbilicus can be seen in edema, which is due to exhaustion of spleen and kidney and is difficult to be cured. It also can be seen in crying baby. If the protruding umbilicus complicated with reddish swelling and exudation, it is the umbilical ulceration, which is caused by accumulation of dampness-heat due to internal attack of water-dampness.

（3）Inspection of lumbus and back

Lumbus is the house of the kidney, and related to bladder meridian of foot taiyang and belt vessel. Governor vessel and bladder meridian of foot taiyang go along the back, so the back disorder is connected with these two meridians.

When observing the lumbus and back, we should pay attention to the morphological abnormalities and restricted activity.

1）Kyphos

The spine is overly protruding, mostly caused by kidney qi deficiency, dysplasia or spinal disease. If a patient's back is bent, two shoulders are drooping, it is usually called "hunchback with feeble arms failing to hold up", and which is the deficiency of the essential qi of the zang-fu viscera.

2）Skoliosis

The spine deviates from the mid-line, bent to the left or right. The condition can be found commonly in children with developmental stage caused by poor sitting posture. It is also seen in patients with hypoplasia, dysplasia, or a disease on one side of the chest.

3）Spinal malnutrition

The patient is so thin that the spine is like the sawtooth and is a manifestation of the essential qi of the zang-fu viscera deficiency overly. It is seen in patients with chronic severe disease.

4）Opisthotonos

Opisthotonos is a state of severe hyperextension and spasticity with the head, neck and spinal column entering into a complete "bridging" or "arching" position caused by spasm of the axial muscles along the spinal column. It is the syndrome of liver wind stirring up internally.

6.1.2.3 Inspection of limbs

The five zang viscera are all related to the limbs, and the relationship between the spleen and the limbs is especially close.

When observing the limbs, we should pay attention to the shapes and the changes of the movement.

（1）Inspection of limb edema

If the lower limbs are pitting edema, it is often seen in the edema disease. If the unilateral limb is swollen, it is often found in the meridian qi stagnation.

（2）Inspection of limb atrophy

The limbs or limb muscles are thin, soft and weak. It can be seen in the patients of liver-kidney depletion or spleen-stomach weakness.

（3）Inspection of lower limb malformation

When upright, two ankles are close together and two knees are separated, called "gonyectyposis"; and two knees are combined and two malleolus separation is called "knock knees". Both of those belong to insufficiency of congenital essence, deficiency of kidney qi, and poor development.

（4）Inspection of finger deformation

Clasping fingers are named chicken-claw-wind, and it is due to the failure of blood to nourish because of wind-cold attack.

Dark purple toes with severe pain, if broken, having exudation, are called "toe ju", which is caused by internal accumulated cold-dampness and transforming into fire.

Swelling and deformed joints of fingers and toes are mostly due to the internal accumulated wind-dampness with liver-kidney yin deficiency.

（5）Inspection of nails

Liver manifests in nails. The normal reddish luster indicates the plenty of qi and blood. Pale nails indicate deficiency of blood, and bluish nails indicate stasis of blood. Dark red nail means the exorbitance of heat.

6.1.2.4   Inspection of skin

Skin is an organization that covers the surface of the body directly with the external environment. It has the function of protecting the body, defending the external pathogen, excreting the sweat and assisting the breathing. It is the outside manifestation of qi and blood, and acts as the protective shield of human body. Skin correlates with the lung internally and is circuited by the defensive qi. Being invaded by exogenous or visceral disease can cause corresponding changes in the skin. The observation of the skin, in addition to the diagnosis of the local skin, can also diagnose the diseases of the zang-fu viscera and the rise and fall of qi and blood.

The normal skin is moist, pliable, smooth, and it is a sign of the ample visceral essential qi visceral and full of qi and blood, fluid and liquid.

The main contents of the inspection of skin are to observe the changes in color and modality.

（1）Inspection of color changes of skin

1）Rubefaction

If the skin is suddenly scorching redness, swollen, sore, and the boundary is clear, at the same time it expands rapidly and heal within a few days but recurrent attacks of several times, it is called "erysipelas"; it is mostly due to the fire toxin in the blood. Erysipelas have different names depending on the incidence of different parts. If it occurs on the head and face, it is called "head erysipelas". If it occurs in the legs and feet, it is called "fire flow". If it occurs in all over the body and wandering, it is called "wandering erysipelas".

2）White maculas on the skin

If the local skin is obviously white, its patch different in size and shape, the boundary is clear, and the progress is slow, which is called "leucoderma". The reasons of this disease are the invasion of wind-dampness and the disharmony of qi and blood.

3）Skin blackening

If the skin is dark, dry-rotten and can't get nutrition, it may indicate the kidney essence insufficiency. If the skin of the body is dark, it can also be caused by the kidney yang deficiency.

4）Dry skin

If the skin is dry and even chapped, it is usually due to the consumption of fluid and the skin can't get nutrition from the inadequate nutrient-blood.

5）Squamous and dry skin

That the skin is dry and rough, like the scale of the fish is often caused by the long time of static blood and failure of skin and muscle to be nourished.

（2）Inspection of changes in skin modality

1）Swelling

If a swelling of the skin which cannot leave a mark on pressure with a finger, this is called "qi oedema" and is not a true oedema. The swelling is caused by qi stagnation.

2）Maculas and papules

Both maculas and papules are symptoms of a systemic disease on the skin, but there is essential difference.

● Macula: It is characterized by carmine or cyanotic patches without swelling on the skin. And the color will not be discoloration due to pressure. The macula is divided into the yang macula and the yin macula.

Yang-macula is characterized by large brocade patches with red or purple color without touchable skin change by palm. It is mostly due to the external contraction of warm pathogen, and forced the camp blood. The case of favorable prognosis is marked by sparse macula with lustrous red color which appear on chest and abdomen first, and then on limbs, accompanying with fever, red facial complexion, rapid pulse and clear consciousness. The case of unfavorable prognosis is characterized by dense macula with dark red or purplish black color which appears on limbs first, and then on chest and abdomen, accompanying with excess heat and coma.

Yin-macula is characterized by irregular macula in different sizes with reddish or blackish purple color, no fixed location. Besides, it usually accompanies fatigued vitality, clear consciousness, cold limbs, and shortness of breath, no thirst, and thready and weak pulse. It is usually due to spleen qi deficiency and failure of spleen to control blood.

● Rash: It has red color, millet-like shape, and is high above surface of the skin. It can be felt by touching. And the red color will disappear by pressing. The papules are divided into measles, wind-rash, and obscure-rash.

Measles: This kind of rash has a pinkish color, and is high above the skin with distinct demarcation. There appears reddish rash behind the ear first, then the rash appears on the hairline and face on the trot, gradually spreading to trunk and limbs. It is sparse at first, and then denser gradually and subside in the order of appearance.

It is due to invasion of seasonal pathogen, which is a common infectious disease in children.

Wind-Rash: The appearance of eruption which is marked by tiny and sparse rash, light protuberance with reddish color and severe itching. The eruption order is from face to neck, trunk and limbs and it erupts completely within a day. Because the rash will disappear after three days, it is also known as "three-day eruption".

It is caused by the heat of the wind-heat, then the qi and blood fight the pathogens, then the pathogens are pushed outwards to skin and muscles, and the wind-rash occurs.

Obscure-rash: It is clinically characterized by severe itching. The skin appears pink or pale color wheal with different sizes and shapes; on scraping, the swollen marks were linked together and are high above the skin. The rashes appear random rapidly.

It is usually caused by wind pathogen attack on meridians or by allergy.

● Blister: The small blisters is clustered or scattered, which can be seen in miliaria alba, chickenpox, pyretic sore, eczema, herpes zoster, etc.

Miliaria alba: There are millet-sized crystalline vesicles on skin, and it is high above the skin. It usually appears in neck and chest, sometimes in limbs, rarely in face and accompanies unsurfaced fever, chest oppression, gastric stuffiness, etc. It is commonly due to attacked by dampness-heat. It can be seen in dampness-heat disease.

There are different cases of favorable and unfavorable prognosis.

The "crystal miliaria" is the case of favorable prognosis, which is characterized by millet-sized and bright crystal vesicles. The "dry miliaria" is of unfavorable prognosis, which is characterized by pale without lustrous, dry and withering vesicles.

Chickenpox: Pink spotted papules arise on the skin, and then become blister with the characteristics of oval-shape, susceptible to be broken, without umbilicus in the top, different sizes and appearances, and occurring in succession. After being cured, there usually no pox-scar left.

It is due to invasion of seasonal pathogen and dampness-heat brewing internally, which is a common infectious disease in children.

Pyretic sore: Blisters on the size of millet appear in clusters on the mouth, lip and other places. It is commonly due to toxic wind-heat and the heat accumulates in lung and stomach.

Eczema: The erythema with itching feeling occurs first, and rapidly swells and forms a papule and blister. There will be exudate after the blister is broken, and then form a red and humid erosive surface. It is usually due to the wind-dampness-heat combination hiding in the skin.

Herpes zoster: The waist skin is bright red, covered with visible clusters of vesicular rash, zonal distribution, and wrapped around the waist. It is usually due to external contraction of fire toxin or dampness-heat in the liver meridian.

● Sore: It is a purulent surgical disorder that occurs between the skin and the muscles of the flesh. Common types are carbuncle, ju, ding, and furuncle, and so on.

Carbuncle: It is characterized by red swelling, higher than skin and pain and scorching sensation and distinct demarcation. It is easy to putrefy and belongs to yang syndrome. It is usually due to dampness-heat and fire toxin combination and qi stagnation and blood stasis.

Ju: It is characterized by boundless swelling without change of skin color or agony. The location of the disease is deep and it belongs to yin syndrome. It is usually due to deficiency of both qi and blood, and congealing yin cold.

Ding: It is characterized by millet-sized boil with white top and hard root. It is numb, itch and ache, which usually occurs in the face, hands and feet. The red line appears from the lesion and extends to the heart direction from distal part is called "red-streak ding", or "deteriorated ding". It is commonly due to external contraction of wind-heat or endogenous fire.

Furuncle: It is characterized by tiny round boil with slight reddish swelling and pain. It is easy to putrefy and heal after the pus out. It is commonly due to external contraction of fire toxin or dampness-heat brewing internally, qi stagnation and blood stasis.

6.1.3　Tongue examination

Tongue examination is also named tongue observation. It is a method of knowing disease by observing the changes of tongue body and tongue coating, which is an important part of inspection of TCM.

6.1.3.1　The relation between tongue and zang-fu viscera, meridians, qi, blood, and fluid

Tongue manifestation is a comprehensive performance of tongue body and tongue coating. Tongue body is the muscular choroid tissue of the tongue nourished by zang-fu viscera qi and blood. Tongue coating is a layer of moss on the tongue surface.

Meridians, for example, three yang meridians of the foot, three yin meridians of the foot, small intestine meridian of hand taiyang, triple energizer meridian of handshaoyang, have connection to the tongue.

Tongue body needs the nourishment of qi, blood and fluid. The color and shape are related to the deficiency or excess of qi and blood. The moist of tongue is related to the profit or loss of fluid.

Tongue is the window of the heart. On the one hand, the heart governs the blood and vessel. The profit and loss of qi and blood can be reflected in the color of the tongue body. On the other hand, the heart governs the vitality light. The movement of the tongue body is controlled by the heart vitality, so the movement flexibility of tongue body and the clarity of the language are closely related to the conscious vitality. In a word, the tongue can show the heart disease.

Tongue is called the out show of the spleen. The spleen governs transportation and transformation. So the tongue is directly related to the function of spleen.

Zang-fu viscera have the representative areas on tongue surface. For example, the tip of tongue belongs to the heart and lungs, the middle to the spleen and stomach, the bilateral margins to the liver and gallbladder, and the root to the kidney. It can also be explained as the tip portion to upper energizer, the middle to the middle energizer and the root to the lower energizer.

6.1.3.2   Significance of tongue examination

The tongue body and coating have their unique significance in diagnosis. Tongue body reflects conditions of yin organs. By inspecting tongue body, so we can judge the deficiency or excess of vital qi and the severity of disease. Tongue coating exhibits the six fu viscera, so we can ascertain the cold or heat of pathogens and the location of disease. Tongue body and coating can show disease in different aspects. To sum up, the significance includes:

(1)To judge qi and blood deficiency or excess

The deficiency or excess of the qi and blood can be shown in tongue. For example, the red and moist tongue means the excess of qi and blood.

(2)To infer the tendency of disease

The rising and falling of vital qi and pathogen, and disease location usually lead to the changes of tongue. We can observe tongue to infer the tendency of disease, especially in exogenous contraction diseases. For example, the turning of coating color from white to yellow, or from yellow to back, is usually due to the transferring of pathogens from cold to heat, or from exterior to interior, which reflects the tendency of disease. If a moist coating turns into dry, it is usually due to loss of body fluid resulting from heat. The change from dry to moister implies the recovery of body fluid.

(3)To detect the location of disease

In exogenous contraction diseases, the deep or shallow of disease location can be shown by the thickness or thinness of the coating. For example, the thin coating suggests that the disease is located shallow part and is in initial stage, while the thick coating suggests that the disease is located in deep part and the pathogens enter into the inner part of the body.

Among the four examination methods, tongue examination is thought to be more reliable than others by some doctors. However, it should be pointed out that the abnormalchanges of tongue can be seen in normal people, and sometimes it is only slightly changed in some severe cases. So the tongue examination should be used in combination with other examinations.

6.1.3.3   Special attentions on tongue examination

In order to guarantee the safety and reliability of the tongue examination, special attention should be paid to some points which can make false changes in tongue manifestations.

(1)Light

It is best to observe tongue in day time under the full natural light. The intensity and tone of light often affect the judgment of the tongue manifestation. For example, in lamp light, the pale tongue is seen as dark purple tongue, and the yellow coating can be seen as a white coating, etc.

(2)Diet or drug

Some food or drugs can make the color of tongue coating changed. After meal, the tongue coating can become thin due to the friction of the chewing. If chewing food in one side of mouth, the coating will be thinner than that of another side. Drinking can make the tongue coating moist. The patient had better to avoid food intake before seeing a doctor to make sure the tongue keeps its true state, as the moist or dry of coating is difficult to be distinguished after meal. If tongue condition is not corresponding to the whole symptoms, one should ask the patient about the diet and drugs to prevent from being confused by the false tongue conditions. Attention should be given to these points.

In addition, certain food or drug can make the tongue coating colorization, which is called as "dyed tongue". For example, drinking milk can dye the tongue coating white, while eating orange can get it yellow. Long-term smoking also can dye the tongue coating gray or black. So the doctor should pay attention on "dyed tongue" affected by food or some factors.

6.1.3.4   The method of tongue examination

(1) The posture of tongue examination

The patient should take a seat or a supine position, and stretch out the tongue in a natural way to expose tongue thoroughly. The tongue should be expanded to two sides without curve. The over extension of tongue with too much strength should be avoided, so as not to affect qi and blood circulation of tongue, which will change the tongue color.

(2) The order of tongue examination

The order to observe the tongue is the tip, the middle, the bilateral and the root. Observing the tongue body and the tongue coating first, then the sublingual vein is observed. In addition, the condition of the tasty and the flexibility of the tongue can be known by acquiring.

6.1.3.5   Normal tongue and its physiological variation

The normal tongue is characterized by medium size, pink color, soft, neither tough nor tender, free movement, covered by thin and white coating with moderate moist, which is briefly summarized as "pink tongue with white and thin coating". It suggests that the zang-fu viscera function is normal, the qi and blood fluid is full, and the stomach qi is exuberant.

The normal tongue is affected by the internal and external physiological variation, such as age, gender, constitution, climatic environment, etc.

(1) Age

Children grow and develop rapidly, but their spleen and stomach are weak. They are often in a state of high metabolism and relatively inadequate nutrition, so the tongue shows pink tongue with thin coating.

While the genuine qi of the aged is weakened, and the function of the zang-fu viscera is decreased with slow circulation of qi and blood.

(2) Gender

The tongue is generally not associated with gender. However, women are affected by menstruation, and the tongue is deep red or purple or spotted in the menstrual period.

(3) Constitution

Differences in constitution can have different tongue manifestation. The tongue of the fat is often enlarged and pale while the tongue of the thin is thin and red.

(4) Climatic environment

The tongue can change according to the changes of seasons and regions.

In term of season, the tongue is thick with yellow coating in summer heat-dampness while the tongue coating exhibits thin and dry in autumn dryness and the tongue is often wet in winter cold. In term of region, the wet and heat in the southeast of China and the cold and dry in the northwest and northeast regions will make certain differences in the tongue manifestation.

Generally speaking, if the abnormal tongue manifestation is constant for a long time but without any symptom, there is a factor that conforms to the variation of the tongue which belongs to physiological variation.

6.1.3.6　Contents of tongue examination

Tongue examination includes observing tongue body and tongue coating. Observing tongue body includes tongue vitality, tongue color, tongue shape, tongue motility and sublingual vein, and it is to diagnose zang-fu viscera qi and blood deficiency or excess. While observing tongue coating includes coating texture and coating color, which is to diagnose the nature and the location of the disease, exuberance and debilitation of pathogenic or health qi. In order to fully understand the disease condition and make the right diagnose, the changes of tongue body and tongue coating should be analyzed comprehensively.

(1) Inspection of tongue body

Inspection of tongue body mainly includes the observation of tongue vitality, tongue color, tongue shape, tongue motility, sublingual vein and so on.

1) Tongue vitality

The observation of the tongue vitality is part of the whole inspection of vitality. Whether the tongue has vitality or not, mainly depends on the flourish or withering of the tongue body.

Lustrous tongue: The lustrous tongue refers to pink tongue with energetic movement and enough fluid. It means full of vitality and suggests the normal stomach qi.

Withered tongue: The withered tongue refers to dark and dry tongue body with sluggish movement. No matter there is coating or not, the disease is in bad condition.

2) Tongue color

Tongue color is the color of the tongue body. There are five colors: pale, pink, red, crimson and green-blue or purple.

● Pink tongue: The tongue is light red and moist. It reflects on the harmony of qi and blood, common in healthy people or in the condition of light illness without injuring qi and blood. Pink tongue mainly reflects in the physiological state of heart blood and stomach qi sufficiency. In the light state of the external disease, the tongue color can still remain normal as the zang-fu viscera qi and blood has not been injured. In internal disease, if the color of the tongue is pink, it indicates that yin, yang, qi and blood are harmony and the disease is not serious.

● Pale tongue: The color of tongue is lighter than that of normal people. The tongue is whiter and less red, and it is called as "pale tongue". If the tongue shows pale, dry and no red at all, it is called as "withered pale tongue". It indicates either yang deficiency or deficiency of both qi and blood and reflects the collapse of qi and blood. If the tongue body is thin and pale, it shows the deficiency of qi and blood. The tongue is usually slightly too wet and swollen due to the deficiency of yang. When the body is in the collapse of qi and blood situation, the tongue is withered and pale.

● Red tongue: Red tongue is redder than normal tongue. It reflects heat syndrome.

A red tip indicates heart fire. Red sides of tongue often indicate liver fire. If the tongue is reddish, or the tip and sides of the tongue is slightly red, it belongs to the initial state of external contraction of wind-heat. The tongue is red and prickly with yellow thick coating, indicating excess heat syndrome. If the tongue is bright red and little moss, or there is a crack, or no moss, it is the syndrome of deficiency heat.

● Crimson tongue: It is deeper than red tongue, or slightly dark red. It indicates the excess of interior heat or hyperactivity of fire due to yin deficiency. Crimson tongue with moss belongs to warm heat disease, because of heat invading nutrient-blood or excess of interior heat in zang-fu viscera. The deeper the crimson, the heavier the heat. Crimson tongue with little moss or no moss, or has a crack, belongs to hyperactivity of fire due to yin deficiency or exhaustion of yin humor in final state of heat disease. In a word, it is usually seen in extreme state of heat disease.

● Green-blue or purple tongue:The whole tongue is pale purple and no red,and is known as "green-blue tongue". The tongue is deep crimson or local stasis spots,and is called as "purple tongue". There are two types of purple color:reddish purple and bluish purple. The green-blue or purple spots can be seen in located tongue body,not higher than the body,which is called as "stasis spots tongue".

Green-blue or purple tongue always indicates stasis of qi and blood. Pale purple tongue develops from a pale tongue,and it is pale purple and moist. Intense internal yin cold obstructs yang qi and congeals blood, or debilitation of yang qi makes stasis of qi and blood.

If the full tongue is blue purplish it usually suggests that the blood stasis is serious and systemic. The tongue with purple spots indicate the blood stasis is not serious and is blocked in a certain part or local veins are damaged.

Reddish purple tongue develops from crimson tongue. The purple and dry tongue with cracks is seen in severe case of yin exhaustion caused by heat. If purple is seen in whole tongue,it is due to extreme heat in zang-fu viscera. If purple is seen only at one part,it is due to stagnated heat in the viscera corresponding to the part.

3)Tongue shape

Tongue shape is the shape of tongue body and it includes tough or tender tongue,enlarged or thin tongue,teeth-marked tongue,spotted tongue and cracked tongue.

● Tough or tender tongue:Tough tongue refers the texture is crude or crapy of the tongue,while tender tongue is that the texture is fine and smooth of the tongue. The tough or tender tongue is one of the important signs to distinguish the deficiency and excess of the disease. Tough tongue indicates excess syndrome, while tender tongue indicates deficiency syndrome.

● Enlarged or thin tongue:The tongue that is larger and thicker than normal,and full of mouth is called as "enlarged tongue". The tongue that is swollen and full of mouth,and cannot even be retracted from the mouth is called as "swollen tongue". The tongue that is thinner and smaller than normal tongue,is called as "thin tongue". Enlarged tongue indicates internal stagnation of fluid-dampness. Swollen tongue indicates alcohol poisoning and toxic heat. Thin tongue indicates dual vacuity of qi and blood or hyperactivity of fire due to yin deficiency.

● Teeth-marked tongue:The pressing marks of teeth on lateral side of tongue are called "teeth-marked tongue". It indicates spleen deficiency or stagnation of fluid-dampness. It is usually due to enlarged tongue pressing on teeth. If it is seen in pale and moist tongue,it belongs to internal cold-dampness syndrome. While in pink and thin tongue,it dues to congenital teeth-marked tongue.

● Spotted tongue:Spotted tongue indicates extreme heat zang-fu viscera or repletion heat of blood level. Spots are frequently seen on the tip(exuberance of heat fire),on the side(effulgent liver-gallbladder fire) and around the centre(exuberant stomach heat).

● Cracked tongue:If there are cracks on tongue surface,it is called "cracked tongue". The size,depth and shape of cracks are different. It indicates either exuberant heat damaging fluid or hyperactivity of fire due to yin deficiency. The tongue,pale white with cracks,indicates blood deficiency. The tongue,red with yellow and dry coating and cracks,indicates injury of fluid due to exuberant heat. Crimson tongue with cracks and no coating indicates hyperactivity of fire due to yin deficiency. Cracked tongue with teeth-marked belongs to dampness-retention due to spleen deficiency.

Cracked tongue can also be seen in normal people and is formed inborn. It can be known by asking.

4) Tongue motility

Tongue motility is the dynamic of the tongue, including flaccid tongue, stiff tongue, deviated tongue, trembling tongue, protruding and waggling tongue and shortened tongue.

● Flaccid tongue: Flaccid tongue is flaccid and weak, and inability to move. It is usually due to either deficiency of qi and blood or injury of fluid due to exuberant heat. The flaccid tongue in pale color is due to deficiency of qi and blood, while in crimson with little or no coating indicates injury of fluid due to exuberant heat. The dry and flaccid tongue in crimson is due to yin depletion of liver and kidney.

● Stiff tongue: Stiff tongue is an inflexible tongue with difficulty in moving or inability of turning. It indicates invasion of pericardium by heat, heat damaging fluid or wind-phlegm obstructing collateral. Stiff tongue in crimson color with little coating is due to blazing pathogenic heat syndrome. Enlarged and stiff tongue with thick coating indicates wind-phlegm obstructing collateral. Stiff tongue with sluggish speech and numbness of the limbs indicates wind stroke.

● Deviated tongue: Deviated tongue is inclined to one side and indicates wind stroke. It is due to wind entering collateral or wind-phlegm obstructing collateral.

● Trembling tongue: Trembling tongue refers to shivering and swaying which is not controlled by the patient oneself. It indicates liver wind stirring up internally. After a chronic disease, trembling tongue in pale color belongs to stirring wind due to blood deficiency while trembling tongue in red color with little coating is due to extreme heat stirring wind or hyperactive liver yang causing wind. It is also seen in alcohol intoxication.

● Protruding and waggling tongue: The tongue stretching out of mouth is called as "protruding tongue". And waggling tongue is that the tongue stretches out and immediately retracts into mouth. Both of them indicate heat in heart and spleen.

Heart opens into the tongue and spleen opens into the mouth. Protruding tongue is due to pestilential toxin invading the heart, and it indicates the impasse of healthy qi in the critical condition.

● Shortened tongue: The tongue is contracted and shortened, and unable to stretch, even cannot reach teeth, which is called "shortened tongue". It is due to cold coagulated in meridians, deficiency of qi and blood, extreme heat stirring wind and liver wind with phlegm. Shortened tongue is a sign of critically ill.

5) Sublingual veins

Sublingual veins are Located in the lower part of the tongue, one on each side. If the sublingual veins are bulging, or purple, they indicate blood stasis. Short and thin sublingual veins and pale tongue are due to deficiency of qi and blood.

(2) Inspection of tongue coating

Inspection of tongue coating includes tongue coating color and coating texture.

1) Coating texture

Coating texture is the texture and form of tongue coating, including thick coating or thin coating, moist coating or dry coating, curdy coating or greasy coating, peeled coating, full coating or part coating, true coating or false coating.

● Thick coating or thin coating: Whether the bottom can be seen or not is taken as the standard of judging thick or thin coating. The thick coating refers to that we cannot see the tongue body through the coating. The thin coating is a coating through which we can see the tongue body.

Thick coating and thin coating can reflect the rising and falling of vital qi and pathogen and the deep and shallow of pathogen. Thick coating indicates interior syndrome, phlegm-dampness or food retention. While thin coating indicates exterior syndrome, and it is often seen in common people.

If thin coating becomes thick, it shows that pathogen qi enters the interior from the exterior and the disease changes from mild to severe, the disease deteriorating. While thick coating turns into thin, it is a sign of pathogen qi being cleared up or expelled, the disease is improving.

- Moist coating or dry coating: Moist coating is that tongue coating is moist with fluid. And dry coating is that tongue coating is dry or even cracked.

They can reflect the situation of the profit and loss of fluid and the distribution of fluid. Moist coating indicates that the fluid is not damaged, and it is often seen in common people. Dry coating suggests consumption of fluid due to intense heat, exhaustion of yin and failure of qi transforming fluid.

- Curdy coating or greasy coating: If the coating looks like coarse mulch granules as putrid bean dregs piling on tongue, and easy to be scraped off, it is called as "curdy coating". The greasy coating is made of fine particles, thicker in middle and thinner in margin and difficult to be scraped off.

Curdy coating is formed by the stomach putrid qi steamed by excessive yang heat, and it indicates food retention or dampness transforming into heat. Greasy coating suggests food retention damp turbidity or phlegm fluid retention.

- Peeled coating: If there is coating on tongue but now coating of some parts or all coating disappears, it is called as "peeled coating". It indicates insufficiency of stomach qi, deficiency of stomach yin or deficiency of qi and blood. The red and peeled tongue suggests deficiency of yin, while the pale and peeled tongue shows deficiency of qi and blood. The crimson and mirror tongue indicates desiccation of stomach yin.

- Full coating or part coating: The coating evenly spreading all over tongue surface is full coating. If the coating is only on some parts of tongue surface, it is called part coating. Full coating is due to the pathogenic qi spreading throughout and the syndrome of phlegm-dampness, while part coating suggests pathogenic qi in the upper part of the tongue corresponding to zang-fu viscera distribution.

- True coating or false coating: The "rooted" or "non-rooted" is taken as the standard to distinguish the true or false coating. The rooted coating refers to the even coating which is closely adhered to the tongue body and is difficult to be scraped off. The non-rooted coating is a thick coating with clear boundary and is easy to be scraped off.

To distinguish whether the coating is true or not is important for judging the state of pathogenic qi, genuine qi and stomach qi. True coating is a sign of sufficiency of stomach qi, and false coating suggests insufficiency of stomach qi.

2) Coating color

There are three main types of the coating color, white coating, yellow coating and gray black coating.

- White coating: White coating indicates exterior syndrome, cold syndrome, and dampness syndrome, and usually is seen in healthy persons. White, thick and greasy coating is due to internal stoppage of dampness turbidity, phlegm fluid retention or food retention. White, thick and dry coating indicates internal retention of phlegm-turbidity and dampness-heat, initial stage of warm heat disease or damp warm disease. White coating is a white, greasy coating like wheat flour over all the tongue body which can be seen in damp warm disease due to the exogenous turbid qi and heat pathogen spread over all triple energizer. White and rough coating like sands on red tongue body is caused by dryness-heat impairing fluid.

- Yellow coating: The tongue coating is yellow. According to the degree of yellowness, there are pale yellow, deep yellow and brown yellow. The pale yellow coating means the heat is not severe, while the deep one means a severe heat. The brown coating shows the heat accumulation. Yellow coating indicates heat syndrome or interior syndrome.

The pale yellow moist coating reflects internal retention of cold-damp due to yang deficiency or phlegm-fluid transforming into heat. Yellow and dry coating indicates exuberant heat damaging fluid or yangming fu viscera excess. Yellow, thick and greasy coating belongs to dampness-heat, internal retention phlegm-heat or food retention.

● Gray black coating: Black coating is deeper in color than gray coating. They indicate intense heat or abundant cold. They usually come from white or yellow coating. If gray black coating is moist, it is mainly due to yang deficiency leading to cold or internal stoppage of phlegm fluid retention. Black and dry coating with red tongue, even prickled tongue, is due to intense heat leading to fluid exhaustion.

6.1.4　Infant's finger examination

The index finger collateral is also called finger veins. It is the superficial vein of the radial side of the medial index of the forefinger. It is a way to understand the disease by observing the changes of color and shape of the infantile index finger collateral, which is suitable for children within 3 years old. It plays an important role in the diagnosis of pediatric diseases.

6.1.4.1　Principle and significance

The infantile finger-vein is a branch of lung meridian of hand taiyin just like cunkou pulse, so observing the finger vein in a manner plays the same role of taking cunkou pulse in diagnosis. And the principle and significance are similar to taking cunkou pulse.

The infantile pulse is short and infant is usually in crying or restlessness when diagnosing, which makes it difficult to take pulse. And the infantile skin is thin and tender and the collateral is obvious to see. The finger-vein observation is used to diagnose disease for infants below 3 years old instead of pulse taking.

6.1.4.2　Methods and precautions

Holding the infant face to the light, the doctor fixes the child's index finger with doctor's left thumb and index finger and puts right thumb on infant index finger and pushes forwards from the fingertip to the root for several times.

The index finger is divided into three parts accordance with the knuckle, and the creases at the metacarpo-phalangeal articulation and interphalangeal articulation are called "pass". The first phalanx of index finger, namely, from the cross striation of metacarpophalangeal to that of the second phalanx, is the "wind pass". The second phalanx, namely, from the cross striation to that of third phalanx, is the "qi pass". The third phalanx, namely from the cross striation to the tip of index finger, is the "life pass".

6.1.4.3　Normal index finger collateral

The normal collaterals are in the medial radial side of the index finger and is indistinct within the wind pass. It is light red, and the shape is mostly oblique, single and medium(Figure 6-1).

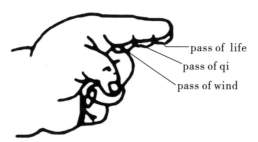

Figure 6-1　**Index finger collateral**

6.1.4.4   Pathologic index finger collateral

Observing infantile index finger collateral should focus on the floating, depth, color and lustre, shape, length and so on.

(1) Floating and deep

The floating and deep of collateral changes can reflect the location of the disease. The floating exposed collateral indicates the exterior syndrome. The deep obscure collateral indicates the interior syndrome.

(2) Color and lustre

The color changes of the collaterals mainly reflect the nature of the disease. If the color is pale, it indicates the deficiency syndrome such as spleen deficiency, deficiency of both qi and blood, and so on. If the color is scarlet, it indicates the exterior syndrome of external heat. Mauve indicates internal heat syndrome. Blueness indicates infantile convulsions and pain syndrome. Purplish black means the static blood blocking collaterals and indicates critical diseases.

In general, the deep and dark color means excess syndrome which is due to the exuberance of pathogenic qi, while the light color usually means the deficiency syndrome which is due to the deficiency of vital qi.

(3) Shape

The growing thick collateral and obvious branching are usually of excessive syndrome, while the decreased thin collateral and unconspicuous branching are usually of deficiency syndrome.

(4) Length

If the collateral appears only beyond the "wind pass", it indicates an invasion by exterior pathogenic factor and a mild disease. If the collateral extends beyond the "qi pass", it indicates an interior and rather more severe disease. If the collateral extends beyond the "life pass", it indicates a serious and life-threatening disease. If the collateral extends into fingertip, it is called "extension through passes toward nail" and is a sign of a dangerous condition.

6.2   Auscultation and olfaction

Auscultation is the method to find the abnormal sound of speech, respiration and cough, etc., by means of auditognosis. Olfaction is the method to know the smell of the patient's body, the secretion and excreta by means of osphresis. Doctors use their auditory and olfactory organs to diagnose disease.

In ancient time, it followed mainly the laws of "five voices and five scales" to distinguish the five zang viscera disease. In Han Dynasty, Zhang Zhongjing regarded the speech, respiration, asthma, and cough, vomiting, hiccup and moan as the main content of the auscultation and olfaction. The later-generation doctor added the odor of mouth, nose, secretion and excreta to the contents.

6.2.1   Auscultation

The production of sound is related to the lung, throat epiglottis, tongue, teeth and nose. The lung plays an important role. The lung dominates the qi of whole body, and controls respiration. The movement of qi leads to sound production. The abnormal change of qi leads to abnormal sound. According to some theories from *Internal Classic*, the abnormal change of sound can reflect condition of five zang viscera.

6.2.1.1   Voices

The voice of normal people is produced naturally and fluently under normal physiologic condition. In condition of disease, if the voice is loud and successive, it belongs to heat or excess syndrome. If the voice is low, weak and non-successive, it belongs to deficiency or cold syndrome, or condition of pathogenic qi being eliminated and genuine qi being injured. The voice is often lower and vague in condition of wind, cold and dampness invasion.

(1) Deep turbid voice

It means the voice is dull and not clear, and also named heavy voice. It is usually due to invasion of wind-cold or turbid phlegm obstructs, and the lung qi failing in dispersion, nasal orifices inhibited.

(2) Hoarseness and Aphonia

Hoarseness, also called as "huskiness", means the voice of speech and cough loses the clear and smooth characters. Aphonia is in a condition of inability to make voice. Both of them have the similar disease mechanism, but the severity is different. The sudden disease often belongs to excess syndrome. It is usually due to invasion of wind-cold, wind-heat or phlegm-dampness accumulated in lung, which lead to lung qi falling in dispersion, purification and descent. It is "obstructed lung not functioning normally". The chronic disease often belongs to deficiency syndrome. It is usually due to loss of essential qi, lung-kidney yin deficiency, deficiency fire burning lung, which lead to fluid deficiency hurt the lung, and the voice was hardly made. It is "damaged lung not functioning normally". In addition, the shouting in fury can also lead to hoarseness. Besides, the aphonia in pregnancy is due to fetus which obstructs the kidney essence and qi to nourish the upper part of body.

6.2.1.2　Speech

Doctors can diagnose disease by listening to the speech. The cold leads to taciturn and the heat to chatter. The deficiency makes speech voice low and inconsistent, and the excess makes the voice loud.

(1) Delirium

The condition occurs in unconscious patients with incoherent, forceful and loud speech. It is excess syndrome and due to heat pathogen disturbing the vitality in heart.

(2) Repeated murmuring

It is the main condition of incoherent speech of deficiency. The speech is in broken sentences, repeated words, vague and feeble voice. It belongs to deficient syndrome of heart qi.

(3) Soliloquy

It is the speech to oneself in murmuring way. It stops when meeting people. The content is incoherent. It is due to insufficiency of heart qi which could not support the vitality, or transformation of qi depression into phlegm, blinded vitality. It is often seen in epilepsy.

(4) Wrong speaking

It is the speech that occurs in conscious patients. But the word or sentence which expresses the wrong meaning is notthe patients want to speak out. The patient can find the mistake by himself / herself at once. The deficiency syndrome is often due to insufficiency of heart qi which could not support the vitality. The excess syndrome is due to turbid phlegm, static of blood, qi depression, etc.

(5) Raving

It is the incoherent speech which is characterized by laughing, cursing, crying or shouting, and is accompanied by irregular running, singing in high place, exposing the naked body. It is seen in affect-vitality dissatisfaction, stagnated qi transforming into fire, phlegm-fire disturbing the heart. It is seen in mania or blood accumulation in cold-attack disease, and so on.

(6) Indistinct speech

It is difficult to make voice with an inflexible tongue, but the speaking can listen clearly. It is due to the wind-phlegm confusing orifice or obstructs meridians.

6.2.1.3　Respiration

Respiration refers to examine the patients' respiratory rate, the strength of breath, the turbid turbidity of breath sounds and examine whether the breath is smooth or not, and so on. Lung is the governor of qi and kidney is the root of qi. Pectoral qi accumulates inside the chest, controlling the breath and running the air. So respiration has close relationship with lung, kidney and pectoral qi.

The rough and fast breath is ascribed to heat and excess syndrome. The faint respiration in slow exhaling and inhaling indicates the deficiency. But in chronic disease of expiring lung and kidney, the breath can also be rough and intermittent, which belongs to false excess. In syndrome of heat in pericardium, the breath can be faint with stupor, which belongs to false deficiency. If the breath is faint, shallow and rapid with dyspnea, it belongs to extreme deficiency and the primordial qi damage.

（1）Dyspnea

The respiration is difficult, short and rapid. In a serious case, there are some symptoms, for example: the patient can express gasping mouth and raising shoulders, flaring nostrils and the patient could not lie flat. The dyspnea can be classified into deficiency syndrome and excess syndrome. The excess dyspnea is characterized by sudden onset, rough and loud voice of breath. The chest is distended. The patient feels a little better when exhaled out. There are strong body movement and forceful pulse. It is often due to exogenous pathogens invasion, excessive heat or phlegm-fluid retention in the lung. The deficiency asthma is characterized by gradual onset, low breathing sound, weak and dimming breath, and qi temerity. The patient feels hardly to inhale and exhale. And the patients feel better when take a deep breath. The body is weak and the pulse is feeble. The deficiency type is caused by kidney yang deficiency or lung qi deficiency, which leads to failure of kidney qi to receive the air.

（2）Wheezing

The breath is rapid like asthma with rough breathing and hasty panting as if phlegm in throat. Wheezing attacks repeatedly and may prolong for years. Due to internal deep-lying phlegm habitually, wheezing is reinduction induced by further contraction of external pathogen. It can also be caused by cold air, irritant gas or over intake of salty, sour, uncooked and cool food.

The differences between dyspnea and wheezing were pointed out clearly in *Orthodox Medical Record* that wheezing is named of sound, and dyspnea is named of breath. So dyspnea is characterized by the difficult, short and rapid respiration, while wheezing is characterized by the sound of phlegm in throat.

（3）Shortness of breath

The shortness of breath is a short, rapid and inconstant respiration. It is similar to asthma but no lifting shoulders, and has no sound in throat. Shortness of breath can be classified into deficiency syndrome and excess syndrome. The deficiency syndrome manifests as short respiration, low voice, and faint breath. The accompanied symptoms are general weakness and fatigued vitality, dizziness and lack of strength. It is due to deficiency of lung qi, or major vacuity of original qi. The excess syndrome manifests as short, rough breath. The accompanied symptoms are stuffiness in the chest, fullness in the chest and abdomen, and so on. It is usually resulted from phlegm-retained fluid, qi stagnation, gastrointestinal stagnant or internal static blood obstruction.

（4）Shortage of qi

It manifests as faint breath, low voice, gas insufficient, and the qi is too less to make speech. The breath and speech sound is low and short. It is not like shortness of breath. It is an emblem of all kind deficiency and declination.

6.2.1.4 Cough

Cough refers to a sound produced by the irritation of the airway due to the adverse rising of lung qi. It is often caused by excess pathogen attacking the lung or lung deficiency. Then the lung fails to diffuse and govern descent and lung qi adversely rise. The sound without phlegm is non-productive cough, and the phlegm without sound is productive cough, and the sound with phlegm is cough. The cough has close connection with the lung, but in *Internal Classic*, it is said, "The five zang viscera and six fu viscera can all make cough, not only the lung". From that we know not only lung disorder, but also other viscera disease can lead to cough.

In addition to listening to the sound of cough, you must also combine the changes of color, quantity and quality of phlegm, time of onset, history and syndrome, and so on. Then doctors can distinguish the cold-heat and deficiency-excess of disease.

The heavy and turbid sound of cough with white clear phlegm, stuffy nose, belongs to invasion exogenous wind-cold. It is due to wind-cold fettering the lung and the lung failing to diffuse and govern descent.

The unclear sound of cough with yellow sticky phlegm which is difficult to be expectorated, belongs to heat syndrome. It is due to heat pathogen invading lung, scorching the fluid of lung.

The muffled sound of cough with quantities of phlegm which is easy to be expectorated, belongs to excess-syndrome. It is due to retention of cold-phlegm and damp-phlegm in lung, leading to failure of lung qi to diffuse.

The low and feeble sound of cough, with panting, often belongs to deficiency syndrome. It is due to the deficiency of lung qi, and the lung failing to diffuse and govern descent. Dry cough with no phlegm or little sticky phlegm that is difficult to be expectorated out, often belongs to dryness pathogen invading the lung or lung yin deficiency.

The paroxysmal cough characterized by uninterrupted cough, and making sound like the crow's echo when ending, and reoccurring after moment, is called "whooping cough". Because the attacks repeatedly and may prolong for a long time, it is also called "hundred-day cough". It is often seen in children. The cause is the wind pathogen in combination with the hiding phlegm obstructing the air tract.

The cough sounds like bark of dog, with hoarse voice, inspiratory dyspnea. It is seen in diphtheria. It is due to yin deficiency of both the lung and kidney and epidemic toxin attacking throat.

6.2.1.5 Vomiting

Vomit indicates ascending counter flow of gastric contents, ejecting stomach contents from mouth. The vomiting is due to impaired harmonious of the stomach, and ascending counter flow of stomach qi. There are many factors leading to the vomit, and doctors can discriminate the cold-heat and deficiency-excess of the disease.

If the sound of vomit is low, the action of vomiting is slow, and the vomitus is clear mucus without acidic odor, it belongs to deficiency cold syndrome. It is often caused by spleen-stomach yang deficiency, breakdown of transportation and transformation, impaired harmonious of the stomach, and ascending counter flow of stomach qi.

While the vomit is yellow sticky phlegm-like with sour or bitter taste, the sound is loud, the action is violent, and it belongs to excessive heat syndrome. It is due to the damage to stomach by the heat pathogen, impaired harmonious of the stomach, and ascending counter flow of stomach qi.

When the vomiting is sprayed, it is a serious condition. It is due to heat disturbs the vitality, or head trauma, craniocerebral hemorrhage.

Evening vomiting of undigested morning meal, or morning vomiting of undigested evening meal is due to stomach yang deficiency or deficiency of both spleen and kidney. It is called "regurgitation". If the patient is thirsty and wants to drink, and when drinking, there is vomiting, it is called "water counter flow", and it is caused by fluid retention.

6.2.1.6   Hiccup

It is the rebellious stomach qi which rushes out through throat involuntarily and the voice is short sound frequently and uncontrolled. It is due to ascending counter flow of stomach. According to the character of the sound, doctors can know the nature of disease when combine the other syndrome.

If the sound is loud and resounding in a new disease, it is due to cold or heal pathogen attacking stomach. The hiccup occurring in prolong disease, with a low voice, weak interrupted hiccup, it means critical condition.

6.2.1.7   Belching

Belching is the stomach qi adversely rises and makes sound when flowing through throat. It is also called "eructation". It is due to the adverse rising of stomach qi. Doctors can discriminate cold-heat and deficiency-excess by the strength and smell of the belching.

Fetid odor of the eructed air, acid regurgitation, accompanied by stomach duct and abdominal fullness and distention, belongs to food stagnating in the stomach dust, ascending counterflow of stomach qi.

If the belching is frequent with loud and clear sound, and stomach duct and abdominal distention are relieved by belching, it belongs to liver qi invading the stomach.

If the belching sound is low without special odor of the air, as well as the appetite is poor, it is due to spleen-stomach weakness, impaired harmonious of the stomach. It is seen in chronic disease or aged patients.

The belching is frequent, accompanied by cold pain in the stomach duct and abdomen, and it will be better when the surroundings are warm. It is due to cold pathogen settling in the stomach, or stomach yang deficiency.

6.2.1.8   Sigh

The sigh is the involuntary sound of melancholic with chest and hypochondrium fullness. It will be better after the sigh. It is due to affect-vitality dissatisfaction, binding constraint of liver qi.

6.2.1.9   Sneeze

The sneeze refers to a sudden burst sound of air from lung to the throat and nose. If it occurs frequently in a new disease accompanied by aversion to cold with fever, running nose with clear snivel, it is caused by exogenous wind-cold, inhibited nose orifices. If it occurs in a prolonged disease, when sneeze suddenly, it is an omen of recovery of yang qi.

6.2.1.10   Snoring

Snoring is a sound that can be emitted by nose and throat when the patient is asleep and coma, indicating an obstruction of airway. If the snoring is loud when asleep, it is due to chronic rhinopathia, or improper sleeping position. If the patient is coma, with snoring continuously, it is seen in heat entering the pericardium, wind stroke in zang-fu viscera. Snoring without other syndrome when the normal person is asleep not belongs to disease.

6.2.1.11   Rumbling intestines

The rumbling intestines, also called "borborygmus", refers to the sound of gastrointestinal motility in the abdomen. In normal condition, it is hardly to hear the sound of rumbling intestines, because the sound is low and weak. When qi movement delayed in abdomen, or qi and water surging in the stomach and intestine, the rumbling intestines can be heard. Doctors can discriminate the location, frequency, tone and accompanied syndrome of disease in clinical practice.

If the voice comes from stomach duct, touching like water in bladder, and the rumbling moves down when patients stand up and walk around or stroke the stomach duct, it is due to collection of phlegm-fluid retention, obstructing the movement of middle energizer of the qi.

If the voice comes from stomach duct and abdomen, rumbling likes hungry intestines, and will be relieved by warming or food, aggravated by cooling and hungry, it is due to insufficiency of middle qi, and deficiency cold of the stomach and intestines.

If the rumbling intestines is loud and sonorous, with stomach duct and abdomen glomus and fullness, sloppy diarrhea, it is due to wind, clod and dampness attacking the stomach and intestines, and disorder of the qi.

If the rumbling intestine is rare, it is due to intestines conduction dysfunction. If the rumbling intestines are disappeared, and the abdomen is too distensible and pain to press, it belongs to severe intestinal gas stagnation.

6.2.1.12　Listening to the child

Hearing is especially useful when dealing with children. Zhou Xuehai said, "When inspecting child, the listening is the first and the observation of color is the second". If the sound is clear, it means survival while the voice is vague and faint, it means dying. Crying with bending body is due to abdominal pain. Crying aggravated by pressing is due to pain in the pressed part. If the child cries but keeps in low voice, it is due to sore throat. If the cry occurred suddenly after awakened from sleep, it is due to abdominal pain or general pain. Crying followed by diarrhea is seen in abdominal pain due to stagnation. If the voice of crying is constant thready, at the same time, the browns are knitted and head is bowed, it is due to headache. In condition of sudden crying in loud sound without other disorders, the child's clothes and whole body should be examined, because it may be caused by foreign body or sores in skin.

6.2.2　Olfaction

Olfaction is to smell the odors to diagnose disease by distinguishing the smell of patient and ward. There is a lot of content in olfaction, such as odors from excreta and secretion including phlegm, sweat, nasal discharge, stool, urine, menstrual blood and vaginal discharge, etc. In healthy body, the qi and blood circulate smoothly, the zang-fu viscera and meridians function well, the body is nourished by pure nutritive essence, and qi movement is normal, so there is no abnormal odor. When disease occurs, due to the pathogens attack the body, the qi and blood movement is abnormal, and the foul and turbid waste could not be cleared away, resulting in the abnormal odors. If the odor is serious, it can spread around the ward.

The foul odor is usually due to excessive heat. If the odor is not heavy, or is only slight stench, it is due to deficiency cold. So doctors can discriminate the cold-heat and deficiency-excess of the disease by olfaction.

6.2.2.1　Odor of mouth

The foul odor of mouth is related to mouth and stomach disorders, and is often due to indigestion. In dental caries, the odor is sour and fetid, because there is cavity in tooth and the food remains in the cavity which rots and produces the fetid odor. The odor will disappear when keeping the mouth clean. In pyogenic gingivitis, the fetid odor is stinking and foul which comes from the rotten gum. In stomach heat syndrome, the heat makes stool dry and filthy qi steaming up, so the odor of mouth is foul. In condition of food retention in stomach, the movement of qi is abnormal in descending and ascending. The food qi flows up. So there is an odor like that of rotten egg. The putrid odor in mouth usually indicates the inner abscess or ulcer.

6.2.2.2 Sweat

The smell of sweat in patients of cold-attack or warm diseases indicates the perspiration. If the sweat is sticky with fishy odor, or in yellow color, it is due to the wind and dampness which accumulate in skin and pollute the body fluids. The foul odor of sweat is smelled in patient of pestilence. In terminal stage of edema, there is an odor of urine in sweat.

6.2.2.3 Phlegm and nasal discharge

The foul odor of turbid pus and bloody phlegm is due to exorbitant heat-toxin. It belongs to lung abscess. The thin phlegm with salt but not fishy odor belongs to cold phlegm. The turbid nasal discharge with foul odor belongs to rhinorrhea due to heat in brain. That without odor is due to wind-cold attack.

6.2.2.4 Vomit

The odorless vomit, with preference to hot drinking, belongs to stomach cold. The sour and foul vomit, with thirst liking cold drinking, is due to stomach heat. If the vomit is undigested food with putrid odor, it is due to food retention. The pus and bloody vomit with fishy and foul odor is caused by internal abscess.

6.2.2.5 Excreta

Odor of excreta includes stool and urine, menstrual blood and vaginal discharge. Doctors should combine the inspection and inquiring to discriminate the disease.

The fetid stool is resulted from heat and the fishy stench of stool is due to cold. Sloppy diarrhea and fishy smell indicates the deficiency cold of spleen and stomach. Diarrhea smelling like rotten eggs, or food retention in the stool, with soar-smelling malodorous flatus, belongs to food damage.

The turbid yellow urine with heavy animal urine odor is due to exorbitant heat in heart and urinary bladder. The incontinent urine without odor means the fire is defeated. The sweet urine, smelling like rotten apples is due to wasting-thirst.

The foul odor of menstrual blood is due to heat while the fishy odor to cold.

When vaginal discharge is foul-smelling, thick and yellow, it is due to dampness-heat, while the odor is fishy and thin, it is due to dampness and cold. When vaginal discharge is cacosmia and mixed colors, it is due to cancer.

6.2.2.6 Odor of ward

The odor of ward means odor forms the body, excreta endocrine of patients. The ward filled with odor that sent forth from patient's body, indicates the disease is serious.

If the odor is offensive in ward, it is usually due to pestilence. In mild case, the smell is just surrounding the bed. While in sever case, the fetid odor fills up the ward. Corpse smell full of the ward indicates decayed zang-fu viscera. The condition is serious.

If putrid smelling surrounds the ward, it is due to sores and ulcers disease. In the ward of patients suffering from massive bleeding, there is blood odor. The urea odor is smelled in the ward of late edema patients. The smell of rotten apple is usually seen in severe case of consumptive wasting-thirst complicated by diabetic ketoacidosis. The garlicky odor smelled in the ward is usually seen in organophosphate poisoning.

6.2.2.7 Odor of body

If there is ulcer or broken sore on patient's body, the odor of the body will be abnormal. For example, odor of the body of the gangrene is described as the odor of rotten field snail in *Golden Mirror of Medicine*.

6.3 Inquiring

Diagnosis by inquiring is a very important part of TCM. And it is the most essential method to collect the clinic data. Inquiring is the interrogation between doctor and patient to find out how the problem arose, the living conditions of the patient, the environment, and so on. The aim of this investigation is to acquire the clinic data and provide evidence of analyzing the disease condition, determining the disease location and character, and the treatment based on syndrome differentiation.

6.3.1 The method of inquiring

The method of inquiring is significant for doctor to get the true message.

6.3.1.1 Selecting a suitable environment

When questioning, the environment should be quiet, so as to avoid the disturbance and make the doctor and patient in a calm mood. The doctor can focus on questioning and the patient can describe the disease in detail.

6.3.1.2 Asking the patient directly

In order to collect the accurate and reliable data, doctor should question the patients oneself. If the patient is in severe case or unconscious, or is a baby, he could not describe the disease in detail, doctor can question the accompanying people.

6.3.1.3 The questioning method

At the beginning, the doctor should listen to patient's complaints, and grasp the main character of the disease from the complaints. Then the doctor should question the main complaint and all aspects should be asked.

6.3.1.4 The attitude to the patient

The doctor should be serious and patient, and be good at thinking and arousing patients.

6.3.2 The content of inquiring

6.3.2.1 General data

The first part in inquiring is the name, age, sex, occupation, birth place, nationality, address and marital status of the patient, and the 24 solar-term of the disease onset, etc. And the visit data and admission data should also be recorded in the medical history.

The age and sex are related to the syndrome of disease. The nationality, occupation and marriage state are closely related to some special disease. For example, hepatic echinococcosis is seen in pastoral area. The birthplace and address could also affect the health. The natural environment and climate are different in difference areas. *Internal Classic* clearly mentioned that in different areas, the disease is not the same.

The data of disease onset is related to syndrome differentiation. And the movement of five elements also affects diseases.

6.3.2.2 Chief complaint

The chief complaints refer to the symptoms the patient feels the most obviously and painfully and the main cause for visiting a doctor.

Though the symptoms of disease are complicate and various, they can be classified into main and secondary symptoms. It is the key point for making correct diagnosis to question the disease condition intensively and purposely according to the main complaints. The onset time should be recorded when recording chief complaints. If the main complaints include several symptoms in different times, the symptoms should be recorded in the order of their occurring time. The record should be done in clear and concise way. Sometimes the main complaint given by patient is not clear, so the doctor should listen to patiently and then ask intensively until getting a clear idea.

6.3.2.3　History of present disease

The history of present disease is the main content of interrogation. It refers to the whole developing course from the onset up to now. It includes three parts: the process of disease, the process of diagnoses and treatment, and present symptoms.

(1) The course of disease

When patient visits doctor, the doctor should ask about the circumstance, time, and symptoms, sudden or not, cause and predisposing cause of the disease, and the development, etc.

(2) The process of diagnoses and treatment

The process of diagnoses and treatment includes time, site that patients went to see a doctor before, which is helpful to diagnose of the disease.

(3) Present symptoms

Present symptoms, as the fundamental basis of syndrome differentiation and disease identification, means the main symptoms and signs of the present diseases. It is main content of inquiring.

6.3.2.4　Family history and anamnesis

The statement about communicable disease has existed since ancient time. The ancients found that some disease could spread among people for a long time. Besides, some diseases are related to hereditary factors. So inquiring family history is significant to diagnose of infectious disease and hereditary disease.

The anamnesis has closely connection with the onset and development of present disease. For example, palpitation usually belongs to the prodromal symptom of heart disease. So it is important to get the past disease history clearly by questioning.

6.3.2.5　Inquiring about personal life style

Internal Classic pointed out that when making a diagnosis, the life history and life style should be asked. The life style, including diet, emotions, lifestyle, working environment, marital history and childbearing history, has connection with disease. What's more, the marital history and childbearing history should also be questioned because they have a close relation with disease.

6.3.3　Present symptoms

The inquiring about present symptoms is the central point of inquiring. It provides the basis for diagnosis. The content of present symptoms inquiring could be summed into the ten-questioning.

The first is to ask the cold and fever, the second the sweat, the third the head and limbs, the fourth the urination and defecation, the fifth the diet, the sixth the chest, the seventh the deafness, the eighth the thirst, the ninth the old disease, the tenth the cause and in women the mense and child bearing. And in children the pox and measles should also be inquired.

6.3.3.1　Inquiring about cold and heat

They are the common symptoms in disease course. Cold means the chilly sensation of patient, the chill which could not be relieved by warming. The heater or putting on more clothes is called as "aversion to cold". The cold sensation which can be relieved by warming or putting more clothes is called as "fear of cold". The fever refers to the higher body temperature than normal body temperature, or the patients feel feverish themselves totally or locally in the body while the body temperature maybe is not higher than normal.

The production of cold and fever is mainly up to the nature of pathogen and the exuberance and debilitation of yin and yang of the body. When questioning cold and fever, one should first answer if there are cold and fever. Secondly, one should ask whether the cold and fever are appeared in the same time or not, then ask the characters of them, such as the seriousness and concomitant symptoms, the occurring time and lasting time, so as to distinguish the nature of disease. For example, the aversion to cold with fever in same time belongs to exterior syndrome while the cold or fever belongs to interior syndrome, and the alternate chill and fever to half-exterior and half-interior syndrome.

(1) Chill and fever

It suggests the condition that patient has a feeling of chill and a high body temperature by measurement in the same time. It belongs to the initial stage of exterior syndrome due to exogenous pathogen. The chill and fever mirrors the struggle between defensive qi and pathogens when pathogens attack the body and stay in skin and muscle. The condition can be divided into three kinds:

1) More chill than fever

It refers to that patient feels obvious aversion to cold with a slight rising of body temperature. It is caused by exogenous cold pathogen invading. The cold pathogen is a yin pathogen and it can wrap the body surface, impair the yang qi, and seal the pore of skin. Then the defensive yang is obstructed and could not disperse.

2) More fever than chill

It is a condition that patient has a feverish sensation and high temperature will mild aversion to cold. It is caused by exogenous heat pathogen. The heat is a yang pathogen and it can make the yang predominant, then the fever is severe. When wind-heat invades the exterior, the radiating nature of heat pathogen makes the pore open.

3) Fever with aversion to wind

The patient has fever and is aversed to wind. It is caused by exogenous wind invading. The wind is a yang pathogen, attributing to opening and releasing. When wind attacks the exterior, it makes the striae and interstitial space open and makes the defensive qi fail to consolidate the body, and then there are sweating and cold sensations when meeting the wind.

The severity of the chill and fever is helpful to discriminate the condition of the genuine qi and the pathogen. In common condition, if the pathogen and the genuine qi is slight, the fever and chill are both slight. When there are strong pathogen and weak genuine qi, the aversion to cold is severe and the fever is mild. If the pathogen and genuine qi are both strong, the chill and fever are both severe.

(2) Fever without chill

There is fever but no sensation of chill. It belongs to interior heat syndrome. It can be divided into the following types according to the nature, time, and concomitant symptoms.

1) Excess heat

The high fever without sensation of cold is called as "excess heat". It is seen in interior heat syndrome which is due to the wind-cold which enters interior and transforms into heat.

2) Tidal fever

The fever waxing and waning in a fixed time like the tide is called as "tidal fever". It can be classified into the following types. The first one is the tidal fever due to yin deficiency. The fever appears in afternoon or at night, without high temperature. It usually caused by yin deficiency which leads to yang prevalent relatively and produces endogenous heat. The second one is the tidal fever of yangming. The fever is high and reaches the highest point at 3 to 5 o'clock in afternoon, which is due to the yangming qi on its duty in afternoon. The third one is the tidal fever due to dampness-warmth. It is frequently seen in dampness-warmth disease caused by the dampness-heat at noon. The dampness obstructs the heat to radiate out, so the fever is hidden. Because the dampness is sticky and hardly cleaned away, it is prolonged and refractory.

3) Low grade fever

It refers to just a feverish sensation with normal temperature, or mild higher temperature in chronic disease. It usually belongs to infant heat stroke syndrome, or yin deficiency, qi deficiency in chronic disease. The fever resulting from qi deficiency has a manifestation of low fever for long time. And it is aggravated in tiredness and relieved by rest. Its accompanied symptoms are shortness of breath, spontaneous sweating, lack of strength, etc. The low fever caused by yin deficiency has similar symptoms as the tidal fever due to yin deficiency.

(3) Intolerance of cold without fever

The patient feels cold without fever or feverish sensation. It is due to interior cold. There are division of deficiency and excess of cold according to the severity, character and concomitant symptoms.

1) The deficiency cold

Because the zang-fu viscera yang and qi are weak and cannot reach the muscle and sink, the limbs are not warmed, and then the patient feels cold. There are concomitant symptoms like pale complexion, lying in curving position, slow and weak pulse, and pale tongue. These symptoms can be relieved by putting on more clothes or warming.

2) The excess cold

Because cold pathogen invades zang-fu viscera directly, the yang and qi are impaired. There is severe pain in the local part where the cold pathogen attacks. The pain is aggravated by pressing and relieved by warming. There may be contraction of limbs, vomiting and diarrhea, taut or tense pulse.

(4) Alternate chill and fever

The aversion to cold and fever occur in turn. It usually belongs to half-exterior and half-interior syndrome. It is classified into two types.

1) Shaoyang syndrome

The alternate chill and fever are irregular of time. It is usually accompanied by bitter taste in mouth, dry throat, distress in chest and hypochondrium and wiry pulse. Its pathomechanism is that the pathogen could not enter the interior completely and the health qi could not drive the pathogen out. The vital qi and pathogen are locked. When the pathogen gets stronger or vital qi is weaker, there is chill, while the predominance of vital qi or declining of pathogen leads to fever. The vital qi and pathogen predominance in turn makes the alternate chill and fever.

2) Malaria

This is a condition of alternate high fever and chill occurring on a fixed time. The accompanied symptoms are severe headache, pain in the whole body, profuse sweating and thirst. The pathomechanism is that after entering the body, the malaria pathogen hides in the mo yuan, the part between the interior and exterior of the body. When entering, the malaria pathogen fights against the yin and makes chill and shiver. When exiting, it struggles against the yang and makes high fever and sweating. So severe chill and high fever always occur alternately.

Doctors should focus on distinguishing the exogenous from endogenous diseases. It is a key point of syndrome differentiation.

6.3.3.2 Inquiring about sweating

As the body fluid, the sweat is evaporate and sent to the skin through the pores of body by yang. *Plain Questions* pointed out, "When the yang puts on yin, it makes the sweating". That explains the mechanism of perspiration.

When people do physical work, take hot or pungent food, or put on too much clothes, or undergo sudden emotional change, there will be sweating and it is a physiological phenomenon. The normal sweat can harmonize the nutrient-defense, enrich and moisten the skin. No sweating when it should sweat, over sweating, and sweating in an improper time are all pathological reactions. No sweating when it should sweat is caused by the following reasons: firstly, the shortage of body fluid which could not produce perspiration; secondly, the yang declination which can not to distill the fluid; thirdly, pathogen in the exterior obstructs the interstitial space between muscle and skin. The improper sweating and over sweating is due to syndrome of excessive pathogen or defensive yang deficiency. When inquiring about sweating, whether there is sweating or not should be asked first, then the time, area of body, quantity, character of sweating should be asked, so as to discriminate the disease location and nature.

(1) No sweating and sweating

In the disease process, especially the externally contracted disease, whether there is sweating or not is the gist to judge the nature of the disease and exuberance and debilitation of defensive yang.

1) No sweating

The condition that in the time that it should sweat, but there is no sweat is named as "no sweating". The condition in exterior syndrome refers to wind-cold in the exterior. Besides, no sweating can be seen in condition of body fluid shortage in endogenous diseases.

2) Sweating

The sweating means abnormal condition of sweat, including sweating in improper time, profuse sweating, or sweating with other pathological reaction.

Many factors are involved in sweating. For example, the visceral yang deficiency, or defensive yang inactivity which results in the interstitial space open and fluid out, makes sweating. Also, the exorbitant interior heat can make profuse sweating.

(2) Special sweating

It refers to many kinds of pathological sweat with character, and it is usually seen in interior syndrome.

1) Spontaneous sweating

The patients sweat in day time and the sweating is aggravated when doing physical work. Because the qi is defensive and yang fails to consolidate the body, the interstice iopen, so the fluid goes out and makes sweating. Physical work consumes qi, and the body fluid flows away, so the sweating is profuse. If it is due to yang deficiency, there is intolerance to cold and cold limbs.

2) Night sweating

The condition that sweating occurs in sleep and stops when awake, it is called as "night sweating". It is mainly caused by yin deficiency. In physiological condition, the defensive qi enters the interior and moves in yin phase with the nutrient yin when sleeping. When the yin is deficient, the defensive qi could not enter the interior and wanders, so construction-yin goes out of the skin following defensive qi. When awaken, the defensive qi goes out of the body and returns to the surface, hence the interstices is tight. Though yin deficiency with internal heat, it could not evaporate the fluid out of the body, hence the sweat stops when awakened. The concomitant symptoms are tidal fever, hectic cheek, dry mouth and throat, red tongue, fine rapid pulse, etc.

The theory that spontaneous sweating is due to yang deficiency while night sweating to yin deficiency should not be followed rigidly.

3) Profuse sweating

It means too much perspiration on skin, and it is a phenomenon of over evaporation of body fluid. The sweating can be divided into two types, the deficiency and the excess.

If there are excess heat and profuse sweating, it is an excess heat syndrome. The exogenous pathogens enter the interior and transform into heat. The exorbitant interior heat distills the body fluid and leads to profuse sweating.

If there is profuse cool sweating, it is yang deficiency syndrome, due to the sudden loss of yang and failing to consolidate the body fluid, leading to the body fluid going out of the body. It is an extreme deficiency condition which indicates a critical situation.

4) Yellow sweating

The perspiration is yellow, which is due to the dampness-heat steaming in the internal. It is often accompanied by edema in head, face and limbs, heavy pain in all body.

5) Fighting sweating

The condition of patient shivers suddenly and then sweats all over the body, which occurs mainly in cold-attack diseases. It is the turning point of disease as the vital qi fights against the pathogens.

6) Dying sweating

The sweating is constant and profuse, because the original qi is escaping and the body fluid follows the original qi. It is a fatal condition of separating yin and yang and the yang escaped. It is also called as "depletion sweating". The dying sweating is usually seen in prolonged and severe disease.

(3) Local Sweating

1) Head sweating

The perspiration emerges only on the head or head and neck, due to the stagnated heat in upper energizer, the dampness-heat in middle energizer, the heat in blood chamber and the upwards floating of yang deficiency.

2) Hemihidrosis

The condition is sweating in half of the body, which is because the wind-phlegm or wind-dampness obstructs the whole or partial meridians of half body and the qi, blood and body fluid could not distribute in the half body. It is usually emerged in apoplexy, atrophy syndrome and paraplegia.

3) Sweating in the palm and sole

The little sweat in palm and sole is normal. If the sweat is profuse, it is due to the yin deficiency with yang hyperactivity, vacuity heat arising internally, or stagnated heat in spleen and stomach, which evaporates body fluid and sends it to four extremities.

4) Chest sweating

The sweating is seen only on the chest, which is due to over strain of heart, or worry impairing the heart and spleen. It leads to deficiency of both the heart and spleen.

5) Genital sweating

The condition of profuse sweating in genital region is due to dampness-heat in lower energizer or kidney yang deficiency.

6.3.3.3 Inquiring about pain

The pain can be divided into deficiency and excess. The excess pain is sudden onset, severe and incessant pain, aggravated by pressing. It is caused by the attacking of exogenous pathogens, qi stasis, blood stasis, phlegm retention, parasitosis or food retention which obstructs the meridians and hinders the qi and blood movement. The deficiency pain occurs gradually and is dull and paroxysmal, and relieved by pressing.

Besides the distinction of deficiency and excess, the pain character is different in accordance with the different cause and mechanism of disease.

(1) Nature of the pain

1) Distending pain

The paroxysmal pain accompanied by distention in the same location is distending pain. It is caused by qi stagnation. The distending pain in epigastrium is due to the qi stagnation resulting from cold attack.

2) Stabbing pain

The pain like being needled or prickled is named as twinge or stabbing pain. It is due to the blood stasis. In the condition, the meridians are obstructed.

3) Colic pain

The severe pain as if the body being strangulated cut is called as "colic pain". It is due to the solid pathogens obstruct vessels suddenly, and qi and blood could not flow in vessel.

4) Retraction pain

The pain as if being pulled is called retraction pain. The pain is caused by the malnutrition of tendons. Because the liver dominants tendons, the retraction pain relates mainly to liver diseases.

5) Scorching pain

The pain just like being burned is called scorching pain or burning pain. The pain is usually resulted from the fire pathogen running in collateral. It can be relieved by cooling.

6) Cold pain

The pain as if being frozen is cold pain or frozen pain. The cold pathogen in meridians or yang deficiency makes the zang-fu viscera and meridians lack of warming and give rise to the pain. It can be aggravated by cold, and be relieved by warming.

7) Hollow pain

The pain with feeling of vacancy is the hollow pain. It is due to the deficiency of essence and blood which could not fill up the meridians.

8) Dull pain

The pain is lingering and mild. It is mainly due to deficiency of both qi and blood.

(2) Location of Pain

1) Headache

This can be distinguished according to onset, time, location, character of pain, condition.

● Onset: The onset of headache can be classified into two types. Recent onset usually refers to exterior attack of wind cold. Gradual onset always means interior syndrome, such as internal damage and vacuity detriment, deficiency of both qi and blood, etc.

● Course: The course of headache can be classified into two types. If the course is short and the pain is serious and incessant, it belongs to excess syndrome. The paroxysmal headache with chronic course belongs to deficiency syndrome.

● Time of day: The time of headache can also be classified into two types: day-time and evening. Day-time headache can be caused by qi or yang deficiency, while evening headache is due to blood or yin deficiency.

● Location: The different location of headache can suggest the meridians of disease.

Nape of neck:The headache can be resulted from exterior invasion of wind-cold, or from interior kidney deficiency. It belongs to taiyang meridian, because the bladder meridian of foot taiyang goes from vertex into brain, then to nape, and goes down along the posterior head and nape to bank.

Forehead:The headache can be resulted from stomach-heat or blood deficiency. It belongs to yangming meridian, because the stomach meridian of foot yangming goes through anterior margin of hair to forehead.

Temples and sides of head:The headache is due to exterior wind-cold or wind-heat in the shaoyang, or from interior liver and gall bladder fire rising. It belongs to shaoyang meridian, because the gallbladder meridian of foot shaoyang stars from lateral canthus and then goes along the bilateral side of head.

Vertex:The headache is usually resulting from deficiency of liver blood. It belongs to liver meridian of foot jueyin.

Whole head:The headache is due to exterior invasion of wind-cold.

2) Dizziness

Dizziness can be caused by four factors which can be summarized as wind, fire, phlegm, and deficiency. The main way to discriminate the various types of dizziness is by integration with the concomitant symptoms and signs.

Severe dizziness is usually caused by internal wind, manifesting when everything seems to sway and the person loses the balance.

Slight dizziness accompanied by a feeling of heaviness and muzziness of the head indicates phlegm obstructing the head and preventing the clear yang from ascending to the head. If the dizziness aggravates when tired, it indicates qi deficiency. A sudden onset of dizziness points to an excess syndrome while a gradual onset points to an deficiency syndrome.

3) Body

● Pain in the whole body:Sudden onset with chills and fever is due to exterior wind-cold. Pain all over the body with feeling of tiredness is usually caused by deficiency of both qi and blood.

For women after childbirth, if the pain is dull, it is due to blood deficiency;if the pain is severing, it is due to blood stasis. It can also be caused by liver qi stagnation.

If pain in all muscles with hot sensation, it is due to stomach heat. If the pain with feeling of heaviness, it is caused by dampness obstructing muscles.

● Pain in joints:The pain wandering from joint to joint is resulted from wind. When the situation is fixed and very painful, it is due to cold. If the situation is fixed with swelling and numbness, the pain is caused by dampness.

● Backache:If the backache is continuous and dull, it is always due to kidney deficiency. The condition of recent onset, severe, with stiffness sprain of back is due to stasis of blood. If the severe pain could be aggravated during cold and damp weather, and alleviated by application of heat, it suggests the invasion of exterior cold and damp to the back meridians. The condition of boring pain with inability to turn the waist, it is due to stasis of blood. If the pain in the back extends up to the shoulders, it is results from exterior pathogen attacking.

● Numbness:The numbness of arms and legs or only hands and feet on both sides is caused by blood deficiency. Numbness of fingers, elbow and arm on one side only, especially of the first three lingers, is caused by internal wind and phlegm. And this may indicate the possibility of impending wind-stroke.

4) Chest

Pain in the chest is often due to stasis of blood in the heart, which, in turn is usually due to deficiency of yang. Chest pain accompanied by cough with profuse yellow phlegm is due to lung heat. Chest pain also can be caused by the phlegm-dampness attacking the lung.

Chest oppression means the patients feel oppressive. Accompanied with palpitation, shortness of breath, the chest oppression is due to insufficiency of heart qi, devitalized heart yang. Accompanied with stabbing pain in heart, green-blue or purple lips and face, it is caused by heart blood stasis. Accompanied with cough and panting, profuse phlegm, it is due to phlegm-dampness obstructing the lung. Accompanied with rib-side distention, frequent sighing, despondency, it is usually due to stagnation of liver qi.

5) Hypochondriac

It is refers to a feeling of distension and stuffiness of the hypochondrium. The distending pain in hypochondrium with frequent sighing, despondency, is usually due to stagnation of liver qi. Scorching pain in hypochondrium with bitter taste in the mouth, dry mouth, nausea, vomiting is due to dampness-heat accumulation in liver and gallbladder. Scorching pain in hypochondrium with vexation, irritability, flushed face and congestive eyes is due to liver fire flaring up. Stabbing pain in a fixed location in hypochondrium, which aggravated in evening, it is due to blood stasis. If hypochondrium pain is in one side with painful distention, aggravated by cough, is due to suspended rheum that is due to fluid retained in chest and hypochondrium.

Stomach: Epigastric pain can be resulted from retention of food in the stomach or stomach heat. If the pain is very dull and not very severe, it is caused by deficient-cold in the stomach. If the pain is relieved by eating, it is the deficiency syndrome. If it is aggravated by eating, it is the excess syndrome.

A feeling of fullness in the epigastrium is due to spleen deficiency or dampness.

Abdominal pain: Lower abdominal pain can be resulted from many different factors, and the most common factors are internal cold, stagnation of liver qi or liver blood, dampness-heat, stasis of blood in the intestines or uterus. These various conditions can only be differentiated on the basis of the accompanying symptoms and signs.

6.3.3.4　Inquiring about stool and urine

It means inquiring about the changes the of stool and urine. The stool is dominated directly by the large intestine, however it is also closely related to transporting and transforming functions of spleen, the conducting function of liver, dispersing and descending function of lung and the warming function of kidney fire. The urine is controlled by urinary bladder, and has connection with the descending of lung, transforming of kidney and the regulating of triple energizer. So the stool and urine are the important aspects for diagnosis.

(1) Stool

The normal people defecate every day or every other day. The defecation is smooth. The stool is moist and in certain form. There is no pus or blood, mucus, undigested food in it. The contents of inquiring about stool are the form and color of stool, the feeling and frequency of defecation.

1) Frequency of defecation

● Constipation: The condition of less frequency of defecation, even several days, accompanied by dry and difficulty to discharge, is called constipation. It is usually due to heat accumulating in intestines or the slowed transportation in intestines resulting from insufficiency of body fluid.

● Diarrhea: It is a condition that the stool is watery and shapeless with frequent defecation. Diarrhea is mainly caused by the attack of exogenous evils, injury due to improper diet, yang deficiency of both spleen and kidney. The fulminant case of diarrhea usually belongs to excess or heat syndrome, and the chronic case to deficiency or cold.

Pain accompanying diarrhea always suggests involvement of the liver or the presence of heat. The presence of a foul smell suggests heat, while the absence of smell suggests cold. The most common cause of chronic diarrhea is either spleen yang, or kidney-yang deficiency or both. Chronic diarrhea occurring every day in the very early morning indicates kidney yang deficiency and is called "cock-crow diarrhea" or also "daybreak diarrhea". Diarrhea with mucus in the stools indicates dampness in the intestines. Loose stools with undigested food indicate spleen qi deficiency. A burning sensation in the anus while passing stools indicates heat.

2) Feeling of defecation

The hot and burning feeling of anus in defecation is due to damp-heat in large intestine.

The stool is loose and sticky, but difficult to be discharged completely, which is due to damp-heat in large intestine. Tenesmus patient feels paroxysmal abdominal pain and heavy sensation in anus, and is always urgent to defecate. It belongs to dysentery, and damp-heat obstructs the qi flow of intestines and leads to tenesmus.

The patient could not control the defecation and the stool is discharged out spontaneously. It is caused by qi deficiency of spleen or yang deficiency.

The patient feels something sagging from the inner body to anus. It belongs to sinking of middle qi.

3) Color of stool

The dark yellow stool is usually due to stagnated heat in intestines.

Black stool like tar is due to blood stasis, and the red(blood) and white(pus) stool pertains to dysentery resulting from damp-heat in large intestine.

The grayish white stool is seen in jaundice of damp-heat.

The color of stool is often affected by the food and drugs, which should be asked carefully.

(2) Urine

A normal people passes urine 4 to 6 times in day time and 0 to 1 time at night. The amount of urine in a day is about 1500 to 2000 mL. The frequency and amount of urination are influenced by the drinking, air temperature, sweating and age. The morbid changes of urine include amount, frequency, color and feeling in urination.

1) Amount of Urine

• Excessive urine: Excessive urine is usually attributed to kidney yang deficiency, which fails to transform body fluid and body fluid flows down. If it is accompanied by thirst, drinking a lot of water, it belongs to consumptive thirst.

• Scanty urination: It is usually due to kidney yin deficiency. It can be caused by exorbitant heat, or over sweating, vomiting and diarrhea. It is also seen in yang deficiency of spleen, lung and kidney.

2) Frequency of Urine

• Frequent urination: The frequent urination with urgency and dark yellow urine in small amount belongs to stranguria, which is caused by the damp-heat in lower energizer.

The frequent urination with clear urine pertains to failure of kidney qi in consolidation.

The increased nocturnal urination with clear urine is seen in late stage of kidney disease or aged people. It is due to kidney yang deficiency.

• Dysuria: The dysuria is a condition of urination in a way of dripping due to difficulty in passing water. The anuria refers to absence of urine discharged even though there is an urge of urination. Those of excess are due to the obstruction of urinary bladder which is caused by damp-heat pouring down to urinary bladder, or by stone and blood stasis. Those of deficiency are due to kidney yang deficiency that leads to dysfunction of urinary bladder.

3) Color of Urine

The normal urine is light yellow and transparent.

Dark urine indicates a heat syndrome.

Pale urine indicates a cold syndrome, usually of the bladder and kidneys.

Cloudy or turbid urine indicates dampness in the bladder.

Copious, clear and pale urination during an exterior invasion of wind cold or wind heat indicates that the pathogenic factor has not penetrated into the interior.

4) Feeling in urination

The urethral pain when urination with feeling of urgency, difficulty and burning belongs to stranguria which is caused by damp-heat.

The hollow pain after urination is mainly due to declining of kidney qi.

The dripping of urine after micturation pertains to kidney qi failing to consolidate urine.

Discharged spontaneously belongs to kidney qi failing to consolidate urine and dysfunction of urinary bladder in containing urine.

The enuresis in children is due to immature or kidney qi insufficiency. That in adults is due to kidney qi failing to consolidate urine, deficient cold in lower energizer or primordial qi deficiency.

6.3.3.5   Inquiring about diet and taste in the mouth

By question the diet and taste in the mouth, we can establish the state of stomach and spleen. The stomach is responsible for receiving food and spleen for transformation and transportation. Three conditions should be known: the food and appetite, thirst and drink, and taste in mouth.

(1) Appetite and food intake

1) Poor appetite

It is also called as "anorexia". The patient don't want to eat at all, even becomes aversion to food. The frequently encountered conditions are as follows:

Poor appetite with little food intake, abdominal distention, loose stool, flaccid pale tongue and weak pulse belongs to qi deficiency of spleen and stomach. It is caused by the dysfunction of spleen and stomach. It is seen in deficiency syndrome in prolong disease or qi deficiency in ordinary time.

Poor appetite with abdominal fullness, lassitude, loose stool and thick greasy tongue coating pertains to spleen encumbered by dampness. The dampness obstructs middle energizer and makes the spleen fail to transports the food, so there is poor appetite. It is also seen in summer heat invading. Lack of appetite suggests spleen qi deficiency. Being hungry ofter is due to stomach heat.

2) Hunger without appetite

The patient feels hungry but loses the desire to eat food or only eat a little. It is usually due to stomach yin deficiency. The concomitant symptoms are upset and burning in stomach, red tongue with little coating, thready and rapid pulse, etc. The stomach yin deficiency results in disturbance of deficient fire inside.

3) Food addiction

The patient is addicted to some food or non-food things. It is called as "food addiction".

If a child is addicted to uncooked rice or soil and so on, accompanyed by distending abdominal pain, moving ball surrounding navel, emaciation, it is caused by parasitosis. The unclean food leads to growth of parasite in body which causes spleen dysfunction and results in special addiction food.

The addiction to sour food in married women after stop of menstruation, with nausea, rapid slippery pulse, is due to pregnancy. It is not a symptom of diseases but a physiological reaction. A preference for hot food(in terms of temperature) indicates a cold syndrome while a preference for cold food indicates a heat syndrome.

Inquiring about the dietary changes in the course of disease can help to know the development and tendency of diseases. If the appetite becomes better and food intake increases, it indicates the stomach qi is recovering gradually. If the appetite turns to bad and the food intake decreases, it shows the stomach qi is declining. If the very poor appetite in a patient of chronic severe diseases turns suddenly to good appetite and eating much, it is an omen of dying stomach qi and is called "removed medial qi". It pertains to false vitality. The stomach qi exhaustion will certainly lead to death. It is a harbinger of death.

(2) Thirst and drink

Thirst means sensation of dryness in mouth. Drinking refers to the quantity of water intake. They are related to each other closely. Generally speaking, if thirst, the patient drinks more than normal; in contrast, the patient does not like to drink. But the relation is not all the same. So the character, degree, quantity of water intake, preference to cold or hot water and the concomitant symptoms should be asked in order to distinguish syndromes. Here are several clinical cases.

Thirst with desire to drink large amounts of cold water indicates an excess heat syndrome. Absence of thirst is caused by a cold syndrome of the stomach or spleen. Thirst but with no desire to drink indicates dampness-heat as the heat gives rise to the thirst, but the dampness makes one reluctant to drink. Thirst with desire to sip liquids slowly, or to sip warm liquids suggests yin deficiency of stomach or kidneys. Desire to drink cold water suggests a heat syndrome while desire to drink warm water suggests a cold syndrome, which can be of any organ.

(3) Taste in mouth

The taste in mouth refers to the morbid taste in disease. Because the morbid taste in mouth is often the reflection of visceral disease, questioning the change of taste is helpful for diagnosing visceral diseases. So according to the diet and taste changes we can ascertain whether the disease is exogenous or endogenous.

A bitter taste indicates a heat syndrome, usually of liver or heart. If it is caused by heart fire, it is accompanied with insomnia, and only present in the morning after a sleepless night, and not after a good night sleep.

A sweet taste indicates either spleen deficiency or dampness heat. A sour taste suggests retention of food in the stomach or disharmony of liver and stomach.

A salty taste indicates deficient cold of lower energizer.

Besides, lack of taste sensation indicates spleen deficiency. It is due to qi deficiency of spleen and stomach, or belongs to deficiency cold syndrome.

6.3.3.6   Inquiring about hearing and vision

Sensation and consciousness are originated from the eye and ear, which can suggest the condition of the meridians and zang-fu viscera. By inquiring about the hearing and vision we can also establish the condition of qi and blood.

(1) Hearing

It mainly refers to inquire about the tinnitus, deafness and hard of hearing.

1) Tinnitus

The patient feels ringing in the ears. Tinnitus can be divided into excess syndrome and deficiency syndrome. A sudden onset suggests an excess syndrome of liver fire or liver wind. A gradual onset suggests a deficiency syndrome of the kidneys. If the noise is aggravated by pressing with one's hands on the ears, it suggests excess syndrome and if it is alleviated, it suggests deficiency syndrome.

The aloud, high-pitch noise like a whistle indicates hyperactivity of liver yang, liver fire or liver wind. A low-pitch noise like rushing water indicates kidney deficiency.

2) Deafness

Deafness refers to patient's dysacousis and even hearing loss. A sudden onset suggests an excess syndrome of liver fire or liver wind and a gradual onset suggests a deficiency syndrome of the kidney.

In chronic cases, besides kidney deficiency, deafness also can be due to heart blood deficiency, deficiency of qi of the upper energizer, and yang qi deficiency.

3) Hard of hearing

Hard of hearing refers to patients with hearing impairment and hearing is not clear and sound repetition. A sudden onset suggests an excess syndrome that is due to wind pathogen and dampness pathogen. A gradual onset suggests a deficiency syndrome and usually can be seen in old and weak people.

(2) Vision

There are so many aspects we can require to evaluate the vision. Here are mainly clinical symptom and significance.

1) Eye pain

The patient feels monocular or binocular pain. It can be seen in a variety of ophthalmological diseases with complex reasons. Generally, the throe belongs to the excess syndrome and the micro pain belongs to the deficiency syndrome. Pain like a needle and with redness of the eye associated with headache indicates fire toxin in the heart meridian. Pain, swelling and redness of the eye indicates either invasion of the eye meridians by exterior wind-heat, or interior liver fire.

2) Dryness of the eye

Dryness of the eye refers to the patient's feeling of dry and unwell discomfort in the eyes, and it indicates liver and /or kidney yin deficiency.

3) Itching of the eye

Itching of the eye refers to the patient's eyelid, eye angle and eyeball pruritus. Tthe eyes itching, photophobia, tears, accompanied by burning, mostly belongs to the wind-heat in liver meridian. If the eyes are slightly itchy and dry, it is mostly due to the blood deficiency and eyes without nourishment.

4) Others

Blurred vision and "floaters" in the eyes indicate liver blood deficiency. Photophobia also indicates liver blood deficiency. A feeling of pressure in the eyes indicates kidney yin deficiency.

6.3.3.7 Inquiring about sleep

The state of sleep is related to the movement of defensive qi and the variation of yin and yang. The yang qi is exuberant in human body in day time and keeps the body awaked and at night the yang qi enters yin meridians and yin qi is exuberant in human body making body asleep. With the disharmony between yin and yang, the prevalent yang and declined yin lead to insomnia while the prevalent yin and declined yang to hypersomnia.

When inquiring about sleep, the sleeping time, state of sleeping and concomitant symptoms are the main points.

(1) Insomnia

It is difficult for the insomnia patients to full asleep, or easy to wake up and difficult to sleep again, even keep awake all the night.

Insomnia in the sense of not being able to fall asleep, but sleeping well after falling asleep, usually suggests deficiency of heart blood. Deficiency of kidney yin usually leads to an insomnia, which in the sense of waking up many times during the night. Liver fire or heart fire can show a dream-disturbed sleep. Restless sleep with dreams indicates retention of food. Waking up early in the morning and failing to fall asleep again indicates deficiency of gallbladder.

It is to some extent normal to wake early with age, due to the physiological decline of qi and blood.

(2)Hypersomnia

Hypersomnia refers that the patient is weary and often involuntary sleep. It is also known as "somnolence".

If one feels sleepy after eating, it indicates spleen qi deficiency. A general feeling of lethargy and heaviness of the body indicates retention of dampness. If there is also dizziness, it indicates phlegm. Extreme lethargy and lassitude with a feeling of cold, indicate deficiency of kidney yang. Lethargic stupor with rattling in the throat, a slippery pulse and a sticky tongue coating, indicate mental confusion by phlegm.

6.3.3.8   Inquiring about gynecological matters

Special questions need to be asked of women regarding menstruation, leucorrhoea, pregnancy and childbirth.

(1)Menstruation

Menstruation refers to the periodic discharge of blood and mucosal tissue from the uterus through the vagina, occurring approximately monthly from puberty to menopause in non-pregnant women. Normally regular menstruation lasts for a few days, usually 2−7 days with a cycle of 28 days. The average blood loss during menstruation is 35 mL with 10−100 mL considered normal and the blood is red, not to thin or thick.

The condition of menstruation gives a very vivid idea of a woman's state of qi and blood. Doctors must ask about the cycle, amount of bleeding, color of blood, quality and pain.

1)Menstruation Cycle

• Advanced menstruation: Advanced menstruation refers to menstrual periods that come 7 days or more ahead of due time, for more than two menstruation cycle. It is usually due to qi deficiency, yang deficiency and heat in blood, or blood stasis

• Delayed menstruation: Delayed menstruation refers to menstrual periods that come 7 days or more after due time, for more than two menstruation cycle. It can be divided into excess syndrome and deficiency syndrome. The excess syndrome is caused by deficiency of qi and blood, insufficiency of kidney essence, kidney yang deficiency. And the deficiency syndrome is often qi stasis due to coagulated cold or phlegm-dampness blocking collaterals.

• Menstruation at irregular intervals: It refers to the periods that come with an irregular cycle, more than 7 days early or later. It is always due to stagnation of liver qi or deficiency of spleen and kidney.

2)Menstruation Amount

• Profuse menstruation indicates heat in the blood or qi deficiency.

• Scanty menstruation indicates either blood deficiency or stagnation of blood or cold.

• Flooding and spotting: It refers to sudden onset of profuse uterine bleeding or incessant dripping of blood, occurring not in the menstruation period.

Sudden onset with profuse uterine bleeding is called as flooding while incessant dripping of blood is named spotting. Flooding and spotting are caused by heat disturbing chong and conception channels, qi deficiency of kidney and spleen, blood stasis blocking in chong and conception channels.

3)Color

A deep red or bright red color indicates heat in the blood. Pale blood indicates blood deficiency. Purple or blackish blood indicates stasis of blood or cold. Fresh red blood indicates deficiency-heat from yin deficiency.

4) Quality

Congealed blood with clots indicates stasis blood or cold. Watery blood indicates blood or yin deficiency. Turbid blood indicates heat in blood or stagnation of cold.

5) Pain

Pain before the menstruation period indicates stagnation of qi or blood. Pain during the menstruation period indicates blood heat or stagnation of cold. Pain after the menstruation period indicates blood deficiency.

These questions and their answers have limited value with regard to women who take the contraceptive pill, or had an intrauterine device fitted, or in multiparous women.

(2) Leucorrhoea

Normal vagina secretes milky, odorless substance for lubricating vagina. is called as "leucorrhoea". It must be distinguished according to color, consistency and smell.

1) Color

A white discharge indicates a cold syndrome, due to spleen or kidney yang deficiency, exterior cold damp, or stagnation of liver qi.

A yellow discharge indicates a heat syndrome, due to dampness-heat in the lower energizer.

A greenish discharge indicates dampness-heat in the liver meridian.

A red and white discharge also indicates dampness-heat.

A yellow discharge with pus and blood after menopause indicates toxic dampness-heat in the uterus.

2) Consistency

A watery consistency suggests a cold-dampness syndrome, whilst a thick consistency suggests a dampness-heat syndrome.

3) Smell

A fishy smell indicates cold-dampness while a leathery smell indicates dampness-heat.

(3) Pregnancy

Infertility can be due to deficiency conditions such as blood or kidney essence deficiency, or to excess conditions such as dampness-heat in the lower energizer or stasis of blood in the uterus. Vomiting during pregnancy indicates stomach and penetrating vessel deficiency.

Miscarriage before three months indicates blood or essence deficiency and is associated with kidney deficiency while after three months it indicates liver blood stasis or sinking of spleen qi.

(4) Childbirth

Nausea and profuse bleeding after delivery indicates exhaustion of the penetrating vessel sweating and fever after delivery indicates exhausting of qi and blood. Post-natal depression is usually due to blood deficiency.

6.3.3.9 Inquiring about infant

Interrogation of infant does not differ substantially from that of adults, except that it needs to be carried out mostly with the child's parents.

According to the infantine zang-fu viscera of delicate, rapid development of physiological characteristics and rapid onset, rapid change, vulnerable to manifestation of deficiency and excess to the pathological features, there are several questions, which are peculiar to infantine problems, such as mother condition during pregnancy, delivery condition, nutrition, any drugs taken, way of feeding, etc.

There are some diseases common seen in morbid condition children.

（1）Infantile cry

Infantile crying refers to incessant crying both in the daytime and night, which can be caused by any disease or uncomfortable conditions, such as hunger, food retention, and pain or frightened.

（2）Five stiffnesses

Five stiffnesses refer to stiffness of the hand, foot, waist, flesh and neck in newborn due to a congenital defect.

（3）Five retardations

Five retardations refer to retarded development in infants covering standing, walking, hair-growth, tooth eruption and speaking usually caused by malnutrition, such as deficiency of kidney essence, or deficiency of the spleen and stomach.

（4）Five limpnesses

Five limpnesses refer to flaccidity of the neck, nape, extremities, muscles and mastication as striking features of delayed growth and mental retardation in infants, often due to deficiency of kidney essence, or postnatal malnutrition.

6.4　Pulse taking

Pulse taking includes pulse diagnosis and body palpation. It is a method for the doctor to use the hand to touch and press some parts of the body surface of the patient, to obtain the information of disease. Pulse diagnosis is to feel the pulse, while body palpation is to touch and press the different parts of patient's body such as skin, hands and feet, chest and abdomen and so on.

6.4.1　Pulse diagnosis

Pulse diagnosis is a method of using doctor's fingers to palpate patient's pulses which are shown in the superficial arteries, to judge diseases. It is a unique diagnostic method of TCM.

6.4.1.1　The formation of a pulse manifestation

The pulse manifestation is the image of the pulsation. The formation of the pulse is directly related to the pulse of the heart, the toning of the veins, and the profit and loss of the blood.

（1）The pulse of the heart is the power to form a pulse manifestation

The heart dominates blood and vessel. The pulse of the heart promotes the normal operation of the blood in the vessel to form impediment. So the pulse of the heart is the power to form a pulse manifestation.

（2）The operation of qi and blood is the basis for the formation of pulse manifestation

Pulse is the house of blood. Vessel is a meridian of qi and blood and depends on the filling of blood. The profit and loss of blood is directly related to the strength of the pulse. Qi is the commander of blood. The operation of blood depends on the promotion and fixation of qi. Blood is the mother of qi. Blood carrying qi can raise the whole body. So, the operation of qi and blood is the basis for the formation of pulse manifestation. The pulse manifestation can reflect the situation of qi and blood under certain circumstances.

（3）The coordination of the zang-fu viscera is the premise of the normal pulse manifestation

The qi and blood circulation also depend on other zang-fu viscera which coordinate the heart. Because the lung dominates qi and it is in charge of breathing. The Blood circulation depends on the dispersing of lung qi. The lung connects all the vessels. The qi and blood circulating all over the body should converge into the lung. The stomach dominates reception and the spleen dominates transportation and transformation.

The spleen and stomach are the source of qi and blood production. The spleen also dominates blood control. The normal flow of blood needs the controlling function of the spleen. The liver stores blood and it dominates free flow and rise of qi. The liver stores the blood and governs the free flow of qi. It can not only regulate the circulation of blood, but also promote the operation of qi and blood. The kidney stores essence and is the root of original yin and yang. The essence can transform itself into blood. It is one of the important sources of blood production. So, the coordination of the zang-fu viscera is the premise of the normal pulse manifestation.

6.4.1.2   Locations for pulse diagnosis

According to the different locations for pulse diagnosis, there are three methods of pulse diagnosis: whole body selection, three-part selection and wrist pulse taking method. Since the Jin Dynasty, wrist pulse taking method has been mainly used while whole body selection and three-part selection have been used less frequently.

(1) Three-part selection

Three-part selection was mentioned in both *Internal Classic* and *Treatise on Cold Damage and Miscellaneous Diseases*. The content of pulse diagnosis is applied to the three parts, the "renying", "cunkou" and "fuyang". Cunkou can show the qi of twelve meridians. Renying and fuyang reflect the qi of stomach and spleen. Some doctors also feel the pulse of Taixi, an acupoint of the kidney meridian of foot shaoyin, to detect whether congenital qi and acquired qi are both exhausted.

The three-part selection is also complicated by comparing with wrist pulse taking method. So it is seldom used except when no pulse in "cunkou" spot, in that time, the fuyang, taixi and renying pulses are felt.

(2) Wrist pulse taking method

Wrist pulse taking method refers to the pulsation place of radical artery behind wrist. The method was first recorded in *Internal Classic* and discussed in detail in *Classic of Difficult Issues*. It was widely used from the *Pulse Classic* by *Wang Shuhe*.

The *Classic of Difficult Issues* established that "The three sections are 'cun', 'guan' and 'chi', and the nine indicators are 'superficial', 'middle' and 'cubit'". In other words, it is a method of feeling the pulse at the radial artery, dividing it into three areas and feeling it at three levels. The three areas of the pulse at the radial artery are called cun, guan and chi, and another name, "front", "middle" and "rear". The three levels of it are called superficial, middle and deep. This can be seen that the three sections and nine indicators of wrist pulse taking method are different from it of whole body selection (Figure 6-2).

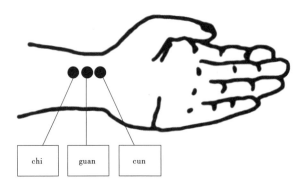

Figure 6-2   **Cun, Guan, Chi**

The principles of exclusive examination of the wrist pulse are as follows:Firstly,wrist pulse is the place where the Taiyuan(LU-9) of the lung meridian of hand taiyin is located. The qi of twelve meridians gather in it,so it is called as meeting point of the vessels. Secondly,the lung connects all the vessels. Wrist pulse can also reflect the state of qi and blood of the five zang viscera and six fu viscera. Finally,wrist pulse is located at the wrist where the muscles are thin and tender,and the veins are easy to expose.

Over the centuries,there have been several different attributions of organs to individual pulse positions. It was first recorded in *Internal Classic*,and follows Table 6-1 in detail.

Table 6-1   **Different attributions of organs to individual pulse positions**

Position	Left	Right
Front	Heart / small intestine	Lung / large intestine
Middle	Liver / gall bladder	Spleen / stomach
Rear	Kidney / bladder	Fire of gate of vitality / lower energizer

It must be pointed out that the "cun", "guan" and "chi" of wrist pulse is divided into zang-fu viscera. It shows the qi of five zang viscera and six fu viscera instead of the meridians of five zang viscera and six fu viscera.

6.4.1.3   Methods for taking the pulse

(1)Time

The pulse diagnosis ought to be done at the time that patient and doctor are both relaxed. *Internal Classic* noted that "The laws of diagnosis are as follows. As a rule,it is at down,before the yin qi has begun its movement,before the yang qi is dispersed,before beverages and food have been consumed,before the conduit vessels are filled to abundance,when the contents of the network vessels are balanced,before the qi and blood move in disorder,that,hence,one can diagnose an abnormal movement in the vessels". So the best time for pulse diagnosis is in the early morning.

Nevertheless,it is impossible to feel the pulse of all patients at dawn in fact. But when the patient is in a calm internal and external environment to be felt the pulse,it can be achieved. Before diagnosing pulse, the patient should rest for a while and breathe well to keep qi and blood calm. In the same time,keep the clinic quiet to help the doctor feel the pulse.

The operation time of the pulse diagnosis is usually 3-5 minutes. In the pulse diagnosis,the doctor's breathing should be natural and uniform,using the rhythm of breath to calculate the patient's pulse rate. It is named as calm breathing. In addition,the doctors must be concentrated and careful to identify the pulse.

(2)Posture

The patient can sit or lie with his forearm stretched on the table or bed at the same level of heart. The palm keeps upwards and the wrist is sustained by a soft pad. Thus the pulse can be felt. The incorrect position can affect the operation of local qi and blood to influence the pulse. It is only by taking the correct position can the more accurate pulse be obtained.

(3)Placing the figures

The best way for doctor to feel the patient's pulse using his fingers is to feel the left pulse in by the right hand,and feel right pulse by the left hand.

When feeling pulse,all of the three fingers,the index finger,the middle finger and the ring finger, should be used. About putting on fingers,first,the middle finger is put on the middle position which is at the medial side of the styloid process of radius; then the index finger is put on the front position which is in front of the middle position; finally the ring finger is put on the rear position which is posterior to middle position.

The general touching is to feeling pulse by three fingers in the same time, which providing us with a whole impression of the pulse. The single touching is to feel pulse by only one single, which gives us the information of visceral conditions respectively.

(4)Considerations

The pulse diagnosis should be performed in quiet clinic environment, to avoid the disturbance to the doctors and patients due to the noise of the environment.

The doctor should pay attention to feeling the pulse. The patient should be calm, and sports, the emotional and other factors should be asked to rest for a moment.

6.4.1.4 Factors to take into account

Several factors should be taken into account in order to evaluate each pulse in its context and in relation to an individual patient.

(1)Season

The change of external environment always affects human life activity. The physiological adjustment that people adapt to this change can be reflected on the pulse. *Internal Classic* noted that "string-like in spring, surging in summer, downy in autumn, deep in winter". The pulse is somewhat taut in spring, is slightly surge in summer, is floating a little in autumn, and is relatively deep in winter. All the changes are within normal range. If pulse changes contrary to those, it is sign of diseases.

(2)Environment

The change of geographical environmental affects the normal pulse. In the south, the terrain is low and the climate is warm and humid. So the pulse in southerner is gentle. In the north, the terrain is high, the air is dry, and the climate is cold. So the pulse in northerner is deep and replete. The different living conditions or constitutions affect the pulse of people.

(3)Sex

Different gender has effect on the constitution and pulse. The pulse of men is naturally slightly stronger than that of women. Also, in men the left pulse should be very slightly stronger than the right one, and in women the right pulse should be slightly stronger than the left. This is in accordance with symbolism of yin and yang, following which the pulse of left side in man is yang and the pulse of right side in woman is yin.

The slippery and rapid pulse is seen commonly during pregnancy.

(4)Age

The younger the age, the faster the pulse. The pulse in infant is 120 times a minute. In a child over 5 years old, the pulse is normal when it beats 90-110 times a minute. The young man has a strong pulse, while the old man has a weak pulse due to the deficiency of qi and blood. The pulse of the younger is strong while that in the aged is a little weaker.

(5)Constitution

The pulse in a body of strong constitution is usually forceful and that in a body of weak constitution is soft. The pulse in a tall person is long and that in a short one is short. The pulse in a fat person is deep and that in a thin one is floating. The pulse of athlete is slow and forceful.

(6)Emotion

A temporary mental stimulus can also cause a pulse. When one is angry, the pulse gets urgent. When one is joyous, the pulse is moderate. When one is in fear, the qi moves down and pulse stirred. When the emotion is calm, the pulse returned to normal.

(7) Occupation

The pulse of those who are engaged in heavy physical work should be stronger than those who are engaged in mental work.

6.4.1.5   The normal pulse

The normal pulse, also called common pulse, is characterized by the pulse in all three portions which is 4−5 beats in one breath (the equivalent of 60−90 times a minute) neither deep nor floating, neither large nor small, neither soft nor forceful, and in equal intervals. The rear pulse has certain strength and the pulse is closely related to the internal and external environment. It often changes along with the change of climatic environment and physiological activity. Only by knowing the normal pulse can the morbid pulse be distinguished.

The characters of normal pulse are presence of stomach qi, presence of vitality and presence of root.

(1) Presence of stomach qi

A pulse is said to be presence of stomach qi when it is felt as "gentle", "clam" and is relatively slow (4 beats in one breath).

Stomach is the reservoir of food and drink and spleen is the root of acquired foundation. The spleen and stomach are the source of qi and blood production. The stomach qi is the root of body. So the body with full stomach qi will live well, that with little stomach qi will be ill, and that without stomach qi will die. The stomach qi is the root of the pulse too. In the same way, the pulse being full of stomach qi is the sign of health, that with little stomach qi indicates the illness, and that without stomach qi means death. Even if it is an abnormal pulse, no matter how slow and rapid, but it is felt as gentle, there is presence of stomach qi.

(2) Presence of vitality

The pulse is said to be presence of vitality when it is soft but with strength, neither big or small and regular.

The heart dominates blood and vessel, and it houses vitality. When qi and blood are abundant, the vitality is vigorous, and the pulse is then full of vitality. Even a weak pulse, a weak one that is not completely weak. Even a wiry and replete pulse, there is a soft feeling in the pulse. They are called as presence of vitality.

(3) Presence of root

The pulse is said to be presence of root in two different statements. On the one hand, it has a root when the deep level can be felt clearly. On the other hand, it reflects when the rear position can be felt clearly.

The kidney is the foundation of congenital constitution. All the activities of the body rely on kidney qi. The kidney qi to the body is the live root to the tree. The tree without leaves is alive only if the root is alive.

To sum up, the pulse of presence of stomach, vitality and root is the essential condition of a normal pulse.

6.4.1.6   Morbid pulse

(1) Floating pulse

1) Feeling

The position of the pulse is shallow and can be easily felt with a light pressure of the fingers, its force decreases slightly in the deeper level.

2) Clinical significance

It often occurs in the early stage of the exterior syndrome. This pulse indicates the battle about healthy and pathogenic qi. If it is floating and tight, it indicates wind-cold. If it is floating and rapid, it indicates wind-heat. If the pulse is floating and forceful, it indicates the exterior excess syndrome. If the pulse is floating and weak, it may indicate the exterior deficiency syndrome.

It may also occur in yin deficiency syndrome of the consumptive disease or declining yang in critical case. If the pulse is floating at the skin layer but empty at the deep level, it indicates deficiency of yin.

(2) Deep pulse

1) Feeling

The pulse only responds to the fingers when heavy pressure and is felt near the bone.

2) Clinical significance

This character indicates the interior syndrome. The forceful deep pulse indicates qi stagnation and blood stasis in the interior or interior cold or heat. The weak deep pulse suggests qi deficiency and yang deficiency.

It also suggests that the problem is in the yin organs. The pathogens accumulate in body and the qi and blood and yang qi are obstructed in the inner part of body and could not rise against the pathogen. If the pulse still beats under the heavy pressing, it may be caused by the abdominal mass. If pulse beating becomes weaker and weaker by pressing, it is due to qi and blood deficiency which is unable to move in vessels.

(3) Slow pulse

1) Feeling

The pulse rate is less than 60 beats per minute and pulsates slowly.

2) Clinical significance

A slow pulse often occurs in cold syndrome. If the pulse is deep and forceful, it is a condition of cold accumulation; but it also can happen when the pathogen transforms into heat and enters the interior and the heat pathogen blocking the circulation of qi and blood and slow the pulse. The slow pulse is forceful, too. If the pulse is deep and weak, it is a condition of deficiency cold.

(4) Rapid pulse

1) Feeling

The pulse rate is rapid and over 90 beats per minute.

2) Clinical significance

This is a situation that often occurs in heat syndrome. The forceful rapid pulse indicates excess heat while the weak one indicates deficiency-heat. A long time disease may lead to the yin deficiency, and the yang is only relatively strong, so the pulse is rapid but weak.

If the pulse is floating and rapid, it indicates the exterior heat. If the pulse is deep and rapid, it may suggest the interior heat. If he pulse is slippery and rapid, it indicates phlegm-fire. If the pulse is thready and rapid. It is a sign of yin deficiency. And the taut and rapid pulse is the sign of the liver fire.

(5) Surging pulse

1) Feeling

The pulse feels wide and powerful and like roaring waves.

2) Clinical significance

The surging pulse often occurs in the syndrome of exuberant heat. It belongs to heat pathogen resulting in expanding vessel wider than the normal. It frequently appears during a fever, but it also can be seen in chronic diseases characterized by interior heat. And it sometimes indicates yang hyperactivity, stomach heat and abscess. The pulse is mostly seen in the fulminant stage of warm diseases.

If the pulse is floating and surge, it means heat in the exterior. If the pulse is deep surge, it indicates heat in the interior. The surge and tight of pulse suggests abscess, the surge and slippery of pulse is due to phlegm-fire, and the strong surge pulse means the epilepsy.

(6) Thready pulse

1) Feeling

The pulse feels thin and soft like a thread, but with quite obvious pulsation.

2) Clinical significance

It often means the deficiency syndrome, especially yin and blood-deficiency as well as dampness syndrome. Yin and blood deficiency cannot completely fill vessel. Moreover, the dampness pathogen can repress the vessel and also make the vessel thin and slow. It may also indicate internal dampness with severe deficiency of qi.

If the pulse is floating and thready, it is present in yang deficiency. If the pulse is deep and thready, it suggests direct invasion of cold into zang-fu viscera, or arthralgia. If the pulse thready and moderate, it means dampness in the middle. If the pulse is rapid and thready, it is the sign of internal heat produced by yin deficiency. If the pulse is thready and weak, it is seen in the case of night sweating. If the pulse is thready and tight, it indicates cold in the body. If the pulse is thready and taut, it shows liver deficiency. If the pulse is uneven and thready, it shows blood deficiency.

(7) Faint pulse

1) Feeling

The pulse is extremely small, soft and weak. It is difficult to feel, and becomes vague when pressing.

2) Clinical significance

The pulse is a sign of heavy deficiency of both qi and blood or decline of yang. The pulse happened due to the condition that yang qi is weak and incapable of agitation, and nutrient-blood cannot completely fill vessel. The pulse presented in a prolonged disease is a sign of dying, while in a newly suffered disease is the sign that the disease can be curable.

If the pulse is faint and floating, it indicates yang deficiency. If the pulse is faint and deep, it suggests yin deficiency or diarrhea with abdominal pain due to visceral yang deficiency. If the pulse is faint and sluggish, it is present in loss of blood. If the pulse is faint and taut, it is seen in the case of convulsion.

(8) Scattered pulse

1) Feeling

This pulse feels very floating, scattered, without root. It is relatively superficial. And the pulse feels as if it is "broken" in small dots instead of feeling like a wave. The pulse will be disappeared if pressing slightly.

2) Clinical significance

This pulse indicates original qi dissociation and zang-fu viscera qi will disappear. It is the decline of both qi and blood, and in particular of kidney qi. It always indicates a serious condition. If the pulse is seen in the second trimester of pregnancy, it may indicate the abortion.

(9) Feeble pulse

1) Feeling

The empty pulse feels rather big but soft when pressed at three regions.

2) Clinical significance

It suggests the deficiency syndrome, especially deficiency of both qi and blood. If qi is insufficient, the pulse cannot move forcefully. While blood is deficient, the vessel is not completely full.

If the pulse presents with moderate pulse in conditions of loss of blood, after delivery and old patient, it means the stomach qi is still in pulse. But if it presents in a physically strong body or sudden onset disease, the prognosis is not good.

If the pulse is feeble and rapid, it suggests loss of sperm or menorrhagia. The feeble and sluggish pulse is the sign of blood deficiency.

(10) Replete pulse

1) Feeling

The pulse feels forceful at all three regions with no matter at what level. And it is also often used to indicate any pulse of the full type.

2) Clinical significance

It suggests the excess syndrome. It means that the conflict between vital and pathogenic qi, results in the blockage of qi and blood. If the pulse is full and rapid, it indicates excess heat, while a full and slow pulse indicates excess-cold.

The pulse sometimes may be seen in deficiency syndrome. If the genuine yin is used up after a long time disease, the solitary yang floats in the out part of body, and the pulse can also be strong. This is a sign of pseudo-excess.

(11) Slippery pulse

1) Feeling

The slippery pulse feels smooth, rounded to the touch, just like a rolling pearl under skin and slides under the fingers.

2) Clinical significance

It suggests the phlegm and fluid retention, indigestion or excess heat. The slippery pulse also can be observed in young adults who have ample qi and blood, and pregnant women.

The slippery pulse in some cases can also be weak, indicating phlegm or dampness with a background of qi deficiency.

If the pulse is floating and slippery, it suggests wind-phlegm. If the pulse is deep and slippery, it indicates phlegm or food retention. The rapid slippery pulse is due to phlegm-fire. If the pulse is slippery and strong, it means heat in the stomach.

(12) Uneven pulse

1) Feeling

The pulse feels unsmooth and sluggish like scraping a piece of bamboo with a sharp knife. Choppy also indicates a pulse that changes rapidly both in rate and quality.

2) Clinical significance

It suggests syndrome of damage of essence, insufficiency of blood, as well as qi stagnation and blood stasis. For deficiency syndrome, the vessel cannot be nourished so that the pulse uneven with powerless. For excess syndrome, qi movement and blood circulation block inside the vessels so that the pulse is uneven but forceful. It may also indicate the depletion of body fluid caused by vomiting and/or diarrhea.

The deep uneven pulse is due to blood stasis and essence insufficiency. If the pulse is uneven and feeble, it means the qi deficiency. If the pulse is faint and uneven, it presents in blood deficiency. If the pulse is thready and uneven, it indicates the exhaustion of body fluid. If the pulse is strong and uneven pulse, it suggests the blood stasis with excessive heat. If the pulse is taut and uneven, it marks the qi stagnation.

(13) Long pulse

1) Feeling

The pulse is straight and basically longer than normal. The pulsation can be felt in not only the three portions but also over the normal position.

2) Clinical significance

The hyperactivity of liver yang, exuberant heat and internal accumulation of phlegm-fire make the meridian qi engorged and vein filling.

If the long pulse is supple and moderately forceful, it is a sign of exuberant qi in normal condition. But if the pulse is too long and forceful, it indicates the excess of yang heat or liver yang hyperactivity, and in that condition, the patient may have a high fever and constipation.

If the pulse is floating and long, it presents in exogenous disease or yin deficiency. If the pulse is surge and long, it is often found in patient of mental disorder. If the pulse is deep and long, it suggests the abdominal lump. If the pulse is long and taut, it indicates liver diseases. If the pulse is slightly uneven and long, it may imply the recovery.

(14) Short pulse

1) Feeling

The pulse is shorter than normal. The pulse in front or rear, or both of them is absent.

2) Clinical significance

The short pulse indicates qi diseases. The forceful short pulse is a sign of qi depression while the weak short pulse is a sign of qi deficiency. Qi deficiency can't push the blood, so the pulse is short and weak. Qi depression or food or phlegm retention obstructs vein, so the pulse is short and forceful.

If the pulse is floating and short, it indicates lung qi deficiency. If the pulse is deep and short, it suggests blood stasis or stuffiness in abdomen. If the pulse is short, slippery and rapid, it is due to phlegm or food retention. If the pulse is short and hollow, it presents in massive bleeding.

(15) Wiry pulse

1) Feeling

The pulse is long and straight, feeling like a string of drown bow under fingers.

2) Clinical significance

The pulse often occurs in liver or gallbladder diseases, pains, or phlegm and fluid retention. Liver cannot normally dominant free flow and rise of qi due to failure in qi transformation, contraction of meridians and vessels, so the vessels become tense making the pulse stretch and straight like a string of drown bow. The pain can lead to qi turbulence. In addition, most aged people also have wiry pulse due to the deficiency of their essence and blood resulting to the vessel lacking of nutrition. This pulse type is likely presented in spring.

If the pulse is floating and taut, it indicates sustained fluid retention. If the pulse is deep and taut, it suggests suspended fluid retention. If the pulse is rapid and taut, it is usually due to heat while the slow one to cold.

(16) Tight pulse

1) Feeling

The pulse is tight and strong, feeling like a stretched and twisted cord under fingers.

2) Clinical significance

A tight pulse indicates cold and pain syndrome. It often occurs in the syndromes of cold, pain and indigestion, which attribute to contract the vessels, so the pulse is tense. If the pulse is floating and tense, it indicates affection by pathogenic cold. If the pulse is deep and tense, it indicates pathogenic cold invading the interior.

If the pulse is floating tight, it is a character of exterior cold. If the pulse is deep tight, it means interior cold. If combined with sluggish pulse, it may indicate cold rheumatism. While with surge, pulse may suggest the abscess.

(17) Moderate pulse

1) Feeling

The pulse rate is close to normal pulse(60 beats per minute), and moves smoothly.

2) Clinical significance

This is generally a healthy pulse or means wind or dampness attack. The pulse occurs in the dampness and spleen-stomach qi deficiency syndrome. The dampness, attributing to viscosity and stagnation, results in hampering the spleen-stomach qi movement. It also can be caused by the spleen-stomach deficiency. If the abnormal people present the pulse, it means the recovery of vital qi.

If the pulse is floating and moderate, it indicates the wind attack, while the deep and moderate pulse is present in cold-dampness syndrome. If the pulse is thready and moderate, it is due to qi deficiency, and if the pulse is moderate and sluggish, it is due to blood deficiency.

(18) Hollow pulse

1) Feeling

The pulse is floating, big and hollow, and the feeling is similar to touch the leaf of green Chinese onion. The pulse can be felt at the superficial level and at the deep level with a stronger pressure but cannot be felt with slightly harder pressure at the middle level. It is empty in the middle.

2) Clinical significance

The pulse usually suggests blood loss and yin depletion. So the pulse is usually seen after the suddenly massive bleeding or dehydration and the blood cannot make the vessels full. If the pulse is rapid and slightly hollow, it may suggest a forthcoming blood loss. If the hollow pulse is rapid, it can be seen in yin deficiency with bleeding. If the hollow pulse is slow, it may be due to deficiency of both qi and blood. If the pulse is hollow, slow and intermittent, it indicates the phlegm retention and blood stasis in combination with deficiency of yin and blood.

(19) Tympanic pulse

1) Feeling

This pulse feels hard and tight at the superficial level but completely empty at the deep level, and the feeling is like pressing drum leather.

2) Clinical significance

The pulse indicates severe deficiency of the kidney essence or yin. It is found in hemorrhages disorder and consumption of essence, abortion, metrorrhagia and metrostaxis.

The hollow character at deep level is a sign of deficiency of both qi and blood. If the pulse is floating, tight and tympanic, it suggests the extremely exorbitant pathogen in the exterior. If the pulse is slow and tympanic, it indicates the dangerous condition.

(20) Firm pulse

1) Feeling

The pulse can be felt only at the deep level and it feels hard, big, long, rather wiry, and the vessel is fixed. By pressing, the pulse can be felt large, taut, long, hard and forceful.

2) Clinical significance

The firm pulse is a sign of interior excess cold syndrome or interior stagnation and pain. It is usually found in abdominal mass and hernia.

The pulse usually cannot be seen in deficiency syndrome, but if the pathogen stays in the body for a long time, the stomach qi may be exhausted by the struggle between the vital and the pathogen, and then firm pulse appears. In this condition, the firm pulse is a dangerous omen.

(21) Weak pulse

1) Feeling

A weak pulse is extremely soft and thin, and can be seen only at the deep level.

2) Clinical significance

The pulse indicates deficiency of both qi and blood and deficiency of yang. Blood deficiency cannot make the vessels full so the pulse is thin. Yang deficiency makes the pulse deep and soft. It can present in all kinds of deficiency syndrome, and also can be seen in summerheat attack.

If the pulse is floating and weak, it means qi deficiency. If the pulse is deep and weak, pulse indicates declination of genuine fire. If the pulse is low and weak, it suggests yang deficiency. If the pulse is rapid and weak, it is due to yin deficiency. If the pulse is sluggish and weak, it presents in blood deficiency. If the pulse is large and weak, it marks the qi depletion.

(22) Soggy pulse

1) Feeling

The pulse feels floating, thin and soft. If a stronger pressure is applied to feel the deep level, it disappears.

2) Clinical significance

This pulse means the deficiency and dampness-syndrome. Failure of qi to control blood makes a floating and soft pulse while insufficient blood makes the pulse thin. In addition, the nature of dampness hampering qi movement can obstruct vessels, so the pulse is thin and soft. The pulse can be usually seen in diarrhea, spontaneous sweating, asthma and weakness.

If the pulse is soggy and sluggish, it indicates the loss of blood. If the pulse is rapid and soggy, it means the dampness-heat in the body.

(23) Hidden pulse

1) Feeling

This pulse is very deep and difficult to feel and it only can be felt when pressing to the muscles and bones.

2) Clinical significance

The hidden pulse indicates pathogen block, syncope and extreme pain.

If the hidden pulse with regular intermittence, it is due to extreme heat which transforms into cold. If the pulse is slow and hidden, it indicates the cold accumulation which is an extremely yin.

(24) Tremulous pulse

1) Feeling

The shape of the pulse just like a bean, which is slippery, rapid and short, and trembles under the finger. It's especially obvious at the guan.

2) Clinical significance

The pulse indicates pain, alarmed and panicky.

The floating and large pulse is an excess syndrome. If the pulse is floating and bouncing, it presents in exterior syndrome. If the pulse is strong and bouncing, it is seen in rheumatism. If the pulse is bouncing and hollow, it means loss of essence.

(25) Rapid intermittent pulse

1) Feeling

The pulse beats rapidly(more than 90 beats per minute) with irregular intermittent. It is the extreme condition of rapid pulse.

2）Clinical significance

This pulse occurs in exuberance of yang, qi and blood stagnation, phlegm and food accumulation, or the decline of five zang viscera qi. For excess syndromes, rapid and powerful pulse is caused by yang exuberance and heat accumulation which stimulates blood circulation. Excessive heat consumes body fluid, and insufficient body fluid causes intermittent in pulse. Qi and blood stagnation, phlegm and food accumulation can obstruct the vessels and cause the intermittent. For deficiency syndrome, rapid and powerless pulse is caused by inadequate body fluid and the decline of five zang viscera qi.

If the pulse is swift and surge, it is present in disease characterized by fidget and chest distress. If the pulse is swift and deep, it is due to disease of abdominal pain. And both of them reflect the yin or yang will be exhausted.

（26）Knotted pulse

1）Feeling

The pulse beats slowly(less than 60 beats per minute) with irregular and intermittent timing of beats.

2）Clinical significance

It occurs in cold, phlegm, and stagnated blood, accumulation of abdominal mass, and deficiency of both qi and blood. For the syndrome of excess, the pathogens are blocked in the vessel and lead to the obstruction in vessel. For the syndrome of deficiency, severely deficiency of qi and blood cause the vessel qi disconnection, causing the slow and irregular pulse. Nevertheless, the pulse can be found in the normal body. This is a congenital variation, but not a disease.

If combined with floating pulse, it indicates cold in meridians. The combined and deep pulse suggests the pathogen retention is in zang-fu viscera. The knotted pulse with slippery pulse indicates the phlegm or fluid retention is in zang-fu viscera. While with weak pulse, it is the sign of deficiency of both qi and blood.

（27）Regular intermittent pulse

1）Feeling

The pulse beats slowly(less than 60 beats per minute) and weak with regular intermittent. And then the pulse will continue beating after a little moment.

2）Clinical significance

This pulse always indicates a serious internal problem of yin organs or spleen qi deficiency. It is a dangerous portent. It occurs in the exhaustion of five zang viscera qi, traumatic injury, pain and fear. The pulse which is powerless and pauses regularly, cannot recover to the normal, indicating the exhaustion of five zang viscera qi. The pulse which is strong and regularly intermittent indicates the obstruction in meridians caused by traumatic injury, fear or pain, etc. It is caused by pathogen blockage and qi stagnation.

（28）Swift pulse

1）Feeling

The pulse is more rapid and beats more than 120 beats per minute. It is the extreme condition of rapid pulse.

2）Clinical significance

The swift and forceful pulse means the unrestrained exorbitant yang. It can be seen in extremely heat condition of cold-attack or warm diseases with exhaustion of yin, and is a critical sign.

The forceful swift pulse indicates exuberance of yang and excessive heat. The weak swift pulse usually suggests the yin deficiency and phthisis.

If the pulse is swift and surge, it is present in disease characterized by fidget and chest distress. If the pulse is swift and deep, it is due to disease of abdominal pain. And both of them reflect the condition that the yin or yang will be exhausted.

The 28 pulse qualities can be grouped into six groups of pulses on the basis of similar qualities in follow Table 6-2.

Table 6-2   **Six groups of pulses**

Groups	Names	Feeling	Clinical significance
The Floating kind	Floating pulse	The position of the pulse is shallow and can be easily felt with a light pressure of the fingers, its force decreases slightly in the deeper level	Exterior syndrome, deficiency syndrome
	Surging pulse	The pulse feels wide and powerful and like roaring waves	Syndrome of exuberant heat
	Soggy pulse	The pulse feels floating, thin and soft. If a stronger pressure is applied to feel the deep level, it disappears	Deficiency and dampness syndrome
	Scattered pulse	This pulse feels very floating, scattered, without root. It is relatively superficial	Original qi dissociation and zang-fu viscera qi will disappear
	Hollow pulse	The pulse is floating, big and hollow, and the feeling is similar to touch the leaf of green Chinese onion	Blood loss and yin depletion
	Tympanic pulse	This pulse feels hard and tight at the superficial level but completely empty at the deep level, and the feeling is like pressing a drum leather	Severe deficiency of the kidney essence or yin
The Deep kind	Deep pulse	The pulse only responds to the fingers when heavy pressure and is felt near the bone	Interior syndrome
	Hidden pulse	This pulse is very deep and difficult to feel and it only can be felt when pressing to the muscles and bones	Pathogen block, syncope and extreme pain
	Firm pulse	The pulse can be felt only at the deep level and it feels hard, big, long, rather wiry, and the vessel is fixed	Interior excess cold syndrome, abdominal mass, hernia
	Weak pulse	A weak pulse is extremely soft and thin, and can be seen only at the deep level	Deficiency of both qi and blood and deficiency of yang

Continue to Table 6-2

Groups	Names	Feeling	Clinical significance
The Slow kind	Slow pulse	The pulse rate is less than 60 beats per minute and pulsates slowly	Cold syndrome
	Moderate pulse	The pulse rate is close to normal pulse(60 beats per minute),and moves smoothly	Damp syndrome, spleen-stomach qi deficiency syndrome
	Uneven pulse	The pulse feels unsmooth and sluggish like scraping a piece of bamboo with a sharp knife	Syndrome of damage of essence,insufficiency of blood
	Knotted pulse	The pulse beats slowly(less than 60 beats per minute) with irregular and intermittent timing of beats	Cold,phlegm,stagnated blood,accumulation of abdominal mass,deficiency of both qi and blood
The Rapid kind	Rapid pulse	The pulse rate is rapid and over 90 beats per minute	Heat syndrome, deficiency syndrome
	Rapid intermittent pulse	The pulse beats rapidly(more than 90 beats per minute) with irregular intermittent. It is the extreme condition of rapid pulse	Exuberance of yang,qi and blood stagnation, phlegm and food accumulation,the decline of five zang viscera qi
	Swift pulse	The pulse is more rapid and beats more than 120 beats per minute. It is the extreme condition of rapid pulse	Extremely heat condition of cold-attack or warm diseases with exhaustion of yin
	Tremulous pulse	The shape of the pulse just like a bean,it is slippery, rapid and short,and it "trembles" under the finger	Pain,alarmed and panicky
The Feeble kind	Feeble pulse	The empty pulse feels rather big but soft when pressed at three regions	Deficiency syndrome
	Faint pulse	The pulse is extremely small,soft and weak. It is difficult to feel,and become vague when pressing	Heavy deficiency of both qi and blood or decline of yang
	Thready pulse	The pulse feels thin and soft like a thread,but with quite obvious pulsation	Yin blood deficiency, dampness syndrome
	Regular intermittent pulse	The pulse beats slowly(less than 60 beats per minute) and weak with regular intermittent	Exhaustion of five zang viscera qi, traumatic injury, pain,fear
	Short pulse	The pulse is shorter than normal	Forceful short pulse means qi depression, weak short pulse means qi deficiency

Continue to Table 6-2

Groups	Names	Feeling	Clinical significance
The Full kind	Replete pulse	The pulse feels forceful at all three regions with no matter at what level	Excess syndrome
	Slippery pulse	The slippery pulse feels smooth, rounded to the touch, just like a rolling pearl under skin and slides under the fingers	Phlegm and fluid retention, indigestion or excess heat
	Tight pulse	The pulse is tight and strong, feeling like a stretched and twisted cord under fingers	Syndromes of cold, pain, indigestion
	Long pulse	The pulse is straight and basically longer than normal	Hyperactivity of liver yang, exuberant heat
	Wiry pulse	The pulse is long and straight, feeling like a string of drown bow under fingers	Liver or gallbladder diseases, pains, phlegm and fluid retention

6.4.2   Palpation

The palpation is to touch and press directly some parts of the patient's body to feel the cold or warm, dry or moist, soft or hard, tender pain, lump or other morbid changes, so as to infer the position, nature and condition of the disease.

6.4.2.1   Significance of palpation

Palpation is an important part of the pulse taking, and is also an indispensable part of the four examinations. It is important for the diagnosis of abdominal disease. It can also enrich and improve clinical data, and provide objective evidence.

6.4.2.2   Method of palpation

The first step is to select the position and then fully expose the location to be examined. According to the different purpose and location of the examination, the patient is required to sit or lie supine. When the patient takes the seat, the doctor needs to sit or stand in front of the patient. The doctor uses the left hand to fix the patient, and the right hand touches and presses on one part of the body. Its purpose is to examine the skin, extremities acupoints and so on. When palpating the chest and abdomen, the patient should lie and keep relaxed with hands laid aside and legs stretched. The doctor ought to stand by the right side of the patient. The right hand or both hands are used for palpating certain parts of the chest and abdomen.

6.4.2.3   Content of palpation

The application range of the consultation is quite extensive, and the commonly used clinical examination is palpating the chest and rid-side, abdomen, skin, extremity, acupoints.

(1) Palpating the chest and rid-side

Chest is from the clavicle to the diaphragm. The bilateral sides of chest from the axillary to the costal margin are rid-side. The chest is the house of the heart and the lung, and the rid-side is the house of the liver and gallbladder. In addition to the diagnosis of local skin and bone, palpating the chest and rid-side are also diagnosed with the heart, lung, liver and gallbladder.

1) Palpating the chest

Palpating the chest is aware of the cardiac apex, chest and breast examination.

● Palpating the cardiac apex: Cardiac apex is located left nipple with apex beating. It is the meeting region of all meridians. So it is an important method for detecting pectoral qi.

In normal condition, the bouncing in cardiac apex is neither rapid nor slow in the moderate force and can be felt with fingers. That is the sign of healthy person of abundant heart qi and pectoral qi in chest.

The feeble beating is caused by the deficiency of pectoral qi, and the too strong beating is sign of escaping pectoral qi. The slow beating is due to the deficiency of heart yang. The extremely forceful beating in a large region and faint beating is sign of heart qi failure and both indicate dangerous. The forceful beating that can be easily seen in women before delivery is not a good sign. The scattered beating with lifted chest and asthma is sign of expiring heart qi and lung qi.

● Palpating the chest: The lifted anterior chest accompanying with asthma occurring by pressing belongs to lung distension. If pain occurs when pressing, it belongs to heart pathogen congesting the lung and retention of fluid in the chest and rid-side.

● Palpating the breast: There are several nodules in the normal breast. There is a sense of particle and flexibility at the time of diagnosis, without pain. If the breast area has tenderness, accompanied by redness and swelling, scorching, it usually indicates acute mastitis.

2) Palpating the rid-side

The liver is located in the right flank, connecting the gallbladder though the meridians. Hypochondriac pain alleviated by pressing is due to liver deficiency. Hypochondriac pain exacerbated by pressing or cough is suspending fluid retention. The swelling below costal margin with red skin and tender pain belongs to liver abscess.

(2) Palpating the abdomen

Palpating the abdomen refers to touch the stomach and abdomen by fingers to acquire the situation of local cold or heat, hard or soft, fullness, mass, tenderness, etc. It is important to speculate about the zang-fu viscera lesions.

The abdomen is the body surface that from epigastrium(xiphoid) to mons pubis(pubic symphysis), generally divided into epigastrium, stomach duct, peri-navel region, lower abdomen and lateral lower abdomen. The lower part of the xiphoid is epigastrium, to reflect the function of heart and diaphragm. Stomach duct is from heart to navel. The surrounding part of the navel is called peri-navel region. Lower abdomen is from navel to mons pubis, and is the house of small intestine, uterus and bladder. The sides of the lower abdomen are called lateral lower abdomen.

1) Cold or heat

If the stomach duct and abdomen is cool and the patient likes to be warmed and pressed, it reflects cold syndrome. While it is warm and the patient likes to be cooled, it is heat syndrome.

2) Distention and fullness

Distention and fullness is divided into excess and deficiency. If there is a persistent abdominal distention which is tense and tenderness in palpation, it belongs to excess. If the abdomen is soft without tenderness in palpation, it is deficiency.

3) Glomus and fullness

Glomus and fullness is referring to the feeling of distending and something clogged up in stomach. If the stomach region is resistance or tender pain when pressing, there is due to excess. While there is soft when pressing, it is a deficiency syndrome.

4) Lump

If the lump is moveable without fixed shape and place, and sometimes it disappears, it is called gathering which is due to qi stasis. While the lump is persistence in a fixed place, and the shape is not changed when pressed, it is called conglomerations which are due to blood stasis. The large lump suggests the disease for a long time. The rapid growth means a bad prognosis. The rough surface or irregular shape also suggests severe condition.

5) Painful

The distending pain in left lateral lower abdomen, if with hard lump in it, is due to dry feces in large intestine. The pain with lump in the right lateral lower abdomen is due to intestinal abscess.

(3) Palpating the skin

Palpating the skin is a method that the doctor touches certain part of skin of patient by hands. It is used to diagnosis the situation of cold or heat, moist or dryness, smooth or rough, pain, swelling, sore and ulcer.

1) Cold or heat

When the skin is cold, it is due to yang deficiency. When the skin is cold with great dripping sweating, accompanied with pale complexion and faint pulse verging on expiry, it is sign of yang collapse. When the skin is heat, it is due to yang excess. If the skins of four limbs are warm with oily sweating and agitated racing but forceless pulse, it is a sign of yin collapse. If the skin is very hot on touching but becomes less hot when palpating for a moment, it suggests exterior heat. While the skin becomes hotter when keeping touching for a little while, it reflects interior heat.

2) Moist, dryness, smooth or rough

It reflects the state of the sweating and qi, blood and fluid. The moist skin shows sweating, while the dry skin reflects no sweating or insufficiency of the fluid. The smooth skin is due to harmony of qi and blood, while the rough skin is the sign of the deficiency of qi and blood.

3) Swelling

The edema and qi swelling can be distinguished by pressing the swelling of skin. When the skin is swollen, if a deep finger shape pitting is formed when it is pressed and returns to flat soon after release the finger, it is qi swelling. If the pitting is formed by pressing but could not return to flat, it is edema.

4) Sore and ulcer

It is diagnosed by whether there is pus or not in the sore. If the sore is hard and warm, there is certainly no pus in it. The hot sore with soft peak and hard root, it is most likely that there is pus. The hot sore with pain pertains belongs to yang syndrome, while the hard, not hot sore with feeling of numb belongs to yin syndrome.

(4) Palpating the extremity

It is a method to judgement the cold, heat, deficiency or excess of the disease by touching the degree of cold and heat of the patient's extremities. If all hands and feet are cold, it belongs to cold syndrome. While all hands and feet are heat, it is heat syndrome. If the forehead or the dorsal part of hand is hotter than palm, it is an exterior heat. While the palm is hotter than the forehead or the dorsal part of hand, it belongs to interior heat.

The cold fingertip of child indicates child fright reversal. The hot middle finger with other normal fingers of child reflects exogenous wind-cold. Only the middle finger is cold, it is a sign of measles.

It is valuable for judging the prognosis to survey the temperature of extremities. If the extremities are still warm in a yang deficiency syndrome, the patient can be saved. While the extremities are cold, the prognosis is bad.

(5)Palpating the acupoints

The acupoint is the place where the qi passes through, it is response point of the visceral lesion in the surface. It is to detect the inner diseases by pressing and watching some acupoints and observing the reaction.

Palpating the acupoints should be noted that there are or not tender pain, sensitive skin and hardened nodule or cold-like nodule on the points.

The frequently used acupoints for diagnosing visceral disease in clinic are following:

For lung diseases:Zhongfu(LU 1),Feishu(BL 13),Taiyuan(LU 9).

For heart diseases:Juque(CV 14),Danzhong(CV 17),Daling(PC 7).

For liver diseases:Qimen(LR 14),Ganshu(BL 18),Taichong(LR 3).

For spleen diseases:Zhangmen(LR 13),Taibai(SP 3),Pishu(BL 20).

For kidney diseases:Qihai(CV 6),Taixi(KI 3).

For large intestine diseases:Tianshu(ST 25),Dachangshu(BL 25).

For small intestine disease:Guanyuan(CV 4).

For gallbladder diseases:Riyue(GB 24),Danshu(BL 19).

For stomach diseases:Weishu(BL 21),Zusanli(ST 36).

For bladder diseases:Zhongji(CV 3).

Wang Xiaoyan,Yuan Xiaoxia,Zhang Jiping

Chapter 7

Differentiation of Syndromes

Differentiation of syndromes is one of essential principles and characteristics in TCM to analyze, differentiate and recognize the syndrome of disease. According to the varieties of clinical data obtained from the four diagnostic methods, we can analyze and summarize the medical data and finally to conclude the current pathological nature. From the above, it is obvious that differentiation of syndromes is the premise and foundation of treatment.

In the theory of TCM, there are a number of methods to differentiate syndromes, such as differentiation of syndromes according to the eight principals; differentiation of syndromes according to the zang-fu viscera theory; differentiation of syndromes according to the theory of qi, blood and body fluid; differentiation of syndromes according to the theory of six meridians; differentiation of syndromes according to the theory of triple energizer; differentiation of syndromes according to the theory of wei, qi, ying and xue; and differentiation of syndromes according to the cause of disease. Each method has its particular aspects and features. They connect with each other and should be applied flexibly and accurately so as to understand a disease comprehensively.

7.1 Differentiation of syndromes by eight principles

The differentiation of syndromes by eight principles is the basic principle of TCM knowledge and treatment of diseases, which is a special study and treatment of TCM. The differentiation of eight principles is under the guidance of TCM theory, a comprehensive analysis of clinical manifestations to determine which treatment method to choose based on the process of thinking, that is the process of syndrome differentiation. Chinese medicine believes that the same disease in different stages of development, there may be different syndromes; and different diseases in its development process may also appear the same syndrome.

Although the disease's manifestation is extremely complicated, it can be basically summed up in eight categories, they are yin syndrome, yang syndrome, cold syndrome, heat syndrome, exterior syndrome, interior syndrome, deficiency syndrome and excess syndrome. The exterior and interior syndromes are two principles to distinguish the depth of the disease severity. Cold and heat are two important conceptions of TCM, which are used to differentiate the nature of diseases. Deficiency and excess are two concepts of TCM to distinguish the ups and downs of the healthy qi and pathogenic qi in the body. Yin and yang are the general principles of differentiation of syndromes, and also the key of eight principles. All in all, the syndromes are not immutable but intertwined, interconnected and mutually transformed. Syndrome is not only a process of understanding the disease, but also the key to opening the treasure chest of Chinese medicine.

7.1.1 Exterior-interior syndrome differentiation

The exterior and interior syndromes are two principles to distinguish the depth of the disease severity. Exterior and interior syndrome is a relative concept, such as skin and bones are relative terms, the skin belongs to the exterior, and the bones belong to interior.

Zang and fu are relative terms, the zang belongs to the exterior, the fu belongs to the interior; meridians and zang-fu viscera, the meridians belong to the exterior, the zang-fu viscera belongs to the interior and so on. Clinically, when the muscular exterior is infected with the exogenous contraction, and the location of the disease is shallow, we call it exterior syndrome; while the zang-fu viscera is infected, and the location of the disease is deep, we call it interior syndrome. This is the concept of exterior and interior. The exterior-interior syndrome differentiation is mainly based on clinical manifestations, so exterior and interior cannot be understood as an anatomical location. For example: a disease may be caused by an exterior pathogenic factor, but if this is affecting the internal organs, the condition will be classified as an interior. Therefore, a disease is classified as "exterior" not because it is derived from an exterior pathogenic factor but because its manifestations are such that they are located in the "exterior" of the body.

Exterior-interior syndrome differentiation is very important for the treatment of disease. Through it we can understand the severity of illness, and predict the trend of disease. The condition of exogenous contraction disease is better than endogenous injury disease in general. With the exterior pathogenic factor non-stop in-depth affects bodies, exterior syndrome will become interior syndrome, and the body's condition is deteriorating.

7.1.1.1　Exterior syndrome

When an exterior pathogenic factor affects the skin, muscles and meridians, we mean that these areas have been invaded by an exterior pathogenic factor through skin, mouth and nose, giving rise to typical "exterior syndrome" clinical manifestations. It is usually seen at the early stage of exogenous contraction disease because it is sudden onset and short-lived.

(1) Clinical manifestations of exterior syndrome

Aversion to cold or wind, fever, head and body ache all over, stiff neck, stuffy and running nose, cough, itching and pain throat, short of breath, light red tongue, thin white coating, floating pulse.

(2) Analysis of exterior syndrome

Exterior syndromes refer to those clinical manifestations caused by six exogenous pathogenic through the skin, mouth and nose. It is the result of healthy qi fighting against the pathogenic qi in the superficial, and this confrontation will disturb the normal diffusion function, so fever and aversion to cold and wind appear. Exogenous pathogenic factor lingers on the superficial portion resulting in the blockage of qi which causes headache, stiff neck and general pain. As the lung is responsible for skin and opens in the nose, so when the superficial portion under attacks, the lung qi would fail to diffuse. As a consequence, stuffy and running nose, cough, itching and pain throat, short of breath, would happen. Since the exogenous pathogenic factors are still in the superficial portion, defensive qi will be affected and cannot rise, so the tongue will manifest as light red tongue with thin white coating. When the combat between the healthy qi and the pathogenic qi is in the superficial portion, the vessel qi will be aroused, so the pulse is floating.

(3)Key points

Aversion to cold or wind, fever, stuffy and running nose, light red tongue, thin white coating, floating pulse.

(4)Treatment methods

Resolve the exterior pathogenic factor.

7.1.1.2   Interior syndrome

Interior syndrome is relative to the exterior syndrome, it refers to the syndrome which appears when the zang-fu viscera , qi and blood, emotion are affected by pathogenic factors as well as improper diet, when the disease is located inside, it also can be classified as interior syndrome. The main features of interior syndrome include long-lived and awfully unwell.

(1)Clinical manifestations of interior syndrome

The manifestations of interior syndrome are complicated and can be covered in a wide range. All the manifestations which do not belong to exterior syndrome are in the category of interior syndrome. Its common symptoms include high fever and aversion to heat, irritability dizziness, or low fever, the coating is not thin and white, the pulse is not floating and so on.

(2)Analysis of interior syndrome

The manifestations listed above are some common symptoms. High fever and aversion to heat are the result of severe interior heat, it may cause constipation, thirsty, irritability dizziness and urethral burning sensation too. When the yang qi is deficiency, as a consequence, low fever, aversion to cold, tired and frequent urination would happen. Since the pathogenic factors are still affecting the interior portion, the pulse will change according to the deficiency and excess of the yang qi and yin qi.

(3)Key points

High fever and aversion to heat, irritability dizziness, frequent urination and other symptoms do not belong to exterior syndrome.

(4)Treatment methods

There are varieties of treatment methods for different kinds of interior syndrome, including reinforcing the immune system, eliminating pathogenic factors and so on.

7.1.1.3   Half-exterior and half-interior syndrome

When an exterior pathogenic factor transmits into an internal portion but not yet completely becomes an interior syndrome, or an internal caused disease heals gradually and the interior pathogenic factors are driven to leave by healthy qi, we mean it is a half-exterior and half-interior syndrome. It is usually seen at the stage of deadlock between healthy qi and pathogenic qi.

(1)Clinical manifestations of half-exterior and half-interior syndrome

The manifestations of half-exterior and half-interior syndrome are representative. Its common symptoms include frequent fever, chest tightness, thirst, dizziness and nausea, poor appetite, the pulse is stiff and so on.

(2)Analysis of half-exterior and half-interior syndrome

The manifestation differs from one syndrome to another since the causes are different. Half-exterior and half-interior syndrome is caused by exterior pathogenic factor which breaks the superficial defense system and transmits into the body. At this time, the healthy qi rises to fight against the exterior pathogenic factor, so frequent fever, chest tightness, thirst, dizziness and nausea, and other symptoms come into being.

(3)Key points

Frequent fever, chest tightness, thirst, dizziness and nausea, the pulse is stiff.

（4）Treatment methods

Resolve the exterior pathogenic factor and reconcile the internal pathogenesis.

7.1.2　Cold-heat syndrome differentiation

Cold and heat are two important concepts of TCM，which are used to differentiate the nature of diseases. Pathogenic qi is divided into two kinds of yang pathogenicity and yin pathogenicity，healthy qi is divided into yang qi and yin qi. Cold syndrome and heat syndrome of diseases are the reflections of the deficiency or excess conditions of yin and yang in the body. Cold can be caused by yin excess or yang deficiency，so cold syndrome reflects yin excess or yang deficiency in the body. Heat can be caused by yang excess or yin deficiency，so heat syndrome reflects yang excess or yin deficiency in the body. Cold-heat syndrome differentiation is extremely important for the treatment of diseases，because cold syndrome and heat syndrome use the opposite treatment，so we must distinguish the right syndrome or the result will definitely turn out to be just the opposite of wish.

There are both similarities and differences between cold syndrome and heat syndrome. Aversion to cold and fever is the symptom of diseases，and the symptom maybe a false signal from the body，however the syndrome reflects the true nature of diseases，so we should make the correct treatment according to the syndrome.

7.1.2.1　Cold syndrome

Cold syndrome refers to the conditions caused by cold pathogenic factors invading body or yang qi deficiency in the body. Cold pathogenic factors include external cold，cold food，cold air，etc. The deficiency of yang qi may due to chronic disease or morbid indulge in sexual pleasures. According to the difference of causes and location of cold syndrome，cold syndrome can be divided into many different types. Such as exterior cold，interior cold，excess cold and so on.

（1）Clinical manifestations of cold syndrome

The manifestations of cold syndrome are complicated and different，but there are some common manifestations such as：aversion to cold and chills with preference for warmth，cold limbs and want to huddle up，facial white expression，tastelessness in the mouth，lack of thirsty，diluted and clear sputum，running nose，cold pain，frequent and clear urination，loose stools，light pale tongue with moist coating，slow or tight pulse.

（2）Analysis of cold syndrome

Cold syndromes refer to those clinical manifestations caused by cold pathogenic factors invading the facial of body or yang qi deficiency in the body. Since the yang qi is deficient or obstructed by exogenous cold，so it cannot play the role of a warming body，and the results of aversion to cold and chills with preference for warmth，cold limbs and want to huddle up，facial white expression，cold pain，etc. appear，Because the cold is preponderant in the body and body fluid cannot be stimulated，so there is tastelessness in the mouth，lack of thirsty，diluted and clear sputum，running nose，frequent and clear urination，loose stools and a light pale tongue with moist coating. Tight pulse is due to the obstruction of yang qi and slow pulse is caused by the deficiency of yang which has less power to stimulate meridian qi circulation.

（3）Key points

Aversion to cold and chills with preference for warmth，cold limbs and want to huddle up，facial white expression，cold pain，frequent urination，light pale tongue with moist coating，slow or tight pulse.

（4）Treatment methods

Supplement the body of yang and disperse the exogenous cold.

7.1.2.2 Heat syndrome

Heat syndrome refers to those diseases with clinical manifestations of heat. It may be caused by exogenous heat out of body, the deficiency of yin in the body, cold and dampness transforming into heat, emotional stress turning into heat or irregular diet result of heat. The heat syndromes can be covered in a wide range including the exterior heat, the interior heat, the deficiency heat and excess heat.

(1) Clinical manifestations of heat syndrome

The manifestations of heat syndrome are different and can be covered in a wide range. The typical symptoms are aversion to heat with a preference for cold, thirsty with a preference for cold drinks, irritability dizziness, flushed complexion, restlessness and insomnia, thick and yellowish and sticky of sputum and nasal mucus, bleeding, dark urine, dry stools, red tongue with a yellow and dry coating, rapid pulse.

(2) Analysis of heat syndrome

Since the heat syndrome is caused by yin deficiency in the body or yang excess, so the body aversion to heat and fever will occur. Excess yang will over stimulate the flowing of blood, so there is a red tongue with a yellow and dry coating, bleeding, flushed complexion and rapid pulse. The heat over stimulates and consumes the fluids in the body, which results in thirsty with a preference for cold drinks, thick and yellowish and sticky of sputum, short and dark urine, nasal mucus and dry stools. The excessive heat affects the heart, so irritability dizziness, restlessness and insomnia will happen.

(3) Key points

Aversion to heat with a preference for cold, thirsty with preference for cold drinks, irritability dizziness, flushed complexion, thick and yellowish and sticky of sputum and nasal mucus, dry stools, red tongue with a yellow and dry coating, rapid pulse.

(4) Treatment methods

Supplement the body of yin and clear away the excessive exogenous heat.

7.1.3 Deficiency-excess syndrome differentiation

Deficiency and excess are two concepts of TCM to distinguish the ups and downs of the healthy qi and pathogenic qi in the body. Deficiency refers to deficient healthy qi, and excess refers to excessive of pathogenic qi. Deficiency means the body immunity is lowered and its function is weak, and excess denotes that the pathogenic factors are hyperactive. Only correct understanding of the patient is deficiency or excess, in order to provide the basis for treatment, and then to make accurate judgments.

Since every disease is caused by the conflict of healthy qi and pathogenic qi, so the deficiency syndrome and excess syndrome refer to the future trends of disease. Likewise, we can treat the disease by adjusting the body's healthy qi and pathogenic qi by making up for its deficiency and undermining its surplus.

7.1.3.1 Deficiency syndrome

Deficiency syndrome refers to the disease of which manifestations are showing that the body lacks of health factor, caused by the congenital deficiency, improper diet, over work, excessive sex or some chronic diseases and so on. Qi and blood are the essential substances of the body, and they are transferred and related to each other in certain conditions. So qi deficiency syndrome is caused by insufficiency of zang-fu viscera or the deficiency of blood, the same to blood deficiency syndrome but external injury may cause blood deficiency immediately.

(1) Clinical manifestations of deficiency syndrome

The manifestations of deficiency syndrome are complicated and different from each syndrome, so it is difficult to be covered in a range, but they have common manifestations. The manifestations of qi deficiency syndrome include short breath, low voices, lassitude, pale complexion, blurred vision, motioning sweat, and symptoms getting worse by physical activity, pale tongue and weak pulse. The manifestations of blood deficiency syndrome include pale or yellowish face, blurred vision, mental sluggishness, pale lips and nails, numbness limbs, irregular menstruation, memory lapses, pale tongue, thin and weak pulse, etc. The manifestations of yang deficiency syndrome include cold limbs and aversion to cold, sensitive to cold weather, cold pain in back, favoured hot water, numbness limbs, lassitude, motioning sweat, edema of limbs after tired, diarrhea, frequent urination at night, hyposexuality, men prone to impotency, menstrual reduction in women, depression, clear and copious urine, pale tongue with white coating, weakness pulse, etc. The manifestations of yin deficiency syndrome include aversion to heat and favoured drink cool, dry mouth and nose and throat, constipation, yellow urine, dry eyes and skin, sleep sweat, fever in the afternoon, flushed cheeks, hot sensation in palm, constipation, insomnia, red tongue with dry coating, rapid pulse, etc.

(2) Analysis of deficiency syndrome

There is a wide range of manifestations of deficiency syndrome, but the etiology can be divided into two parts, yang deficiency and yin deficiency. If the yang is deficient, so the body and zang-fu viscera cannot be warmed, and symptoms like cold limbs and aversion to cold, frequent urination at night, hyposexuality, sensitive to cold weather, cold pain in back, favoured hot water will appear. When the yang qi has less power to promote blood to the upper and further portion of the body, the pale tongue with white coating, lassitude, and motioning sweat will occur. When yang qi fails to flow in the meridian, people will feel tired easily and their pulse becomes weakness. If the yang qi fails to warm and transform the body fluids, edema of limbs after tired and diarrhea appear. If the yin is deficient, the symptoms are different from yang deficiency syndrome, and flushed face and red tongue will appear. When the yin qi is not enough to compete with the yang qi, the excessive yang qi will force the yin fluids out of the body, so the sleep sweat, aversion to heat and favoured drink cool, dry mouth and nose and throat, dry eyes and skin will appear. When the excessive yang qi is burning the yin-fluid of the body, flushed cheeks, hot sensation in palm, constipation, insomnia, red tongue with dry coating, rapid pulse and so on will occur.

(3) Key points

Qi deficiency: short breath, low voices, lassitude, motioning sweat, symptoms getting worse by physical activity, pale tongue and weak pulse. Blood deficiency: pale or yellowish face, blurred vision, pale lips and nails, numbness limbs, irregular menstruation, memory lapses, pale tongue, thin and weak pulse. Yang deficiency: cold limbs and aversion to cold, sensitive to cold weather, cold pain in back, favouredhot water, motioning sweat, edema of limbs after tired, diarrhea, frequent urination at night, hyposexuality, men prone to impotency, menstrual reduction in women, pale tongue with white coating, weakness pulse. Yin deficiency: aversion to heat and favoureddrink cool, dry mouth and nose and throat, constipation, dry eyes and skin, sleep sweat, fever in the afternoon, flushed cheeks, hot sensation in palm, constipation, insomnia, red tongue with dry coating, rapid pulse.

(4) Treatment methods

Supplement the human body with the corresponding lack of materials like yin, yang, qi or blood, and clear away the pathological products.

7.1.3.2 Excess syndrome

Excess syndrome is a generalization of the wide range of clinical manifestations of body affected by the exterior pathogenic factor or over-accumulation of pathological products in the body. There are two main causes of excess syndrome, exterior pathogenic factor affects external of the body, or the dysfunction of zang-fu viscera internal of the body.

(1) Clinical manifestations of excess syndrome

The clinical manifestations vary with the difference types of excess syndrome due to the different of pathogenic factors and affected regions. There are some common symptoms included mostly are acute diseases, high fever, chest tightness, restlessness even coma delirium, constipation, coarse breathing, excessive phlegm, pain and aggravated by pressure, difficulty and yellow urine, red tongue with thick and greasy coating, excess and powerful pulse, etc.

(2) Analysis of excess syndrome

As the excessive of the pathogenic factors affect body, which cause the body healthy qi to rise up to fight against it. Excess syndrome can be covered in two ranges. Firstly, it occurs when the exterior pathogenic factors including wind, cold, summer heat, dampness, dryness, hot and pestilence, invades the body. Secondly, there are functional disorders of the zang-fu viscera, and which produce some pathological products in the body, like sputum, dampness, blood stasis, undigested food, excessive water, etc. Because of the effect of the pathogenic factors in vivo the healthy qi will fluctuate. If the yang is excess, high fever, constipation, difficulty and yellow urine will appear. If the movement of qi is obstructed by pathogenic factors, the liquid absorption and metabolism would be stagnated and cause chest tightness, coarse breathing, excessive phlegm, difficulty urine, tongue with thick and greasy coating. Pain and aggravated by pressure indicates that there are something pathological products blocking the meridian. And if there are excessive qi and blood flowing in the vessel, the pulse will become powerful and rapid.

(3) Key points

Acute diseases, high fever, chest tightness. restlessness and even coma delirium, constipation, coarse breathing, excessive phlegm, pain and aggravated by pressure, difficulty and yellow urine, red tongue with thick and greasy coating, excess and powerful pulse.

(4) Treatment methods

Eliminate the extra yang qi and clear away the pathological products.

7.1.4　Yin-yang syndrome differentiation

Yin and yang are the general principles of differentiation of syndromes, and also the key of eight principles. In the diagnosis, according to the clinical manifestations of the pathological nature of the symptoms, all diseases can be divided into two main aspects of yin and yang. Thus, syndromes of the exterior, heat and excess are classified as the yang syndrome, and the other syndromes of interior, cold and deficiency are classified as the yin syndrome.

Clinically, due to the syndromes of interior, exterior, deficiency, excess, cold and heat are sometimes interwoven with each other and cannot be completely divided. In this case the yin syndrome and yang syndrome sometimes intereact, causing complex syndromes as disussed in the coming chapters, such as false appearance of syndromes, interchange of syndromes and combination of syndromes. In addition to the yin syndrome and yang syndrome named with the yin and yang, there are some other conditions such as the deficiency of true yin, yang prostration or yin prostration, etc.

7.1.4.1　Yin syndrome

Yin syndrome refers to those syndromes of negative clinical manifestations, including deficiency syndrome, interior syndrome and cold syndrome. It is caused by congenital deficiency, improper diet, over work, excessive sex and long lasting disease.

(1) Clinical manifestations of yin syndrome

Different diseases, the performance of the negative symptoms are not the same, they all have their own focus, and there are some common manifestations as follows: pale complexion, lassitude, low voice, aversion to cold and chills with preference for warmth, cold limbs and want to huddle up, diluted and clear sputum, loss of appetite, frequent and clear urination, loose stools, pale tongue with moist coating, slow or weak pulse.

(2)Analysis of yin syndrome

Yin syndrome is caused by the deficiency of yang and qi. When there is less qi to promote the normal function of zang-fu viscera, it will result in pale complexion, lassitude, loss of appetite, low voice. If there is no enough yang to warm the zang-fu viscera, aversion to cold and chills with preference for warmth, cold limbs and want to huddle up, diluted and clear sputum, frequent and clear urination, pale tongue with moist coating will appear. When the yang has less power to promote blood and qi flow in the meridian and to the upper or further portion of the body, the pulse will become slow and weak.

(3)Key points

Pale complexion, lassitude, low voice, aversion to cold and chills with preference for warmth, cold limbs and want to huddle up, diluted and clear sputum, loss of appetite, preference for hot water, dull eyes, slow movement, frequent and clear urination, loose stools, pale tongue with moist coating, slow or weak pulse.

(4)Treatment methods

Supplement the human body with the corresponding lack of materials like yin, yang, qi or blood, eliminate the exterior pathogenic factor and clear away the pathological products in the body.

7.1.4.2　Yang syndrome

Yang syndrome refers to those syndromes of active clinical manifestations, including excess syndrome, exterior syndrome and heat syndrome. The symptoms of yang syndrome are characterized by excitation, hyperactivity, brightness, which is caused by excessive heat or yang pathogenic factors, or the conflict between strong health qi and exterior pathogenic factor.

(1)Clinical manifestations of yang syndrome

Different diseases, the performance of the yang symptoms are not the same, there are some common manifestations as follows: mostly are acute diseases, aversion to heat with preference for cold, thirsty with preference for cold drinks, dry stools, irritability dizziness, flushed complexion, restlessness and insomnia, high fever, chest tightness, restlessness even coma delirium, constipation, coarse breathing, excessive phlegm, pain and aggravated by pressure, difficulty and yellow urine, red tongue with thick and greasy coating, excess and powerful pulse, etc.

(2)Analysis of yang syndrome

Yang syndrome is a summary of exterior syndrome, heat syndrome and excess syndrome. It is caused by the excessive heat pathogenic factors. When the body is affected by a pathogenic factor, whose location is exterior, and the nature is heat or excess, it will show many symptoms which belong to yang syndrome. Fever and aversion to cold and mostly acute diseases are the representative characteristics of exterior syndrome. There are some typical symptoms of heat and excess syndrome as follows: aversion to heat with preference for cold, thirsty with preference for cold drinks, dry stools, irritability dizziness, flushed complexion, restlessness and insomnia, high fever, chest tightness, restlessness even coma delirium, constipation, coarse breathing, excessive phlegm, pain and aggravated by pressure, difficulty and yellow urine, red tongue with thick and greasy coating, excess and powerful pulse, so it also belongs to yang syndrome.

(3)Key points

Aversion to heat with preference for cold, thirsty with preference for cold drinks, dry stools, flushed complexion, restlessness and insomnia, high fever, restlessness even coma delirium, constipation, coarse breathing, excessive phlegm, pain and aggravated by pressure, difficulty and yellow urine, red tongue with thick and greasy coating, excess and powerful pulse.

(4)Treatment methods

Harmoniz qi and blood in the body and clear away the pathological products.

7.2　Differentiating syndromes according to zang-fu viscera

Differentiating syndromes according to zang-fu viscera theory is a differential method by which symptoms and signs are analyzed to clarify the cause, and location and nature of disease as well as the conditions between vital qi and pathogens in light of the theories of viscera manifestation, yin-yang and five elements. It is an important component part of all differential systems in TCM, including differentiating syndromes according to zang viscera diseases, fu viscera diseases and complicated diseases of both zang viscera with fu viscera.

7.2.1　Syndromes differentiation of heart and small intestine

Heart, situated in the chest and protected on the outside by the pericardium, is internally-externally connected with small intestine and related closely with vessels in tissues. And it takes tongue as its orifice and manifests in complexion. Its physiological functions include: dominating blood and housing the spirit. So it is the center of mental, conscious and emotional activities. The physiological functions of small intestine are to clear from the turbid and to absorb the decomposed food.

The main pathologies of heart and small intestine manifests as disorder in governing the blood vessel, abnormality in governing the spirit-mind. As a consequence, the common symptoms and signs include: chest pain, palpitations, restlessness, insomnia, poor memory, unconsciousness, irregular or intermittent pulse, pain and ulceration of the tongue. The differentiation syndromes of heart can be classified generally into deficiency and excess. The details are as follows: heart qi deficiency, heart blood deficiency, heart yang deficiency, sudden prostration of heart yang, heart yin deficiency, heart fire flaming, phlegm-fire disturbing heart, mind confusion by phlegm, heart blood stagnation and obstruction and excess-heart in small intestine.

7.2.1.1　The syndrome of heart qi deficiency

The syndrome of heart qi deficiency refers to the condition of heart qi weakness in pushing blood flow. The main symptoms include: palpitations, mental fatigue and general symptoms of qi deficiency syndrome.

The clinical manifestation as follows: chest oppression, palpitations, shortness of breath, spontaneous sweating, mental fatigue, symptoms worsening with physical exertion and a pale complexion. The tongue is pale and the pulse is deficient.

7.2.1.2　The syndrome of heart-blood deficiency

The syndrome of heart-blood deficiency refers to the condition of general weakness such as dizziness, chest oppression, palpitations, insomnia, dream-disturbed sleep and the general symptoms of blood deficiency syndromes.

The clinical manifestation as follows: chest oppression, palpitations, dizziness, blurred vision, insomnia, poor memory, dream-disturbed sleep, pale or sallow complexion. The tongue is pale and the pulse is deficient.

7.2.1.3　The syndrome of heart yang deficiency

The syndrome of heart yang deficiency refers to the condition of heart yang failing to warm and circulate blood, resulting in producing deficient cold internally. The main symptoms include: chest oppression, palpitations and general symptoms of deficient-cold syndrome.

The clinical manifestation as follows: chest oppression and pain, palpitations, shortness of breath, aversion to cold, cold limbs, a bright white complexion and a purple face and lips. The tongue can be pale, swollen or dark-purple and the pulse can be deficient or irregular.

7.2.1.4　The syndrome of sudden prostration of heart yang

The syndrome of sudden prostration of heart yang refers to a critical condition. The heart-yang qi suddenly collapses. The main symptoms include: severe chest pain, palpitations, cold sweats, cold limbs and a weak pulse.

The clinical manifestations include: severe chest pain, palpitations, sudden cold sweats, cold limbs, a pale complexion, sudden fainting or coma and purple lips and weak respiration. The tongue is purple and the pulse is extremely faint.

7.2.1.5　The syndrome of heart yin deficiency

The syndrome of heart yin deficiency refers to the condition of yin-fluid consumption failing to nourish heart, leading to deficient heat internally. The main symptoms include: restlessness, palpitations, insomnia and general symptoms of deficient heat syndrome.

The clinical manifestations include: restlessness, palpitations, insomnia, dream-disturbed sleep, dry mouth and throat, emaciation, a feverish sensation in the palms, soles and chest, a tidal fever or low fever, night sweats and red cheeks. The tongue is dry and red with a scanty coating and pulse is thready and rapid.

7.2.1.6　The syndrome of rampancy of heart fire

The syndrome of rampancy of heart fire refers to the condition of internal accumulation of fire and heat, which would go upward to the mouth and tongue or go downward to affect the normal function of small intestine or the urinary bladder. The main symptoms include: fever, restlessness, vomiting blood, mouth ulceration and dark-yellow urine with burning pain.

The clinical manifestations include: fever, restlessness, thirst, insomnia, constipation, yellow urine, a red face, a red tip of the tongue with yellow coating, and a rapid and powerful pulse. Such manifestations may also present as mouth or tongue ulceration, scanty urine with a burning sensation, vomiting blood, mania, delirium and unclear consciousness.

7.2.1.7　The syndrome of mind confusion by phlegm

The syndrome of mind confusion by phlegm refers to the condition of turbid-phlegm disturbing the heart-mind. The main symptoms include: mental confusion, depression, dementia and loss of consciousness and general symptoms of turbid-phlegm syndromes.

The clinical manifestations include: mental confusion, dementia, inability to recognize acquainted people, muttering to oneself, sudden coma, loss of consciousness, vomiting of phlegm, a grey-dark and lusterless complexion, chest oppression, nausea and vomiting. The tongue coating is white and greasy and the pulse is slippery.

7.2.1.8　The syndrome of phlegm-fire disturbing heart

The syndrome of phlegm-fire disturbing heart refers to the condition of fire, heat and turbid-phlegm disturbing the heart-mind together. The main symptoms include: mania, delirium, loss of consciousness and general symptoms of "internal obstruction of phlegm-heat" syndrome.

The clinical manifestations include: fever, chest oppression, fast respiration, yellow sputum wheezy phlegm in the throat, thirst, restlessness, insomnia, coma, delirium, manic agitation, inability to recognize relatives or acquainted people, nonsensical talking, abnormal laughing and crying and a red face. The tongue is red with yellow and greasy coating and the slipper and rapid.

7.2.1.9 The syndrome of heart blood stagnation and obstruction

It is the syndrome due to obstruction of heart vessels brought about by stagnant blood, turbid-phlegm, accumulated yin cold and qi. The main symptoms include: mild or severe palpitation, chest oppression and pain.

The clinical manifestations include: mild or severe palpitation, distress and pain in the chest with the shoulder back and medial aspect of the arm involved.

The tongue is dark-grey with purple ecchymosis spots and the pulse is thread, hesitant and intermittent pulse. Because of obstruction of the heart vessel by phlegm, other manifestations may appear: chest oppression, obesity, fatigue, general heaviness, a white greasy coating and a deep and slippery pulse or a deep and hesitant pulse. Because of obstruction of the heart vessel by yin cold, other manifestations may appear: the pain in the chest aggravated with cold and relieved with warmth, aversion to cold, cold limbs, a pale tongue with a white coating and a deep slow or a deep and tense pulse. Because of stagnation of qi, the patients may present with a distending pain relating to emotional fluctuation, frequent sighing and a pale-red tongue and a wiry pulse.

7.2.1.10 The syndrome of excess-heart in small intestine

The syndrome of excess heat of the small intestine refers to the downward transmitting of the heart heat in the small intestine.

The clinical manifestations include: restlessness, thirsty, mouth and tongue ulceration and dark-yellow, difficult and painful urination, or bloody urine. The tongue is red with yellow coating and the pulse is rapid.

7.2.2 Syndrome differentiations of lung and large intestine

Lung resides in the chest and connects with the trachea and throat. It governs qi and manages breathing. In addition, lung governs dispersing, descending and regulates waterways. Opening into the nose, lung connects with the skin and body hair externally and it is internally-externally connected with large intestine. The physiological function of large intestine is to govern the transmission and to discharge wastes.

The main pathologies of lung lie in dysfunction of the lung in governing respiration or disturbance of the lung in regulating the water metabolism. The common symptoms and signs include: cough, spitting of phlegm, chest oppression or chest pain, and panting or fast respiration. The abnormal transmitting function of large intestine manifests as constipation and diarrhea.

7.2.2.1 The syndrome of lung qi deficiency

The syndrome of lung qi deficiency refers to the condition of declined function of lung in governing qi and defending the exterior.

The clinical manifestations include: weak cough, spitting of clear and thin phlegm, panting, lack of qi, laziness in speaking, a low voice, spontaneous sweating worse with physical exertion, aversion to wind, easily catches a common cold, fatigue and a pale complexion. The tongue is pale with white coating and the pulse is weak.

7.2.2.2 The syndrome of lung yin deficiency

The syndrome of lung yin deficiency refers to the condition of lung yin failing to disperse and descend an internal production of deficient-heat.

The clinical manifestations include:either dry and unproductive cough or cough with scanty and sticky sputum or even with blood-streaked sputum,a dry mouth and throat,emaciation,a feverish sensation in the palms,soles and chest,tidal fever,night sweats,red cheeks and a hoarse voice. The tongue is red with scanty coating and the pulse is thready and rapid.

7.2.2.3　The syndrome of dryness injuring lung

The syndrome of dryness injuring lung refers to the condition of consumption of fluids in the respiratory system. The dryness can be classified into warm dryness and cool dryness by its characteristics of more heat or colder.

The clinical manifestations include:either dry and unproductive cough or cough with scanty or sticky sputum,and sometimes even with blood-streaked sputum,chest pain,nasal bleeding,hemoptysis,dry lips, nose and throat,fever,slight aversion to wind and cold,dry stool,scanty urine and no or scanty sweating. The tongue is dry with thin coating and the pulse is superficial and rapid or superficial and tense.

7.2.2.4　The syndrome of wind-cold attacking lung

The syndrome of wind-cold attacking lung refers to the condition of the defensive qi of lung failing to disperse.

The clinical manifestations include:cough with thin and white sputum,nasal obstruction,running nose, slight aversion to cold and fever,scratchy throat,headache,general body aches and no sweating. The tongue coating is thin and white and the pulse is superficial and tense.

7.2.2.5　The syndrome of wind-heat invading lung

The syndrome of wind-heat invading lung refers to the condition of wind-heat attacking the respiratory system and affecting the lung defensive.

The clinical manifestations include: cough with yellow and sticky sputum, nasal obstruction, turbid nasal discharge,fever,slight aversion to wind-cold,a little thirst and sore throat. The tongue tip is red with thin and yellow coating and the pulse is superficial and rapid.

7.2.2.6　The syndrome of turbid phlegm obstructing lung

The syndrome of turbid phlegm obstructing lung refers to the condition of the lung failing to disperse and descend due to the retention of turbid-phlegm.

The clinical manifestations include:shortness of breath,cough with profuse sputum,and the sputum can either be thin,white and clear or sticky,easy to be expectorated,possible wheezy phlegm in the throat,cold limbs and chest oppression. The tongue is pale with a white and greasy or white and glossy coating and the pulse is either slow and soft or slippery.

7.2.2.7　The syndrome of phlegm-heat accumulating in the lung

The syndrome of phlegm-heat obstructing lung refers to the condition of excessive syndrome of the lung meridian due to the mixture of heat and phlegm being retained in the lung.

The clinical manifestations include:cough with yellow and sticky sputum,shortness of breath,panting, a red and swollen throat,a burning sensation of the nostrils and chest pain. Other symptoms may include wheezy phlegm in the throat,spitting of purulent bloody sputum,a high fever,thirst,yellow and scanty urine and constipation. The tongue is red with a yellow or yellow and greasy coating and the pulse is rapid or slippery.

7.2.2.8　The syndrome of liquid insufficiency of large intestine

The syndrome of liquid insufficiency of large intestine refers to the condition of the liquids failing to moisten the large intestine.

The clinical manifestations include: constipation, the bowel movement usually occurs once several days and other complications may include foul breath, a dry mouth and throat. The tongue is red and the pulse is thready and hesitant.

7.2.2.9 The syndrome of large intestine qi deficiency

The syndrome of large intestine qi deficiency refers to the condition of declined function of large intestine in governing transmission and discharging wastes.

The clinical manifestations include: diarrhea, dull abdominal pain, fecal incontinence, or even rectal prolapse. The tongue is pale with white and slippery coating and the pulse is weak.

7.2.2.10 The syndrome of dampness-heat in large intestine

The syndrome of dampness-heat in large intestine refers to the condition of downward transmission of dampness-heat to large intestine.

The clinical manifestations include: diarrhea, a burning sensation of the anus, dark or white sticky stool, sometimes sudden severe diarrhea with yellow and a very bad odor to the stool, abdominal pain, tenesmus, scanty and yellow urine, thirst and aversion to cold and fever or fever without aversion to cold. The tongue is red with yellow and greasy coating and the pulse is either soft and rapid or slippery and rapid.

7.2.3 Syndrome differentiations of liver and gallbladder

The liver is situated in the right-side hypochondriac area, with the gallbladder attached to it. And they are internally-externally connected through meridians. The liver opens into the eyes, its tissue shows in tendons and its luster manifests in the nails. The liver meridian of the foot jueyin starts from the dorsal hairy region of the big toe, curves around the external genitalia, goes up to the lower abdomen, spreads over the hypochondriac region, connects with the gallbladder and reaches the eye system and the vertex. The liver stores blood, maintains free flow of qi, discharges bile, and promotes the digestion and absorption of the spleen and stomach. In addition, it regulates emotion and helps to regulate irregular menstruation and seminal emission; the physiological functions of the gallbladder are to store and discharge bile and to govern decision-making.

The main pathologies of the liver manifest lie in dysfunction of liver in maintaining free flow of qi or disorder in storing the blood. The common symptoms include: pain in the hypochondriac area and lower abdomen, depression, irritability, dizziness, distending pain of the head, tremor of limbs, convulsion of both hands and feet, eye problems, irregular menstruation and genital symptoms. The main pathologies of gallbladder manifest as an abnormal function in storing and discharging the bile. The common symptoms include: jaundice, a tendency to panic, a bitter taste in the mouth, palpitations, timidity and restlessness.

7.2.3.1 The syndrome of liver blood deficiency

The syndrome of liver blood refers to the condition of liver blood failing to nourish the eyes, tendons, and finger nails and general symptoms of blood deficiency syndrome.

The clinical manifestations include: blurred vision or night blindness, dry finger nails, numbness and tremor of the limbs, muscular twitch, joint contracture, pale-color and scanty menstruation with delayed periods, possible amenorrhea, dizziness and pale and lusterless face and lips. The tongue is pale and the pulse is thready.

7.2.3.2 The syndrome of liver yin deficiency

The syndrome of liver yin deficiency refers to the condition of liver yin failing to nourish the eyes, tendons and hypochondriac area and general symptoms of deficient-heat syndrome.

The clinical manifestations include: dry eyes, declined eyesight, dull and burning pain in the hypochondriac area, twitching of hands and feet, dizziness, blurred vision, red cheeks, tidal fever, night sweats, a feverish sensation in the palms, soles and chest, dry mouth and throat. The tongue is dry and red and the pulse is wiry, thready and rapid.

7.2.3.3 The syndrome of liver qi stagnation

The syndrome of liver qi stagnation refers to the condition of an abnormal function of the liver in maintaining free flow of qi and the obstructed qi flow of the liver meridian.

The clinical manifestations include: depression, irritability, chest oppression, a distending or wandering pain in the hypochondriac area and lower abdomen, frequent sighing, a distending pain of the breast, dysmenorrhea, irregular menstruation and amenorrhea. The coating is thin and white and the pulse is wiry. Other symptoms may include: sensation of foreign body in the larynx, thyroid adenoma, scrofula and masses in the hypochondriac area. All of the disease conditions closely relate to emotional changes.

7.2.3.4 The syndrome of liver fire flaming

The syndrome of liver fire flaming refers to the condition of hyperactivity of liver fire, manifesting as an excessive fire or heat in the liver meridian and the adverse flow of liver qi and liver fire.

The clinical manifestations include: dizziness, a distending pain of the head, a red face and eyes, restlessness, irritability, a possible burning pain of the hypochondriac area, a bitter taste in the mouth, a dry throat, constipation and scanty and yellow urine. The tongue is red with a yellow coating and the pulse is wiry and rapid. Other symptoms may include: tinnitus or deafness, swollen and painful ears with an outflow of pus, insomnia, dream-disturbed sleep, hemoptysis and non-traumatic hemorrhage.

7.2.3.5 The syndrome of dampness-heat in liver and gallbladder

The syndrome of dampness-heat in liver and gallbladder refers to the condition of either dampness-heat in liver and gallbladder affecting the normal function in maintaining free flow of qi or downward dampness-heat in liver meridian.

The clinical manifestations include: a distending pain in the chest and hypochondriac area, a bitter taste in the mouth, poor appetite, abdominal distention, nausea, vomiting, irregular bowel movement and scanty and yellow urine. The tongue is red with a yellow and greasy coating and the pulse is wiry and rapid or slippery and rapid. Other symptoms may also include yellow sclera and body, and alternating chills and fever.

7.2.3.6 The syndrome of cold stagnating in the liver meridian

The syndrome of cold stagnating in the liver meridian refers to the condition of an attack by pathogenic cold, manifesting as cold stagnating and qi stagnation in liver meridian.

The clinical manifestations include: a cold pain in the lower abdomen, radiating to the external genitals, exogenous pathogenic cold, scrotum contraction, dysmenorrhea, dark-color menstruation with blood clots, a cold pain aggravated by cold and relieved with warmth and cold limbs. The tongue is pale with a white and moist coating and the pulse is deep and slow or wiry and tense.

7.2.3.7 The syndrome of ascendant hyperactivity of liver yang

The syndrome of ascendant hyperactivity of liver yang refers to the condition of yin deficiency of both liver and kidney and hyperactivity of liver yang, manifesting as excessive symptoms in the upper body and deficient symptoms in the lower body.

The clinical manifestations include: a distending pain of head and eyes, vertigo, tinnitus, a red face and eyes, irritability, insomnia, dream-disturbed sleep, soreness and weakness in the lower back and knee joints. The tongue is red and the pulse is wiry or wiry and thready.

7.2.3.8 The syndrome of internal stirring of liver wind

The syndrome of internal stirring of liver-wind generally refers to the pathological state of "moving and shaking" caused by the internal wind, such as dizziness, possible fainting, convulsion, tremor and tic. In clinical, this syndrome includes the following four subtypes: liver yang transforming into wind, extreme heat producing wind, yin deficiency stirring wind and blood deficiency producing wind.

(1) The syndrome of liver yang transforming into wind.

The syndrome of liver yang transforming into wind refers to the condition of liver and kidney yin failing to control yang and hyperactivity yang transforming into wind.

The clinical manifestations include: headache, vertigo, possible fainting, shaking of the head, tremor of limbs, unclear speech, numbness of both hands and feet, and an abnormal gait. Other symptoms may include: unconsciousness, a sudden collapse, deviation of the mouth and eyes. Hemiplegia, a stiff tongue and wheezy phlegm in the throat. The tongue is red with a white or greasy coating and the pulse is wiry and powerful or wiry and thready.

(2) The syndrome of extreme heat producing wind

The syndrome of extreme heat producing wind refers to the condition of excessive heat in liver meridian stirring the liver wind

The clinical manifestations include: a high fever, convulsion, superduction or even opisthotonus, trismus and restlessness or even coma. The tongue is dark-red with a dry and yellow coating and the pulse is wiry and rapid.

(3) The syndrome of yin deficiency stirring wind

The syndrome of yin deficiency stirring wind refers to the condition of yin fluids failing to nourish the muscles and vessels. The clinical manifestations of this syndrome can refer to the syndrome of liver yin deficiency.

(4) The syndrome of blood deficiency producing wind

The syndrome of blood deficiency producing wind refers to the condition of blood failing to nourish the muscles and vessels. The clinical manifestations can refer to the syndrome of liver blood deficiency.

7.2.3.9 The syndrome of gall bladder stagnation and phlegm-disturbance

The syndrome of gallbladder stagnation and phlegm-disturbance refers to the condition of internal disturbance of phlegm-heat, manifesting as restless gallbladder qi and general symptoms of phlegm-heat syndrome.

The clinical manifestations include: distention in the chest and hypochondriac area, palpitation, insomnia, timidity, restlessness, frequent sighing, dizziness, a blurred vision, a bitter taste in the mouth, nausea and vomiting. The tongue is red with a yellow and greasy coating and the pulse is wiry, slippery and rapid.

7.2.4 Syndrome differentiations of spleen and stomach

The spleen and stomach both reside in the middle energizer, and they are related to each other in the exterior and interior by the meridians. The physiological functions of the spleen include: dominates transportation and transformation of water, food and the body fluids; dominates rise of the clean; controls blood and the muscles of the four limbs. And it opens into the mouth and manifests in lips. The stomach is the sea of water and food, its physiological function is to dominate reception and decomposition, so the spleen and stomach work cooperatively to complete the digestion, absorption and distribution of water and food, they are also named as "the root of the acquired essence".

The main pathologies of the spleen lie in abnormal function in transportation and transformation or failure to control blood and dominate rise of the clear, resulting in water and food retention, disturbance in digestion, absorption and distribution, insufficient supply of producing and transforming qi and blood, internal phlegm-dampness. The common symptoms include: poor appetite, abdominal distension and pain, loose stool, diarrhea, edema, and possible prolapse and bleeding of the internal organs.

The main pathologies of the stomach manifest either as a dysfunction in receiving and decomposing food or failure of stomach qi to descend. The common symptoms include: a reduced appetite, gastric distension and pain, belching, nausea, vomiting and hiccup.

7.2.4.1　The syndrome of spleen qi deficiency

The syndrome of spleen qi deficiency refers to the condition of spleen qi deficiency and weakness in transportation and transformation.

The clinical manifestations include: a reduced appetite, an abdominal fullness and distension after eating food, loose stool, mental fatigue, emaciation or edema, lassitude, laziness in speaking, a sallow or pale complexion, weakness in bowel movements or a gurgling sound in the intestine, a lingering dull pain in the abdomen. The tongue can be pale, tender or swollen with teeth marks and white and moist coating and the pulse is moderate and deficiency or deep and thready.

7.2.4.2　The syndrome of spleen yang deficiency

The syndrome of spleen yang deficiency due to the failure of spleen-yang's warming function. It can often develop from the syndrome of spleen qi deficiency.

The clinical manifestations include: a poor appetite, a gastric and abdominal fullness and distension, clear and loose stool with undigested food, a cold pain in the abdomen which can be relieved with warmth and pressure, aversion to cold, cold limbs, tastelessness and no thirst. Other symptoms may present as a general edema, scanty urine, and thin and profuse leucorrhea for women. The tongue is pale and swollen with teeth marks and a white and slippery coating. The pulse is deep, slow and weak.

7.2.4.3　The syndrome of spleen qi sinking

The syndrome of spleen qi sinking refers to the condition of the spleen qi failing to ascend.

The clinical manifestations include: distension of the stomach and abdomen worsening after eating food, and a frequent and urgent sensation of defecation. Other complications include: fatigue, laziness in speaking, a low and weak voice, lassitude, dizziness and blurred vision, a sallow complexion, emaciation, a poor appetite and loose stool. The tongue is pale with thin and white coating and the pulse is moderate and weak.

7.2.4.4　The syndrome of spleen failing to control blood

The syndrome of spleen failing to control blood refers to the condition of spleen qi deficiency and blood seeping out of the vessels, mainly manifesting as chronic bleeding.

The clinical manifestations include: Bloody stool and urine, purpura, gum bleeding, nasal bleeding, profuse menstruation, metrorrhagia and metrostaxis. Other complications include fatigue, a reduced appetite, an abdominal distension, loose stool, a sallow or lusterless complexion, lassitude, and laziness in speaking. The tongue is pale with white coating and the pulse is thready and weak.

7.2.4.5　The syndrome of cold-dampness encumbering the spleen

The syndrome of cold-dampness encumbering the spleen refers to the condition of internal cold-dampness affecting the normal function of spleen yang.

The clinical manifestions include: a gastric and abdominal fullness, distension and pain, greasy taste, a poor appetite, an abdominal pain, loose stool, nausea, vomiting, tastelessness, no thirst, heaviness sensation of the head and whole body, sallow complexion, lusterless dark-yellow skin, possible edema of the limbs, scanty urine, and thin and profuse leucorrhea. The tongue is pale and swollen with white and greasy coating and the pulse is soft and moderate.

7.2.4.6   The syndrome of spleen-stomach dampness-heat

The syndrome of retention of spleen-stomach dampness-heat in spleen refers to the condition of dampness-heat accumulating in middle energizer, and affecting the function of spleen-stomach in transportation and transformation.

The clinical manifestations include: a gastric and abdominal fullness, a poor appetite, nausea, vomiting, sick of greasy food, a bitter and sticky mouth, either constipation or loose stool and unsmooth defecation, heaviness of the head and body, a bright-yellow body skin and eyes, yellow urine, possible itching of the skin, alternating high and low fever and remained fever after sweating. The tongue is red with yellow and sticky coating and the pulse is soft and rapid.

7.2.4.7   The syndrome of stomach yin deficiency

The syndrome of stomach yin deficiency refers to the condition of stomach yin failing to moisten stomach and then affecting the abnormal function of stomach.

The clinical manifestations include: a dull and burning pain in stomach, hunger but no appetite, an empty sensation in stomach, retch and belching, a dry mouth and throat, thirst with a desire for water, constipation, scanty urine. The tongue is dry and red with a scanty or geographic coating. The pulse is thready and rapid.

7.2.4.8   The syndrome of cold-retention in stomach

The syndrome of cold-retention in stomach refers to the condition of stomach dysfunction due to pathogenic yin cold retention.

The clinical manifestations include: a sudden cold pain in stomach, relieved after vomiting and worsening with cold, tastelessness, no thirst, a gastric and abdominal fullness and distention, and vomiting of thin saliva. Other symptoms may include nausea and vomiting, cold limbs, a pale complexion and bluish lips. The tongue is pale with a white and moist coating and the pulse is wiry or deep and tense.

7.2.4.9   The syndrome of intense stomach fire

The syndrome of intense stomach fire refers to the condition of the heat or fire affecting the function of stomach in receiving and decomposing food.

The clinical manifestations include: a burning pain and an empty sensation in the stomach, acid regurgitation, a good appetite and a bitter mouth and foul breath. Other symptoms may include swelling, pain and erosion of the gum, mouth and tongue ulcerations, hemoptysis, non-traumatic bleeding, bloody stool, thirst with desire for cold drinks, scanty and yellow urine and dry stool. The tongue is red with a yellow coating and the pulse is slippery and rapid.

7.2.4.10   The syndrome of food retention in stomach

The syndrome of food retention in stomach refers to the condition of the stomach failing to decompose and digest food.

The clinical manifestations include: a distention, fullness, pain and tenderness of stomach, belching, acid regurgitation, no appetite, nausea and vomiting. Other symptoms may include vomiting of sour and rotten food, relief of the distention and pain after vomiting, passing flatus, loose stool with sour, rotten and foul feces, or constipation. The tongue coating is thick and greasy and the pulse is slippery or deep and excessive.

7.2.5 Syndrome differentiations of kidney and bladder

Kidney, called the congenital source, resides in the lumbar region. It opens into the ears and urinogenitals and anus, internally-externally connected with the urinary bladder through meridians. Its tissue shows in the bone and its luster manifests in hair. The physiological functions include: stores essence, governs reproduction, dominates bone and produces bone marrow, dominates water metabolism and reception of qi. And the physiological function of bladder is to dominate fluid storage.

The main pathologies of kidney manifest either as an abnormal function in governing human growth, development and reproduction or as a functional disorder in dominating water metabolism. The common symptoms include: soreness and pain in the lower back and knee joints, tinnitus, deafness, premature greying or loss of hair, loose teeth, impotence, nocturnal emissions, sterility and infertility, scanty menstruation, amenorrhea, edema, abnormal urine and bowel movement and shallow breath. The dysfunction of bladder in storing and discharging urine manifests as frequent, urgent and painful urination, enuresis and incontinence.

7.2.5.1 The syndrome of kidney yang deficiency

The syndrome of kidney yang deficiency refers to the condition of kidney yang failing to warm the body and affecting the transformation of kidney qi.

The clinical manifestations include: soreness and weakness in the lower back and knee joints, a pale or dark facial complexion, dizziness, a blurred vision, lassitude and cold limbs. Other symptoms may include: impotence, infertility, dawn diarrhea, edema, fullness and distension in abdomen, palpitations, cough and shortness of breath. The tongue is pale and swollen with a white coating, and the pulse is deep and thready.

7.2.5.2 The syndrome of kidney yin deficiency

The syndrome of kidney yin deficiency refers to the condition of yin essence failing to nourish kidney and production of internal deficient heat.

The clinical manifestations include: soreness and weakness in the lower back and knee joints, dizziness, tinnitus, insomnia or dream-disturbed sleep, frequent sex desire with nocturnal emissions, scanty menstruation, amenorrhea, possible metrorrhagia and metrostaxis, emaciation, a feverish sensation in the palms, soles and chest, tidal fever, night sweats, a dry throat, red cheeks, yellow urine and dry stool. The tongue is dry and red and the pulse is thready and rapid.

7.2.5.3 The syndrome of kidney essence insufficiency

The syndrome of kidney essence insufficiency refers to the condition of a declined function of the kidney in governing growth, development and reproduction.

The clinical manifestations include: a retardation of development, a delayed closure of the fontanel, microsoma, underdevelopment of intelligence, slow action and weakness of bones. And the above symptoms occur in children; for adults, either sterility or infertility, and decline sexual function. Other symptoms may also include: premature senility, loss of hair and loose teeth, tinnitus, deafness, poor memory, mental trance, weakness of feet and slow reaction. The tongue is pale and the pulse is thready and weak.

7.2.5.4 The syndrome of kidney qi deficiency

The syndrome of kidney qi deficiency refers to the condition of kidney qi failing to store and hold essence.

The clinical manifestations include: soreness and weakness in the lower back and knee joints, lassitude, a declined hearing, nocturnal emissions, premature ejaculation, clear leucorrhea, and possible miscarriage. The symptoms on urination may include: frequent urination, clear and profuse urine, dribbling, enuresis, incontinence and frequent urination at night. The tongue is pale with white coating and the pulse is deep and weak.

7.2.5.5　The syndrome of dampness-heat in bladder

The syndrome of dampness-heat in bladder refers to the condition of dampness-heat in bladder affecting the transformation of bladder qi.

The clinical manifestations include: frequent and urgent urination, a burning sensation and painful micturition, scanty and yellow urine and a fullness and distension of the lower abdomen. Other symptoms may also include fever, pain in the lower back, bloody urine. The tongue is red with a yellow and greasy coating and the pulse is rapid.

7.2.6　Syndrome differentiations of concurrent syndromes of zang-fu viscera

As we mentioned above, zang-fu viscera are physiologically complementary and affect each other pathologically, the concurrent syndromes of zang-fu viscera refer to the syndromes involving at least two zang-fu viscera. In clinical, syndromes in which more than two organs are affected at the same time are known as concurrent syndromes. Generally, so long as the organs are interrelated and complementary to each other, concurrent syndromes are likely to appear. On the contrary, it seldom occurs.

The rule of differentiation of concurrent syndromes of the zang-fu viscera involves three steps: to be familiar with the key points of syndrome differentiation on one zang or fu viscera; to analyze the physiological relationships among the zang-fu viscera; and then to investigate the cause and result, and major and minor changes of the pathological mechanism. For the concurrent syndromes of the zang-fu viscera are very common and complicated, we'll only discuss the most common syndromes.

7.2.6.1　The syndrome of disharmony between heart and kidney

The syndrome of disharmony between heart and kidney refers to the condition in coordination between the kidney water and heart fire, caused by heart and kidney yin deficiency and hyperactivity of yang qi.

The clinical manifestations include: palpitations, restlessness, insomnia, poor memory, dizziness, tinnitus, soreness in lower back and knee joints, nocturnal emissions, a feverish sensation in the palms and chest, tidal fever, night sweats and a dry mouth and throat. The tongue is red with a scanty coating or no coating and the pulse is thready and rapid.

7.2.6.2　The syndrome of deficiency of both heart and spleen

The syndrome of deficiency of both heart and spleen refers to the qi and blood deficiency condition of both heart and spleen, and heart-blood failing to nourish the heart-mind and spleen qi failing to transport, transform and control the blood.

The clinical manifestations include: palpitations, dizziness, dream-disturbed sleep, poor memory, a poor appetite, an abdominal distention and loose stool, purpura, pale-color and scanty menstruation, fatigue and a sallow complexion. The tongue is pale and tender and the pulse is weak.

7.2.6.3　The syndrome of blood deficiency of both heart and liver

The syndrome of blood deficiency of both the heart and liver refers to the condition of the heart and liver blood failing to nourish the heart, liver and their related tissues and orifices.

The clinical manifestations include: palpitations, dream-disturbed sleep, poor memory, dizziness, a blurred vision, numbness and tremor of the limbs, pale scanty menstruation and possible amenorrhea, a pale and lusterless complexion and dry nails. The tongue is pale-white and the pulse is thready.

7.2.6.4 The syndrome of yang deficiency of both heart and kidney

The syndrome of yang deficiency of both heart and kidney refers to the deficient-cold condition of obstructed blood circulation and water retention, manifesting as palpitations and edema.

The clinical manifestations include: palpitations, chest oppression, panting, edema, difficult urination, soreness and coldness in the low back and knee joints, fatigue, aversion to cold, cold limbs and bluish-purple lips and nails. The tongue is pale-purple with white and slippery coating and the pulse is weak.

7.2.6.5 The syndrome of qi deficiency of both heart and lung

The syndrome of qi deficiency of both heart and lung refers to the deficient and weak condition, manifesting as palpitations, cough and panting.

The clinical manifestations include: palpitations, worsening with physical exertion, chest oppression, cough with thin and clear sputum, panting, fatigue, low voice, laziness in speaking, spontaneous sweating and a pale complexion and purple lips. The tongue is pale or pale-purple with a white coating and the pulse is weak or intermittent.

7.2.6.6 The syndrome of qi deficiency of both heart and gallbladder

The syndrome of qi deficiency of both heart and gallbladder refers to the condition of heart qi failing to nourish the heart-mind and gallbladder qi failing to make decisions.

The clinical manifestations include: palpitations, easily panics, insomnia and dream-disturbed sleep, easily wakes up with a startle, restlessness, shortness of breath and lassitude. The tongue is pale with a thin and white coating and the pulse is wiry and thready or slippery and rapid.

7.2.6.7 The syndrome of qi deficiency of both spleen and lung

The syndrome of qi deficiency of both spleen and lung refers to the condition of spleen failing to transport and transform and the lung failing to disperse and descend.

The clinical manifestations include: a poor appetite, an abdominal distention, loose stool, edema, panting, shortness of breath, cough with thin and clear sputum, laziness in speaking, fatigue and a pale and lusterless complexion. The tongue is pale with a white and slippery coating and the pulse is weak.

7.2.6.8 The syndrome of yang deficiency of both spleen and kidney

The syndrome of yang deficiency of both spleen and kidney refers to the condition of yang qi of spleen and kidney failing to warm and transform, manifesting as either diarrhea or edema.

The clinical manifestations include: a cold pain in the lower back, knee joints and lower abdomen, aversion to cold, cold limbs, chronic diarrhea or dysentery, dawn diarrhea with undigested food, edema, difficult urination and a bright pale complexion. The tongue is pale and swollen with a white and slippery coating. The pulse is deep, slow and weak.

7.2.6.9 The syndrome of qi deficiency of both lung and kidney

The syndrome of qi deficiency of both lung and kidney refers to the condition of qi deficiency, and both lung and kidney failing to disperse, descend, receive and hold qi.

The clinical manifestations include: weak cough with thin and clear sputum, more exhalation and less inhalation, shortness of breath and panting, the symptoms worsening with physical exertion, a low voice, lassitude, spontaneous sweating, tinnitus, soreness and weakness in the lower back and knee joints. The tongue is pale and the pulse is weak.

7.2.6.10   The syndrome of yin deficiency of both lung and kidney

The syndrome of yin deficiency of both lung and kidney refers to the condition of an internal disturbance of yin deficiency, and lung failing to disperse and descend.

The clinical manifestations include: cough with less sputum or blood streaked sputum, soreness and weakness in the lower back and knee joints, nocturnal emissions, scanty menstruation and emaciation. In addition, accompanying with the symptoms and signs of yin deficiency, such as a dry mouth and throat, tidal fever, night sweat and red cheeks, the tongue is red with a scanty coating and the pulse is thready and rapid.

7.2.6.11   The syndrome of yin deficiency of both liver and kidney

The syndrome of yin deficiency of both liver and kidney refers to the condition of yin failing to control yang and leads to internal deficient heat.

The clinical manifestations include: dizziness, a blurred vision, tinnitus, hypochondriac pain, soreness and weakness in the lower back and knee joints, a dry mouth and throat, insomnia, poor memory, dream-disturbed sleep, a low fever or feverish sensation in the palms, soles and chest, red cheeks, nocturnal emissions and scanty menstruation. The tongue is red with a scanty coating and the pulse is thready and rapid.

7.2.6.12   The syndrome of disharmony between liver and spleen

The syndrome of disharmony between liver and spleen refers to the condition of the liver failing to dominate free flow and rise of qi, and the spleen failing to transport and transform, manifesting as a distending pain in the chest and hypochondriac area, an abdominal distention and loose stool.

The clinical manifestations include: a distention, fullness and wandering pain in the chest and hypochondriac area, no appetite, frequent sighing, mental depression or restlessness, irritability, an abdominal distention, unsmooth defecation, loose stool, an abdominal pain with the sensation of defecation, relieved after the bowel movement, and loose and sticky stool. The tongue coating is white and the pulse is wiry or moderate.

7.2.6.13   The syndrome of disharmony between liver and stomach

The syndrome of disharmony between liver and stomach refers to the condition of liver qi affecting stomach, and the stomach qi failing to descend, manifesting as a gastric distention, belching and hiccup.

The clinical manifestations include: a distention, fullness and wandering pain in the gastric and hypochondriac area, no appetite, belching, acid regurgitation, hiccup, depression, frequent sighing, restlessness and irritability. The tongue is pale-red with a thin and yellow coating and the pulse is wiry.

7.2.6.14   The syndrome of liver fire invading lung

The syndrome of liver fire invading the lung refers to the excess heat condition of lung failing to disperse and descend due to the ascending of liver meridian fire.

The clinical manifestations include: a burning pain in the chest and hypochondriac area, head distention and dizziness, restlessness, irritability, a red face and eyes, a dry and bitter mouth, cough with yellow and sticky sputum and possible hemoptysis. The tongue is red with thin and yellow coating and the pulse is wiry and rapid.

Yang Zongbao, He Lingling, Yao Zengyu

Chapter 8

Health-Preservation, Prevention and Treatment Principles

TCM has always been playing an important role on health preservation and prevention. Health preservation, originally known as "Shesheng", "Daosheng", and "Baosheng" in ancient times, means nursing and taking good care of one's own health. Prevention is to take certain measures in order to prevent the occurrence and development of diseases. TCM had put forward the thought of prevention as *preventive treatment* in the *Internal Classic*. It is pointed out in the *Plain Questions* that "the sage does not cure but prevent the disease, and does not suppress but prevent the revolt…It is too late to treat the disease when it occurs and to suppress the revolt after it happens, that's exactly as to dig a well when feeling thirsty and to cast an awl when the fight starts. Isn't it too late?" In the process of the long-term clinical practice, this idea of "preventing the disease before its occurrence" is embedded throughout the medical treatment of TCM in every aspect, and serves as a key component of preventive medicine in TCM.

TCM recognizes various body constitution differences existing among individuals, and these differences result from the differences in zang-fu, qi and blood of the individuals. Hence, fundamental principles of clinical treatment, health preservation and disease prevention are put forward according to different types of body constitution. Furthermore, ancient physician generalized and summarized the "Eight Methods" which was the basic treatment method generalized from the syndrome differentiation of eight principles and the main function of formulas. However, the practical application in modern clinics has gone beyond the scope of the "Eight Methods", with the progress of society, the development of medical science and the need for medical practice. This chapter only introduces the treatment principles which are shared in commonality and widely practised in clinics.

8.1　Health-preservation

Health-preservation, known as "Yangsheng" and also as "Shesheng", primarily refers to a kind of self-preventive health care activity when people have not been involved in illness yet. "Yang" means to maintain, to nurse, to take care and to cultivate; "Sheng" means life, living and growth. Thus, health preservation is a method to keep the balance between yin and yang, and to enhance the body's resistant qi and body constitution, in order to keep the body in an optimal state physically and mentally. It can improve the adaptability to the external environment and the ability of resistance to the disease, and reduce or avoid the occurrence of diseases, thereby delaying senescence through various health care and maintenance measures.

There is an incisive discussion on the basic principles of health preservation in *Plain Questions* as which the saying goes, "the ancients, who knew about the meaning of health preservation, could achieve the right standard by following the laws of the natural changes occurring on the world, between yin and yang and combining with adaptive methods of health preservation. Furthermore, these ancients kept a proper diet and regular living routine, and never undertook excessive work or sexual intercourse so that they could possess a good condition physically and mentally, and then to live until the natural death and even pass away over 100 years old". Health preservation has a great significance to prevent diseases, strengthen body constitution, and prolong life. The idea of prevention "do not cure but prevent the disease" emphasized in the book is the essence of the TCM theory.

According to following the natural law, the health-preservation study in TCM comes up with the theory of "nourishing yang in spring and summer while nourishing yin in autumn and winter". In spring and summer, all things are thriving, so people should comply with the trend of venting yang qi, getting up early to do outdoor activities, walking in the fresh air and stretching the body to store plentiful yang qi in body. In autumn and winter, the weather turns cool and the wind rushes, and yin qi is on convergence, so people have to pay attention to preventing cold and keeping warm, in order to hide the yin essence inside the body and do not leak the yang qi. This principle of preserving yin and yang in accordance with the four seasons is the concrete embodiment of the health-preservation principle of "correspondence between nature and human" and "conforming to nature".

TCM underlines the great importance of the relationship between emotions and activities of human health. Under normal circumstances, the changes of spirit and emotions are the "responsive reaction" produced by the body to various external stimuli. It reflects the normal mental activity in the process of life. A good mental state helps us to improve the body adaptability to the environment and resistance to disease, strengthen body constitution, prevent disease and prolong life. If regulation range of normal physiological function of human body is exceeded, the self-regulation ability of human body will be reduced, the qi movement in zang-fu viscera will result in disorders and the imbalance among yin, yang, qi, and blood, and consequently the onset of different of diseases.

TCM has always emphasized the importance of the kidney on human vital activities, which regards the kidney as the root of innate endowments, the house of the fire and water, the storage of the essence from five zang and six fu viscera, the origin of the yuan(original) qi and yin essence, as well as the regulation center of the vital activities. The exuberance and debilitation of the yin and yang of the essential qi in the kidney have a direct and close relationship with the growth and aging process of human beings. The essence can be transformed into qi, and then qi can produce the energy which can affect spirits, and thus the essence is the basis of qi, energy and spirits. Shown in health preservation, there is a proposition of protecting the kidney and preserving the essence. Otherwise, TCM considers sexual exhaustion is one of the main ausos of diseases.

Modern medicine has proved that exercise can strengthen the cardiac functions, power the contraction of the cardiac muscle, improve blood supply, increase vascular elasticity, and delay or reduce the pathological changes of atherosclerosis. Exercise is able to improve cardio-pulmonary function, increase lung capacity, have good effect on lung tissue elasticity, as well as aeration and ventilation function of lung. Exercise can improve digestive system, facilitate the metabolism of nutrients in the body, and maintain a good appetite. Exercise can also enhance the muscular contraction and relaxation, improve the blood circulation of skeleton, make the muscles stronger and the joints movement more flexible, so as to prevent such kind of diseases like arthritis and osteoporosis effectively.

It was said in *Internal Classic* that human beings were fed on water and food, so people would die without water and food. When the water and food entered the stomach, the essence and qi were full and moved around and transferred upward to the spleen. Sequentially the essence and qi in the spleen would emanate from it. Those words indicate that the spleen and stomach function is the source of acquired constitution, depending on which the essence of food and water can be absorbed and transferred to nourish zang-fu viscera, so that the functions and activities of zang-fu viscera can be maintained.

After nourished with nutrition, the spleen delivers the essence to tissues and organs, such as skin and body hair, muscles, sinew and bones in order to maintain the normal physiological functions. Thus, the spleen is regarded as the source of the engender transformation of qi and blood, on which all the five zang and six fu viscera, limbs and skeletons rely to be nourished. The strength of spleen and stomach is an important factor to determine the life span.

8.2 Body constitution

8.2.1 The concept of body constitution

Body Constitution is known as "Ti Zhi" in TCM. It means the figure and body constituent, which can be extended to the body and physiology. Body Constitution is an inherent characteristic with relative stabilization in function and morphous, which is formed by human body on the basis of congenital heredity and acquired characters. And a certain shape and structure will inevitably produce and show its specific physiological functions and psychological characteristics, which are interdependent and inseparable with each other, also synthetically embodied in the inherent characteristics of constitution. In other words, the constitution is a stable individuality and characteristic united by human shape and structure, physiological function and psychological factors, which is formed in the progress of growth and development under the impact by endowments and acquired conditioning and maintenance.

Besides, it is also featured with the capability of adaptation to the nature, society and environment. On the physical level, the body constitution shows up as the individual differences in function, metabolism and response to external stimuli. In pathology, it manifests as the susceptibility or vulnerability to certain pathogenic factors and diseases, and the type of disease lesion the tendency of the progress and outcome of disease. In the case of individuals, the constitution has obvious particularity and always consists in the process of health or disease. Therefore, the constitution is actually the physiological particularity possessed by different individuals on the basis of shared physiological commonality by human.

Ideal healthy constitution means the human body is in a relatively good condition, namely the united states of body and spirit, which allows an integrated development of the body in all aspects, such as the morphological structure, physiological function, psychological state and adaptability to the environment, through acquired active cultivation and on the basis of a full use of the innate endowment.

8.2.2 Classification of constitution

The classification of constitution in TCM is guided by the concept of holism, and the determination on the differences of constitution of diverse individuals among the population mainly accords to the basic theories of yin-yang, five elements, visceral manifestations, and essence, qi, blood, and body fluids.

8.2.2.1　Classification methods of constitution

The classification methods of constitution are an important way to recognize and master the constitutional differences. Ancient doctors classified the constitution from different views, such as yin-yang classification, five element classification, and zang-fu viscera classification, etc. And the yin-yang classification is the basic method of constitutional classification.

8.2.2.2　Common classification and characteristics of constitution

(1) Neutral type

Individuals have a strong physique, stable emotional or mental state and feel optimistic. They often present with lustrous complexion and hair, bright eyes, proper senses of smell and taste, red and moisture lips, uneasy to feel fatigue, good sleep and appetite, normal bowel and urinary habits. They are adaptable to environmental changes.

(2) Qi deficient type

Individuals tend to have flabby muscles, and are introvert and timid in personality. They often present with feeble voice, shortness of breath, fatigue, catching cold or flu easily, sweating and teeth marks in the tongue margin. They are sensitive to environmental changes. Since individuals are relatively weak in immune functioning, it usually takes a longer time for them to recover from illnesses.

(3) Yang deficient type

Individuals tend to have flabby muscles, and are quiet and introvert in personality. They often complain about cold hands and feet, cold feeling in stomach, sensitive to low temperatures or noises, sleepiness, discomfort after eating cold foods, and a pale and bulky tongue. They often feel uncomfortable in windy, cold and humid environments. They are susceptible to health problems such as puffiness, diarrhea and excess throat secretions.

(4) Yin deficient type

Individuals usually have a thin physique, and are outgoing and impatient in personality. They like to complain about warm palms and soles, mouth dryness, dry nose, preference for cold drinks, dry stools or constipation. They often feel uncomfortable in hot and dry environments. They are susceptible to cough, fatigue, seminal emission, insomnia, and some chronic conditions.

(5) Phlegm-dampness type

Individuals are usually overweight and have tummy, with a mild temper, steady and patient personalities. They often present with oily face, sticky or sweet taste in the mouth, excessive throat secretion, sweating, chest stuffiness, preference for sweet and greasy foods, and a thick tongue coating. They often feel uncomfortable in humid and rainy environments. They are susceptible to diabetes, metabolic syndrome or cardiovascular diseases.

(6) Dampness-heat type

Individuals are either with a normal or thin physique, they tend to be irritable and short-tempered. They often present with an oily face that erupts acne or pimple frequently, a bitter or strength taste in the mouth, fatigue or heaviness of the body, uncompleted feeling after defecation or dry stools, yellow urine, excess vaginal discharges in female, wet scrota in male, and a yellow and greasy tongue coating. They are sensitive to humid and hot environments especially in late summer or early autumn. They are susceptible to skin problems and urinary difficulties.

(7) Blood stasis type

Individuals tend to be impatient and forgetful. They often present with a dull complexion, spots on the face, dark-red lips, dark circles under eyes, lusterless or rough skin, unknown bruise on the body surface, and varicose veins. They often feel uncomfortable in cold environments. They are susceptible to bleedings, painful conditions, and abnormal growths.

(8) Qi stagnation type

Individuals are mostly thin, and tend to be emotional unstable, melancholy or suspicious. They often present with a depressed mood, being nervous or anxious, timid, frequent sighing, and heart palpitations. They respond relatively poor to stressful situations, especially in winter and autumn and also rainy days. They are susceptible to insomnia, depression, anxiety disorder and breast lumps.

(9) Special constitution type

Individuals usually have inborn weakness, they are very sensitive to drugs, foods, smells, pollens or other environmental allergens. They often develop nasal congestion, sneezing, runny nose, panting, wheals, itchiness and even purple spots or patches under the skin. Common health problems among individuals are drug allergies, hay fever, eczema and asthma. They respond relatively poor to external influences, and their health problems can easily be induced by seasonal changes.

8.3 Prevention

Prevention means taking certain measures to prevent the occurrence and development of the diseases. TCM has always been attaching great importance to prevention. The idea of "preventive treatment" was early put forward in *Internal Classic. Plain Questions* which pointed out, "the sage does not cure but prevent the disease, and does not suppress but prevent the revolt…It is too late to treat the disease after it occurs and to suppress the revolt after it happens, that's what exactly as someone to dig a well when he feels thirsty and to cast an awl when fighting is already on. Isn't it too late?" For healthy people prevention can strengthen the constitution and prevent the occurrence of disease; for the sick one, it can prevent the development and transmission.

The so-called preventive treatment includes two aspects, preventive treatment and prevention of progress of disease.

"Preventive treatment" means taking a variety of measures before diseases appearing in human bodies to protect the healthy qi, to improve the resistance to diseases, to prevent the invasion of pathogens as well as the occurrence of disease. The occurrence of diseases relates not only to healthy qi of the body but also to the invasion strength of external pathogens. TCM believes that pathogen is an important condition of resulting in the occurrence of a diseases; yet healthy qi deficiency is the inherent reason and basis to the occurrence of diseases. External pathogen functions through internal reason. Hence, prevention treatment should be commenced from health preservation and prevention.

Prevention of progress of disease means that early diagnosis and early treatment are supposed to be taken as soon as the disease onset in order to prevent the development and progress of the disease.

After the onset of illness, people should receive early diagnosis and treatment as soon as possible in order to prevent the deterioration of disease from disorder to serious disease. Destroying pathogens before they become menacing is an important principle of disease prevention and treatment. The book *Medical Insights* said, "The reason why we should observe the disease at the first beginning. Following this, then we can find out how things develop and destroy dangers before its emergence. This is what we call skillful treatment".

Pathological changes can be controlled by carrying out predictive therapy according to the progress law of different disease lesions. As *Synopsis of Golden Chamber* has said, "spleen is to be infected when liver is in disorder, so we had better strengthen spleen first when we find the disease of liver". In clinical treatment to liver diseases, the medicine to regulate the spleen and stomach is often used together so that the spleen qi can be vigorous without pathogens, and it can obtain good effect in this way. For instance, when the warm-heat disease harms stomach yin, its pathological development trend will consume kidney yin. According to this progress law of disease, Ye Tianshi, a master physician in Qing Dynasty suggested that the salty and cold medicine of nourishing kidney yin should be added in sweet and cold medicine of nourishing the stomach yin so as to prevent the consumption of kidney yin. These are all effective application of the prevention of progression of disease principle. Prevention of progress of disease should be used to not only cut off the progress path of pathogens but also to make sure "the unaffected area must be treated at first. "

Generally, diseases have certain laws and paths of progress. In disease prevention and control, the progress of diseases can be prevented only by mastering the law of disease development and the path of its progress, such as six meridians transmission, transmission of defense qi, nutrient and blood, triple energizer transmission, mutual restraint rules of five elements generation and restriction of internal damage miscellaneous diseases, progress of meridians and collaterals, and progress between interior and exterior. With the six-meridian progress of typhoid fever as an example, its initial phase more occurs in taiyang meridian of the muscle surface, and its development of lesion is inclined to progress toward other meridians.

Therefore, the stage of taiyang pathogenesis is the key to the early diagnosis and treatment of typhoid fever. Adopting correct and effective treatments at this stage is the best measure to prevent the development of typhoid fever. For another example, warm disease usually starts with defense syndrome, and thus the stage of defense syndrome is the key to early diagnosis and treatment of warm disease. Accordingly, we can apply timely and appropriate measures of disease prevention and control if we can understand and grasp the path and laws of the progress of diseases so as to prevent the development or deterioration of disease.

8.4   The principles and methods of treatment

The therapeutic principles serve as the basic principles by which the treatment of diseases must follow. It is the disease treatment criteria which possess a general guiding significance on clinical legislation, prescription and medicinal administration and is formulated according to the objective documents obtained based on four diagnostic methods(inspection, inquiring, auscultation and olfaction, and pulse taking and palpation) and on the basis of an all-sided analysis, integration and judgment, under the guidance of the concept of holism and the spirit of syndrome differentiation and treatment.

The methods of treatment are the specific common treatments and methods which are formulated to and aim at diseases and the signs under the guidance of the therapeutic principle. The common methods are established for the disease with the same pathogenesis, such as the eight methods therapeutic methods including diaphoresis, emesis, harmonization, purgation, warming, clearing, and supplement and dispersing. With a relatively broad range of adaptation, it is in the higher level among methods of treatment. And the specific remedy, within the limited range of common methods, is aimed at specific disease syndrome, such as using acrid-warm herbs relieving superficies to release the exterior with pungent-warm, calm the liver to extinguishing wind, fortify the spleen and drain dampness, etc.

There are both differences and correlations between the therapeutic principles and the methods of treatment. The therapeutic principles are the general principles guiding the treatment of disease, of principle and universal significance. The methods of treatment are the specific common treatment, therapeutic method and therapy measure, subordinating a certain therapeutic principle, and they are featured with strong pertinence and maneuverability, specific and flexible. For example, for the relations between healthy qi and pathogenic qi, it can be known that the various diseases are nothing more than the conflict between healthy qi and pathogenic qi, and changes of waxing-waning and of exuberance or decline.

Hence, reinforcing healthy qi with eliminating pathogens is the basic principle in treatment. Under the guidance of this basic principle, the specific methods of strengthening healthy qi are tonifying qi, nourishing blood, enriching yin, and supplementing yang based on specific conditions; while methods inducing diaphoresis, emesis are the specific methods of eliminating pathogens.

8.4.1 The principles of treatment

Chinese medicine believes that: "treatment aiming at its pathogenesis. " (*Plain Questions*). Pathogenesis means the nature, property, root, and source. Treatment with seeking for the pathogenesis is to find out the root cause of the disease and treat it based on the nature of the disease in the treatment.

It is a fundamental principle of treatment upon syndrome differentiation in TCM, and also the most basic principle in the treatment of TCM. Its core is to grasp the pathogenesis of the disease and the treatment should be targeted to it, which is the principle that must be followed in the treatment of any disease. Hence, treatment aiming at pathogenesis is the treatment principle of the highest level in the theory system of therapeutic principle of TCM. It is playing a guiding role in all kinds of treatment rules, and all other treatment principles subordinate to this very principle.

The disorder between yin and yang is the root cause of the occurrence of pathological changes resulted from human losing the physiological state in clinical diseases. When treating diseases, we need to rebalance yin and yang, namely, the contradiction of preponderance and decline of yin or yang, so that the body can regain the dynamic balance between yin and yang.

Hence, tracing the root of the disease in treatment refers to the tracing to the nature of yin and yang. It means that, treating diseases must find out the root cause of the disease and examine the yin and yang routine to determine the treatment method.

But the pathological changes of a disease are very complicated, and the process of lesion can divide into being primary, secondary, urgent or less urgent. Thus, we need to be familiar with the common status and then we can realize the flexible use of treatment rules. Should not cling to one principle or stick to one rule. For example, for some pathogenic syndromes, we often induce them with employing nearby principle according to the status and the location of the pathogen, and then discharge them out of the body so as to avoid the injury of healthy qi.

To sum up, the TCM believes we should seek for the pathogenesis of the disease to make the body in balance, know the commons status and changes and guide the pathogen in the light of its general trend.

8.4.2 Symptom, root-cause, chronic and acute condition

Symptom is like the branch, the top of a tree, but not the root; root-cause is like the root of grass which is fundamental. In terms of the relations of pathogenic factors and healthy qi, the latter is the root cause and the former is the symptom; from the perspective of the cause of disease and symptom, the former is the root and the latter is the symptom.

For the sequence of the occurrence of diseases, the previous one is root and the latter one is the symptom; in the case of the locations where the disease exists, interior and lower portions are the roots and the exterior and upper portions part are the symptoms; in respect to appearance and nature, nature is root and appearance is symptom.

From comparisons above, it can be seen that the root and symptom are not absolute, but relative and conditional. To the point of the priority of root cause and symptoms in clinical syndromes, the rule of "treating the symptom for acute condition and treating the root cause for chronic condition" should be adopted to achieve the aim of treating diseases with seeking for root cause. This is the basic rule of the treatment sequence of symptom and root-cause. The theory of root and symptom is of guiding significance in analyzing diseases correctly, distinguishing the primary and secondary syndromes, causes and results, mild and severe syndromes, and urgent of non-urgent syndromes as well as applying correct treatment.

8.4.2.1   Symptomatic treatment in acute condition

It is generally applicable to acute and very serious diseases or to some of the symptoms that threaten life in the disease development. In the early phase of a disease, the pathogens have not penetrated deep yet and thus a treatment with instant effect should be applied to the dispelling of those pathogens. Afterwards, the healthy qi will not be hurt, and the patient will recover easily.

Hence, it is said, "When treating chronic disease and emergency, we should treat the emergency at first." (*Synopsis of Golden Chamber*) Take the disease of massive hemorrhage as another example. In this case, bleeding should be regarded as the symptom and the cause of bleeding as the root. But the situation of this disease is risky and urgent, and hence stopping bleeding should be taken as priority. After the bleeding stopped, the cause of bleeding can be treated with, then, for curing the root.

Additionally, it is emphasized in *Plain Questions* that there are two syndromes, resulted by former reasons, should be treated firstly, stomach fullness and obstruction of both urination and defecation.

If there is a serious stomach fullness, then the transportion and transform of food and drinks cannot be obtained, and sequentially, all the zang-fu viscera will lose their nourishment. Under such an urgent situation the symptom should be treated firstly.

For the patient with serious obstruction of both urination and defecation, which is called as "guan ge" in TCM, the dangerous stage, the symptoms must be treated firstly though they are the manifestations. If it is just a common obstruction, not so emergency, the treatment should be determined at the discretion and the symptoms may not be treated firstly.

8.4.2.2   Radical treatment in chronic condition

It is applicable to chronic disease, or on the occasion when the disease is about to heal, healthy qi is deficient, and pathogen has not been destroyed utterly yet. The chronic condition means the symptoms are not urgent. At the moment, symptom does not endanger the life or the body can still cope with the symptom.

Thus, we should treat its root cause directly. When the root cause is dispelled, the symptoms will disappear accordingly. Or we can treat its root cause firstly and then the symptom. Its clinical application mainly includes two kinds of cases: the first one is to analyze the root cause and symptom from the nature and appearance, of which the former is root cause and the latter is symptom. At this moment, the root cause of the syndrome is resulted from the competition between healthy qi and pathogenic qi, while its reflected manifestations and signs are the symptoms.

Generally, symptoms are not urgent. Therefore, we should treat the disease from the root cause. Once the root cause of disease is eliminated, the symptoms will disappear naturally. For example, when treating wind-cold headache, the pathogenesis of wind-cold pathogenic blockage of the meridians is considered to be the root cause, and headache is the symptom. The method of dispelling pathogens with dispersing wind and dissipating cold should be adopted.

Once the pathogens of wind-cold are dispelled, accordingly the headache will gone. For another example, when treating coughing caused by deficiency syndrome of the lung, the pathogenesis of lung yin deficiency should be the root and the cough should be the symptom. Thus, methods of nourishing yin and moisturizing lung should be taken to strengthen healthy qi. When the lung yin is sufficient, the cough will disappear, too. Secondly, the onset sequence of diseases should be analyzed. The former disease should be the root cause and the latter one should be the symptom. All the diseases with onset later are urgent.

Thus, it is general to firstly treat the disease with onset first and then the later onset one. In *Plain Questions*, it is said, "as for root and symptom, we should treat the former firstly then coming to the latter". For instance, when people have exogenous contraction cough firstly, then palpitation and insomnia, we should treat cough firstly if the syndromes of palpation and insomnia are not urgent. After the pathogens of exogenous contraction are dispelled and cough is cured, we can treat palpitation and insomnia.

8.4.2.3 Treating both manifestation and root cause of disease

It means to treat both symptom and root concurrently. It is applicable to the time when root-cause and symptom are both urgent. Take diarrhea as an example. The poor appetite is the deficiency of healthy qi (root), and non-stop diarrhea is because of the excessiveness of pathogenic qi(symptom). In this case, the root-cause and symptom are both urgent, and hence, the methods of drug strengthening healthy qi and clearing heat should be used together. It is treating both symptom and root-cause.

For another example, when treating patients with spleen deficiency and qi stagnation, spleen deficiency is the root cause and qi stagnation is the symptom. The medicine for fortifying the spleen and replenish qi, such as Renshen, Cangzhu, Fuling, Gancao, should be used to cure the root, and the medicines for regulating qi to move stagnation for activating stagnancy, such as woody, fructus amomi, and tangerine peel, should be used to cure the symptom.

The principle of treating both root cause and symptom is widely used. For example, Shensu Yin are used for both supplement and dispelling, Zhizhu Wan are used for supplement and dispersion, and Zengye Chengqi Tang are used for treating both elimination and reinforcement and so on. Based on the condition, the method of treating both root cause and symptom is not contradictory but mutually beneficial.

It must be pointed out that the principle of "treating the symptom for acute condition, and treating the root-cause for chronic condition" should not be absolutized. The root cause should also be treated even if the disease is urgent.

For example, as there is yang depletion collapse and deficiency in the body, methods of restoring yang from collapse should be adopted which is treating the root; after massive hemorrhage, the qi is collapsed along with blood loss, and thus pure ginseng decoction should be used to replenish qi and prevent exhaustion which is also treating the root.

Treating for acute condition at first is a fundamental principle for no matter it is root cause or symptom. Meanwhile, symptom can also be treated even if the disease is non-urgent. For instance, we should use drugs for regulating qi flow for the patients with spleen deficiency with qi stagnation, which is different from supplementing spleen purely. In conclusion, generally, we should treat the root cause for disease with slow development; when treating acute disease, we should treat the symptom firstly; when treating disease with both urgent root and symptom, both root-cause and symptom should be treated.

To sum up, we should deal with diseases from a point of view of "moving", and be good at grasping the main contradictions to determine the treatment priorities.

Hence, it is said, "when the disease goes deep, we should take a targeted treatment measure. Treating the symptoms or root is the key to solve the disease." (*Plain Questions*)

8.4.3   Orthodox treatment and retrograde treatment

Guided by the basic principle of "treatment aiming at its epathogenesis",orthodox treatment and retrograde treatment are two treatment principles aimed at whether the disease has false appearance or not. The natures of various diseases are different,and the external phenomenon reflected from the nature of the disease is also very complex. The nature of most diseases is consistent with the reflected phenomenon. But in some cases,the nature of the disease is inconsistent with the reflected phenomenon,which is called the false appearance.

The so-called orthodox treatment and retrograde treatment are in fact two kinds of manifestations of the reflected relations between the nature of treatment and the disease appearance based on the principle of "treatment aiming at its pathogenesis" orthodox treatment is the most common clinical therapeutic principle. While routine treatment is used for reverse disease movement,retrograde treatment is used for normal movement. These two treatment methods are the concrete application of the treatment principle of seeking the root of the disease.

8.4.3.1   Orthodox treatment

It refers to the the rapeutic principle which is against the nature of the syndrome,and thus it is also called "counteracting treatment". "Counteracting" means that the nature of the adopted formula is contrary to the nature of the disease,such as "treating cold syndrome with heat", "treating heat syndrome with cold", "treating deficiency syndrome with tonifying",and "treating excess syndrome with purgative". It is applicable to the disease whose symptoms are consistent with the nature of the disease. The commonly used routine methods are as follows.

(1)Treating coldness with heat

Disease with cold syndrome shows a sign of coldness and should be treated with a formula with warm-heat nature. For example,prescription of releasing the exterior with pungent-warm should be used for exterior cold syndrome,and prescription of warming interior and dispelling cold should be used for interior cold syndrome.

(2)Treating heat with coldness

Disease with heat syndrome shows a sign of heat and should be treated with a formula with cold nature. For example,prescription of relieving the exterior syndrome with pungent in flavor and cool in property should be used for exterior heat syndrome,and prescription of bitter cold and attacking interior should be used for interior heat syndrome.

(3)Treating deficiency with reinforcement

Syndrome of deficiency shows a sign of weakness and should be treated with prescription of replenishing. For instance,prescription of warming and supplement yang qi should be used for the syndrome of deficiency of yang qi,and prescription of nourishing yin and blood should be applied for the syndrome of deficiency of yin liquid.

(4)Treating excessiveness with expelling

Pathogenic excessiveness syndrome shows the sign of excessiveness,and it can be treated with prescription of attacking the pathogen and inducing diarrhea. Prescription of clearing heat and detoxifying and reducing fire should be applied for syndrome of prosperity in fire,heat,toxin and interior heated. Prescription of relieving bowels and expelling heat should be used for syndrome of Yangming fu-viscera excess and interior retention. Prescription of activating blood and resolving stasis should be used for pain syndrome of blood stasis.

8.4.3.2　Retrograde treatment

It is a therapeutic principle to treat disease with complying with its false signs, which is also known as "following-treatment". "Following" means the nature of the adopted prescription should follow the false signs of the disease.

Under the guidance of the principle of searching for the root cause of disease, it is a method aiming at the nature of the disease, and thus, it is also "treating disease with searching for its root cause". The commonly used methods include "treating pseudo-heat with heat", "treating pseudo-cold with coldness", "treating obstructive syndrome with tonifying" and "treating incontinent syndrome with dredging". It is feasible for the syndromes with the signs inconsistent or contrary with its root cause. This is a method targeting at the root cause of the disease under the guidance of treating disease with searching for its root cause.

(1) Treating coldness with coldness

It means treating false cold syndromes with cold nature medicine. It is applicable to true heat with false cold, namely to the syndromes of disease with a cold sign of true heat interior and false cold exterior, exuberant yang interior and repelling yin exterior. Although cold signs can be seen from the exterior, excessive heat is its nature.

Thus, cold and cool medicine should be used for treating heat and dispelling false cold. For example, when treating the heat exhaustion syndrome with false cold symptom on the extremities caused by exuberant yang and repelling yin exterior. But the natures of these are high fever, thirst, dry stool, reddish urine and other heat syndromes.

Hence, cold and cool medicine should be used for treating its true heat, and then the false cold will disappear naturally. This is the paradoxical treatment of treating cold with cold medicine for false cold symptoms.

(2) Treating heat with heat

It means treating heat cause with heat medicine, using hot drug to treat false heat symptoms. It is applicable for true cold with false heat, namely the syndrome of true cold interior and false heat exterior caused by yin cold interior excessiveness and repelling yang exterior. Albeit the heat sign can be seen in clinics, its nature is true cold. Targeting at the true cause when treating the disease, the hot medicine should be used for treating the true cold. The false heat will disappear once the true cold goes away. The method is "treating heat with heat" for its false signs.

For example, the nature of the patient with yang depletion collapse belongs to internal cold and yang debilitation. Due to the exuberance of internal yin cold, yang qi is repelled external. In clinics, the disease shows true cold syndromes, such as watery diarrhea with indigested food in the stool, extremities inverses, and feeble and impalpable pulse, and the false heat signs, such as general fever, and flushing face. The cold syndrome is the nature of the disease, and the heat signs are false.

Thus, instead of the method of heat being treated with cold medicine, the warm medicine should be applied to it. Once the interior cold disappears, yang qi will be regained, and the external signs of false heat will disappear, too. This is the specific application of "treating heat with heat".

(3) Treating stuffiness with tonics

It means opening obstruction with supplement, namely using nourishing and replenishing drugs to treat symptoms of obstruction. It is applicable to a syndrome of true weakness and false excess that is to the symptoms of obstruction caused by the decrease of functions of viscera and bowels, qi movement due to the weakness of the constitution. For the syndromes like constipation, abdominal fullness and distention resulted from weak spleen and stomach and the dysfunction of rising and falling of qi movement. When treating them, methods of nourishing spleen and benefiting stomach should be used to restore the function of spleen qi rising and stomach qi falling. Once the qi falling and rising turns to normal, abdominal fullness and distention will disappear normally.

For another example, when treating the decline of kidney yang, in order to improve the retention of urine caused by powerless evaporation, kidney yang should be warmed and replenished to promote the formation and excretion of urine, and then the urination will be smooth naturally. Such method of opening obstruction with supplement is treating obstruction with tonics, mainly aiming at the disease nature of deficiency syndrome.

(4) Treating diarrhea with purgative

It means treating symptoms of excessive catharsis with purgatives, which is used for true excess with false deficiency, namely the syndromes of catharsis raised by internal block of excessive pathogens.

Normally, the symptoms of diarrhea, metrorrhagia, and frequent urination can be treated with methods of relieving diarrhea, strengthen thoroughfare vessel, arresting polyuria and other methods. But when these symptoms of catharsis appear in some syndrome of excessive diseases, the symptoms of real catharsis should be treated with purgatives. For instance, when treating food stagnation, gastrointestinal tract blockage lead to abdominal pain and diarrhea, and stool as stinky as rotten eggs, the catharsis should not be stopped and methods of digestion, relieving stagnation, inducing purgation, and removing gastrointestinal accumulation and stagnation should be used to remove the food stagnation and then the diarrhea will stop naturally.

For another example, when treating blood stasis of internal obstruction, and metrorrhagia caused by blood failing to circulate in the vessels, the blood stasis will be more severe and blood is difficult to flow along the vessels, and then metrorrhagia is difficult to stop if we use hemostatic. So, at this moment, we should activate blood circulation to dissipate blood stasis. Then as the stagnation disappears, the blood will return to vessels and bleeding will stop naturally. Such method is treating diarrhea with purgative, this is a very common therapeutic method with the aim of treating pathogen by root.

With shared commons, both orthodox treatment and retrograde treatment are aiming at the root of disease, and thus they belong to the method category of searching for the primary cause of diseases in treatment. The difference between those two is that orthodox treatment is applicable to the disease where root and external manifestations are consistent, while retrograde treatment is applicable to the disease where root and external manifestations are inconsistent.

8.4.4　Strengthening healthy qi and eliminating pathogens

Strengthening healthy qi means the therapeutic principle of nourishing healthy qi to cure the disease. Namely, the therapies of the medicine for supporting healthy qi, acupuncture or qigong are used with complementary methods of proper diet regulation and mental adjustment to invigorate health effectively and improve the resistance to diseases so as to eliminate pathogens and then to defeat the diseases and getting well.

Eliminating pathogens is the therapeutic principle of curing disease through eliminating pathogens, namely, using the medicine of expelling pathogenic qi to alleviate or remove the poisonous function of pathogenic qi, and allowing the dispelling of pathogens and protection of healthy qi so as to get well. Purgative methods are mainly used for eliminating pathogens. Different treatments should be taken due to different pathogenic qi and where they locate.

Though strengthening healthy qi is different from eliminating pathogens, they are mutually related to each other. Strengthening healthy qi is of benefit to resistance and elimination of disease and pathogen.

Eliminating pathogens helps to remove the impairment brought by pathogenic factors so as to protect healthy qi and get well. This is so-called "pathogenic qi away and healthy qi secure". Strengthening healthy qi and elimination of pathogen are two aspects of complementing each other.

Therefore, when applying the therapeutic methods of strengthening healthy qi and eliminating pathogenic qi, we should analyze the contrast between them. We should draw a clear distinction on the primary one and the secondary one of them. And we should also decide whether to support healthy qi or to eliminate pathogen or the applying order of those two methods. Normally, strengthening healthy qi can be used for deficiency syndrome while eliminating pathogens can be used for excessiveness syndrome. If the disease has deficiency syndrome mingling with excessiveness syndrome, strengthening healthy qi and elimination of pathogen should be used together rather than half strengthening healthy qi and half dispelling pathogenic qi.

We should distinguish the priority of deficiency and excess in order to decide the priority of strengthening healthy qi or eliminating pathogenic qi. In a word, we should take "strengthening healthy qi without remains of pathogenic qi, and eliminating pathogenic qi without hurting healthy qi" as the standard. The specific details are as follows.

8.4.4.1 Strengthening healthy qi

It is applicable to deficiency syndrome of healthy qi deficiency as primary one accompanied with non-exuberance or excess of pathogenic qi. Methods of nourishing qi and strengthening yang should be used for qi and yang deficiency. Methods of nourishing yin and blood should be used for yin and blood deficiency.

8.4.4.2 Eliminating pathogen

It is applicable to excess syndrome in which the pathogenic qi takes the domination and healthy qi has not been weak and declined yet. Guided by this principle, methods such as diaphoresis, emesis, harmonization, purgation, clearing, drain dampness disperse, regulating qi and blood, are formulated based on different situation of pathogenic qi.

8.4.4.3 Reinforcement after elimination

It means eliminating pathogenic qi before strengthening healthy qi, which is applicable to the disease with a syndrome where the pathogenic qi is vigorous, healthy qi is deficient but resistant to the reinforcement, the exuberance of pathogenic qi is the main contradiction, and the pathogenic qi will be benefited if taking strengthening healthy qi into account. For example, when treating uterine bleeding syndrome caused by blood stagnation, we should activate firstly, then enrich the blood because bleeding will not be stopped if the blood stagnation cannot disappear.

8.4.4.4 Elimination after reinforcement

It means strengthening healthy qi before eliminating the pathogenic qi. It is applicable to the syndromes of healthy qi deficiency and pathogenic qi excessiveness resulting in a mix of excessiveness and deficiency and the situation poor attack resistance of healthy qi. If we eliminate pathogen at the same time, we will hurt body resistance more. Hence, we need to strengthen the healthy qi with tonifying methods. Until the body resistance recovers and can withstand attack, then we can treat pathogenic factors. For example, when treating distension of abdomen, the main contradiction is the healthy qi deficiency. When healthy qi has intolerance of attack, we must strengthen healthy qi firstly. Till healthy qi recovers and can withstand attack, we can eliminate pathogenic qi in case of the occurrence of an incident.

8.4.4.5 Simultaneous elimination and reinforcement

It means we need to use the two methods of strengthening healthy qi and eliminating pathogenic qi together. It is applicable to syndromes with deficient healthy qi and excessive pathogenic qi while both not severe. We need to distinguish the primary and secondary syndromes between healthy qi deficiency and pathogenic qi excessiveness and apply a flexible use.

If healthy qi deficiency is the main contradiction, we should mainly strengthen healthy qi with eliminating pathogenic qi secondary. Because if we take the reinforcement method alone it will cause the remaining of pathogenic qi and if we attack the pathogenic qi alone, it will impair healthy qi easily. For example, when treating a cold with qi deficiency, we should regard replenishment of qi as the primary method and releasing the exterior as the secondary. If the excess of pathogenic qi is the dominated contraction, we should eliminate pathogens mainly with strengthening healthy qi secondary because if we attack pathogen alone, healthy qi might be hurt, and if we strengthen healthy qi alone, the pathogen might not be removed.

8.4.5　Coordinating yin and yang

No matter how complicated the pathological changes are, the occurrence and development of the disease are essentially the results of the disharmony of yin and yang in the body caused by the destruction of the relative balance between yin and yang.

Therefore, it is one of the fundamental laws to cure the disease with coordination of the exuberance and decline of yin and yang by decreasing the excessive one and supplementing the deficient one to recover the relative balance between yin and yang in order to realize the purpose of healing the disease.

8.4.5.1　Impair the preponderance

Impairing the excess is also known as impairing the surplus, which is applicable to disease with the preponderance of yin or yang, namely to the syndromes of yin or yang excessiveness. Such diseases require a method of treating excess by purgation. When treating excess heat syndrome with yang excessiveness, the method of clearing and purging yang heat should be used with following the rules of "treating heat syndrome with cold". Clearing away yang heat is to treat the excess heat syndrome with excess yang heat; as for excess cold syndrome of cold by yin excessiveness, the method of warming and dispelling cold should be used with following the rules of "treating cold syndrome with heat" to warm and dissipate yin cold and treat syndrome of excess cold yin caused by the cold and interior excessiveness of yin.

Owing to the interdependence between yin and yang, "yin is exuberant and then disease featured by yang will occur" and "yang is exuberant and then disease featured by yin will occur". In the pathological changes of yin or yang preponderance, if either side is in deficiency we need to consider it with a method of strengthening yang or nourishing yin.

8.4.5.2　Tonifying the decline of yin or yang

Tonifying the decline of yin or yang means tonifying the insufficient one which mainly aims at the disease with one of yin and yang deficiency. The method of supporting the deficiency should be used. Because of the distinguishing between yin deficiency, yang deficiency and both yin and yang deficiency, we should apply the methods of nourishing yin, tonifying yang or supplementing both yin and yang.

(1) Mutual restraint between yin and yang

According to the principle of mutual restriction between yin and yang, the treatment of yin for the yang disease is applicable to yin deficiency syndrome, and the treatment of yang for the yin disease is applicable to yang deficiency syndrome.

When treating deficiency heat disease with relative hyperactivity of yang due to yin deficiency, that is, "yin deficiency causing heat", we need to nourish yin to restrain yang based on the principle of "treating yang for the yin disease". Here, "yang disease" means yin deficiency leading to relative hyperactivity of yang and treating yin means supplementing yin. When treating disease that the yang is too deficient to restrain yin then leading to relative hyperactivity of yin, that is "deficiency of yang causing cold syndrome", we need to nourish yang to prohibit yin based on the principle of "treating yin for the yang disease". "Yin disease" means yang deficiency leading to relative hyperactivity of yin and yang treatment means to nourish yin.

(2) Mutual assistance between yin and yang

According to the principle of interdependence between yin and yang, the method of mutual assistance between yin and yang as "treating yang for reinforcing yin" and "treating yin for reinforcing yang" should be used in meditation. The "yang" in "treating yin for reinforcing yang" refers to yang-tonifying medicinal and "treating yin" means to obtain the effect of supplementing yin. The whole phrase means supplementing yin with an assistance of proper yang-tonifying medicine so as to promote the production and resolving of yin fluid. In "treating yin for reinforcing yang," the "yin" refers to yin-tonifying medicine and "treating yang" means to acquire the effect of supplementing yang. Together, it means that supplementing yang requires an assistance of proper yin-tonifying medicine so as to promote the production and resolving of yang qi. In clinical treatment of yin deficiency syndrome, yang-tonifying medicine should be added into yin-nourishing formula, which is so-called "treating yin for reinforcing yang."

While in the treatment of yang deficiency syndrome, yin-tonifying medicine should be added in yang-nourishing formula, that is, "treating yang for reinforcing yin." yang obtains the assistance from yin and then its production and resolving are unlimited while yin fluids will not be run out with the help of the raising yang. Hence, we need to add medicine of qi-tonifying into blood-tonifying formula to treat blood deficiency syndrome in clinics; in treatment of qi deficiency syndrome, the blood-tonifying medicine are added into qi-tonifying formula.

(3) Supplement of both yin and yang

Due to the interdependence between yin and yang, if yang deficiency is resulted from yin deficiency, then it belongs to yin injury with yang involved; if yin deficiency is resulted from yang deficiency, then it belongs to yang injury with yin involved. In the treating of the syndrome of deficiency of both yin and yang caused by yin-yang mutual injury, we should take methods of supplement of both yin and yang. But we need to distinguish the priority.

If it is yang injury with yin involved, we need to take yang deficiency as primary syndrome, and add yin-nourishing medicinal as secondary based on yang reinforcement. If it is yin injury with yang involved, we need to take yin deficiency as primary syndrome, and add medicinal of nourishing yang as secondary based on yin reinforcement.

In conclusion, the ultimate goal is to select targeted measures of coordinating yin and yang so as to restore the abnormal state of disharmony between yin and yang back into the normal balance of yin and yang, with the theory of yin and yang to guide the determination of therapeutic principles.

8.4.6　Regulating essence, qi, blood and fluids

Essence, qi, blood and fluids are material basis of functional activities of zang-fu viscera, meridians and collaterals. In physiology, they have diverse functions and reinforce each other.

Therefore, there are disharmony in their mutual-use relations and respectively in essence, qi, blood and fluids itself in pathogen. Regulating essence, qi, blood and fluids is the therapeutic principle established to the point of treatment on the above disorders.

8.4.6.1　Regulating qi and blood

It is a therapeutic principle formulated to the point of the deficiency, malfunction of qi and blood itself as well as the imbalance between qi and blood. Qi and blood are interdependent and mutual used with each other; hence they often mutually affect each other in pathology. The lesion results of qi disease with blood involved and blood disease with qi involved are diseases involving both qi and blood. Thus, when treating qi and blood diseases, we cannot treat either of them alone.

It is necessary for us to take into account that the disharmony of their mutual relation. The normal harmony of relations between them can be promoted as a whole through regulation. When treating patient with blood deficiency caused by qi deficiency which is unable to generate blood, we should primarily tonify qi with the assistance of blood supplement, or tonify both qi and blood; when qi deficiency resulted from blood deficiency which is unable to nourish qi, we should primarily supplement blood with the assistance of tonifying qi.

8.4.6.2   Regulating qi and fluids

There is also a mutual-use relation between qi and fluids in physiology. Hence, they often affect each other in pathology. Deficiency of production and transformation of fluids can occur due to qi deficiency, thus we should suppl qi and produce fluids. When treating a patient with water dampness and retained phlegm due to qi failing to form fluids, the method of supplementing qi to move fluids should be adopted. For the patients with fluids loss due to qi failing to control fluids, they should be treated with supplementing qi.

Regard to the patients with qi stagnation caused by fluids retention, their water dampness and retained phlegm should be treated with a secondary treatment of moving qi and removing stagnation; for those with qi collapse following fluids, we need to tonify qi in order to secure collapse assisted by supplementing fluids.

8.4.6.3   Regulating the relation between qi and essence

Qi can disinhibit and induce essence movement, while qi and essence can generate and be transformed into each other in physiology. Qi stagnation can cause essence blockage which leads to defecate dysfunction, hence we need to disinhibit and induce essence and qi. Essence loss and failing to generate qi can cause qi deficiency while qi deficiency and failing to generate essence can cause essence loss, and thus we need to tonify qi and replenish essence concurrently.

8.4.6.4   Regulating the relation between essence, blood and fluids

Based on "homogency of essence and blood", when treating people with blood deficiency, we need to enrich blood and concurrently replenish essence and supply bone marrow; when treating people with damage of essence, and we need to replenish essence and tonify bone marrow with enriching blood at the same time. According to "body fluids and blood are derived from the same source", the syndromes of disease of both fluids and blood causing depletion of fluids and blood or fluids consumption and blood dryness can be observed commonly in pathology, and thus, the treatment method of supplementing blood and nourishing fluids or nourishing blood and moisten dryness should be applied.

8.4.7   Treatment in accordance with three factors

Three factors are a general term for treatments in accordance with seasons, local conditions, and individuality. Human is the product of nature. The movement and change of yin and yang in the natural world is closely related to the human body. Thus, such factors as seasons, climate, rhythm, and regional environment, must affect human physiological activities and pathological changes. The individual differences in gender, age, physical feelings, and dietary habits of the patient also have a certain impact on the occurrence, development and outcome of the diseases.

Hence, when treating diseases, we should make an analysis on the basis of these specific factors and treat them differently so as to formulate appropriate treatment methods and prescriptions. Namely, the so-called treatment in according to seasons, local condition and individual are basic principles that must be followed in disease treatment.

8.4.7.1 Treatment in accordance with seasons

We should consider the principle of treatment based on the climatic characteristics of different seasons, which is called treatment in according to time. The year has four different seasons, and the climate is distinguished by cold, hot, warm and cool, and then these differences will lead to diverse impact on physical activities and pathological changes in human body. Therefore, when treating the disease, we should be guided by characteristics of different seasons and climates to administrate the medicines. In spring and summer, the climate changes from being warm to hot, yang qi tends to ascend and accumulate, and the striae and interstitial spaces of the skin become loose and open. Thus, even if people are affected by exogenous wind-cold, we should be cautious to use pungent-warm dispersing medicinals with strong perspiration such as ephedrine, cassia twig in case of over purging hurting yin. There is much rain in summer and the climate is humid, hence, there are many dampness diseases. We should treat them with medicine of resolving and penetrating dampness. While in autumn, the climate changes from being cool to cold, and the yin becomes exuberant and yang turns to deficiency. The skin striae and interstitial spaces are tight and yang qi hides in the interior. At this time, if people have heat syndrome, we should be cautious to use cold and cold medicine such as gypsum, and mint etc. in case of bitterness and coldness injuring yang.

8.4.7.2 Treatment in accordance with local condition

Formulating the principle of treatment medication according to the environmental characteristics of different regions, this method is called "treatment in accordance with local conditions". Due to the differences in geographical environment, climate, and living habits of different regions, people living in different regions have different body constitutions. In addition, their living and working environment, living habits and ways are all different, and these differences will cause the diverseness in their physiological and pathological changes.

Consequently, there should be differences in the treatment and meditation. For example, for the people living in northwest because of its high sea level and cold weather, their yang qi will be inward astringency and muscular interstices are blocked, and thus, they often have dry and cold diseases. Medicine with the function of moisturizing should be used while cold medicine should be cautious to use. While southeast places in China have low sea level with warm and humid climate, thus, yang qi of the people is easy to release and the skin striae are loosen. Consequently, people living there often have warm-heat or humid heat disease. Medicine with the function of clearing and resolving should be used instead of warm and moisten agents.

In addition, people are vulnerable to local diseases, such as local goiter and Kaschin-Beck disease, due to geological soil and water factors. Therefore, we should take local conditions as a concern when treating them.

8.4.7.3 Treatment in accordance with individuality

Determining the treatment principle according to the different characteristics in ages, genders, constitutions, lifestyle and others of patients is called treatment in accordance to individuality.

Due to differences in ages, physiological conditions, the excess and depletion of qi and blood, the treatment and medication should be different. The elderly have qi and blood deficiency, and then they have more of deficiency syndrome or syndrome of healthy qi deficiency and excessive pathogenic qi. In their treatment, deficiency syndrome should be tonified. We should pay attention to the formula and medication adopted for one with excessive pathogens acquiring attack in case of injuring healthy qi.

Children have vigorous vitality, but they have hyperactivity of qi and blood and delicate zang fu viscera. Besides,they are unable to look after themselves so the young often suffer from diseases and have uneven diet with disharmony in cold and warm. Therefore,when treating them,we should be cautious to use formula of drastic purgation and supplement. In general,the dosage should also be distinguished according to their ages.

Due to different genders,males and females are different in their physiological characteristics. Especially for female,they have physiological characteristics of such as menstruation,leucorrhea,pregnancy,and delivery,etc. When treating them,we should consider the treatment according to their syndromes of diseases.

For example,medicine of drastic purgation,blood breakage,dispelling and diffusion and poison are prohibited to use during their pregnancy. After the childbirth,medicines for treating the consumption and depletion of qi and blood and lochia should be taken into consideration. Males have more diseases such as impotence,emission,and premature ejaculation,and thus the medicine adopted for treating excessiveness syndromes should be primarily of dispelling pathogen,while for deficiency syndromes should in line with the therapeutic principle of tonifying the kidney and regulating and tonifying related zang-fu.

Due to the diverse natural endowment and acquired nursing,individuals are different in figures of being strong or weak,shapes of fat or slim,and in coldness or heat and preponderance of yin or yang. Hence,we should distinguish themedia in treatments. Cool medicinals should be used for the one with yang heat constitution or with appetite preference to spicy food,while the warm or heat medicinals should be cautious in administrating. For people with constitution of yang deficiency,or people who love cold food,we should use warm medicine and be cautious about the bitter and cold one. Besides,we should consider different situations that fat people have more of phlegm,thin people have more of fire,and some people have chronic and occupational diseases and other situations. Thus,we need to take the specific situation of each individual case into consideration.

In a word,the principle of three factors fully embodies the principles and flexibility of the practical application of the holism concept and treatment according to syndrome differentiation in TCM. We should not regard each syndrome as one independent disease in the diagnosis and treatment,but should consider them as a whole from all sides and analyze them based on specific situation.

8.5   Treatment methods

Therapy includes the general therapy and concrete therapy. The general therapy is also called as the basic therapeutic method,including many common features of the concrete therapeutic method,which have the common significance in the clinic. *Internal Classic* records the theory of the therapeutic method,which firstly and exactly proposes the root treatments of "treatment of yin for yang diseases and treatment of yang for yin disease". Through the continuous supplement and choices by the following medical schools,it makes many therapies during the long medical practice period and gradually forms systems,among which the most representative,generalized and systemic is "eight methods" of Cheng Guopeng. In the preface of *Medical Insights*, he said that the origins of disease were internal damage and external contraction. The presentations of disease were cold,hot,deficiency,excess,internal,yin and yang. And the therapeutic methods were diaphoresis, emesis, harmoniztion, purgation, clearing, warming, tonifying and dispersing. The "eight methods" deeply influences the latter clinic therapy. The following sections are the brief introduction.

8.5.1 Diaphoresis

Diaphoresis is also called releasing the exterior or releasing the flesh, which is the method of promoting sweat and solving the pathogen with the sweat through opening the interstices, harmonizing qi and blood also defusing the lung qi. The main function is to get to the purposing of promote sweating to release the exterior. The therapy position is shallow and proper for the beginning of the disease and the disease on the surface with the symptoms of cold fever, headache and body-ache, the thin tongue coating and pulse floating. The application of diaphoresis is divided into releasing the exterior with pungent-warm and releasing the exterior with pungent-cool according to the different features of external contractions, external heat and external cold.

Pungent-warm exterior-releasing medicine is applicable to exterior syndromes, such as exogenous wind-cold exterior syndrome, aversion to cold syndrome and mild fever, whereas pungent-cool medicine is used for heat syndromes, such as exogenous wind-heat exterior syndrome, and heat syndromes of severe fever or mild aversion to cold.

Besides, sweating method can be used for outthrusting pathogens which means to outthrust some pathogenic qi out of the body through dispersing. Although the disease is not caused by exogenous pathogens, its pathogens have the tendency to go outward. We can improve the occasion through diaphoresis to alleviate the disease. For example, diaphoresis can be used for measles at its early phase, when the rashes have not been erupted yet or the outthrusting is obstructed, so as to dispell the measles toxin along with sweating out of body. Then all the symptoms will disappear naturally.

Diaphoresis medication should be different in accordance with seasons, individual and disease. The medication should also be changed corresponding to the properties of different syndromes and the features of different seasons such as warm of spring, hotness of summer, coolness of autumn, and coldness of winter.

Additionally, diaphoresis cannot be used for blood depletion, patient who suffers from strangury disease or person with sores. We should also be cautious to use diaphoresis for the people who are during menstruation and after delivery. According to specific syndromes of the patient, such as yin deficiency, yang deficiency, qi deficiency, blood deficiency or phlegm retention, medicines of nourishing yin, reinforcing yang, tonifying qi, enrich blood, or resolving phlegm can be properly added in exterior-releasing medicine so as to achieve the purpose of strengthening healthy qi and dispelling pathogenic qi. These are some methods of nourishing yin diaphoresis, reinforcing yang diaphoresis, tonifying qi diaphoresis, enriching blood diaphoresis, and eliminating-rheum and resolving-phlegm diaphoresis.

The application of diaphoresis should consider the sweating with pathogens expelled as the rule. Over sweating will cause the consumption and dissipation of fluids, then impairing healthy qi. This method is not applicable for those people whose exterior pathogen has been resolved, measles has been outthrusted, sores and ulcers have been ulcerated as well as the ones with spontaneous perspiration, night sweat, hemorrhage, vomiting and diarrhea, and fluids depletion at the later phase of heat syndrome disease. When administrating the sweat-relieving formula, wind cold, greasy and spicy food should be avoided after taking medicine.

8.5.2 Emesis

Emesis is also called emetic therapy, which is a method of inducing emesis of substantial pathogenic factor and poisonous substance retaining in throat, chest and diaphragm, stomach phlegm, and indigestion out of mouth with the performances of the medicinals. The pathogenic location of the disease is in the upper part of body with pathogens more of tending to go upwards. Therefore, emesis is often used in accordance with the condition to induce the pathogen out of mouth for the purpose of curing the disease. It is applicable to symptoms of food stagnation in stomach, stubborn phlegm retention in chest and diaphragm, sputum blockage in trachea with pathogen moving upwards, or poisonous food remaining in the stomach. In addition, emesis can replace qi supplement lifting method for retention of urine, and pregnancy resistance.

Emesis is usually used for severe and urgent illnesses in which stagnation or poison must be spat out quickly. However, there are cold and hot pathogens and different syndromes of healthy qi impaired or not impaired by pathogen excessiveness. Hence, the specific application of emesis method can be divided into four categories. Cold-medicinal emetic method is used for syndrome of upper heat pathogen stagnation; heat medicinal emetic method is used for syndrome of upper cold pathogen stagnation; drastic medicinals is used for urgent syndromes with upper pathogenic excessiveness; while slow-acting medicinal emetic method is used for syndrome of pathogen excessiveness and healthy qi deficiency, disease at upper energizer, and that must be treated with emesis.

When using emesis, we should note that emesis is an emergent treatment which will have good effect with proper use; while it will hurt healthy qi most easily with improper use. Hence, we must be cautious to use it. In clinics, this emesis method should not be used for the patients who have critical illness, old and weak patients with qi deficiency, blood loss syndrome, and dyspnea. Neither should it be used for children, nor pregnant women or patients with postpartum deficiency of qi and blood.

After being treated with emetic method, patient should have porridge for autotrophic nutrition, but should not have spicy or tough food. Besides, patients should avoid seven emotional stimulation, sexual fatigue, and wind-cold. Emesis, generally, is applied to quick spit, thus repeated use should be avoided.

8.5.3   Harmonization

Harmonization, also known as mediation method, is a treatment with applying harmonizing and releasing formula to realize the dispelling of pathogens, adjustment on the functions of zang fu viscera, and reinforcement of healthy qi. It is featured with low-acting effect, peaceful nature, comprehensiveness, prevalent application, and complicated indications.

Initially, harmonization was designed for harmonizing and release the shaoyang, focusing on the treatment to shaoyang disease which possesses various symptoms of alternating chills and fever, fullness and distention of chest and hypochondria, poor appetite, vexation, nausea, vomiting, bitter taste in the mouth, dry throat, dizzy vision, thin and yellow fur, and string pulse. Take minor decoction of bupleurum as the representative formula. To treat this disease, it requires not only to resolv the semi-exterior pathogen but also to discharge the semi-interior pathogen, but also to achiev the concurrent dissipation of pathogen out of both interior and exterior area. With no other proper method, harmonization was formulated to treat it. Except for the disease with shaoyang, harmonization can also be used for syndromes with complicated pathogenesis, such as liver-stomach disharmony, incoordination between the liver and the spleen, intestine-stomach disharmony, irregular menses caused by liver qi depression, pain diarrhea caused by over restriction of liver wood and spleen earth and other diseases resulted from disharmony among zang-fu viscera. Due to the disability of pure elimination, pure reinforcement, pure warming, or pure clearing on these syndromes, only can the harmonization treatment comprehensively solve them all.

The main purpose of harmonization is eliminating pathogens and simultaneously taking care of healthy qi into consideration. For the features of releasing exterior with treating interior, expelling stagnation with lowering adverse qi, no obvious cold or hot preference, peaceful nature and slow-acting effect, the method of harmonization allows a wide range of practice and is applicable to complicated syndromes. Although it is generalized into one character "harmonization", it embraces various treatments in fact.

Under common situations, harmonization is feasible at the time the disease condition is not severe, the methods of diaphoresis, emesis and purging are not applicable and healthy qi is not deficient. In specific utilization, based on the syndromes of preponderance in exterior, interior, cold, or hot and the excessiveness and deficiency of pathogenic or healthy qi, treatment of harmonization with diaphoresis can be adopted for diseases with exterior preponderance and demand of harmonization; treatment of harmonization with purgation is able to cure diseases with interior preponderance and excessiveness as well as acquiring harmonization; treatment of harmonization with warming is accessible to diseases with cold preponderance and need of harmonization; treatment of harmonization with clearing is applicable for diseases with hot preponderance and requiring harmonization; treatment of harmonization with dispersing is efficacious for diseases with internal stagnation and calling for harmonization; treatment of harmonization with supplementing can heal diseases with healthy qi tending to deficiency and requesting harmonization.

The application of harmonization method should be applied with caution to the diseases with pathogen in exterior and not yet penetrated into shaoyang. And it is not applicable to those three syndromes including syndrome of pathogenic qi penetrating interior, excessive syndrome of intense yang and hot exuberance, and cold syndrome of three yin.

8.5.4　Purgation

Purgation, also known as reducing method, is a method of dispelling the substantial pathogenic factor such as indigestion, accumulation, blood stasis, phlegm and retained fluid out of body through actions of purging, cleansing, attacking and expelling so as to resolve excess heat accumulation. The main function of purgation is to relieve constipation. Thus, it primarily treats the diseases with excessive syndromes and interior and lower onset location, such as indigestion, accumulation and stagnation in intestine and stomach, with symptoms of constipation, fullness, distention and hard pain in stomach and abdomen.

Due to the differences of coldness, heat, water, blood, phlegm and worm in stagnation and the distinctions of latter, former, urgent and chronic diseases, purgation can be divided into cold, warm and moistening purgation in clinical application. Cold purgation is used for constipation and heat accumulation, and applicable to interior sthenic heat syndromes, such as heat dry constipation, heat retention with watery discharge, and dysentery caused by stool stagnation in intestinal. Warm purgation is mainly used to treat cold-accumulation constipation, and applicable to syndromes of cold phlegm stagnation, gastrointestinal cold accumulation, cold-excess accumulation in chest and constipation. Moistening purgation is used for constipation resulted from deficiency of fluid and liquid, applicable to the constipation syndromes of intestinal fluid deficiency, and yin depletion and lesser blood.

Promoting blood stasis method is applicable to blood amassment and blood stasis stagnating internal. Attacking phlegm is used for syndromes of stagnation and obstruction of phlegm. Expelling worms is used for severe accumulation of worms in intestines. Attacking stasis is used for the excessive constitution with stasis-heat binding in the lower energizer. Purgation can also be efficacious for initial-phase dysentery or excessive dysentery with syndromes of blood and pus watery discharge and tenesmus, though it mainly focuses on constipation. The aforementioned are all purging methods. For the methods of promoting blood stasis, attacking phlegm and expelling worm, however, there are primary medicinals to their indications, while purgation serves as an auxiliary method for them.

Additionally, all the methods above require divisions as slow acting or quick acting. Drastic purgation can be used only in urgent conditions where the patient has strong body constitution. Slow purgation is used in a mild and slow conditions where the patient has a weak body constitution. Purgation, in particular the drastic diuretics formula, is extremely easy to impair the healthy qi. Hence, it is important to note that the application of this method should only purge or dispelpathogens at the certain degrees, no overuse or long-term use, in case of the impairment of healthy qi. When the constipation is smooth after the medicine is taken, the disease is cured and the medication should be ceased. Drastic purgation shall not be used for patients with advanced age, fluids consumption and constipation, or with weak body constitution, debilitation in yang and qi, as well as with constipation due to postpartum insufficiency of blood. For the patients in menstruation and gestation period or with weak spleen and stomach, the utility of this method should be cautious or prohibited.

8.5.5   The warming method

The warming method, also named as method of dissipating cold which is a treatment to dispel internal cold with warm-nature medicinal herbs and to dissipate the interior cold and restore yang through warming. It can be used for cold syndrome with cold pathogen invading zang-fu and yin-cold excessiveness; also, be used for asthenia cold syndrome with yang and qi deficiency and internal cold.

The warming method in clinics can be divided into methods of warming interior to dispel cold, warming the meridian to dissipate cold, and restoring yang from collapse according to the differences of cold pathogenic locations and patients' constitution. Cold dispelling by warming interior is applicable to deficiency-cold in middle energizer syndromes including cold pathogen invading middle energizer or yang-deficiency and cold middle energizer, in which the signs are vomiting, diarrhea, abdominal pain, inappetence, lack of warmth in the limbs. Warming the meridian to dissipate cold is applicable to cold arthromyodynia with cold pathogen stagnating meridian or obstructed blood and pulse, often accompanied with blood deficiency or yang deficiency. The signs include cold limbs, faint pulse verging on expiry, or painful and numb limbs. Restoration of yang from collapse is applicable to critical syndromes such as exhaustion and collapse of yang, and internal excessiveness of yin cold. With a drastic effect, it is used for first aid in clinics by breaking yin by expelling cold, and controlling and floating yang to recover the declined or collapse yang. It also is applicable for dangerous and severe syndromes like deficient yang with exuberant yin or exuberant yin repelling yang which is featured with curling due to aversion to cold, vomiting without being thirsty, abdominal pain with diarrhea, incessant cold sweating, cold limbs, and faint pulse verging on expiry.

Warming method is usually adopted with tonifying methods because of the occurrence of interior cold syndrome usually ascribed to the coexistence of yang deficiency and cold pathogen. Besides, the treatment methods commonly applied in clinical diagnosis such as warming lung to resolve fluid retention, warming and resolving cold phlegm, warming kidney for diuresis, warming liver and meridian, and warming stomach with regulating qi also pertain to warming methods.

When using warming method, it is worth noting that medicine of warming method is hot and easy to hurt and consume yin, blood and fluids, thus its application to those with yin deficiency, blood deficiency and bleeding syndrome with blood-heat frenetic movement, hot internal fire, dysentery with heat, or to pregnant women and parturient should be cautious or prohibited.

8.5.6   The clearing method

Clearing method is a treatment using cold medicine to clear poisonous pathogen such as dampness-heat toxin by purging intense heat, detoxifying and cooling blood. It is especially used for interior heat syndrome with a wide treatment range. It can be used for patients with heat exterior diseases whether heat is accumulated in qi aspect, nutrient aspect or blood aspect, as long as the exterior pathogen is expelled with the hot interior, we can use it.

Interior heat syndrome includes warm-heat disease, fire-toxicity syndrome, dampness-heat syndrome, summer-heat syndrome, and deficiency heat syndrome. In the light of the disease stage, level and the nature, clearing method can be divided into clearing heat and purge fire, clearing heat and cool blood, clearing heat and detoxify, clearing heat of zang-fu, and clearing deficiency heat and so on.

Clearing heat and purge fire is mainly used for clearing the heat pathogen in qi aspect, it mainly treats qi aspect heat syndrome. Clearing heat and detoxify is used for pestilential disease, heat toxin sore. Clearing nutrient and cool blood can clear heat pathogen in nutrient and blood aspects. It can be used for heat in nutrient aspect and blood aspect syndrome. Based on the aspects of qi, nutrient and blood where pathogen enter, the following method is used in clinical treatment.

Clearing heat with pungent cool-natured drugs is used for heat in qi aspect, and hot hurting fluid syndrome; clearing heart with bitter and cold medicine is used for heat in qi aspect, and patient with excess-heat syndrome. Clearing nutrient and outthrusting heat is used for heat entering nutrient aspect; clearing heart with salty and cold medicine is used for heat entering blood aspect; clearing heat while nourishing yin is used for heat hurting yin and syndrome with water failing to restrain blazing fire; and clearing heat and opening the orifices are used for high fever, and patients in delirium. The method is used to clear heat pathogen in zang-fu if heat pathogen enters. Therefore, there are different treatments such as purging the lung and clearing the heat, clearing the heart and putting out the fire, clearing liver and purging fire, and clearing and purging stomach fire and so on.

When using clearing method, it must be mentioned that all prescriptions of clearing method are cold and easy to hurt yang qi of spleen and stomach, thus it should not be used for long time. Plus, it cannot be used for those patients with weak body constitution, spleen and stomach deficiency and coldness, unresolved exterior pathogen, stagnated yang qi and fever, and those with asthenia fever due to qi and blood deficiency.

8.5.7   The tonifying method

Tonifying method also known as nourishing and replenishing method is a treatment using prescription with tonic effect to replenish body qi, blood yin and yang and eliminate weakness. Asthenia syndrome is caused by healthy qi deficiency, deficiency of yin and yang of qi and blood in viscera and bowels are included.

Tonifying method can enhance or improve physiological function of organs, with the purpose of improving body weakness, and improving disease resistance ability by supplementing qi, blood, yin and yang. It is applicable to syndrome caused by zang-fu, yin and yang deficiency or syndrome of deficiency of certain zang-fu viscera. Due to the qi, blood, yin and yang deficiency and syndrome of dual deficiency of qi and blood, tonifying method can be divided into tonifying qi, tonifying blood, tonifying yin, tonifying yang and both qi and blood supplement or inter-supplement of yin and yang.

Tonifying qi method is applicable for spleen and lung qi deficiency, fatigue and lack of strength, lack of qi, spontaneous sweating, and vacuous and large pulse. Tonifying blood method is used for patient with blood deficiency and blood loss, and medication should be different due to hot and cold blood. Tonifying yin method is used for syndrome caused by deficiency of yin essence and fluids. Tonifying yang method is used for spleen and kidney yang deficiency. It is featured with cold pain in the waist and knees, cold pain in lower abdomen, frequent micturition, impotence and premature ejaculation.

Except the four above, the application of tonifying zang-fu viscera in clinics based on the deficiency in zang-fu viscera such as tonifying heart and blood, tonifying the heart qi, nourishing blood and emolliate liver, enriching yin and moisturizing the lung, tonifying qi and spleen, enriching yin and tonifying kidney, and tonifying kidney yang, etc. When there is deficiency of qi, blood, yin and yang of viscera and bowels, the treatments of supplement need to balance spleen and kidney, nourish liver and kidney, and nourish qi and yin.

It is required to distinguish "true excess with false deficiency pattern" when using tonifying method. In other words, when treating "excessive sthenia with pseudoasthenia", tonification should be absolutely prohibited. For those with excessive pathogen with deficient healthy qi and exuberant pathogen as the primary syndrome, this method should be used with caution in case of the adverse outcome of "keeping burglar at home". Medicinals for regulating qi flow should be added in when using tonic in order to avoid qi stagnation due to the intolerance of deficiency to supplementing.

8.5.8   The dispersing method

The dispersing method, known as digestant method, is a treatment of gradually resolving or dissipating stagnation or stuffiness caused by retention of food, qi, blood, phlegm and dampness by medicinal for promoting digestion, moving qi, resolving phlegm and inducing diuresis. It can be divided into several methods, containing promoting digestion, moving qi, activating blood, resolving stasis and dispelling dampness.

Promoting digestion and removing food stagnation is used for dietary predilection due to dietary intemperance, uncomfortable spleen and stomach. Activating qi to resolve stasis is used for qi stagnation and blood stasis, while the substantial pathogenic factors such as accumulation and stagnation, static blood, phlegm and retained fluid, dampness all obstruct the movement of the qi. It is often accompanied with fullness; thus, the method is the most commonly used.

Activating blood method can promote blood circulation and resolve blood stasis. If the syndrome is mild, the blood will not be smooth. If severe, there will be stagnation of blood stasis. Thus, we should activate blood circulation and resolve blood stasis for the light one, while we need to break blood and expel stasis for the severe one.

Resolving phlegm and retained fluid is used for syndrome of phlegm retained. Dispelling dampness method is used for various water-dampness syndromes to remove the water and dampness pathogen by resolving dampness, draining dampness and drying dampness. The pathogen can be treated with dissolving, drying or draining in accordance with the location, disease nature and clinical manifestation of water dampness syndrome. Softening hardness and dissipating binds are used for stagnation of phlegm, dampness, qi and blood, syndrome with a lump in the abdominal mass, aggregation accumulation. Besides, it can also be used for syndromes with worm accumulation and internal and external abscess.

Aggregation-accumulation disease experiences three stages which is early, middle and last stages, different treatments using resolve, resolve and harmonization, resolve and supplement should be taken based on the healthy qi condition.

Though dispersing method is not as drastic as purgation, it still injures the healthy qi if used improperly. It should not be used for those patients who suffer from heat disease of yin-deficiency, or abdominal distension, diarrhea and undigested food resulted from deficient spleen, or for women with menstrual block due to blood depletion. Dispersing method is created for dispelling pathogen. Thus, reinforcing healthy qi should be concurrently adopted in the process of dispelling pathogen for all the patients with deficient healthy qi with excessive pathogen.

With the need of medical practice, among the "eight methods" except emesis method barely used, the rest of treatments are still widely used clinically. From them there are more treatments, such as methods of stopping endogenous wind, calming and suppressing the hyperactive yang, inducing securing and astringing, and activating blood and resolving stasis, which have derived according to actual clinical demand, allowing a far more plenteous content for the theory and treatment methods of the TCM.

Liu Yanling, Huang Huanlin

Chapter 9

Basic Knowledge of Chinese Materia Medica

For thousands of years, Chinese materia medica as the main weapon in the prevention and treatment of disease of the human body and mind has made great contributions to the prosperity of Chinese. Chinese materia medica is a major aspect of traditional Chinese medicinal, which focuses on restoring a balance of yin-yang and qi-blood to maintain health rather than treating a particular disease or medica condition.

The vast majority of Chinese medicinals are originally produced in China, but even a natural medicine coming from China can't be called Chinese materia medica. The understanding and application of the Chinese materia medica have a unique theoretical system and application form, which must be based on the theory of traditional Chinese medicinal.

Chinese medicinals mainly come from natural medicine and its processed products, including plants, animals, mineral medicine and some chemical and biological drugs. Plants medicines are the most of the Chinese medicinals, as a result, Chinese materia medica has often been called "Bencao" from ancient times.

9.1 Properties and effects

The properties and effects of Chinese medicinal also referred to as "medicinal preferences" by predecessors, which were highly summarized from the basic natures and characteristics of their effects relating to treatment, are the essential basis of the analyses and clinical usage of Chinese medicinal. The basic principle of TCM treatment is to use medicinal preferences to rebalance the excess or deficiency of yin and yang, as well as the re-establish the functions of zang-fu viscera and meridians of the body, so as to achieve the therapeutic effects.

Properties and effects of the Chinese medicinal include the five important aspects: four properties, five flavors, four directions (ascending, descending, floating and sinking), meridian entry and toxicity, which are of great significance in TCM practice.

9.1.1 Four natures and five flavors

9.1.1.1 Four natures

Four natures refer to the four properties of Chinese medicinals, cold, hot, warm and cool, and are also called the "four xing" in TCM. Cold and cool or hot and warm are only varying in intensity, and cold-cool and warm-hot are two completely different categories of nature. Cool is inferior to cold, and cold-cool belonging to yin, whereas warm is inferior to hot, and warm-hot belonging to yang. In addition, sometimes some medicinal are marked as extremely cold or hot, cold or hot, and slightly cold or hot.

Four natures are summarized mainly from the body's response after different Chinese medicinals are taken, which can reflect the properties, cold or hot of the diseases treated. Medicines with cold-cool property can clear heat, purge fire and remove heat toxin, which are mainly used for heat-syndrome. On the contrary, medicinals with warm-hot property can disperse cold, warm the middle and assist yang, which are mainly used for cold-syndrome.

When you apply medicinal herbs to treat heat or cold syndromes respectively with hot or cold medicinal, you can't achieve desired results of treatment and even bring about harmful results if you don't consider the properties of Chinese medicinals, cold or hot.

In addition, there are herbs also some Chinese medicinals of neutral nature, medicinal preference of which for cold or hot are not so remarkable, and their properties and effects are relatively mild. But actually, they still have differences in the tendency to cool or warm, so they are still in the range of four natures.

9.1.1.2   Five flavors

Five flavors refer to the five different Chinese medicinal tastes in a prescription—sour, bitter, sweet, pungent, and salty. As the characteristic of Chinese medicinals, five flavors are summarized by ancient people not only from the actual and true taste of the Chinese medicinal by the tongue, but more importantly from the clinical effect of Chinese medicinal. So five flavors demonstrate the basic range of effects of the medicinal. Chinese medicinals with same flavor mostly possess similar effects while the Chinese medicinals with different flavors show different effects in the treatment.

(1) Pungent

It has the functions of dispersing and promoting the circulation of qi and activating blood. Pungent medicinals are generally indicated for exterior syndromes, syndromes of qi stagnation and syndromes of blood stasis. For example, Shengjiang(Rhizoma Zingiberis Recens) and Bohe can produce the effects of inducing sweating to expel the exogenous pathogenic factors from the exterior, and Muxiang(Radix Aucklandiae) and Chenpi can circulate qi, and Chuanxiong and Honghua(Flos Carthami) can activate blood circulation.

(2) Sweet

It has the effects of nourishing, harmonizing and moderating. Sweet medicinals are generally ultilized for deficiency syndromes, spasm or pain of epigastric abdomen and limbs, and spleen-stomach disharmony sydrome. It can moderate toxic and violent property of other medicinal and blend taste. So it is widely used in many prescriptions. For example, Huangqi(Radix Astragali seu Hedysari) and Renshen have nourishing effect, while Fengmi(Mel) and Gancao(Radix Glycyrrhizae) can moderate emergency and relieve spasm and pain, and moderate toxic and violent property of many medicinal.

(3) Sour

It has the effects of consolidating, contracting and astringing. Sour medicinals are often used to treat collapse syndromes which are for the loss of essence due to deficiency of right qi, such as spontaneous sweating, night sweating, chronic cough, chronic diarrhea, seminal emission, enuresis, etc. For example, Wumei (Fructus Mume) and Wuweizi are used to relieve cough and diarrhea, Shanzhuyu(Fructus Corni) are used to relieve emission and enuresis.

(4) Bitter

It has the effects of purging and drying. Purging medicinals are often used for clearing heat and purging fire, descending and purging, and purging and rushing down the bowels, heat syndromes, cough, vomit and hiccup due to adverse rising of lung qi or stomach qi and constipation. For example, Huanglian, Huangqin (Radix Scutellariae) and Zhizi(Fructus Gardeniae) can clear heat away, Kuxingren(Armeniacae Semen Amarum) and Banxia can lower and disperse lung qi or stomach qi, Dahuang and Mangxiao(Natrii Sulfas) can cause downward discharge. And drying means drying dampness and is used for damp syndromes, including cold-damp syndrome and dampness-heat syndrome. For example, Cangzhu(Rhizoma Atractylodis) and Yinchen(Herba Artemisiae Scopariae) are able to remove dampness.

(5)Salty

It has the effects of purging and softening. Purging means that it is able to relieve constipation, while softening means that it can soften hardness and dissipate nodules. Salty medicinals are often used to treat constipation and hard nodes or masses syndromes, such as scrofula, goiter, and phlegm nodule. For example, Mangxiao can relieve constipation by purgation, and Muli and Kunbu(Thallus Eckloniae) can disperse scrofula.

Five flavors are the basic tastes of medicinal, and actually the tastes are more than five kinds. There are also astringent and bland flavors. Astringent flavor has the same effects with sour flavor. Bland flavor has the effects of promoting urination and draining dampness. But they are still included in the range of five flavors. People in ancient times held that bland flavor falls under the sweet and astringent flavor falls under the sour flavor category, for the purpose to integrate the five flavors with five elements theory. In five flavors, they can be divided into two parts: pungent, sweet and bland belong to yang property, while bitter, sour and salty to yin property.

Due to the fact that both the four properties and the five flavors can only reveal one of the basic characteristics of Chinese medicinal herbs from different angles, the relationship between four properties and five flavors is very close. in order to obtain a comprehensive and correct understanding. The clinical application of medicinal must combine their specific individual property with flavor.

9.1.2 Four directions(ascending, descending, floating and sinking)

Ascending, descending, floating and sinking are the four directions that the specific embodiment of qi movement, which is presented as the activities of ascending, descending, exiting and entering. They indicate the directional effects of medicinals on the human body when they are taken.

Different diseases often appear to show a tendency to move upward, downward, towards the exterior or the interior because of various pathogenic factors. To correct the disorder of the body functions and restore them to the normal, the directions of effects of Chinese medicinals on human body also have the ascending, descending, floating and sinking distinction. When treating diseases, doctors should select corresponding Chinese medicinals and make the best use of their ascending, descending, floating or sinking effects to help dispel pathogenic factors.

The four directions of medicinal are opposite to the pathogenic tendencies and correspond with syndrome locations. Generally speaking, for syndromes in the upper and superficial part of the body, it is appropriate to choose medicinals of ascending or floating direction. For the syndromes in the lower and interior part of the body, medicinals of descending or sinking direction should be used. Medicine of descending direction are more suitable for syndromes of upward tendency, while medicinal of ascending for syndromes of sinking tendency.

Chinese medicinals of "ascending" have the effect toward the upper parts, which are utilized for the diseases in lower and deeper parts. For instance, Huangqi and Shengma(Rhizoma Cimicifugae) are able to raise splenic qi and are indicated for syndrome of visceroptosis with hyposplenic qi such as chronic diarrhea and lingering dysentery, prolapse of the rectum, prolapse of uterus and gastroptosis. Chinese medicinals of "descending" have the function toward the lower parts and possess the effect of descending adverse qi and are utilized for the disease due to adverse ascending of pathogenic factors. For example, Daizheshi, Xuanfu-hua(Flos Inulae), Banxia and Kuxingren can descend adverse flow of qi, subdue exuberant rang of the liver and descend adverse qi of the lung and stomach and are indicated for dizziness due to hyperactivity of liver yang, cough and dyspnea due to adverse rising of lung qi, nausea and vomiting and eructation due to adverse rising of stomach qi. Chinese medicinals of "floating" have the function toward the upper and outward parts, generally exert the effects of sweating and dispersing and are indicated for the disease in the upper and superficial parts. For example, Mahuang, Fangfeng(Radiax aposhnikoviae) and Qianghuo(Rhizoma et Radix Notopterygii) can dispel wind-cold and dampness from the exterior and are indicated for syndrome of exterior tightened by wind-cold, wind-dampness type of impediment disease, etc. Chinese medicinals of "sinking" have the function toward the lower and inward parts, have the effects of lowering the adverse flow of qi and relaxing bowels and promoting diuresis and are indicators for the disease in the lower and interior. For instance, Dahuang and Mutong(Caulis Akebiae) separately have the effects of relaxing the bowels and promoting diuresis and are used to treat constipation, abdominal distention and pain, dysuria, etc.

The ascending and descending, floating and sinking of Chinese medicinal are often mentioned as two opposite pairs. Ascending and floating, descending and sinking are respectively similar in their effects and often mentioned concurrently. The former belongs to yang and the later belongs to yin. The ascending and floating Chinese medicinals move in ascending and outward directions, generally exert the effects of elevating yang, relieve superficies, dispell wind and cold, cause vomiting, move qi and relieve depression, induce emetic, etc. The descending and sinking Chinese medicinals move in descending and inward directions generally have the effects of lowering the adverse flow of qi, clear heat, purg, promot diuresis, uppress the hyperactive yang, stop wind, etc.

The ascending, descending, floating and sinking of Chinese medicinals arehaving a close relationship with the four properties, five flavors, medicinal parts and qualities. Generally speaking, Chinese medicinals of pungent and sweet in flavor, of warm or heat in property are mostly ascending and floating in their effects. While those of bitter, sour and salty in flavor, and of cold or cool in property are mostly descending and sinking in their effects. Chinese medicinals of flowers, leaves, branches, etc., which are light in quality are mostly ascending and floating in their effects while those of fruits, seeds, minerals, etc., which are heavy in quality are mostly descending and sinking. But it should be noted that this is not always the case. There is an additional small number of Chinese medicinal, for instance, Houpo(Cortex Magmoliae Officinalis), a bark kind, pungent, bitter and warm in its flavor and nature can lower qi and relieve dyspnea. Xuanfuhua, a flower kind, can lower qi.

In addition, the ascending, descending, floating and sinking effects of Chinese medicinal can be affected or even altered by some medicinal processing or medicinal combination. For example, the descending or sinking Chinese medicinal can turn into the ascending and floating ones when they are stir-baked with wine. In the same way, the ascending or floating Chinese medicinal will turn into the ascending or sinking ones, which enter the kidney when they are stir-baked with a salt solution. And when they are used in combination with a variety of strong descending or sinking ones, and their ascending or floating effects are changed into obscurity.

9.1.3 Meridian entry

Meridian entry refers to that Chinese medicinal may often produce their therapeutic effects on some portion of a human body in preference, in other words, their therapeutic effect is mainly related to some specific zang-fu viscera or meridians or some meridians in predominance, while it may seem to produce fewer effects on or seem not related to the other zang-fu viscera and meridians.

Meridian entry takes the theory of zang-fu and meridians and the indication of syndromes as bases. So generally speaking, meridian entry has close relations with defining the location of the syndromes, in a word, what meridian or meridians a Chinese medicinal herb is attrilbuted to is just related to the certain meridian or meridians on which the Chinese medicinal herb may work. For example, Mahuang and Xingren effective to syndromes of the disorder of the lung meridian marked by cough and dyspnea are attribated to the lung meridian. Chaihu(Pericarpium Citri Reticulata), Qingpi(Pericarpium Citri Reticulatate Viride) and Xiangfu(Rhizoma cyperi) indicated for syndromes of the disorder of the liver meridian of foot jueyin marked by distending pain of breast and hypochondrium and hernia pain are attributed to the liver meridian. From above, we can see that meridian entry of Chinese medicinal is summerized from the therapeutic effects through a long time of clinical observation, and being practiced repeatedly, gradually develops into a theory. In addition, when the theory of meridian entry is used, the relationships between zang-fu viscera and meridians must be taken into full consideration.

Mastery of meridian entry is essential for improving clinical practices, because the theory of meridian entry plays an important role in clinical selection of Chinese medicinal herbs according to syndromes, improving the pertinence of direction and strengthening the therapeutic effects. For instance, Chinese medicinals which are cold in nature all have effects of clearing away heat, but with the differences in tendency towards clearing away heat in the heart, lung, stomach, liver or kidney. Those hot in nature can all warm the interior to expel cold, but their effects also have the differences in warming the lung, spleen, stomach or kidney. Medicine for tonifying yin is sweet in flavor and cold in nature, Shashen(Radix Adenophorae, Radix Glehniae) is attributed to lung meridian, while Guiban(Carapax et Plastrum Testudinis) is attributed to kidney meridian. So when we prescribe medicinals, we should select those that work on the diseased zang-fu viscera or meridian or some zang-fu viscera or meridians in the light of their properties of meridian entry to achieve desired therapeutic effects.

The theories such as meridian entry, four natures and five favors, ascending, descending, floating and sinking all explain the properties of Chinese medicinal from various points of view, which jointly constitute their properties and effects.

Therefore, when we apply Chinese medicinal in clinic, we must combine their various properties and effects to give them an allround consideration so that we can select and apply them correctly and avoid one-said.

9.1.4 Toxicity

There are different implications of toxicity of Chinese medicinal between ancient time and today. In the ancient, times toxic medicinal was the general name for all of the medicinal, because the toxicity of medicinal was regarded as medicinal deflection, by which pathological deflection could be treated. The basic principle of treating diseases was to revise the deflection of diseases with the deflection of medicinal. Meanwhile, the ancients also took toxicity as an index to judge how the toxic and side effect was, which was caused by medicinal. In modern times, toxicity only indicates the degree of toxic and side effects, and refers to the harmful effects and injuries of a medicinal on organism. The so-called toxicant refers to the material drastic or poisonous in nature that can do harm to the human body for the light and can cause death for the severe if used improperly. Close observation of the potential side effect of toxic reaction during the therapeutic process is beneficial to the early diagnosis and treatment of poisoning.

In addition, TCM always held that there is a theory of "treating virulent pathogen with poisonous agents", that is, some poisonous Chinese medicinal with obvious therapeutic effects, under the safety of administration, may be used properly for such serious intractable diseases as malignant boil with swelling, scabies, scrofula, goiter, cancer tumor and abdominal mass.

Factors with close relation with toxic reaction can be summarized into the following five aspects. Dosage of poisonous Chinese medicinal in the treatment is close to or the same as poisoning dosage, so the safety margin is small and poisoning is easily resulted. Whereas the dosage of nonpoisonous Chinese medicinal in treatment is much farther from the poisoning dosage, and the safety margin is also larger. But it is not absolute whether they can result in poisonous reaction or not. Toxicity also has a close relationship with processing, combination, preparation of medicinal, ways, mount and the period of using them, the physical condition, age and syndromes of the patient. Therefore, in order to ensure the safety in the use of Chinese medicinal and bring therapeutic effects into play and avoid poisonous reaction, toxic medicinal must be controlled according to the above facts to avoid poisoning when be used. In particularlly, we should pay more attention to the follows.

9.1.4.1 Strictly processing

The toxicity of Chinese medicinal can be weakened by being processed. Therefore, we must strictly follow the process principles to minimize or eliminate the toxicity or side effects before use. For example, Badou(Fructus Crotomis), a kind of drastic purgatives that is poisonous, easily results in poisoning if not processed into Badoushuang(Semen Crotonis Pulzerataum) which is taken orally. After Fuzi is prepared through soaking, its toxicity decreases and it can be widely used.

9.1.4.2 Control of dosage

Poisoning occurrence is related to the excessive dosage of treatment. So the dosage of toxic Chinese medicinals especially those with extreme toxin must be controlled strictly and can not be increased at will. Toxic medicinal such as Pishuang (Arsenicum), Banmao (Mylabris), Maqianzi (Semen Strychni) and Fuzi should be used from small dose and increased according to the syndromes and reaction of the patient after they are taken. At the same time, administration time of medicinals should be controlled strictly too. If Chinese medicinals have been taken for a long time, the body will be poisoned due to accumulation of toxicity.

9.1.4.3 Notes of application

The poisonous Chinese medicinals may be used in different ways. Some can't be taken orally and can only be applied exteriorly, such as Shengyao(Coarsely prepared mercuric oxide) and Tianxianzi(Semen Hyoscyami); some can only be added to pill or bolus and powder, and not to decoction, such as Banmao and Chansu(Venenum Bufonis); others can't be prepared into pill or tablet with wine, such as Chuanwu. And still others should be decocted longer(about 0.5–1 hour) and the toxins of which can be destroied, such as Fuzi. If the boiling time is short, it will cause poisoning.

9.1.4.4 Reasonal combination

If being put into a complex prescription, the toxicity of some medicinals often can be reduced. And if taken singly, the toxicity will be severer. For instance, Banxia has a toxin if being taken singly, but its toxicity will decrease if being taken with Shengjiang. On the other hand, using medicinals with prohibited combinations may cause a strong side-effect, for example, when the incompatible medicinal Gancao and Gansui (Radix Euphorbiae Kansui) used together.

9.2　Compatibility and contraindication

9.2.1　Compatibility

Compatibility refers to the combination of more than two Chinese medicinals to lighten of the clinical requirement such as specific syndromes and medicinal properties and effects. It is the main method of medicinal application and the basis of making up formulae of Chinese medicinal.

In clinical practice, if a disease is simple and light, we can use a single medicine to treat it and achieve the therapeutic purpose. While a disease is complicated, accompanied by other diseases, with exterior and interior syndromes appearing simultaneously, or asthenic syndrome complicated with sthenic syndrome, or cold syndrome accompanied by heat syndrome, single-medicinal formula will fail. Furthermore, some medicinals used in single form may produce toxic and side effects and be harmful to patients. Therefore, Chinese medicinals are usually used in combination according to their specific properties so as to decrease or eliminate their toxic side effects, reinforce or increase their effects and gain better therapeutic effects, whereas unreasonal combination may produce toxicity and poor reactions.

The relationship between medicinals was generalized by the ancients as seven aspects, namely, singular application, mutual reinforcement, mutual assistance, mutual restraint, mutual detoxication, mutual inhibition and incompatibility.

9.2.1.1　Single application

It means the use of a single Chinese medicinal to treat a disorder and fulfill its therapeutic purpose. Usually the case condition is simple and light, but sometimes is serious. For example, Dushen Tang uses Renshen to treat the syndrome of qi collapse. Strictly speaking, singular application means using a medicinal alone, not denoting the relationship of compatibility between Chinese medicinals.

9.2.1.2　Mutual reinforcement

It means that two or more Chinese medicinals with similar properties and effects are combined to reinforce each other's effect. For example, Dahuang and Mangxiao are both purgative and can reinforce each other's original purgating effect when they are used in combination. Mahuang and Guizhi are both pungent and warm-natured and are combined to reinforce their effect of sweating and relieving exterior syndrome.

9.2.1.3　Mutual assistance

It means Chinese medicinals that are not certainly similar but have some relationship in the aspect of medicinal properties and effects are used in combination, in which one medicine is taken as the dominating factor and the others as its assistant to raise its therapeutic effects. For example, Huangqi with the effect of tonifying qi and promoting the flow of water is used in combination with Fangji (Radix Stephaniae Tetrandrae) with the effects of promoting the flow of water and permeating the dampness, the latter reinforcing the former's effect of promoting the flow of water, so their combination can be used for edema due to spleen deficiency. Gouqizi and Juhua are combined to treat blurred vision due to liver and kidney deficiency. Gouqizi, able to nourish liver and kidney yin, supplement blood and essence, and improve vision, is the major medicinal, while Juhua, which can remove liver heat, dispel wind-heat and improve vision, acts as the assistant medicinal.

The similarities between mutual reinforcement and mutual assistance are that by combination, medicinals can cooperate to enhance the overall medicinal effect. The differences lie in the fact that the medicinals in mutual reinforcement relationship are of equal importance, while in mutual assistant relationship, which are comprised of a major medicinal and an assistant one.

9.2.1.4 Mutual restraint

It means a combination in which one Chinese medicinal's toxicity or side effects are reduced or removed by another one. For instance, the poisonous effect of Banxia or Nanxing(Rhizoma Arisaematis) may be decreased or eliminated by Shengjiang. Therefore, we say that there is mutual restraint between Banxia or Nanxing and Shengjiang.

9.2.1.5 Mutual suppression

It means that one Chinese medicinal can relieve or remove toxic properties and side effects of the other. A common example is that Shengjiang can be used to relieve or eliminate the toxicity or side effects of Banxia or Nanxing. Therefore, we say that Shengjiang can detoxicate the toxicity or eliminate the side effects of Banxia or Nanxing.

From the above, we can see that mutual restraint and mutual suppression actually refer to the same thing, but they are expressed in two different ways.

9.2.1.6 Mutual inhibition

It means that when two Chinese medicinals are used in combination, their original therapeutic effects or even their medicinal effects are weakened or losed. For instance, the effect of tonifying qi of Renshen can be weakened by Laifuzi. Therefore, we say that there is mutual inhibition between Renshen and Laifuzi.

9.2.1.7 Mutual antagonism

It means that when two incompatible Chinese medicinals are used in combination , toxic reaction or side effects may result. There are eighteen antagonisms of incompatible medicaments which are believed to give rise to serious side effects if given in combination. For instance, Gancao antagonizes Haizao(Sargassum), Daji(Radix Euphorbiae Knoxiae), Gansui, and Yuanhua(Flos Genkzwa).

In conclusion, in clinical application of Chinese medicinals, mutual reinforcement and mutual assistance medicines can improve their therapeutic effects; while mutual restraint and mutual suppression can suppress or neutralize each toxicity or side effect, and make medicinal safe and effective, so we should make the widest possible use of them. While mutual inhibition and incompatibility can decrease or lose the therapeutic effects and producing toxin and side effects, so we should avoid using them as much as possible.

9.2.2 Contraindication of medicine

Chinese medicinals have not only effects of treating and preventing diseases, but also harmful effects on human body. So when learning medicinal properties, we should not only know their therapeutic efects but also master their harmful effects produced after being taken, which is essential to understanding the contraindications of Chinese medicinal.

The properties of those medicinals which have an unfavorable aspect on human body should be corrected or avoided. In order to decrease the risk of side effects and increase treatment efficacy, doctors must pay close attention to the contraindication of Chinese medicinals. The contraindications mainly include prohibited combination, contraindication during pregnancy, syndrome medication contraindications and dietary incompatibility.

9.2.2.1 Prohibited combination

Prohibited combination means that medicinal in specific combinations in a prescription that can reduce and neutralize efficacies, or reinforce toxicity and increase side effects should be avoided. The prohibited combinations mainly include mutual inhibition and mutual antagonism, especially denotes "eighteen antagonisms" and "nineteen incompatibilities".

Eighteen antagonisms are as follows: Wutou (Radic Aconiti) being incompatible with Banxia, Gualou (Fructus Trichosanthis), Beimu (Bulbus Fritilariae), Bailian (Radic Ampelopsis) and Baiji (Rhizoma Bletinae); Gancao with Haizao, Daji, Gansui and Yuanhua; Lilu (Rhicoma et Radix Veratri) with Renshen, Shashen, Danshen, Xuanshen (Radic Scrophulariae), Kushen (Radix Sophorae Flavescentis), Xixin and Shaoyao (Radic Paeoniae).

Nineteen incompatibilities are as follows: Liuhuang (Sulfur) being antagonistic to Poxiao (Mirabilite), Shuiyin (Hnydrargyrum) to Pishuang, Langdu (Stellera chamaejasme Linn) to Mituoseng (Lithargyrum), Badou to Qianniu (Semen Pharbitidis), Dingxiang (Rlos Caryorphglli) to Yujin (Radic Curcumae), Yaxiao (Crstallised Mirabilite) to Sanleng (Rhicoma Sparganii), Chuanwu and Caowu to Xijiao (Coral Ehinocerotis Asiatici), Renshen to Wulingzhi, Rougui (Corter Cimnamomi) to Chishizhi (Faeces Traopteroram).

As to "eighteen antagonisms" and "nineteen incompatibilities", they are regarded as medicinal which are incompatible, but some of them were still used in combination by some doctors. The conclusion of "eighteen antagonisms" and "nineteen incompatibilities" got in modern experiments and research is not completely similar. Therefore, the conclusion has not been confirmed and further research will be made. So we should use them cautiously and generally avoid using them in combination.

9.2.2.2   Contraindication of drugs in pregnancy

Some medicinals that are regarded as contraindicated should be used with cautions in pregnant women. Otherwise, negative effects on mother, fetus or the growth and development of the born and the unborn child may occur, or induced abortion or miscarriage may be brought about.

Contraindication of medicines in pregnancy can be classified into two types according to the intensity of the medicinals effect as follows: to be avoided completely or to be given cautiously. The medicines to be avoided usually have severe toxicity and drastic property, such as Daji, Gansui, Shanglu, Badou, Qianniuzi, Banmao, Shuizhi (Hirudo), Wugong (Scolopendra), Sanleng, Ezhu (Rhizoma Curcumae), Yuanhua, Shexiang (Moschus Artifactus), Shuiyin, Chansu, and Xionghuang (Realgar). On the other hand, the medicinals pertain to blood-activating and stasis-dispelling, qi-moving, purgative, and part of pungent-warm medicines should be given cautiously, such as Taoren (Semen Persicae), Honghua, Ruxiang (Olibanum), Moyao (Myrrha), Wangbuliuxing (Semen Vaccariae), Dahuang, Zhishi, Fuzi, Ganjiang and Rougui.

No matter whether the medicinals are regarded as forbidden herbs or cautiously used ones, they should be avoided in pregnancy if there is no special need so as to avoid unexpected results. But if the pregnant woman is dangerously ill, and no other choices are available, those mentioned above may be used with great care. If the patient in pregnancy has blood stasis, the medicinal for blood-activating and stasis-dispelling regaining like Taoren may be still used.

9.2.2.3   Contraindication of drugs in syndrome

As it is said, "every medicinal contains toxicity in a certain degree". On account of the different properties and meridian entry of the Chinese medicinal, one kind of Chinese medicinal is only suitable to one certain or some specific syndromes, while invalid to other syndromes, even counteractive sometimes, and it is contraindication to the syndromes at the moment. Actually, each medicinal has its prohibited syndrome. Most of the medicinals have medication contraindications, which will be referred to below the category "prohibitions for use". For example, cold or cool medicinals with the effect of clearing away heat may be likely to damage yang. For example, Huanglians cold in nature and bitter in flavor is indicated for diarrhea due to dampness-heat, but it is not suitable for diarrhea due to spleen yang deficiency. Warm or hot ones with the effect of dispersing pathogenic cold may damage yin. For example, Ganjiang hot in nature and pungent in flavor is indicated for cough due to lung cold, but contraindicated for dry cough due to lung heat.

9.2.2.4 Contraindication of diet

In the period of medicine being taken, some foods are forbidden or limited to be eaten for therapeutic purpose during the treatment of illness, and this is known as forbidden food. Those foods have a negative influence on the absorption of stomach and spleen or decrease efficacies, and reinforce toxicity side effects.

Generally speaking, while taking Chinese medicinals a patient should abstain from raw, cold, greasy and spicy foods and foods with a smell of fish or mutton. In addition, dietetic restraint differs in different diseases. Some foods should be avoided based on certain disease conditions. For example, for warm febrile disease, pungent, greasy or fried foods are prohibited. For cold disease, raw and cold foods should be avoided. Fatty or greasy foods, smoking and drinking should be prohibited while a patient with such syndromes as retention of phlegm in the chest, chest distress and cardiac pain. Pungent foods should be avoided in a patient with syndromes of headache and dizziness due to hyperactivity of liver yang. Fried and greasy foods should be prohibited in a patient with deficiency of the stomach and spleen. Fish, shrimp, crab and pungent foods should be prohibited in a patient with pathogenic infection and ulcerous disease of skin and other skin troubles.

Moreover, some foods are incompatible during medicine taking, and not beneficial to the cure of a disease and even toxic effects can be brought about. For example, Renshen with radish, Guanzhong(Rhizoma Dryopteris Crassirhizomatis) with greasy, Dihuang, Heshouwu(Radix Polygoni Multiflori) with onion, garlic and radish. We should take all the above for reference when we take Chinese medicinals.

9.3 Dosage and usage of medicine

9.3.1 Dosage of medicine

Dosage refers to the amount of each Chinese medicine to be taken. Now we take the metric system(g) as the unit of measurement, which is now stipulated in the Mainland of China. Exact dosage is an important factor to ensure the safety and efficacy of medicinal administration.

Exact dosage is based on the specific features of each medicine, its properties, aimed disease and application methods, as well as consideration of the individual differences of patients.

Generally speaking, the medicine moderate in nature such as Gouqizi and Shanyao can be used in a large dose. Those drastic or toxic in nature such as Banxia and Gansui must be used in a small dose. Those light in property such as flowers and leaves should be used in a small dose. Those heavy in property, such as metals stones and shells but without toxin can be used in a large dose. Fresh plant medicine, since they contain water, should be used in a large dose. Medicine which is bitter and cold in nature cannot be used in a long time and large dosage to avoid injuring the spleen qi and stomach qi.

In clinic, the dosage of one medicine varies according to the combination, formula and aimed disease. Generally speaking, the dosage of a medicine used alone is usually larger than that applied in a prescription. While the dosage of a main medicine in a prescription is larger than that of an accessory one. Under the same condition, the dosage of a medicine used in decoction is larger than that in pills or powder.

The dosage varies greatly with differences of disease, ages, and gender of the patients. Generally speaking, based on disease trends, the dosage used in the treatment of the mild or chronic disease is comparatively smaller, while the dosage of a medicine used in the treatment of serious or acute disease must be fairly larger. Based on patients' constitution, the dosage used for those with strong physique must be larger while for those with weak physique, such as children, delivery women and the elders, the dose is generally smaller. Based on patients' ages, the dosage for children over 5 years old is half of that given to an adult; for children below 5 years old the dose is one fourth of that for adult; for an infant, the dose should be much smaller.

9.3.2   Usage of medicine

The common administration of Chinese medicine may be oral, external or local. Forms of decoction, pill, powder, soft extract, wine, etc. , are prepared for oral use, while application, moxibustion, pigmentum, lotion, laryngeal insufflation of medicinal powder, eye drops, thermotherapy, suppository, etc. , are used exteriorly. Whereas decoction is the most widely used form in clinic, which are generally prepared by patients. The correct method for decoction and administration is very important to ensure high quality of decoction and desired curative effect, and medication safety, therefore doctors should tell their patients or patient's relatives how to decoct medicine.

9.3.2.1   Methods of decocting Chinese medicine

First of all, choose an appropriate decocting utensil, such as a clay pot or earthen jar or a piece of enamelware as metal utensils such as iron and copper are forbidden to decoct medicinal, because metal tends to take chemical reactions with medicinal ingredients, which can reduce the treatment effect and may even cause toxicity or side effects. And then the decocting water must be clean without peculiar smell.

Secondly, the decocting methods must be mastered. Put Chinese medicine into the enamelware and pour the water in it, the water being usually over the surface of the medicine. Before being decocted, the Chinese medicinal need immerse in water for about half an hour in order to make their active ingredients easily dissolve in the solution. Usually fire used in decocting the medicine should be controlled in the light of medicinal properties and qualities, because the method for decoction depends on the properties qualities and effect of the medicine. For example, the medicine with aromatic smell should be decocted with strong fire until the solution is boiled for several minutes, then mild fire is used until the decoction is finished. Otherwise, the medicine effects will reduce. These nourishing medicinal should be decocted with mild fire for a long time because of their greasy qualities, or the effective factors are not easily to dissolve out.

Because their properties and qualities are usually obviously different, different medicinal should be given different decocting methods and time. When a prescription is made out, the decocted methods of some Chinese medicinal should be noted. The chief methods in clude to be decocted earlier, to be decocted later, to be wrap-decocted, to be decocted separately, melting and infusions for oral taking. These methods will be introduced with detail in specific medicine's "Usage and dosage"9. 6.

9.3.2.2   Methods of taking Chinese medicine

Generally speaking, decoction must be taken warm. A dose of Chinese medicine in a prescription is usually decocted twice daily, while nourishing medicine may be decocted three times. And the decocted juice is about 150−200 mL every time. When the decocting is finished, squeeze the Chinese medicine in order to obtain all the liquid of the decoction, then mix the decoction and divide into two or three parts for daily use.

An acute patient must take twice a day or even three times, that is, once for every four hours. A chronic patient may take a dose a day or two days. Those used for stopping vomiting should be taken frequently in small amount. The decoction should be fed through nose for the patients who are in unconsciousness or trismus. Diaphoretics should be taken warmly and after taking medicine patients should tuck in the quilt or drink some hot porridge in order to promote the medicinal effects until sweating. Purging medicine must be taken until reducing diarrhea or vomiting. Wan or powder can be taken with warm water. As far as treatments are concerned, Chinese medicinal warm in nature should be taken in cold or those cold in nature should be taken in warm. As for the time of taking medicinal, tonics that are greasy and tend to be digested and absorbed should be taken before meals in the morning and evening, those irritant to the stomach and intestine should be taken after meals. Paraciticides and purging medicinal should be taken when stomach is empty, those for calming the mind should be taken before sleeping and those for stopping malaria should be taken two hours ahead when the disease has an attack. Medicine should be taken at a regular time for chronic diseases, while a patient with an acute and severe disease can take medicine at any time. In addition, when disease is in the chest and diaphragm above such as headache, dizziness and sore throat, it should be taken after meals. When disease is below chest and stomach such as liver, kidney, and stomach, it should be taken before meals.

Pills can be delivered directly with warm water. The big honeyed pill can be divided into small ones. Powder can be mixed with honey or encapsulated to avoid stimulating the throat. Paste should be taken after mixing with water.

9.4 Classification and common used medicine

9.4.1 Exterior-releasing medicine

Exterior-releasing medicines refer to the medicines with the main effects of releasing the exterior and treating the exterior syndrome. They are also considered to be diaphoretic medicine herbs. These kinds of medicines mainly have the pungent taste and the quality of lightly floating, and they are mainly attributed to the lung and bladder meridians, with the function of promoting sweating and dispersing exogenous pathogenic factors. They are mainly used for the treatment of exterior syndrome, manifested as aversion to cold, fever, headache, no sweat, floating pulse etc. Parts of the medicine also can be used for the edema, cough, measles, rubella, rheumatic pain at the early stage with the exterior-syndrome.

Exterior-releasing medicines are divided into two kinds: wind-cold-dispersing medicinal and wind-heat dispersing medicinal. The former are used for the treatment of wind-cold syndrome and the later are used for the wind-heat syndrome. When we use these kinds of medicines, the dosage shouldn't be too large to avoid excessively sweating and consumption of yin. The application should be stopped as soon as the syndrome disappears. Therefore, these kinds of medicines do not apply to the interior deficiency syndrome, strangury and blood lost patients. Most exterior-releasing medicines have active volatile oil. If added to decoction, they should not be decocted for a long time to prevent effective constituents from volatilizing and decrease the clinical efficacy.

In addition, they can dry dampness and harmonize stomach, so they are effective for disharmony of stomach and restlessness when combined with Shumi in Banxia Shumi Tang.

In addition, they can be used to treat gastroptosis, prolapse of rectum and uterus, but in order to get good therapeutic effect, they must be combined with Chaihu, Shengma, and Huangqi, and they has the effect of raising blood pressure as well.

In addition, they could also be used in the treatment of coronary heart disease with angina pectoris and various stagnant blood syndromes of gynecology.

In addition, they can replenish qi and strengthen yang and it is used to treat impotence. When combined with pathogen-expelling such as exterior-releasing, cathartic drugs, they have the efficacy to reinforce the healthy and dispel the pathogenic. They are used to treat excessive pathogens with healthy qi being deficient, such as in the case of qi deficiency with external contraction, or with heat accumulation of interior-excess.

Mahuang(Ephedra, Herba Ephedrae)

Properties and Tastes: pungent, slightly bitter and warm.

Meridian Entry: lung and bladder meridians.

Effects: ①Promote sweating to release the exterior. ②Diffuse the lung to calm panting. ③Induce diuresis to alleviate edema.

Application:

(1)The common cold due to wind-cold

The medicinal herb has the nature of pungent and warm, and attributive to the lung meridian, therefore, it can diffuse the lung qi and strongly promote sweating. It is often used for superficial sthenia-syndrome due to wind-cold, which is manifested as aversion to cold, fever without sweating, headache and pain all over the body, nasal obstruction, a floating and tense pulse. It is often used in combination with Guizhi in order to strengthen the work of promoting sweating to releasing the exterior, such as Mahuang Tang.

(2)Cough and dyspnea

It is majorly used for the cough and dyspnea due to stagnation of lung qi which belongs to excessive syndrome. But after combination, it can be used in all kinds of cough and dyspnea. For example, when it is combined with Gancao and Xingren, it can be used to treat cough and dyspnea due to wind-cold attacking lung. When it is combined with Shigao, Xingren and Gancao, it can be used to treat the cough and asthma due to lung heat. The former is called Sanao Tang and the latter is called Mahuang Xingren Shigao Tang.

(3)The wind edema

The wind edema is a type of edema especially of the face and head, ascribed to attack on the lung by pathogenic wind, manifested by sudden onset of edema accompanied by fever with aversion to wind, aching joints, and oliguria. The medicinal herb can promote sweating and diffuse the lung qi, so it can be used to treat the wind edema. Such as Yuebi Jiazhu Tang, which is consisting of Mahuang, Shengjiang and Baizhu.

Usage and dosage: 2-10 g for decoction. When it is used to relieve exterior, the herb is fresh. When used to control asthma, the honey-Mahuang is often used.

Guizhi(Cassia Twig, Ramulus Cinnamomi)

Properties and Tastes: pungent and sweet in flavor, warm in nature.

Meridian Entry: heart, lung and bladder meridians.

Effects: ①Promote sweating to release the flesh. ②Warm and free the meridian. ③Reinforce yang and promote the flow of qi.

Application:

(1)The common cold due to wind-cold

The medicinal herb has the nature of pungent, sweet and warm, and it can disperse yang qi and promote blood to flow in the body surface and muscles. Therefore, it has the function of promoting sweating to release the flesh. It is used for the exterior syndrome due to wind-cold whether the syndrome is deficiency or sufficiency. It is often used in combination with Mahuang in order to strengthen the work of promoting sweating to releasing the exterior, such as Mahuang Tang. For the wind-cold syndrome with spontaneous perspiration due to superficial deficiency, it is often used in combination with Baishao, such as Guizhi Tang.

(2)The stomach duct cold pain, blood cold amenorrhoea, joint pain caused by impediment

The medicinal herb can warm and free the meridian, so it can be used in all kinds of pain resulted from the syndrome of congealing cold with blood stasis. When it is used in combination with Zhishi and Xiebai, it can treat the patient with chest impediment and heart pain, such as Zhishi Xiebai Guizhi Tang. When it is used in combination with Baishao and Yitang, it can warm spleen and stomach for dispelling cold and relieving pain, such as Xiaojianzhong Tang. If a woman has the syndrome of congealing cold with blood stasis and the symptoms of dysmenorrhea, amenorrhea, irregular menstruation and postpartum abdominal pain, it can be used in combination with Danggui, Wuzhuyu, such as Wenjing Tang. When it is used in combination with Fuzi, it can be beneficial to the patient with impediment, such as Guizhi Fuzi Tang.

(3)Phlegm syndrome and edema

Because of the nature of pungent, sweet and warm, it can not only warm spleen yang to promote the transportation of water, but also warm kidney yang to promote the qi transformation of bladder. It is often used in the phlegm, fluid-retention and edema, such as Wuling San.

(4)Palpitation and renal mass due to retention of fluids

Because of the nature ofpungent, sweet and warm, it warms heart yang and promotes blood circulation to stop throb. Such as Zhigancao Tang, in which combined with Gancao, Renshen, and Maidong.

Usage and dosage: 3–10 g for decoction.

Bohe(Peppermint, Herba Menthae)

Properties and tastes: pungent and cold.

Meridian Entry: lung and liver meridians.

Effects: ①Disperse wind-heat. ②Clear heat from the head and eyes. ③Soothe the throat. ④Outthrust rashes. ⑤Soothe the liver and move qi.

Application:

(1)The common cold due to wind-heat and early stage of seasonal febrile disease

For the syndrome manifested as fever and anhidrosis, slight aversion to wind and cold and headache, it is often combined with Jingjie, Niubangzi, Jinyinhua, Lianqiao, etc., such as Yinqiao San.

(2)Headache and redness of eyes, swollen and painful throat

The drug has light texture and fragrant odour, so it is usually for the syndrome of wind and heat attacking up-wards manifested as headache and redness of eyes, it is used together with Sangye, Juhua and others that can clear away heat from head and eye. For the swollen and painful throat, it is often used with Jiegeng, Gancao and Jiangcan, such as Liuwei Tang.

(3)Unsmooth eruption of measles and itching due to rubella

It is usually used together with Chantui, Niubangzi, etc. So as to promote eruption of measles, such as Zhuye Liubang Tang. It can be combined with Kushen, Baixianpi, Fangfeng, etc., to expel wind and relieve itching and treat rubella with itching, too.

(4)The syndrome of stagnation

Especially for stagnation of liver qi, oppressed feeling in the chest and hypochondriac pain, or swollen pain of breast and irregular menstruation, it can be used together with Chaihu, Baishao, and Danggui, such as Xiaoyao San.

Usage and dosage: 3–6 g for decoction and decoct later.

Niubangzi(Great Burdock Achene, Fructus Arctii)

Properties and tastes: pungent, bitter and cold.

Meridian Entry : spleen and stomach meridians.

Effects : ① Disperse wind-heat. ② Diffuse the lung and outthrust rashes. ③ Detoxify and soothe the throat.

Application :

(1) The Chinese common cold due to wind-heat and the early stage of seasonal febrile disease

The medicinal has the nature of cold, and the taste of pungent and bitter. Therefore, it can be used for exterior syndrome of wind and heat type with sore and swollen throat, together with Bohe, Jinyinhua and Lianqiao, etc. , such as Yinqiao San. For those with sore and swollen throat, usually used together with Dahuang, Huangqin and other herbs that can clear away heat and remove toxic materials.

(2) Itching due to rubella

Also it can be used for unsmooth eruption of measles. At this time, usually combined with Bohe, Jingjie, Chantui, etc.

(3) The urticaria and sores

It is often used together with Dahuang, Mangxiao, and Zhizi, etc. It is combined with Xuanshen, Huangqin, Banlangen, etc. to treat mumps and pharyngalgia.

Usage and dosage : 6-12 g for decoction. It is pounded into pieces that are used in decoction, and the stir-baked one can reduce its cold nature.

Simple list of other exterior-releasing medicinals see Table 9-1.

Table 9-1   **Simple list of other exterior-releasing medicinals**

Name	Properties and Tastes	Meridian entry	Effects	Application	Dosage
Zisu(Folium Perillae)	Pungent and warm	Lung and spleen meridians	(1) Release the exterior and dissipate cold (2) Move qi and smooth the middle (3) Prevent abortion	(1) The common cold due to wind-cold (2) Stagnation of spleen qi and stomach qi and vomitus gravidarum (3) Poisoning from fish and crabs	5-10 g for decoction. Do not overcook
Shengjiang (Rhizoma Zingiberis Recens)	Pungent and slightly warm	Lung, spleen and stomach meridians	(1) Release the exterior and dissipate cold (2) Warm the middle energizer to arrest vomiting (3) Warm the lung to suppress cough	(1) The common cold due to wind-cold (2) Spleen and stomach cold syndromes (3) Vomiting due to stomach cold (4) Cough caused by lung cold (5) Poisoning of fish and crabs	3-10 g for decoction

Continue to Table 9-1

Name	Properties and Tastes	Meridian entry	Effects	Application	Dosage
Xiangru (Herba Moslae)	Pungent and slightly warm	Lung, spleen and stomach meridians	(1) Promote sweating to release the exterior (2) Eliminate dampness and regulate the function of the spleen and stomach (3) Induce diuresis to alleviate edema	(1) The affection of exotenous wind-cold and internal injury by summer-damp, aversion to cold with fever, vomiting and diarrhoea (2) Edema, inhibited urination	3-10 g for decoction
Jingjie(Herba Schizonepetae)	Pungent and slightly warm	Lung and liver meridians	(1) Release the exterior and dissipate wind (2) Outthrust rashes (3) Disperse wounds (4) Stop bleeding	(1) The common cold and headache (2) The early stage of measles, urticaria and sores (3) Blood disease	5-10 g for decoction. Do not overcook.
Fangfeng (Root Radix Saposhnikoviae)	Pungent, sweet and slightly warm	Bladder, liver and spleen meridians	(1) Dispel wind and release the exterior (2) Dispel dampness and relieve pain (3) Relieve convulsive disease	(1) The exterior syndrome (2) Wind-cold-dampness impediment (3) Itching due to rubella (4) Urticaria	5-10 g for decoction
Qianghuo (Rhizoma et Radix Notopterygii)	Pungent, bitter and warm	Bladder and kidney meridians	(1) Release the exterior and dissipate cold (2) Dispel wind and dampness (3) Relieve pain	(1) The common cold due to exogenous wind-cold (2) Wind-dampness impediment and pain of back and shoulder	3-10 g for decoction

Continue to Table 9-1

Name	Properties and Tastes	Meridian entry	Effects	Application	Dosage
Baizhi(Radix Angelicae Dahuricae)	Pungent and warm	Lung, stomach and large intestine meridians	(1)Release the exterior and dissipate cold (2)Dispel wind and relieve pain (3)Relieve the stuffy nose (4)Dry dampness and stanch vaginal discharge (5)Disperse swelling and expel pus	(1)The common cold due to wind-cold (2)Headache, toothache caused by wind-cold-dampness (3)The allergic rhinitis, sinusitis and stuffy running nose (4)Vaginal discharge	5-10 g for decoction
Gaoben (Rhizoma Ligustici)	Pungent and warm	Bladder meridians	(1)Release the exterior and dissipate cold (2)Dispel dampness and relieve pain	(1)The common cold due to wind-cold (2)Wind-cold-dampness impediment	3-10 g for decoction
Xinyi(Flos Magnoliae)	Pungent and warm	Spleen, and stomach meridians	(1)Release the exterior and dissipate cold (2)Relieve the stuffy nose	(1)The common cold due to wind-cold (2)The allergic rhinitis, sinusitis and stuffy running nose	3-9 g for decoction. Wrap-decoction
Congbai (Fistular Onion Stalk)	Pungent and warm	Lung and stomach meridians	(1)Promote sweating to release the exterior (2)Dissipate cold and promote the yang qi	(1)The common cold due to wind-cold (2)The exuberant yin repelling yang	3-10 g for decoction
Sangye (Folium Mori)	Sweet, bitter cold	Lung and liver meridians	(1)Disperse wind-heat (2)Clear lung fire and moisten dryness (3)Pacify the liver yang (4)Clear the liver and improve vision	(1)The common cold due to wind-heat and early stage of seasonal febrile disease (2)The cough with lung heat or dryness-heat (3)The hyperactivity of liver yang, headache and dizziness (4)For the red eyes and dim-sight	5-10 g for decoction

Continue to Table 9-1

Name	Properties and Tastes	Meridian entry	Effects	Application	Dosage
Chantui (Periostracum Cicadae)	Sweet and cold	Lung and liver meridians	(1) Dispersing wind-heat (2) Soothe the throat (3) Outthrust rashes (4) Remove nebula and improve vision (5) Relieve convulsion	(1) The wind-heat syndrome, seasonal febrile disease at the early stage, sore throat (2) Itching due to rubella and unsmooth eruption of measles (3) Conjunctivitis and pterygium (4) Tetanus and infantile convulsion	3-6 g for decoction
Juhua (Flos Chrysanthemi)	Pungent, bitter, sweet and slightly cold	Lung and liver meridians	(1) Dispersing wind-heat (2) Clear the liver and improve vision (3) Clear heat and detoxify	(1) The common cold due to wind-heat and early stage of seasonal febrile disease (2) Dizziness and headache due to hyperactivity of liver yang (3) Red, swollen and painful eyes and blurred vision (4) Furuncle and especially for furunculosis	5-10 g for decoction
Manjingzi (Fructus Viticis)	Pungent, bitter, and slightly cold	Bladder, liver, and stomach meridians	(1) Disperse wind-heat (2) Clear heat from the head and eyes	(1) The common cold due to wind-heat (2) Red eye, obscure eyes (3) For dizziness	5-10 g for decoction
Chaihu (Radix Bupleuri)	Pungent, bitter and slightly cold	Liver, gallbladder and lung meridians	(1) Release the exterior and discharge heat (2) Soothe the liver and alleviate mental depression (3) Elevate yang qi	(1) Fever caused by exogenous pathogenic factors and alternating chills and fever (2) The liver qi stagnation, fullness and pain in chest and hypochondrium, irregular menstruation (3) Prolapses due to deficiency of qi, such as uterine prolapse and archoptosis	3-10 g for decoction

Continue to Table 9-1

Name	Properties and Tastes	Meridian entry	Effects	Application	Dosage
Shengma (Rhizoma Cimicifugae)	Pungent and slightly sweet	Lung,spleen,stomach and large intestine meridians	(1)Release the exterior and outthrust rashes (2)Clear heat and detoxify (3)Uplift yang qi	(1)The common cold due to wind-heat (2)For itching due to rubella or unsmooth eruption of measles (3)Toothache and aphtha, swollen and throat pain (4)Prolapse due to qi deficiency manifested as shortness of breath, fatigue, prolapse of rectum due to chronic diarrhea, prolapse of uterus, flooding and spotting	3–10 g for decoction
Gegen (Radix Puerariae)	Sweet,pungent and cold	Spleen, stomach and lung meridians	(1)Release the flesh and bring down a fever (2)Engender fluid and relieve thirst (3)Outthrust rashes (4)Uplift yang and check diarrhea	(1)Fever,headache caused by exogenous factors (2)Thirst during febrile disease and internal heat with diabetes (3)For itching due to rubella with unsmooth eruption (4)Dampness-heat dysentery and spleen deficiency diarrhoea	10 – 15 g for decoction
Dandouchi (Semen Sojae Preparatum)	Bitter,pungent and cold	Spleen and stomach meridians	(1)Release the exterior (2)Relieve restlessness (3)Disperse stagnated heat	(1)The common cold (2)For irritability,chest tightness	6–12 g for decoction

9.4.2　Heat-clearing medicine

Heat-clearing medicines refer to the medicinal herbs that has the main effect of clearing away interior heat.

These kinds of medicines are mostly cold and cool in nature, have sinking effect and working toward the inward parts. They have the effects of clearing away heat, draining dampness, cooling the blood, detoxifying, relieving malnutrition fever, etc. They are often used for various internal heat syndromes, manifesting as high fever, excessive thirst and dampness-heat diarrhea and dysentery, jaundice with dampness-heat pathogen, carbuncle, maculae due to warm-toxin and fever due to yin deficiency.

According to different effects and on different types of qi aspect, xue aspect, ying aspect, sthenia and asthenia of the internal heat syndrome, these kind of medicinals are divided into five types, that is, heat-clearing and fire-purging medicinal, heat-clearing and dampness-drying medicinal, heat-clearing and detoxicating medicinal, heat-clearing and blood-cooling medicinal, and deficiency heat-clearing medicinal.

Heat-clearing medicinal herbs are cold and cool in nature, so can they easily injure the spleen and stomach qi. When heat-clearing medicinals are applied, we must pay attention to the patients with deficiency of spleen and stomach or yin deficiency. Firstly, we must distinguish the exterior from the interior and be sure of the position of heat. If the heat is at qi aspect with high fever, thirst, sweat, restlessness, heat-clearing and fire-purging medicinal should be applied. If the heat in blood aspect, manifesting high fever at night, restlessness and insomnia, heat-clearing and blood-cooling medicinal should be used. There are differences in application of these five kinds of medicinals. Secondly, we must distinguish the asthenia from sthenia. For the sthenic heat-syndrome, those medicinal herbs of clearing away heat and purging fire, or clearing away heat from both qifen and xuefen, or clearing away heat from yingfen and cooling blood are used. For deficient heat-syndrome, those medicinal herbs of cooling blood and clearing away heat, or cooling blood to remove steaming fever or nourishing yin to clear away heat. In the meantime, according to syndromes accompanying with or following the above syndromes, antipyretic herbs must be used in combination with others. For example, for heat syndrome with exogenous pathogenic factors, exterior-releasing medicinal and heat-clearing medicinal are used together.

Shigao(Gypsum, Gypsum Fibrosum)

Properties and Tastes: sweet, pungent and extremely cold.

Meridian Entry: lung and stomach meridians.

Effects:

(1) Hydrated gypsum: ①Clear heat andpurge fire. ②Relieve restlessness and thirst.

(2) Calcined gypsum: ①Induce astringent. ②Promote tissue regeneration and close wound.

Application:

(1) High fever and excessive thirst

The medicinal herb has the nature of sweet, pungent and extremely cold, and is attributed to the lung and stomach meridians. Therefore, it is most suitable to be used for clearing away heat and fire of the lung and stomach, which is manifested as high fever, excessive thirst, perspiration, and large and bounding pulse. It is often used in combination with Zhimu in order to strengthen the work of clearing away heat and fire such as Baihu Tang. For syndrome involving both xuefen and qifen with coma, high fever, maculae and delirium, it is usually combined with Mudanpi, Shengdihuang, and others that can cool blood.

(2) Cough and dyspnea due to heat in the lung

It is attributed to the lung meridian and it can clear away heat and fire of the lung. Therefore, when it is used in combination with Mahuang, Guizhi, Gancao, etc., we will get a very good curative effect on such a kind of disease as Mahuang Xingren Gancao Shigao Tang.

(3) For excessive stomach fire, headache and toothache, internal heat dispersion-thirst

Shigao can be used for clearing away heat and fire in the stomach. In clinical practice, it is often used in combination with Huanglian, Shengma, Zhimu, Shengdihuang, Maidong etc., such as Qingwei San and Yunv Tang.

(4) For the anabrosis, eczema, scald and bleeding wound

Calcined gypsum has the function of promoting tissue regeneration and closing wound. It is often used in combination with Shengyao for the treatment of anabrosis, such as Jiuyi Dan. When it is used with Huangbai, it can treat eczema, such as Shihuang San. Shigao together with Qingdai can used for scald.

Usage and dosage: Hydrated gypsum, 15 – 60 g, decoct first. Calcined gypsum for external using, spread the affected area with appropriate amount powder.

Zhimu(Commom Anemarrhena Rhizome, Rhizoma Anemarrhenae)

Properties and Tastes: bitter, sweet, cold.

Meridian Entry: lung, stomach and kidney meridians.

Effects: ①Clear heat and purge fire. ②Nourish the yin and moisturize dryness.

Application:

(1) For high fever and excessive thirst

The medicinal herb has the nature of bitter and cold. Therefore, it can be used for clearing away heat and fire, which is manifested as high fever, excessive thirst, perspiration and large and bounding pulse. It is often used in combination with Shigao in order to strengthen the function of clearing away heat and fire, such as Baihu Tang.

(2) The cough due to lung heat, dry cough due to yin deficiency

The medicinal herb is attributed to the lung meridian, and has the nature of bitter, sweet and cold, and it can clear away heat and purge fire from the lung as well as nourish yin and moisten the lung. Therefore, it can clearing away heat and fire of lung meridian, which is manifested as cough or dry cough. For cough with yellow sputum due to lung heat, it is often used in combination with Huangqin, Zhizi, Gualou, etc. , such as Qingjin Huatan Tang. For dry cough due to yin deficiency in lung, it is used together with Maimendong, Beishashen and others that can nourish yin and moisten the lung.

(3) For osteopyrexia and fever

The medicinal herb is attributed to the kidney meridian, and has the nature of bitter, sweet and cold. Therefore, it can nourish the kidney yin, clear away heat and fire of kidney meridian. It can be used for such diseases as hectic fever, night sweat and restlessness. It is often used in combination with Huangbai, Di Huang, etc. , such as Zhibai Dihuang Wan.

(4) Internal heat dispersion-thirst

It is often used in combination with Tianhuafen, Gegen to clear away heat and fire and nourish the yin and moisturize dryness, such as Yuye Tang.

(5) For the constipation due to intestinal dryness

The medicinal herb can nourish the yin and moisturize dryness to purge. It is often used in combination with Shengdihuang, Xuanshen, Maidong etc.

Usage and dosage: 6 – 12 g for decoction. When it is used to clear away heat and fire, the herb is fresh. When used to nourish the yin and moisturize dryness, the herb is often processed with brine.

Zhizi(Cape Jasmine Fruit, Fructus Gardeniae)

Properties and Tastes: bitter and cold.

Meridian Entry: heart, lung, and triple energizer meridians.

Effects: ①Purge fire and relieve dysphoria. ②Cool the blood and detoxify. ③Clear heat and drain dampness. ④Cool the blood to stop bleeding.

Application:

(1) Febrile disease with irritability

It can clear away fire from the triple energizer and heart, and relieve vexation. For febrile diseases with irritability, it is often used combined with Dandouchi, such as Zhizichi Tang. For overabundance of heart heat with high fever, irritability, coma and delirium, it is usually used together with Huanglian, Huangqin,

Huangbai and others that can clear away heat and purge fire, such as Huanglian Jiedu Tang.

(2)Jaundice of dampness-heat syndrome

For stagnation of dampness and heat in the liver and gallbladder manifested as jaundice, fever and oliguria with brownish urine, it is often combined with Yinchen, Dahuang, etc. , such as Yinchenhao Tang.

(3)Strangury disease due to dampness-heat

The medicine can cool the blood to stop bleeding, so it is mostly used for blood strangury. It is often used with Mutong, Cheqianzi, Huashi and so on, such as Bazheng San.

(4)Hematemesis, epistaxis caused by blood heat

For bleeding due to blood heat manifested as hematemesis, epistaxis, hematuria, etc. , it is often combined with Baimaogen, Dahuang, Cebaiye, etc. , such as Shi Hui San. Also it can be used together with Huangqin, Huanglian, Huangbai, such as Huanglian Jiedu Tang.

(5)Red, swollen and painful eyes

It can be used for such symptoms due to heat of liver and gallbladder, usually with Dahuang, such as Zhizi Tang.

Usage and dosage: 5 – 10 g for decoction.

Huangqin(Baical Skullcap Root, Radix Scutellariae)

Properties and Tastes: bitter, cold.

Meridian Entry: lung, gallbladder, spleen, large intestine and small intestine meridians.

Effects: ①Clear heat and dry dampness. ②Clear fire and detoxify. ③Stop bleeding. ④Prevent abortion.

Application:

(1)Dampness-warmth, summerheat-dampness, epigastric fullness due to dampness-heat, diarrhea and jaundice

The medicinal herb has the nature of bitter and cold, and is attributed to the lung, gallbladder, spleen, large intestine and small intestine meridians. Therefore, it can clear heat and eliminate dampness of them, especially effective in clearing away dampness-heat of the middle and upper energizers. For dampness-warmth manifested as perspiration, fever, chest oppression, greasy fur, it is often combined with Tongcao, Huashi, Baidoukou, etc. For jaundice due to dampness-heat, it is used together with Zhizi, Yinchen, Dahuang, etc. For the treatment of diarrhea of dampness-heat type, it is often used in combination with Huanglian, Banxia, Ganjiang, etc, such as Banxia Xiexin Tang.

(2)For cough due to heat in the lung and high fever and excessive thirst

The medicinal herb as attributed to the lung meridian, so it can be used for clearing heat in lung and good at clearing away sthenic-heat of the upper energizer. It is the important herb for cough caused by lung heat. It is often used in combination with Gualou, Sangbaipi, Kuxingren, etc, such as Qingqi Huatan Wan. On the other hand, it is suitable for clearing heat in qifen, which is manifested as high fever and excessive thirst, such as Liangge San. For shaoyang syndrome of alternating episodes of chills and fever, it is often used in combination with Chaihu, and the representative formula is Xiaochaihu Tang having the effect of regulating the function of shaoyang.

(3)For sore and ulcer, swollen sore

The medicinal herb has the effect of clearing fire and detoxicating, so it can be used to treat sore and ulcer. For example, Huanglian Jiedu Tang consists of Huanglian, Huangbai and Zhizi.

(4)Hemopyretic bleeding

It can be used alone(Huangqin San), or combined with Dahuang(Dahuang Tang) for hemopyretic bleeding, which is manifested as hematemesis, hemoptysis, hematochezia, hemafecia and metrorrhagia.

(5) For threatened abortion

It can be used for excessive fetal movement and gravid vaginal bleeding due to heat-syndrome in pregnancy together with Baizhu, Danggui, such as Danggui San.

Usage and dosage: 3-10 g for decoction. When it is used to clear heat and eliminate dampness and clear fire and detoxicate, the herb is fresh. When used to prevent miscarriage, the herb is often processed with wine.

Huanglian(Coptis chinensis Franch, Coptis Rhizome)

Properties and Tastes: bitter and cold.

Meridian Entry: heart, spleen, stomach, liver, gallbladder and large intestine meridians.

Effects: ①Clear heat and dry dampness. ②Clear fire and detoxify.

Application:

(1) The stuffiness and fullness, vomiting and acid regurgitation

The medicinal herb has the nature of bitter and cold, and it has a stronger effect of clearing heat and eliminating dampness than Huangqin, especially specializes in clearing away dampness-heat of middle energizers. And it serves as an essential medicinal herb for the treatment of diarrhea and dysentery of dampness-heat type. It can be combined with Muxiang for the patients with abdominal pain due to qi stagnation, such as Xianglian Wan. Gegen Qinlian Tang, combined with Gegen for the case with general fever. Shaoyao Tang, combined with Baishao, Muxiang, Binlang, etc. , for dysentery with pus and blood. For dampness-heat stagnation in the middle energizer, it is used together with Ganjiang, Huangqin, Banxia, etc. , such as Banxia Xiexin Tang.

(2) High fever and coma, heart fire hyperactivity, vexation and sleeplessness, palpitation and lusterless

It can clear heat, and is especially good at removing heart fire. Therefore, it can be used for the diseases with excessive fire and heat, which is manifested as high fever and restlessness, such as Huanglian Jiedu Tang, which is combined with Zhizi and Huangqin. For heart fire hyperactivity, manifested as vexation and sleeplessness, it can be used together with Danggui and Shichangpu, such as Huanglian Anshen Wan. For vexation and sleeplessness due to insufficiency of yin and blood, it can be used together with Ejiao and Baishao, such as Huanglian Ejiao Tang.

(3) For vomiting blood due to blood heat

It has the effect of clearing fire and detoxicating, and it can be used together with Dahuagn and Huangqin, such as Xiexin Tang.

(4) Vomiting due to stomach heat and toothache due to stomach fire

It can be used together with Zhuru, Banxia, Jupi, etc. , such as Huanglian Jupi Zhuru Tang, which can clear away stomach heat and relieve vomiting. To treat vomiting with acid regurgitation due to liver fire attacking the stomach, it is often used together with Wuzhuyu, such as Zuojin Wan. When used together with Shengdihuang, Shengma and Mudanpi, it can treat the toothache due to stomach fire. For the syndrome of excessive stomach fire with polyorexia and diabetes manifested as excessive thirst and frequent drinking, it can be used together with Tianhuafen, Dihuang, and others that can clear away heat and promote the production of the body fluids.

Usage and dosage: 2-5 g for decoction. The herb stir-baked with wine is especially effective in clearing away dampness-heat of the middle energizers. And the one stir-baked with ginger is especially good at clearing away stomach heat and relieving vomiting.

Huangbai(Amur Cork-Tree, Cortex Phellodendri)

Properties and Tastes: bitter and cold.

Meridian Entry: kidney and bladder meridians.

Effects: ①Clear heat and dry dampness. ②Clear fire and detoxify. ③Relieve malnutrition fever and hectic fever due to yin deficiency.

Application:

(1)Syndrome of dampness-heat in the lower energizer.

The medicinal herb has the nature of bitter and cold, and is attributed to the kidney and bladder meridians, so it is effective in clearing away dampness and heat of the lower energizer. For dysentery due to dampness-heat, it is usually combined with Baitouweng, Huanglian and Qinpi to clear heat and eliminate dampness, such as Baitouweng Tang.

When combined with Zhizi, it can be used for jaundice and brownish urine due to dampness and heat, such as Zhizi Baipi Tang. For yellow and thick leukorrhea due to dampness and heat, often combined with Shanyao, Qianshi, Cheqianzi, etc., such as Yihuang Tang. For the oliguria and brownish urine due to dampness-heat in bladder, it is usually combined with Cheqianzi, Fuling, Bixie, etc., such as Bixie Fenqing Yin. For beriberi, swelling and pain of foot and knees due to dampness-heat in the lower energizer, it is usually combined with Cangzhu, Niuxi, such as Sanmiao Wan.

(2)Hectic fever, night sweat and spermatorrhea

The medicinal herb is attributed to the kidney meridian, and can relieve malnutrition fever and hectic fever due to kidney yin deficiency and excessive kidney fire. At this time, it is usually comobined with Zhimu, Shengdihuang, Shanyao, such as Zhibai Dihuang Wan.

(3)Carbuncle and swelling and sore of dampness type due to heat toxin

It is often used orally and combined with Huangqin, Huanglian, Zhizi, etc., such as Huanglian Jiedu Tang.

Usage and dosage: 3–12 g for decoction. A suitable amount used externally.

When it is used to clear heat, eliminate dampness, clear fire and detoxicate, the herb is fresh. When used to relieve malnutrition fever and hectic fever due to yin deficiency, the herb is often processed with brine.

Jinyinhua(Honeysuckle Flower, Flos Lonicerae)

Properties and Tastes: sweet and cold.

Meridian Entry: lung, heart and stomach meridians.

Effects: ①Clear heat and detoxify. ②Disperse wind-heat.

Application:

(1)Carbuncle and pyocutaneous disease, pharyngitis and erysipelas

It is the essential medicine to clear away heat and detoxify, so it is used for excessive yang syndrome, such as carbuncle, whether the carbuncle is ripe or not or the beginning of rupture, and pyocutaneous, pharyngitis and erysipelas. It can be used orally or the fresh is pounded for external application. For carbuncle and pyocutaneous, it is often used in combination with Danggui, Chishao, Baizhi, etc., such as Xianfang Huoming Yin. Also combined with Yejuhua, Pugongying, etc., for the treatment of deep-rooted boil. When it is used in combination with Danggui, Diyu and Huangqin, it can treat the abdominalgia with intestinal abscess, such as Qingchang yin. For abscess of lung, it is often combined with Yuxingcao, Lugen, Yiyiren, etc.

(2)The common cold due to wind-heat and seasonal febrile disease, no matter whether the heat of seasonal febile diseases is in weifen, qifen, or involving yingfen and xuefen

For early stage of seasonal febrile disease which manifested as generalized heat, headache, sore throat and thirst, it is often used in combination with Lianqiao, Bohe and Niubangzi, such as Yinqiao San. For pathogenic factors being in weifen manifested as strong heat and polydipsia, it is combined with Shigao, Zhimu,etc.

When the heat of seasonal febile disease involves yingfen and xuefen,it is often used in combination with Shengdihuang,Xuanshen,etc. ,to clear heat and cool blood,such as Qingying Tang.

(3)For blood and epidemic dysentery

The medicinal herb has the nature of cold,and it can be used for clearing away heat and detoxicating, combined with Huanglian,Huangqin and Baitouweng to strengthen the effect of relieving dysentery.

(4)For summerheat syndrome

Manifested as excessive thirst,sore throat,summer carbuncle,heat rash,etc. ,it can be steamed with water into Jinyinhua Distillate for oral or external use.

Usage and dosage:6-15 g for decoction. The fresh is better for clearing away heat and detoxicating; the carbonized one is used for dysentery;distillate medicinal water is used for heat polydipsia.

Lianqiao(Weeping Forsythia Capsule,Forsythia Forsythiae)

Properties and Tastes:bitter and slightly cold.

Meridian Entry:lung,heart and small intestine meridians.

Effects:①Clear heat and detoxify. ②Disperse swelling and nodules. ③Disperse wind-heat.

Application:

(1)Carbuncle,crewels,acute mastitis and erysipelas

The medicinal herb has the nature of bitter and slightly cold,and it is similar to Jinyinhua in effects. It can also clear away heat and toxin,and is accompanied with expelling wind and heat as well,so it is usually used for heat syndrome due to exogenous attack. It is often used in combination with Chuanshanjia and Zaojiaoci in order to strengthen the work of clearing away heat and detoxicating,such as Jiajian Xiaodu Yin. When combined with Mudanpi and Tianhuafen,it can be used for carbuncle appeared red swollen,ulceration,such as Lianqiao Jiedu Tang. For eryslpelas,it is often combined with Xiakucao,Beimu and Xuanshen. Since it is good at clearing away heart fire,it can also be used for febrile disease involving the pericardium with restless fever,coma or delirium.

(2)For the common cold due to wind-heat and early stage of seasonal febrile disease

The medicinal herb has the nature of bitter and slightly cold,and its effects are similar to Jinyinhua. For early stage of seasonal febrile disease manifested as fever,sore throat and thirsty,it is often used in combination with Bohe,Niubangzi,etc. ,such as Yinqiao San. For pathogenic factors being in xuefen manifested as high fever polydipsia,god faint spots,it is often combined with Shengdihuang,etc. Because it specializes in clearing away heart fire,it can also be used for febrile disease involving the pericardium manifested as fever,coma or delirium.

(3)For dysuria or dribbling urination with pain

Usually,it is combined with Cheqianzi,Baimaogen and Zhuye for the treatment of dysuria or dribbling urination with pain,such as Rusheng San.

Usage and dosage:6-15 g for decoction.

Shengdihuang(Fresh Rehmannia Root,Radix Rehmaniae Recens)

Properties and Tastes:sweet and cold.

Meridian Entry:heart,liver and kidney meridians.

Effects:①Clear heat and cool the blood. ②Nourish yin and promote the production of body fluid.

Application:

(1)Seasonal febrile disease involving xuefen and yingfen

The medicinal herb has the nature of sweet and cold, it is good at clearing away heat in yingfen manifested as fever, restlessness and crimson tongue, often combined with Xuanshen, Lianqiao and Huanglian and others that can cool the blood, promote the production of the body fluids and clear away heat, such as Qingying Tang. If the heat in xuefen manifested asmacules, it can be used in combination with Shuiniujiao, Chishao, Mudanpi, etc. , such as Xijiao Dihuang Tang.

(2) For hemorrhage due to blood heat

The medicinal herb is effective inclearing away heat in yingfen and has the effect of cooling blood and hemostasis. For hematemesis and epistaxis, it is often used in combination with Cebaiye, Heye and Aiye, etc. , such as Sisheng Wan. For hemafecia and hematuria, usually combined with Diyu, Yimucao, etc.

(3) Febrile disease consuming yin

The medicinal herb has the nature of sweet and cold, and has the effect of clearing away heat and nourishing yin and promoting production of body fluid. When manifested as red tongue and oral dryness, it is combined with Maidong, Shashen and Yuzhu to promote the production of body fluid, such as Yiwei Tang.

(4) For constipation due to dryness of intestine

It is usually used together with Xuanshen and Maimendong, such as Zengye Tang.

Usage and dosage: 10–15 g for decoction. The fresh amount is doubled or the fresh being pounded into juice that is put in decoction. The fresh is very cold and with plenty of juice, it can clear away heat and promote the production of the body fluids, and has effect of cooling blood and arresting bleeding, so the fresh is suitable for seasonal febrile diseases and bleeding due to blood heat. The cold nature of the dry is slightly-weak while its effect of nourishing yin is better, so the dry is especially suitable for yin deficiency with interior heat.

Simple list of other heat-clearing medicinals see Table 9–2.

Table 9–2　Simple list of other heat-clearing medicinals

Name	Properties and Tastes	Meridian Entry	Effects	Application	Dosage
Lugen(Rhizoma Phragmitis)	Sweet and cold	Lung and stomach meridians	(1) Clear heat and purge fire (2) Engender fluid and relieve thirst (3) Relieve dysphoria (4) Check vomiting (5) Promote diuresis	(1) Fever with restlessness, thirsty (2) Cough due to lung heat and pulmonary abscess (3) Vomiting due to stomach heat (4) For pyretic stranguria with pain	15–30 g for decoction, 30 – 60 g of the fresh
Zhuye(Herba Lophatheri)	Sweet, pungent, and cold	Heart, stomach, small intestine meridians	(1) Clear heat and purge fire (2) Engender fluid (3) Relieve dysphoria (4) Promote diuresis	(1) Fever with restlessness, thirsty (2) For tongue sore, dysuria, edema and oliguria	6–15 g for decoction, 15 – 30 g of the fresh

Continue to Table 9-2

Name	Properties and Tastes	Meridian Entry	Effects	Application	Dosage
Tianhuafen(Radix Trichosanthis)	Sweet,slightly bitter and slightly cold	Lung and stomach meridians	(1)Clear heat and purge fire (2)Engender fluid and relieve thirst (3)Resolve swelling and drain pus	(1)Febrile disease with thirst, diabetes and frequent drinking (2)Dry cough due to lung heat (3)Pyocutaneous disease of heat type whether the infection is ulcerous or not	10-15 g for decoction
Xiakucao(Spica Prunellae)	Bitter,pungent and cold	Liver and gallbladder meridians	(1)Clear the liver and purge fire (2)Disperse swelling and nodules (3)Improve the vision	(1)Hyperactivity of liver fire with conjunctivitis, headache and dizziness (2)Scrofula and goiter (3)Acute mastitis and lump in breast	9-15 g for decoction
Juemingzi (Semen Cassiae)	Sweet, bitter, salty, and slightly cold	Liver and large intestine meridians	(1)Clear the liver and improve the vision (2)Moisten the intestines and relax the bowels	(1)Redness,swelling and pain of the eyes due to liver heat or wind-heat (2)Headache and dizziness (3)Constipation due to dryness of the intestine	9-15 g for decoction
Longdan(Radix Gentianae)	Bitter,and cold	Liver, and gallbladder meridians	(1)Clear heat and dry dampness (2)Clear fire of liver and gallbladder	(1)Jaundice,brownish urine, pudendal swelling, vaginal discharge, eczema,etc. (2)For headache caused by liver fire,deafness,hypochondriac pain and bitter taste in the mouth	3-6 g for decoction
Kushen(Radix Sophorae Flavescentis)	Bitter and cold	Heart,liver,stomach, large intestine and bladder meridians	(1)Clear heat and dry dampness (2)Kill worms (3)Promote urination	(1)Dampness-heat diarrhea and jaundice (2)For vaginal discharge disease, eruption caused by dampness	5-10 g for decoction
Baixianpi(Cortex Dictamni)	Bitter and cold	Spleen, stomach and bladder meridians	(1)Clear heat and dry dampness (2)Dispel wind and detoxify	(1)Eruption caused by dampness (2)For dampness-heat jaundice,wind-heat-dampness impediment	5-10 g for decoction

Continue to Table 9-2

Name	Properties and Tastes	Meridian Entry	Effects	Application	Dosage
Chuanxinlian (Herba Andrographis)	Bitter and cold	Heart, lung, large intestine, and bladder meridians	(1) Clear heat and detoxify (2) Cool the blood (3) Disperse swelling (4) Drain dampness	(1) The common cold due to wind-heat and seasonal febrile disease at the early stage (2) For sore throat, mouth sores (3) For abscess of lung (4) For stranguria due to heat and dribbling urination with pain	6-9 g for decoction
Daqingye (Folium Isatidis)	Bitter, and cold	Heart, stomach meridians	(1) Clear heat and detoxify (2) Cool the blood and disperse maculae	(1) It is indicated for seasonal febrile diseases with fever, maculae and papules (2) Abscess, erysipelas, aphtha, and mumps	9-15 g for decoction
Qingdai (Indigo Naturalis)	Salty and cold	Liver meridian	(1) Clear heat and detoxify (2) Cool the blood and disperse maculae (3) Purgefire and relieve convulsion	(1) For maculae due to warm-toxin (2) Hematemesis, epistaxis due to blood heat	5-3 g for pill or powder
Pugongying (Herba Taraxaci)	Bitter, sweet, and cold	Liver, and stomach meridians	(1) Clear heat and detoxify (2) Disperse swelling and nodules (3) Drain dampness and promote urination	(1) Carbuncle, furuncle, erysipelas, scrofula, and lung abscess (2) For dampness-heat jaundice and urination with pain	10-15 g for decoction
Zihuadiding (Herba Violae)	Bitter, pungent and cold	Heart and liver meridians	(1) Clear heat and detoxify (2) Cool the blood and disperse swelling	(1) carbuncle toxin (2) Acute mastitis (3) For jaundice caused by heat-damp and heat strangury	15-30 g for decoction
Baitouweng (Radix Pulsatillae)	Bitter, and cold	Stomach and large intestine meridians	(1) Clear heat and detoxify (2) Cool the blood and relieve dysentery	(1) Heat-blood dysentery (2) For vaginal discharge	9-15 g for decoction

Continue to Table 9-2

Name	Properties and Tastes	Meridian Entry	Effects	Application	Dosage
Banlangen (Radix Isatidis)	Bitter, and cold	Heart, stomach meridians	(1) Clear heat and detoxify (2) Cool the blood andsoothe the throat	It is indicated for seasonal febrile diseases with fever, sore throat, maculae and papules, carbuncle, sore toxin, etc.	9 - 15 g for decoction
Yuxingcao (Herba Houttuyniae)	Pungent, and slightly cold	Lung meridian	(1) Clear heat ⋯ and detoxify (2) Disperse swelling and nodules (3) Disperse abscess and expel pus	(1) It is indicated for cough due to lung heat, pulmonary abscess (2) For carbuncle toxin (3) For stranguria due to heat and dribbling urination with pain	15-25 g for decoction
Baijiangcao (Herba Patriniae)	Pungent, bitter and slightly cold	Stomach, large intestine, and liver meridians	(1) Clear heat and detoxify (2) Disperse swelling and nodules (3) Dissipate blood stasis and relieve pain	(1) For intestinal abscess and lung's abscess (2) For postpartum abdominal pain and dysmenorrhea due to blood stasis	6 - 15 g for decoction
Lvdou(Green Gram)	Sweet and cold	Heart and stomach meridians	(1) Clear heat and detoxify (2) Release summerheat (3) Promote urination	(1) Swollen sore and ulcer (2) For thirst caused by summerheat (3) For drug and food poisoning (4) For edema	15-30 g for decoction

9.4.3   Purgative medicine

Purgative medicines refer to the drugs that can cause diarrhea or lubricate the intestine, helping the bowels move and relieve constipation.

These kinds of medicines mainly have the functions of relaxing the bowels and purgation. Therefore, they are mainly used to treat constipation, various interior excess syndromes due to food and water retention, interior excess heat-syndrome etc. According to the difference of the purgating drug's effects and application, they can be classified into three categories, that is, offensive purgative medicinal, laxative medicinal and drastic water-expelling medicinal. All these three kinds of medicines should be used with caution in cases of injuring healthy qi, especially for the pregnancy, menstruation, postpartum, and old and weak patients. As long as the conditions of disease get better, their application must be stopped and the large dosage must be avoided.

Dahuang(Rhubarb, Radix Et Rhizoma Rhei)

Properties and Tastes: bitter and cold.

Meridian Entry: spleen, stomach, large intestine, liver and pericardium meridians.

Effects: ①Remove accumulation with purgation. ②Clear heat and purge fire. ③Cool the blood and detoxify. ④Break blood and expel stasis, unblock the meridian. ⑤Drain dampness and remove jaundice.

Application:

(1)Constipation due to stagnation of heat

With strong effects of removing stagnation by purgation, Dahuang is an essential medicine for the treatment of constipation. And the medicinal herb has the nature of bitter and cold, so it is especially effective in treatment of constipation due to stagnation of heat. In order to strengthen the work of purging heat and removing accumulation, it is often used in combination with Mangxiao, Houpo and Zhishi, such as Dachengqii Tang. If the constipation is accompanied with deficiency of qi and blood, Danggui, Renshen are always combined with, such as Huanglong Tang. For yin deficiency due to stagnation of heat, Maimendong and Shengdihuang are added to the prescription mentioned above, such as Zengye Chengqi Tang. For constipation due to insufficiency of spleen yang and stagnation of cold, Ganjiang and Fuzi are combined with, such as Wenpi Tang.

(2)For redness of eye, sore throat and haematemesis due to blood heat

With significant effects of removing heat from the blood, clearing away heat and purging fire, it is combined with Huanglian and Huangqin for blood heat syndrome manifested as redness of eye, sore throat, oral ulcer and haematemesis, such as Xiexin Tang.

(3)Pyocutaneous disease due to toxic heat and abdominalgia with intestinal abscess

It is often used in combination with Jinyinhua, Pugongying, Lianqiao, etc., for carbuncle due to toxic heat, such as Banxia Xiexin Tang. For abdominalgia with intestinal abscess, combined with Mudanpi, Taoren, Mangxiao, etc. such as Dahuang Mudan Tang.

(4)For menischesis and postpartum abdominal pain caused by blood stasis

With the effects of promoting blood circulation to relieve blood stasis, it can be used as a common medicine for syndrome of blood retention. For menischesis due to blood stasis, it is often used in combination with Taoren, Guizhi, etc., such as Taohe Chengqi Tang. For postpartum abdominal pain due to blood stasis, it is used combined with Taoren, Tubiechong, etc., such as Xiayuxue Tang.

(5)Dysentery, stranguria due to dampness-heat

It can be used alone, or combined with Huanglian, Huangqin and Baishao for dysentery due to stagnation. For stranguria resulting from dampness-heat, it is often used in combination with Mutong, Cheqianzi, Zhizi, etc., such as Bazheng San.

(6)For burn and scald

It can be used alone, or combined with Diyu. When it is used for this kind of disease, it should be made into the type powder, then mixed with sesame oil for external application.

Usage and dosage: 3–15 g for decoction, just right amount for external use, and the crude one with stronger purgative effect is used for downward discharging. It is later added to decoction or soaked in boiling water for oral use, and it is not decocted for a long time. That prepared with wine is suitable for blood stasis because of its better effect of circulating blood. The carbonized form is usually used for bleeding syndrome.

Mangxiao(Sodium Sulfate, Natrii Sulfas)

Properties and Tastes: salty, bitter, and cold.

Meridian Entry: stomach and large intestine meridians.

Effects:①Relax the bowels with purgation. ②Moisten dryness and soften hardness. ③Clear heat and disperse swelling.

Application:

(1)Constipation due to accumulation of heat in the stomach and intestine

The medicinal herb has the nature of cold and is an essential medicinal herb to treat the constipation. It is especially effective in the treatment of constipation caused by dryness and usually used in combination with Dahuang in order to strengthen the work of relaxing the bowels, such as Dachengqi Tang

(2)Abdominalgia with intestinal abscess

Usually, it is used combined with Dahuang, Mudanpi, Taoren, etc. , such as Dahuang Mudan Tang. For the early stage of intestinal abscess, it is often used in combination with Dahuang and Dasuan.

(3)For acute mastitis, hemorrhoids, sore throat, aphthae, swelling and pain of the eyes

For the early stage of mastiffs, it can be dissolved in water for external application and wrapped with gauze. It also can be used alone for decoction to rinse for hemorrhoids. And it is usually combined with Zhusha, Pengsha and Bingpian to treat the sore throat and aphthae, such as Bingpeng San. For swelling and pain of the eyes, the solution form of Xuanmingfen can be used.

Usage and dosage:6-12 g dissolved in decoction or in boiling water for oral using. Just appropriate amount is for external use application.

Yuliren(Chinese Dwarf Cherry Seed, Semen Pruni)

Properties and Tastes:Pungent, bitter, sweet and medium.

Meridian Entry:spleen, large intestine and small intestine meridians.

Effects:①Moisten the intestines to relax the bowels. ②Induce diuresis to alleviate edema.

Application:

(1)Constipation due to deficiency of blood and dryness of intestine

The medicinal can not only moisten the intestines, but also promote the circulation of large intestine qi. It is usually combined with Huomaren, Baiziren and Xingren, such as Wuren Wan.

(2)For edema, abdominal fullness, beriberi and dysuria

It can be used together with Sangbaipi, Chixiaodou and so on, such as Yuliren Tang.

Usage and dosage:6-12 g is used in decoction for oral use, broken and then added to decoction.

Songziren(Pine Nut, Pinus Pinea)

Properties and Tastes:sweet and warm.

Meridian Entry:lung, liver and large intestine meridians.

Effects:①Moisten the intestines to relax the bowels. ②Moisten the lung to suppress cough.

Application:

(1)Constipation due to dryness of intestine

The medicine has the function of moistening the intestines, so it can be used for the constipation caused by intestine-dryness due to consumption of fluid. It also can be used for the old man's constipation. Usually, it is used with Huomaren, Yuliren and Baiziren, which are made into the type of powder, taken with Huangqi Tang.

(2)Dry cough due to lung dryness

The medicine can moisten the lung, so it is better for the dry cough. It can be used with Hutaoren, mixed with honey, taken with rice-water.

Usage and dosage:5-10 g for decoction.

Simple list of other purgative medicinals see Table 9-3.

Table 9-3　**Simple list of other purgative medicines**

Name	Properties and Tastes	Meridian Entry	Effects	Application	Dosage
Fanxieye (Folium Sennae)	Sweet, bitter and cold	Large intestine meridian	(1) Cool purgation and relax the bowels (2) Promote diuresis	(1) Constipation due to stagnation of heat (2) For edema	2-6 g for decoction and decoct later or soaked in warm boiled water for oral use
Luhui(Aaloe)	Bitter and cold	Liver, stomach, large intestine meridians	(1) Relax the bowels (2) Clear fire of the liver (3) Kill worms	(1) Constipation due to heat stagnation (2) Overabundance of fire in the liver meridian (3) Infantile malnutrition and convulsion	2-5 g is added to pill or powder for oral using

9.4.4　Wind-dampness-dispelling medicine

Wind-dampness-dispelling medicinals refer to the drugs that mainly dispel the pathogens of wind and damp, which is for the treatment of impediment diseases.

These kind of medicinals are mainly pungent and bitter in nature. The pungent taste not only can dispel wind and damp, but also unobstructed meridians, therefore, they can dispel the wind-dampness staying in the muscles, meridians and muscles. Wind-dampness-dispelling medicinals mainly treat the impediment diseases caused by wind-dampness, manifesting as limb pain, swollen joints, and tendon spasm.

According to the difference of the natures and effects, the wind-dampness-dispelling medicinals can be classified into three categories: wind-cold-dampness dispelling medicinals, wind-heat-dampness dispelling medicinals, wind-dampness-dispelling and strengthening the bones and muscles medicines. The medicines with pungent taste and warm mature should be used carefully in cases of injuring blood and body fluid.

Most impediment diseases belong to chronic disease. Therefore, this kind of medicine can be made into the type of pills or powder, and processed with wine.

Duhuo(Doubleteeth pubescent angelica root, Radix Angelicae Pubescentis)

Properties and Tastes : pungent, bitter and slightly warm.

Meridian Entry : kidney and bladder meridians.

Effects : ①Dispel wind and dampness. ②Relieve pain of impediment diseases. ③Release the exterior.

Application :

(1) Impediment diseases of wind-cold-dampness type

The medicinal herb has the nature of pungent and warm, and it serves as an essential medicinal herb for wind-cold-dampness type of impediment diseases. And it is attributed to the kidney meridian, so it is especially effective in the back and the lower half of the body with soreness and pain due to dampness. For the symptoms as muscle pain, back pain, hand and foot pain, it can be used together with Danggui, Baizhu, Niuxi, etc. , such as Duohuo Tang. For prolonged impediment diseases due to deficiency of qi and blood and insufficiency of the liver and kidney, it is often combined with Sangjisheng, Duzhong, Niuxi, etc. , such as Duhuo Jisheng Tang.

(2) For headache caused by wind-cold and dampness

The medicinal herb has the effect of relieving exogenous pathogenic factors, therefore, it can be used together with Qianghuo, Gaoben and Fangfeng to treat the exterior syndrome, which is manifested as headache, general heavy sensation of body, such as Qianghuo Jisheng Tang.

Usage and dosage: 3–10 g for decoction. Just appropriate amount is for external using.

Qinjiao(Largeleaf Gentian Root, Radix Gentianae Macrophyllae)

Properties and Tastes: pungent, bitter and medium.

Meridian Entry: stomach, liver and gallbladder meridians.

Effects: ①Dispel wind and dampness. ②Relieve pain of impediment diseases. ②Relieve asthenia heat. ③Clear heat and dampness.

Application:

(1) Impediment diseases, spastic muscles

Qinjiao has the nature of pungent and bitter, but it isn't dry. Therefore, it can be used for all kinds of impediment diseases and spastic muscles, especially for the heat impediment together with Fangji and Rendongteng. It also can be used together with Tianma, Qianghuo and Chuanxiong to treat the impediment diseases of wind-cold-dampness type, such as Qinjiao Tianma Tang.

(2) Jaundice with damp-heat pathogen

The medicinal herb is attributed to the liver and gallbladder meridians, so it is better at clearing the heat and dampness of these two organs. When it is used for the jaundice, it can be alone or together with Yinchen, Zhizi and Dahuang, such as Shanyinchen Wan.

(3) Bone-steaming tidal fever

The medicinal is vital to the osteopyrexia and fever, usually together with Qinghao, Digupi, Zhimu and so on, such as Qinjiao Biejia Tang.

Usage and dosage: 3–10 g for decoction.

Wujiapi(Acanthopanax, Cortex Acanthopanax Radicis)

Properties and Tastes: pungent, bitter and warm.

Meridian Entry: liver and kidney meridians.

Effects: ①Dispel wind and dampness. ②Nourish the liver and kidney. ③Strengthen tendons and bones. ④Promote urination and disperse swelling.

Application:

(1) Impediment diseases

It is mostly used for the old people and the people with aeipathia because of its function of nourishing the liver and kidney. It can be soaked alone in wine, or used together with Danggui, Niuxi etc. , or with Mugua and Songjie.

(2) Weakness of waist and knees or retarded ambulation of children

The medicine can nourish the liver and kidney, so it can be used for yin deficiency of the liver and kidney with weakness of waist and knees or retarded ambulation of children, usually combined with Duzhong, Niuxi and others that tonify the kidney and liver.

(3) Edema

It is usually in combination with Fulingpi, Dafupi and Shengjiangpi, such as Wupi San.

Usage and dosage: 5–10 g for decoction.

Simple list of other wind-dampness-dispelling medicinals see Table 9–4.

Table 9-4 Simple list of other wind-dampness-dispelling medicines

Name	Properties and Tastes	Meridian Entry	Effects	Application	Dosage
Weilingxian (Radix Clematidis)	Pungent, salty and warm	Bladder meridian	(1) Dispel wind and dampness (2) Free the collateral vessels and relieve pain of impediment diseases (3) Remove fishbone stuck in the throat	(1) Impediment disease due to wind-cold-dampness (2) Fishbone stuck in the throat	6-9 g for decoction
Mugua (Fructus Chaenomelis)	Sour, warm	Liver and spleen meridians	(1) Relax sinews and activate collateral (2) Resolve dampness and harmonize the stomach	(1) Wind-dampness impediment (2) Swelling of the foot (3) Vomiting, diarrhea and twitch	6-9 g for decoction
Qingfengteng (Caulis Sinomenii)	Bitter and pungent	Liver and spleen meridians	(1) Dispel wind and dampness (2) Free the collateral vessels (3) Promote urination	(1) Wind-dampness impediment (2) Swelling of the foot	6 - 12 g for decoction
Fangji (Radix Stephaniae Tetrandrae)	Bitter, and cold	Bladder and lung meridians	(1) Dispel wind and relieve pain (2) Promote urination and disperse swelling	(1) Wind-dampness impediment manifested as painful joints and stiffness (2) Edema, ascitic fluid and dysuria (3) Eczema and carbuncle and sore toxin	5 - 10 g for decoction
Sangzhi (Ramulus Mori)	Slightly bitter and medium	Liver meridian.	(1) Dispel wind and dampness (2) Disinhibit the joints	Wind-dampness impediment with pain of general joints	9 - 15 g for decoction
Sangjisheng (Herba Taxilli)	Bitter, sweet and medium	Liver and kidney meridians	(1) Dispel wind and dampness (2) Nourish the liver and kidney (3) Strengthen tendons and bones (4) Prevent abortion	(1) Wind-cold-wetness type of arthralgia (2) For habitual abortion due to yin deficiency of the liver and kidney (3) Dizziness caused by yin deficiency of the liver and kidney	9 - 15 g for decoction
Gou Ji (Rhizoma Cibotii)	Bitter, sweet, and warm	Liver and kidney meridians	(1) Dispel wind and dampness (2) Nourish the liver and kidney (3) Strengthen waist and knee	(1) Wind-dampness impediment (2) For weakness of waist and knees and flaccidity of extremities due to yin deficiency of the liver and kidney	6 - 12 g for decoction

9.4.5　Dampness-resolving medicines

The medicinals that resolve dampness, with fragrant odor, warming and drying belong to dampness-resolving medicinals.

The spleen does not function well with dampness. If turgid dampness blocks the middle energizor internally, the transformation and transportation functions of the spleen become impaired. Dampness-resolving medicinals are warm and dry. They facilitate the movement and functional activities of qi, dissipate turgid dampness, strengthen the spleen and stimulate the stomach. They are especially useful when the spleen is blocked by dampness and its functions impaired, leading to such symptoms as abdominal distention, vomiting, acid regurgitation, diarrhea, anorexia, weariness, a sweet taste in the mouth with much salivation and a white greasy tongue coating. They are also useful for treating illnesses due to dampness-heat and heatstroke.

Illnesses of dampness may be of cold-dampness or heat-dampness. When treating an illness caused by dampness it is important to select an appropriate combination of herbs. For cold-dampness supplement with medicines that warm the interior. For heat-dampness supplement with herbs that cool heat and dry dampness.

The nature of dampness is viscous and impeding. When it invades the meridians, qi movement becomes impeded. For this reason, when treating with dampness-resolving medicinals it is common to supplement them with mecicinals that promote qi movement. Also, weakening of the spleen can generate dampness. Treatment of dampness generated when the spleen is weakened should include medicinals that nourish the spleen.

Some of the medicinals are warm and dry in nature so they easily consume yin and blood. Therefore, we must pay attention to these medicinals to avoid insufficiency of yin, deficiency of blood or consumption of the body fluids.

Huoxiang(Herba Agastaches, Wrinkled Gianthyssop Herb)

Properties and Tastes: pungent and slightly warm.

Meridian Entry: spleen, stomach and lung meridians.

Effects: ①Resolve dampness with aroma. ②Stop vomiting. ③Release summerheat.

Application:

(1) The obstruction of dampness in the middle energizer

The syndrome is manifested as fatigue of the body and spirits, loss of appetite and nausea, fullness in the chest and epigastrium. It is often combined with Houpo, Cangzhu, etc. , such as Buhuanjin Zhengqi San.

(2) Vomiting

It serves as an essential medicinal herb for the treatment of dampness-retention syndrome with vomiting. It is often used in combination with Banxia and Dingxiang, etc. , such as Huoxiang Banxia Tang. For the vomiting caused by dampress heat, it is used with Huanglian and Zhuru. For the vomiting caused by pregnancy, often with Sharen and Sugeng. If the vomiting is caused by weakness of the spleen and the stomach, it is used with Dangshen, Baizhu and so on.

(3) Superficial syndrome of summerheat and dampness type and early stage of seasonal febrile disease

For the former, which is manifested as headache, fever, fullness and pain in the chest and epigastrium, vomiting and diarrhea, it is often combined with Huangqin, Huashi, Yinchen, etc. , such as Ganluxiaodu Dan. And also combined with Zisuye, Houpo, etc. , such as Huoxiangzhengqi San.

Usage and dosage: 3－10 g for decoction. The amount of the fresh is doubled.

Cangzhu(Rhizoma Atractylodis, Atractylodes rhizome)

Properties and Tastes: pungent, bitter and warm.

Meridian Entry: spleen, stomach and liver meridians.

Effects: ①Dry dampness to fortify the spleen. ②Dispel wind and dissipate cold. ③Improve vision.

Application:

(1) Dampness-retention syndrome involving the middle energizer

For such a syndrome manifested as abdominal fullness and distention, nausea and vomiting and poor appetite, it is usually combined with Chenpi, Houpo, etc., such as Pingwei San. For the damp-retention due to deficiency of the spleen, it is often with Fuling, Zexie and Zhuling, such as Zhuling Tang.

(2) Wind-dampness type of arthralgia and wilting disease

The medicinal herb has the nature of pungent and bitter, it is especially suitable for arthralgia with domination of dampness. It is often used in combination with Yiyiren, Duhuo, etc., such as Yiyiren Tang.

For arthralgia of dampness-heat type, it is usually combined with Zhimu, Shigao, etc., such as Baihu Jia Cangzhu Tang. For wilting disease due to damp invasion of the lower energizer manifested as beriberi and swelling and pain of foot and knees, limp wilting, it is usually combined with Huangbai, Yiyiren and Niuxi, such as Simiao San.

(3) The common cold due to wind-cold, especially suitable for affection of exogenous wind-cold-dampness

It is usually combined with Baizhi, Qianghuo, Fangfeng, etc., such as Shenzhu San.

(4) Night blindness

It can be used alone or combined with lamb liver and pork liver.

Usage and dosage: 3–9 g for decoction.

Houpo(Officinal magnolia bark, Cortex Magnoliae Officinalis)

Properties and Tastes: bitter, pungent and warm.

Meridian Entry: spleen, stomach, lung and the large intestine meridians.

Effects: ①Promote circulation of qi and dry dampness. ②Remove stagnation and relieve fullness. ③Descend qi, remove phlegm and asthma.

Application:

(1) Abdominal distention and fullness due to stagnation of dampness or food

It is often used in combination with Dahuang and Zhishi to remove the stagnation and relieve fullness, such as Houpo Sanwu Tang.

(2) Cough, asthma and profuse sputum

It is often used in combination with Zisuzi, Chenpi and Banxia in order to strengthen the work of descending qi, removing phlegm and relieving asthma, such as Suzi Jiangqi Tang. For cough due to wind-cold, it is usually combined with Guizhi, Xingren, etc., such as Guizhi Jia Houpo Xingzi Tang.

Usage and dosage: 3–10 g for decoction.

Simple list of other dampness-resolving medicinals see Table 9–5.

Table 9–5　**Simple list of other dampness-resolving medicines**

Name	Properties and Tastes	Meridian Entry	Effects	Application	Dosage
Peilan(Herba Eupatorii)	Pungent	Spleen, stomach and lung meridians	(1) Resolve dampness (2) Release summer-heat	(1) The obstruction of dampness in the middle energizer (2) Affection of exogenous summerheat and dampness, the early stage of damp febrile disease	3–10 g for decoction. 6–20 g of the fresh
Sharen(Fructus Amomi Villosi)	Pungent and warm	Spleen, stomach and kidney meridians	(1) Resolve dampness and move qi (2) Warm the middle to check diarrhea (3) Prevent abortion	(1) The obstruction of dampness in the middle energizer and stagnation of spleen qi and stomach qi (2) Vomiting and diarrhea due to asthenia-cold of the spleen and stomach (3) Vomiting due to pregnancy and threatened abortion due to stagnation of qi	3–10 g for decoction and decoct later
Doukou(Semen Myristicae)	Pungent and warm	Lung, spleen, and stomach meridians	(1) Resolve dampness and move qi (2) Warm the middle to check vomiting	(1) The obstruction of dampness in the middle energizer (2) Vomiting and hiccup due to cold and dampness	3–6 g for decoction and decoct later

9.4.6　Dampness-draining diuretic medicine

Dampness-draining diuretic medicines are herbs that have their principal actions of unblocking the water pathways and the dissipation of dampness(diuresis). They can increase the amount of urine, so that retained water and accumulated dampness can be excreted as urine.

Some of these medicines also act to clear dampness-heat, and are especially suitable for conditions such as difficult and painful urination, edema, accumulated rheum and phlegm, jaundice and exudative dermatitis. Dampness-draining diuretic medicines are sweet or bland in flavor and neutral, slightly cold or cold in nature. Bland flavor is associated with ability to drain water and dissipate dampness. Cold nature is associated with the ability to cool heat. In addition to increasing the amount of urine dampness-draining diuretic medicines of cold nature are especially effective in cooling heat and eliminating dampness from the lower energizer. They are often prescribed for dysuria. When prescribing these medicinals, pay attention to the character of the illness and add medicines as appropriate. For example, for acute edema associated with symptoms of the exterior, add medicines that soothe the lung and induce sweating. For chronic edema due to deficiency of spleen and kidney yang, add medicines that warm and nourish the spleen and the kidney. For illnesses of simultaneous dampness and heat, add medicinals that cool heat and purge fire. For heat injury to blood vessels and hematuria, add medicinals that cool blood and stop bleeding. When dampness-draining diuretic medicines are used inappropriately, they can easily damage yin fluids; hence great care must be exercised when treating patients with yin deficiency or fluid insufficiency.

Fuling(Indian Bread,Poria)

Properties and Tastes：sweet and medium.

Meridian Entry：heart,lung,spleen and kidney meridians.

Effects：①Induce diuresis to drain dampness. ②Fortify the spleen. ③Nourish the heart to tranquilize.

Application：

(1)Edema and dysuria

It is an essential medicine to treat all kinds of edema. For edema caused by retention of water in the body,it is usually combined with Zexie,Zhuling,Baizhu,etc.,such as Wuling San. For that with deficiency of spleen yang and kidney yang,it is usually combined with Ganjiang,Fuzi,etc.,such as Zhenwu Tang. For accumulation of water with heat,manifested as anuresis and edema,it is often used with Huashi,Ejiao and Zexie,such as Zhuling Tang.

(2)Phlegm-fluid retention

For that manifested as dizzy and palpitation,it is usually combined with Guizhi,Baizhu,Gancao,etc., such as Linggui Zhugan Tang. For that manifested as vomit,usually combined with Banxia and Shengjiang, such as Xiaobanxia Jia Fuling Tang.

(3)Spleen deficiency syndromes

The medicinal herb has the effect of invigorating the spleen and stopping diarrhea,which is especially effective in spleen deficiency with dampness. It is usually combined with Shanyao,Baizhu and Yiyiren,such as Shenling Baizhu San. And it is also combined with Renshen,Gancao and Baizhu,such as Sijunzi Tang.

(4)Restlessness,palpitation and insomnia caused by deficiency of both the heart and spleen

It is often combined with Huangqi,Danggui,Yuanzhi,etc.,such as Guipi Tang. If it is caused by heart qi deficiency,usually with Renshen,Longchi,Yuanzhi and so on,such as Anshen Dingzhi Wan.

Usage and dosage：10-15 g for decoction.

Yiyiren(Coix Seed,Semen Coicis)

Properties and Tastes：pungent and cold.

Meridian Entry：spleen,stomach and lung meridians.

Effects：①Induce diuresis to drain dampness. ②Fortify the spleen to to stanch diarrhea. ③Treat impediment manifested. ④Expel pus. ⑤Detoxify and disperse nodules.

Application：

(1)Dysuria,edema,beriberi

The medicine has the function of inducing diuresis to drain dampness and fortifying the spleen. Therefore,it is used for spleen deficiency syndrome with accumulation of dampness manifested as dysuria,edema, and beriberi. For edema,it is usually combined with Fuling,Baizhu,Huangqi,etc. For spleen deficiency with loss of appetite and diarrhea,it is usually used together with Dangshen and Baizhu.

(2)Diarrhea due to Spleen deficiency

It is often used with Renshen,Fuling and Baizhu,such as Shenling Baizhu San.

(3)Impediment disease

For impediment disease with dominant dampness manifested as bodily heaviness and soreness and rigidity of limbs,it is often used together with Mugua. For that with heat,it is combined with Dilong,Fangji. For the one with cold,combined with Mahuang and Guizhi. For that with heavy dampness,usually combined with Cangzhu.

(4)Pulmonary and intestinal abscess

For the former that with cough and thick sputum,it is usually used with Weijing,Dongguaren,Taoren, etc. , such as Weijing Tang. For the later, it is used together with Baijiangcao, Mudanpi, Fuzi, etc. , such as Yiyi Fuzi Baijiang San.

Usage and dosage : 9-30 g for decoction.

Zhuling(Chuling, Polyporus Umbellatus)

Properties and Tastes : sweet and medium.

Meridian Entry : kidney and bladder meridians.

Effects : Induce diuresis to drain dampness.

Application : Edema, dysuria, diarrhea and turbid strangury.

It can be used alone to treat edema caused by retention of water in the body. For dysuria and edema, it is often used in combination with Zexie, Fuling and Baizhu, such as Siling San. For diarrhea due to cold and dampness in the stomach and intestine, usually combined with Roudoukou, Huangbai, etc. , such as Zhuling Wan. For dysuria and turbid strangury due to yin-deficiency, it is usually combined with Ejiao, Zexie, etc. , such as Zhuling Tang. In addition, it doesn't have the effect of invigorating the spleen. So for edema syndrome due to spleen deficiency, it must be combined with other herbs of invigorating the spleen, such as Fuling, Baizhu, etc.

Usage and dosage : 6-12 g for decoction.

Zexie(Oriental Waterplantain Rhizome, Rhizoma Alismatis)

Properties and Tastes : sweet and cold.

Meridian Entry : kidney and bladder meridians.

Effects : ①Induce diuresis to drain dampness. ②Discharge heat. ③Eliminate turbid and reducing blood lipida.

Application :

(1) Dysuria and edema

It is often used with Fuling, Zhuling and Guizhi, such as Wuling San. It also can be used for the diarrhea due to the cold of spleen and stomach, with Houpo, Cangzhu, Chenpi an so on, such as Weiling Tang. For the phlegm retention manifested as dizzy, it is used with Baizhu, such as Zexie Tang.

(2) Stranguria caused by heat

Zexie is especially effective in dampness-heat type in the lower energizer, usually with Mutong, Cheqianzi. For seminal emission, tidal fever caused by deficiency of kidney yin, it is used with Shudihuang, Shanzhuyu, Mudanpi and so on, such as Liuwei Dihuang Wan.

(3) Hyperlipidemia

Studies have shown that the medicine can reduce blood lipida. It can be used in combination with Juemingzi, Heye, Heshouwu and so on.

Usage and dosage : 6-10 g for decoction.

Cheqianzi(Plantain Seed, Semen Plantaginis)

Properties and Tastes : sweet and cold.

Meridian Entry : liver, kidney, lung and small intestine meridians.

Effects : ①Clear heat and induce diuresis. ②Drain dampness to stanch diarrhea. ③Improve vision. ④Dispel phlegm.

Application :

(1) Edema and stranguria

It is especially suitable for stranguria of damp-heat types manifested as oliguria with reddish urine, difficulty and pain in micturition, and it is usually combined with Mutong, Huashi and Bianxu, such as Bazheng San. For the edema caused by retention of water-damp, it is used with Zhuling, Fuling, Zexie. For the kidney deficiency caused by aeipathia, it is used with Niuxi, Shudihuang, Shanzhuyu and so on, such as Jisheng Shenqi Wan.

(2) Diarrhea due to summerheat-dampness

It can promote the diuresis so does to make defecation forming. Therefore, it can be used for diarrhea due to domination of dampness. It can be used alone or with Baizhu, Fuling, Zexie, etc.

(3) Conjunctivitis due to flaring up of liver fire

It is usually used combined with Juhua and Juemingzi. For deficiency of liver yin and kidney yin manifested as dim eyesight and nebula, often used together with Shudihuang, Tusizi and Gouqizi.

(4) Cough caused by lung heat

It is usually combined with Gualou, Zhebeimu, Pipaye, etc.

Usage and dosage: 9–15 g for decoction. Wrap-decoct.

Huashi (Talc, Talcum)

Properties and Tastes: sweet and cold.

Meridian Entry: bladder, lung, and stomach meridians.

Effects: ①Induce diuresis to treat stranguria. ②Release summerheat.

Application:

(1) Strangury disease caused by heat

Huashi is a commonly used medicine for the treatment of strangury, often used with Mutong, Cheqianzi, Qumai and so on, such as Bazheng San. For the stone strangury, it is often used with Haijinsha, Jinqiancao, Mutong and so on.

(2) Summerheat syndrome with excessive thirst, dysuria. It can be used with Gancao, such as Liuyi San. For the early stage of damp febrile disease manifested as headache, aversion to cold, heavy body, chest tightness, it is used with Yiyiren, Baikouren, Xingren and so on, such as Sanren Tang.

(3) Diarrhea due to dampness and heat

It can promote the diuresis to make defecation forming, often used with Zhuling, Cheqianzi, Yiyiren.

Besides, Huashi can astring dampness and furuncle when it is being external used, so it can be used for eczema, miliaria and so on.

Usage and dosage: 10–30 g for decoction. Just appropriate amount of fresh for external using.

Yinchen (Virgate wormwood Herb, Herba Artemisiae Scopariae)

Properties and Tastes: bitter, pungent and slightly cold.

Meridian Entry: spleen, stomach, liver and gallbladder meridians.

Effects: ①Clear heat and dampness. ②Normalize gallbladder to cure jaundice.

Application:

(1) Jaundice and dysuria

It is an essential medicine to treat all kinds of jaundice. For that due to dampness and heat manifested as yellow tint of sclera and skin, it is usually combined with Zhizi, Dahuang, etc. , such as Yinchenhao Tang. For that due to cold-dampness of spleen and stomach, it usually combined with Fuzi, Ganjiang, etc. , such as Yinchen Sini Tang.

(2) Dampness-warmth syndrome and summer febrile disease, which is manifested as fever, malaise, stuffy chest, vomiting and dysuria

It is usually combined with Huashi, Huangqin, Mutong, etc. , such as Ganlu Xiaodu Dan.

（3）Eczema pruritus

It can be used combined with Huangbai,Kushen,Difuzi,etc.

Usage and dosage:6-15 g for decoction. Just right amount is for external using.

Simple list of other dampness-draining diuretic medicinals see Table 9-6.

Table 9-6　**Simple list of other dampness-draining diuretic medicines**

Name	Properties and Tastes	Meridian Entry	Effects	Application	Dosage
Dongguapi(Exocarpium Benincasae)	Sweet and cool	Spleen and small intestine meridians	(1)Induce diuresis to disperse swelling (2)Release summerheat	(1)Dysuria,edema (2)For summerheat syndrome with excessive thirst, dysuria	9-30 g for decoction
Tongcao(Medulla Tetrapanacis)	Sweet and slightly cold	Lung and stomach meridians	(1)Clear heat and promote urination (2)Promote lactation	(1)Dysuria,edema and stranguria caused by heat (2)For oligogalactia or agalactia	3-5 g for decoction
Qumai(Herba Dianthi)	bitter and cold	heart and small intestine meridians	(1)Induce diuresis to treat stranguria (2)Activate blood and unblock the meridian	(1)Heat stranguary,blood strangury, stone strangury and dysuria (2)Menstrual irregularities and amenorrhea caused by blood stasis	9-15 g for decoction
Bianxu(Herba Polygoni Avicularis)	Bitter and slightly cold	Bladder meridians	(1)Induce diuresis to treat stranguria (2)Kill worms (3)Relieve itching	(1)Heat strangury and oliguria with reddish urine (2)Abdominal pain due to parasitic infestation,eczema,pruritus vulvae	9-15 g for decoction
Haijinsha(Spora Lygodii)	Sweet,salty, and cold	Bladder and small intestine meridians	(1)Clear heat and drain dampness (2)Induce diuresis to treat stranguria	various stranguria	6-15 g for decoction. Wrapdecoction
Bixie(Rhizome Dioscoreae Hypoglaucae)	Bitter	Kidney and stomach meridians	(1)Eliminate dampness and turbidity (2)Expel wind	(1)Chyloid stranguria and whitish turbid urine (2)Wind-dampness impediment manifested as bodily heaviness,sore and painful waist and knees	9-15 g for decoction
Jinqiancao(Herba Lysimachiae)	Sweet and slightly cold	Liver, gallbladder,kidney and bladder meridians	(1)Eliminate dampness to treat jaundice (2)Induce diuresis to treat stranguria (3)Detoxify and relieve swelling	(1)Jaundice due to dampness-heat (2)Strangury disease (3)Eczema and damp sore	15-60 g for decoction

9.4.7 Interior-warming medicine

These are herbs that have as their principal action the warming of and dispelling cold from interior. They are of pungent flavor and hot nature. These are the properties that make them so suitable for treating illnesses of interior cold.

There are two types of interior cold illnesses: those of exogenous cold invading the interior and suppressing yang qi of the spleen and the stomach, and those of endogenous cold arising out of deficiency of yang qi or injury of yangqi by excessive sweating. In either case, interior-warming medicinals are appropriate treatment.

When prescribing interior-warming medicinals it is appropriate to modify the combination of medicinals depending on the clinical condition. For exogenous cold invading interior but associated with symptoms of exterior, add medicinals that release the exterior. For qi stagnation due to congealing by cold, add medicinals that mobilize qi. For accumulation of cold and dampness in interior, add medicinals that strengthen the spleen and dissolve dampness. For yang deficiency in the spleen and the kidney, add warming medicinals that strengthen the spleen and the kidney. For yang collapse and qi depletion, add medicinals that can vigorously augment and support genuine qi.

The medicinals in this group are pungency and hot, and they are drying. If applied improperly they can easily injure body fluids. In illnesses of heat or yin deficiency and in pregnancy they must be used with great care or be contraindicated.

Fuzi(Lateralis Preparata, Radix Aconiti Lateralis Praeparata)

Properties and Tastes: pungent, sweet, extremely hot, toxic.

Meridian Entry: heart, kidney and spleen meridians.

Effects: ①Recuperate the depleted yang for resuscitation. ②Supplement fire and strengthen yang. ③Expel cold to relieve pain.

Application:

(1)Syndrome of yang exhaustion

It is used for yang exhaustion syndrome. It is an essential drug for the treatment of yang exhaustion syndrome manifested as clammy perspiration, faint breath, cold clammy limbs, indistinct and faint pulse. It is usually used in combination with Ganjiang and Gancao, such as Sini Tang. For exhaustion of qi due to yang deficiency, it can be combined with Renshen to supplement qi to prevent collapse of qi, such as Shenfu Tang.

(2)Syndrome of yang deficiency

It is used to treat all kinds of syndromes of yang deficiency. For insufficiency of kidney yang with impotence, cold and painful waist and knees, and frequent micturition, it is usually combined with Rougui, Shanzhuyu, and Shudihuang, such as Yougui Wan. For insufficiency of spleen yang and kidney yang and interior domination of cold and dampness with coldness and pain in epigastric abdomen, loss of appetite and diarrhea, it is combined with Dangshen, Baizhu, and Ganjiang, such as Fuzi Lizhong Tang. For yang deficiency resulting in edema, and dysuria, it is usually used together with Baizhu, Fuling and Shengjiang, such as Zhenwu Tang. For exogenous affection due to yang deficiency, it is combined with Mahuang and Xixin, such as Mahuang Fuzi Xixin Tang.

(3)Syndrome of cold-pain

It is used to treat all pain syndromes of cold type. For arthralgia of wind-cold-dampness type, pain of general joints due to domination of cold and dampness, it is combined with Guizhi, Baizhu and Gancao, such as Gancao Fuzi Tang. For abdominal pain due to cold accumulation and qi stagnation, it is combined with Dingxiang and Gaoliangjiang.

Usage and dosage: 3-15 g is used in decoction for oral use and decocted at first for about a half to one hour until its narcotic-pungent taste is lost when its decoction is tasted by mouth. The raw medicinal material has a stronger toxicity, and is generally used for external application.

Precautions: Contraindicated in a case with yin deficiency leading to hyperactivity of yang and pregnant women because of its pungent, hot, dry and violent properties. It is incompatible with Banxia, Gualou, Beimu, Bailian and Baiji. It must be soaked for oral use, decocted for longtime, and over dosage and long-term treatment must be avoided.

Ganjiang(Zingiber Dried Ginger, Rhizoma Zingiberis)

Properties and Tastes: pungent and hot.

Meridian Entry: spleen, stomach, kidney, heart and lung meridians.

Effects: ①Warm the middle energizer to expel cold. ②Restore yang and dredge meridians. ③Warm the lung to resolve phlegm.

Application:

(1) Stomachache, vomiting, diarrhoea

It is used to treat spleen cold and stomach cold syndromes whether they are deficiency syndrome or excess syndrome. For stomach cold with vomiting and cold and painful epigastric abdomen, it is usually used in combination with Gaoliangjiang, such as Erjiang Wan. For deficiency and coldness of the spleen and stomach, it is usually combined with Dangshen, Baizhu, such as Lizhong Wan.

(2) Syndrome of yang exhaustion

For syndrome of yang exhaustion, it is usually combined with Fuzi for maximal effect to decrease the toxicity of Fuzi as well as to strengthen the effect of Fuzi in recuperating the depleted yang and rescuing the patient from qi collapse, such as Sini Tang.

(3) Cough and asthma due to cold accumulation in the lung

For cold accumulation in the lung manifested as cough and asthma, body's coldness and profuse thin sputum, it is usually combined with Xixin, Wuweizi and Mahuang, such as Xiaoqinglong Tang.

Usage and dosage: 3-10 g is used in decoction for oral use.

Precautions: It must be used with caution when treating pregnant women, internal heat of yin deficiency and blood heat. It is not suitable to be taken in large dosage and for a long time.

Simple list of other interior-warming medicinals see Table 9-7.

Table 9-7　**Simple list of other interior-warming medicines**

Name	Properties and Tastes	Meridian Entry	Effects	Application	Dosage
Rougui(Cortex Cinnamomi)	Pungent, sweet and extremely hot	Spleen, kidney, liver and heart meridians	(1) Supplement fire and strengthen yang (2) Expel cold and alleviate pain (3) Warm the meridians to promote the circulation of the blood	(1) It is used for insufficiency syndromes of kidney yang (2) It can be used to treat all pains due to accumulation of cold and stagnation of qi or stasis of the blood (3) Deficiency and coldness of lower energizer, and upfloating of deficiency yang (4) Yin abscess, carbuncle and sore that without being healed before suppuration or after rupture for a long time	1-5 g for decoction
Wuzhuyu (Fructus Evodiae)	Pungent, bitter, hot and mild toxic	Liver, spleen, stomach and kidney meridians	(1) Expel cold and relieve pain (2) Warm the spleen and stomach to stop vomiting (3) Strengthen yang and arrest diarrhea	(1) It is used to treat all syndromes due to cold accumulation in the liver meridian (2) Incoordination between the liver and stomach with acid regurgitation and vomiting (3) Diarrhea due to deficiency and cold	2-5 g for decoction
Xiaohui xiang (Fructus Foeniculi)	Pungent and warm	Liver, kidney, spleen and stomach meridians	(1) Expel cold to alleviate pain (2) Regulate the stomach qi	(1) Colic of cold type, orchidoptosis and dysmenorrhea (2) Qi stagnation due to stomach cold with epigastric distention and pain, vomiting and loss of appetite	3-6 g for decoction
Huajiao(Pericarpium Zanthoxyli)	Pungent and warm	Spleen, stomach and kidney meridians	(1) Warm the middle energizer to alleviate pain (2) Kill worms to relieve itching	(1) It is used to treat syndrome of epigastric and abdominal cold pain, vomiting and diarrhea (2) It is used to treat abdominal pain due to worms (3) Eczema and pruritus vulvae	3-6 g for decoction
Dingxiang (Flos Caryophylli)	Pungent and warm	Spleen, stomach, lung and kidney meridians	(1) Warm the middle energizer and descend adverse-rising (2) Expel cold to alleviate pain (3) Warming the kidney and supporting Yang	(1) Vomiting, hiccup due to stomach cold (2) Cold pain in epigastric abdomen (3) Impotence due to kidney deficiency	1-3 g for decoction

9.4.8　Qi-regulating medicinal

These are medicinals that have their principal actions of promoting the functional activities of qi and of facilitating qi movement. Qi-regulating medicinals are generally aromatic and have pungent and bitter flavor and warm nature. They are efficacious in normalizing qi activities and movement, strengthening the spleen, unblocking the liver and releasing stagnation, and are particularly suitable for treating qi stagnation or suppressing abnormally ascending qi caused by impedance of qi movement.

Impedance of qi movement is manifested mainly through effects on the functions of the lung, the liver, the spleen and the stomach. Qi stagnation generally shows tightness or an oppressed sensation, distention and pain. Abnormal qi ascent generally shows hiccups, vomiting or labored breathing.

Because of differences in location, progression and severity, the actual symptoms may also differ. Hence, when prescribing qi-regulating medicinals the physician must choose them to suit the actual illness and supplement them appropriately. For example, for obstruction of qi caused by exogenous pathogenic evils, add medicinals that ventilate the lung, dissolve sputum and stop cough. For cough and dyspnea due to phlegm and heat in the lung, add medicinals that cool heat and dissolve phlegm. For stagnation of spleen and stomach qi with associated dampness and heat, add herbs that cool heat and dissipate dampness. For cold and dampness blocking the spleen, add medicinals that warm the middle energizer and dry dampness. For food retention and indigestion, add medicinals that promote digestion and relieve retention. For insufficiency of the spleen and the stomach, add medicinals that augment qi and strengthen the spleen.

Many symptoms can accompany the stagnation of liver-qi. Depending on the specific associated symptoms, it may be necessary to add medicinals that nourish the liver, soften the liver, promote blood circulation, regulate the nutritive level, stop pain or strengthen the spleen.

Most qi-regulating medicinals are pungent and drying and can easily consume qi and injure yin. They must be used with great care in deficiency of both qi and yin.

Chenpi(**Dried Tangerine Peel Pericarpium**, **Citri Reticulatae**)

Properties and Tastes: pungent, bitter and warm.

Meridian Entry: spleen and lung meridians.

Effects: ①Regulate qi and invigorate spleen. ②Eliminate dampness and resolve phlegm.

Application:

(1) Stagnation of spleen qi and stomach qi

It is used especially suitable for stagnation of spleen qi and stomach qi due to accumulation of cold and dampness in the middle energizer manifested as distention and fullness of epigastric abdomen, belching, nausea, and vomiting. It is usually used in combination with Cangzhu and Houpo, such as Pingwei San. For vomiting due to phlegm heat, it is combined with Zhuru, Huanglian. For deficiency of spleen qi and stomach qi with abdominal pain that is reduced by pressure, fullness after meal, loss of appetite, it is usually combined with Dangshen, Baizhu, and Fuling, such as Yigong San.

(2) Retention of dampness, cough with profuse sputum

It is used to treat cough with profuse sputum caused by dampness phlegm and cold phlegm. In the treatment of cough and dyspnea due to dampness phlegm, it is usually combined with Banxia and Fuling to deprive dampness and resolve phlegm, such as Erchen Tang. For cough due to cold phlegm, it is usually combined with Ganjiang, Xixin and Wuweizi, such as Linggan Wuwei Jiangxin Tang.

Usage and dosage: 3-10 g is used in decoction for oral use.

Zhishi(Immature Orange Fruit, Fructus Aurantii Immaturus)

Properties and Tastes: bitter, pungent, sour and warm.

Meridian Entry: spleen, stomach and large intestine meridians.

Effects: ①Break stagnation of qi and remove food retention. ②Resolve phlegm and eliminate mass.

Application:

(1) Food retention syndromes

It is indicated for the treatment of indigestion, constipation due to accumulation of heat and dysentery. For indigestion and fullness and pain in the chest and upper abdomen, it is used together with Shanzha, Maiya and Shenqu, such as Qumai Zhizhu Wan. For constipation due to accumulation of heat, abdominal mass, and fullness and pain in the epigastrium, it can be combined with Houpo, Dahuang, Mangxiao, such as Dachengqi Tang. For stagnation of dampness and heat with dysentery and tenesmus, it is combined with Dahuang, Huanglian, and Huangqin, such as Zhishi Daozhi Wan.

(2) Chest impediment, epigastric stuffiness

It is used for turbid phlegm obstructing qi activity with fullness in the chest and epigastrium. For the syndrome due to deficiency of stomach yang and accumulation of cold phlegm, it can be combined with Xiebai, Guizhi, and Gualou, such as Zhishi Xiebai Guizhi Tang. For stagnation of dampness phlegm in the middle energizer, fullness in the epigastric abdomen, poor appetite, it is combined with Houpo, Banxia and Baizhu, such as Zhishi Xiaopi Wan.

In addition, it can be used to treat gastroptosis, prolapse of rectum and uterus, but it must be combined with Chaihu, Shengma, and Huangqi, in order to get good therapeutic effect, and it has the effect of raising blood pressure as well.

Usage and dosage: 3-10 g is used in decoction for oral use and a large dosage is 30 g.

Precautions: It is used with caution in the cases with deficiency of the spleen and stomach and pregnant women.

Simple list of other qi-regulating medicinals see Table 9-8.

Table 9-8　Simple list of other qi-regulating medicines

Name	Properties and Tastes	Meridian Entry	Effects	Application	Dosage
Qingpi (Pericarpium Citri Reticulatae Viride)	Bitter, pungent and warm	Liver, gallbladder and stomach meridians	(1) Soothe the liver to break qi stagnation (2) Eliminate mass and relieve dyspepsia	(1) It is indicated for liver qi stagnation manifested ashypochondriac distending pain, breast distending pain, and pain due to hernia (2) Distention and pain of the epigastrium due to indigestion	3 - 10 g for decoction
Muxiang (Radix Aucklandiae)	Pungent, bitter and warm	Spleen, stomach, large intestine, triple energizer and gallbladder meridians	(1) Move qi to relieve pain (2) Regulate the middle energizer	(1) syndromes of stomach and spleen qi stagnation (2) Dysentery due to dampness and heat with tenesmus (3) Syndromes of liver and gallbladder qi stagnation	3 - 6 g for decoction

Continue to Table 9–8

Name	Properties and Tastes	Meridian Entry	Effects	Application	Dosage
Xiangfu (Rhizoma Cyperi)	Pungent, slightly bitter, slightly sweet and neutral	Liver, spleenand triple energizer meridians	(1) Soothe the liver and regulate qi (2) Regulate menstruation to relieve pain	(1) The syndromes of stagnation of liver qi with pain in the hypochondrium, distention and pain in epigastric abdomen and pain due to hernia (2) Irregular menstruation, dysmenorrhea and distension and pain of the breast	6 – 10 g for decoction
Foshou (Fructus Citri Sarcodactylis)	Pungent, bitter and warm	Liver, spleen and lung meridians	(1) Soothe liver to regulate qi flow (2) Harmonize stomach (3) Resolve phlegm	(1) Liver depression and qi stagnation (2) Spleen and stomach qi stagnation (3) Cough with profuse sputum	3 – 10 g for decoction
Wuyao (Radix Linderae)	Pungent and warm	Lung, spleen, kidney and bladder meridians	(1) Promote the circulation of qi to relievepain (2) Warm the kidney to disperse cold	(1) It is indicated for stagnation of cold and qi manifested as oppression and pain in the chest, fullness andpain in the epigastrium, hernia of cold type and dysmenorrhea (2) Insufficiency of kidney yang, frequent urination and enuresis due to deficiency and coldness of the bladder	6 – 10 g for decoction
Xiebai (Bulbus Allii Macrostemonis)	Pungent, bitter and warm	Lung, stomach and large intestine meridians	(1) Activate yang and disperse lumps (2) Promote qi circulation and relieve the stagnation	(1) It is used to treat turbid phlegm and thoracic fullness due to deficiency of thoracic yang (2) Qi stagnation in the stomach and intestine manifested as dysentery with tenesmus	5 – 10 g for decoction
Shidi (Calyx Kaki)	Bitter, astringent and neutral	Stomach meridian	Lower the adverse rising qi and relieve hiccup	It is used to treat syndrome of hiccup, and can be combined with relevant medicinal herbs according to symptoms and signs	5 – 10 g for decoction

9.4.9　Digestant medicine

Any medicinal herb that acts to improve appetite and digestion or remove food stagnation is named digestant medicine.

These medicinals mainly have the sweet taste and are mainly attributed to the spleen and stomach meridians, with the function of improving appetite and digestion and removing food stagnation. Besides, some of the medicines have the functions of regulating flow of qi and blood, etc.

They are mainly used for removing food stagnation, manifested as abdominal distension, eructation, acid regurgitation, nausea, and vomiting, irregular bowel movements.

Modern studies indicate that most of this category can promote gastrointestinal peristalsis, increase digestive juice, which helps digestion.

Shanzha(Hawthorn Fruit, Fructus Crataegi)

Properties and Tastes: sour, sweet and slightly warm.

Meridian Entry: spleen, stomach and liver meridians.

Effects: ①Promote digestion and invigorate the stomach. ②Move qi and dissipate blood stasis. ③Eliminate turbid and reduce blood lipida.

Application:

(1) Food stagnation

It is especially effective in meat-type food accumulation, which is manifested as abdominal fullness and distention, belching and acid swallowing, abdominal pain and diarrhea. It can be used alone or used in combination with Laifuzi, Shenqu and so on.

(2) Diarrhea and bellyache

For this kind of syndrome, it is usually combined with Muxiang and Binglang.

(3) Menischesis and postpartum abdominal pain due to blood stasis, chest stuffiness and pains

Shanzha is usually used combined with Danggui, Xiangfu, Honghua, etc. to move qi and dissipate blood stasis, such as Tongyu Jian.

(4) Hyperlipidemia studies have shown that the medicine can reduce blood lipida

The medicine can be used alone or combination with Danshen, Sanqi and Gegen.

Usage and dosage: 9-12 g for decoction. Charred Shanzha has stronger digestion-promoting effect than Shanzha.

Shenqu(Medicated Leaven, Massa Medicata Fermentata)

Properties and Tastes: sweet, pungent and warm.

Meridian Entry: spleen and stomach meridians.

Effects: Promote digestion and harmonize the stomach.

Application: Indigestion and retention food.

It is often used in combination with Shanzha, Maiya and Muxiang for sydromes manifested as abdominal fullness and distention, poor appetite, borborygmus and diarrhea. This medicine also can relieve exterior syndrome, so it is more suitable for the dyspeptic retention with exterior syndrome in exopathy.

Usage and dosage: 6-15 g for decoction.

Maiya(Germinated Barley, Fructus Hordei Germinatus)

Properties and Tastes: sweet.

Meridian Entry: spleen, stomach and liver meridians.

Effects: ①Promote digestion and and fortify the stomach. ②Terminate lactation.

Application:

(1) Food indigestion and retention

The medicine can promote the circulation of qi and promote digestion, fortify the spleen and stomach. It is better at promoting the digestion of starchy foods. So it is mainly used for the retention of rice, noodles and yam, often used with Shanzha, Shengqu, Jineijin and so on. For the anorexia caused by insufficiency of the spleen, it is usually used with Baizhu, Chenpi, such as Jianpi Wan.

(2) Stagnation of qi

Maiya can smooth the liver and regulate the flow of qi, so it is used for the liver qi stagnation, marked by pain of lateral thorax and abdomen, often used together with Chaihu, Xiangfu, and Chuanlianzi and so on.

(3) Milk stasis and breast pain

The medicine can terminate lactation, therefore, it can be used for the women's delactation and breast pain.

Usage and dosage: 10-15 g for decoction. Stir-baked Maiya is used for delactation and the dosage is 60 g. Raw Maiya is used for promoting digestion and and fortifying the stomach.

Simple list of other digestant medicinals see Table 9-9.

Table 9-9　**Simple list of other digestant medicinals**

Name	Properties and Tastes	Meridian Entry	Effects	Application	dosage
Jineijin (Endothelium Corneum Gigeriae Galli)	Sweet and medium	Spleen, stomach, small intestine and large intestine meridians	(1) Promote digestion and invigorate the stomach (2) Arrest seminal emission	(1) Dyspepsia, vomiting, diarrhea, especially effective in food accumulation of rice and noodles (2) Spermatorrhea, enuresis (3) Stone stranguria	3-10 g for decoction
Laifuzi (Semen Raphani)	Pungent, sweet and medium	Lung, spleen and stomach meridians	(1) Promote digestion and relieve fullness (2) Descend qi and resolve phlegm	(1) Retention of indigested food and stagnation (2) Cough and dyspnea of retention of phlegm	5-15 g for decoction

9.4.10　Hemostatic medicine

These are medicines that have their principal action of stopping bleeding. They are used mainly to treat bleeding conditions such as hemoptysis, epistaxis, hematemesis, hematuria, metrorrhagia, ecchymosis and traumatic bleeding.

Hemostatic medicines come with a variety of associated properties, such as blood cooling, astringent, clot dissolving and channel warming. When prescribing, the physician must select the most suitable medicinals for the whole body and combine it with appropriate supplementary medicinals to enhance the therapeutic effect. For example, if the bleeding is due to heat in the blood driving it to flow erratically, add medicines that cool heat and blood. If it is due to yin deficiency with hyperactive yang, add medicines that nourish yin and suppress yang. If it is due to blood stasis, add medicines that mobilize qi and blood. If it is due to deficiency cold, add medicines that warm yang, augment qi or strengthen the spleen as appropriate for the clinical condition. If excessive bleeding has depleted qi and brought it to the verge of collapse, medicinals that stop bleeding used alone are too slow in action for such an urgent situation. It is necessary to add medicines that augment genuine qi vigorously to avoid prostration.

When applying hemostatic medicines, the physician must take note whether there is blood stasis. If the clots that result from the stasis have not been completely reabsorbed, the physician must add medicines that mobilize blood and eliminate clots to avoid leaving residual clots.

Sanqi(Sanchi, Notoginseng Radix)

Properties and Tastes: sweet, slightly bitter and warm.

Meridian Entry: liver and stomach meridians.

Effects: ①Remove blood stasis to stop bleeding. ②Promote blood circulation and alleviate pain.

Application:

(1) Bleeding syndromes

It is used for various kinds of internal and external bleedings, especially for bleeding with blood stasis, for it has the advantage of arresting bleeding without stasis and removing blood stasis while keeping healthy qi. For hematemesis, emptysis, metrorrhagia and metrostaxis, it can be ground singly into powder to be swallowed or combined with Huaruishi, Xueyutan, such as Huaxue Wan. For bleeding due to trauma, its powder is applied externally on local area alone or combined with Longgu and Xuejie, such as Qibao San.

(2) Trauma and painful swelling with blood stasis

It is the primary medicinal material for wounds, for it has the effects of promoting blood circulation to remove blood stasis, relieving swelling and alleviating pain. It could be taken orally or applied externally alone or combined with blood-activating, trauma-treating and pain-relieving medicinal materials.

In addition, it could also be used in the treatment of coronary heart disease with angina pectoris and various stagnant blood syndromes of gynecology.

Usage and dosage: 3-9 g for decoction. 1-3 g of the powder to be taken orally. Appropriate amount for external application.

Precautions: It is used with caution for pregnant women.

Baiji(Common Bletilla Rubber, Rhizoma Bletillae)

Properties and Tastes: bitter, sweet, astringent and slightly cold.

Meridian Entry: lung, stomach and liver meridians.

Effects: ①Stop bleeding by astringency. ②Remove swelling and promote regeneration.

Application:

(1) Bleeding syndromes

It is the primary astringent hemostatic and is used for various internal and external bleedings, especially for bleedings in the lung and stomach. It can be powdered and used alone or mixed with rice soup for oral use, or in combination with other medicinal materials. For insufficiency of lung-yin with dry cough and hemoptysis, it is usually combined with Pipaye, Oujie, Ejiao. For bleeding of stomach, it is combined with Haipiaoxiao; while for bleeding due to trauma, it can be ground into powder or combined with Duanshigao for external application.

(2) Sores and carbuncle, and rhagadia of hands and feet

It is suitable for both oral and external uses. For the early stage of carbuncle, its powder could be used alone for external application, or combined with Jinyinhua, Tianhuafen to clear off carbuncle. For ulcerated and unhealed carbuncle, it is usually ground into powder together with Huanglian, Qingfen, and Wubeizi for external application. For rhagadia of hands and feet, the powder can be mixed with sesame oil and then applied to the local area.

Usage and dosage: 6-15 g. 3-6 g of the powder is used per time. Appropriate amount for external application.

Precautions: It is incompatible with Wutou.

Simple list of other hemostatic medicines see Table 9–10.

Table 9–10   Simple list of other hemostatic medicines

Name	Properties and Tastes	Meridian Entry	Effects	Application	Dosage
Xiaoji(Herba Cirsii)	Bitter and cold	Heart and liver meridians	(1)Cool blood and stop bleeding (2)Eliminate toxic material to treat carbuncle	(1)Blood heat causing bleeding (2)Toxic-heat causing sores and carbuncles	5 – 12 g for decoction
Diyu(Radix Sanguisorbae)	Bitter, astringent and slightly cold	Liver, stomach and large intestine meridians	(1)Cool the blood and stop bleeding (2)Eliminate toxic material and treat pyogenic infection	(1)Blood heat causing bleeding (2)Scald,eczema,sores and ulcers,swollen pains	9 – 15 g for decoction
Huaihua(Flos Sophorae)	Bitter and slightly cold	Liver and large intestine meridians	(1)Cool the blood and stop bleeding (2)Clear away liverheat and lower the fire	(1)Blood heat causing bleeding (2)Conjunctivitis and headache	5 – 10 g for decoction
Cebaiye(Cacumen Platycladi)	Bitter, astringent and slightly cold	Lung, liver and intestine meridians	(1)Cool the blood and stop bleeding (2)Eliminate phlegm and relieve cough	(1)Blood heat causing bleeding (2)Lung heat causing cough with sputum	6 – 12 g for decoction
Qiancao(Radix Rubiae)	Bitter and cold	Liver meridian	(1)Remove blood stasis and stop bleeding (2)Cool the blood and circulate the meridians	(1)Bleeding caused by blood stasis or blood heat (2)Stagnant-blood syndromes	6 – 10 g for decoction
Puhuang(Pollen Typhae)	Sweet and neutral	Liver and pericardium meridians	(1)Stop bleeding and remove blood stasis (2)Promote diuresis	(1)Bleeding syndromes (2)Blood stasis causing pain (3)Blood stranguria	5 – 10 g for wrapped decoction
Xianhe cao(Herba Agrimoniae)	Bitter, astringent and neutral	Liver meridian	(1)Stop bleeding by astringing (2)Relieve dysentery and kill trichomonad	(1)Bleeding syndromes (2)Chronic dysentery,sores and carbuncles (3)Trichomoniases	6 – 12 g for decoction
Aiye(Folium Artemisiae Argyi)	Bitter, pungent and warm	Liver, spleen and kidney meridians	(1)Stop bleeding by warming meridians (2)Expel cold and alleviate pain	(1)Deficiency and cold causing bleeding (2)Irregular menstruation, menstrual pain and abdominal pain and cold	3–9 g for decoction
Paojiang(Rhizoma Zingiberis)	Bitter, astringent and warm	Spleen and liver meridians	(1)Warm meridians to stop bleeding (2)Warm the middle energizer to alleviate pain	(1)Deficiency and cold causing bleeding (2)Abdominal pain and diarrhea	3–9 g for decoction

9.4.11 Blood-activating and stasis-resolving medicinal

These are medicinals that have their principal action of stimulating blood circulation and of removing blood stasis. They are especially efficacious at dispersion, including reversing stasis, dissolving hematomas, stimulating blood circulation, restoring menstrual flow, ameliorating rheumatism, reducing swelling and stopping pain.

The main application of these medicinals is the condition of blood stasis. This is a commonly seen condition with four major presentations: ①aches, pain or numbness; ②masses in the interior or the exterior, or traumatic hematomas; ③internal hemorrhage with dark purple blood clots; ④ecchymosis on the skin, mucous membranes or the tongue. Blood stasis develops in the course of many illnesses, and itself is also the cause of further disease.

Since there are many causes of blood stasis, when prescribing medicines that stimulate blood circulation and remove blood stasis the physician must form a firm diagnosis and select and add medicines appropriate to the clinical requirements. For example, if the blood stasis is due to cold gelling qi and impeding blood flow, add medicinals that warm the interior and dispel cold. If it is due to heat consuming yin and blood, add medicinals that cool heat and blood. For rheumatism with pain due to wind-dampness, add medicines that dispel wind and dissipate dampness. For blood stasis associated with deficiency of genuine qi, add medicines that restore the deficient.

Qi and blood are intimately interrelated. When qi moves, so does blood, and when qi becomes impeded, then blood becomes static. Hence, when prescribing medicinals that stimulate blood circulation and relieve stasis, it is appropriate to include medicinals that stimulate qi movement. Doing so enhances the ability of the medicinals to stimulate blood circulation and relieve stasis.

Chuanxiong(Szechwan Lovage Rhizome, Rhizoma Ligustici Chuanxiong)

Properties and Tastes : pungent and warm.

Meridian Entry : liver, gallbladder and pericardium meridians.

Effects : ①Activate blood and move qi. ②Expel wind and alleviate pain

Application :

(1)Stagnation of blood and qi

For irregular menstruation, dysmenorrheal and amenorrhea, this medicinal material is usually combined with Danggui and Xiangfu. In case of postpartum abdominal pain due to blood stasis, it is often combined with Yimucao and Taoren. For hypochondriac pain due to unsmooth circulation of blood caused by stagnation of liver qi, it is combined with Chaihu, Xiangfu. In the case of physical trauma, it is used with Chishao and Honghua. Also, for carbuncle, sore, purulence without ulceration, it is usually combined with Danggui and Chuanshanjia, such as Tounong San.

(2)Headache and Impediment disease pain of wind and damp

For headache due to external contraction of wind-cold, it is usually combined with Baizhi, Fangfeng and Xixin, such as Chuanxiong Chatiao San. If the headache is due to wind-heat, it should be combined with Juhua, Shigao and Jiangchan, such as Chuanxiong San. If headache is due to wind-dampness, it is often used with Qianghuo, Gaoben and Fangfeng, for example, in the Qianghuo Shengshi Tang. If headache is due to blood stasis, it is usually combined with Chishao, Honghua and Danshen. For headache due to blood deficiency, it is often combined with Danggui and Baishao. For painful joints due to impediment disease blockage, it is usually combined with Qianghuo, Duhuo and Sangzhi.

Usage and dosage :3-9 g. For powder form, 1.5 g is used and taken each time.

Precautions：It is pungent，warm，ascending and dispersing，so it is contraindicated in cases with a reddish tongue and dryness of the mouth，caused by yin-deficiency with hyperactivity fire. It should be used with caution in cases of excessive menstruation and with conditions with hemorrhagic disease.

Danshen(Danshen Root, Radix Salviae Miltiorrhizae)

Properties and Tastes：bitter and slightly cold.

Meridian Entry：heart and liver meridians.

Effects：①Promote blood circulation to remove blood stasis. ②Clear heat from the blood and resolving swelling. ③Remove annoyance and tranquilize the mind.

Application：

(1)Blood stasis Syndromes

It is especially effective for women's syndromes of blood stasis with heat，such as irregular menstruation，amenorrhea and postpartum abdominal pain. It can be taken in powder form together with aged wine，or combined with Danggui and Yimucao. For angina pectoris and epigastric pain，caused by blood stasis and stagnation of qi，it is usually combined with Tanxiang and Sharen，such as，in the Danshen Tang. In cases of abdominal masses，it is combined with Sanleng，Ezhu and Biejia. For trauma with pain due to blood stasis，it is combined with Danggui，Honghua and Chuanxiong. In addition，for heat heat impediment with reddish，swollen and painful joints，it should be combined with Rendongteng，Chishao and Sangzhi.

(2)Breast abscess with swelling and pain

To treat breast abscess with swelling and pain，it is usually combined with Ruxiang，Jinyinhua and Lianqiao，such as Xiaoru Tang.

(3)Restlessness and insomnia

For heat invading the Yingfen and Xuefen in the seasonal febrile disease，it is usually combined with Dihuang and Xuanshen，such as in the Qingying Tang. For blood failing to nourish the heart，it is usually combined with Suanzaoren and Yejiaoteng.

Usage and dosage：9−15 g. The stir-baked with wine form has the ability to strengthen the medicinal function of promoting blood circulation.

Precautions：It is incompatible with Lilu.

Yanhusuo(Yanhusuo, Rhizoma Corydalis)

Properties and Tastes：pungent，bitter and warm.

Meridian Entry：liver，spleen and heart meridians.

Effects：①Activate blood. ②Move qi. ③Relieve pain.

Application：

Syndromes of stagnation of qi and blood stasis causing pain

For pain in the epigastric abdominal area，it can be taken orally alone，or ground into a powder，and mixed with warm liquor. Also，it can treat the problems above when combined with Chuanlianzi，such as，in the Jinglingzi San. In cases of abdominal pain during menstruation，it should be combined with Danggui，Chuanxiong and Xiangfu. If stuffiness and pains in the chest，it should be used together with Gualou，Xiebai and Yujing. In cases of hypochondriac pain，it is usually combined with Qingpi and Xiangfu. For pain due to hernia，it is used with Xiaohuixiang and Wuzhuyu. In addition，for pain in the limbs，or general pain due to blood stasis，it is combined with Danggui，Guizhi and Chishao. To treat physical trauma，it should be combined with Danggui，Ruxiang and Moyao.

Usage and dosage：3−9 g. 1. 5−3 g of the powder to be swallowed per time.

Yimucao(Motherwort Herb,HerbaLeonuri)

Properties and Tastes:pungent,bitter and slightly cold.

Meridian Entry:liver,pericardium and bladder meridians.

Effects:①Activate blood and dispel stasis. ②Induce diuresis to alleviate edema.

Application:

(1)Syndromes of blood stasis

To treat blood stasis causing irregular menstruation,dysmenorrheal,amenorrhea,postpartum abdominal pain,lochiorrhea,and trauma pain,it can be decocted alone into a paste,or combined with Danggui,Chuanxiong and Chishao,such as Yimu Wan.

(2)Dysuria and edema

It can be decocted alone or combined together with Xianmaogen and Zelan.

In addition,it can clear heat and relieve toxicity,for which it may be used for ulcer and carbuncle,and itchy skin rash.

Usage and dosage:9-30 g. In the fresh form 12-40 g. It can be used decocted into a paste or processed into pills. The appropriate amount of the pounded fresh form is utilized for external application.

Precautions:It is contraindicated in pregnant women.

Simple list of other blood-activating and stasis-resolving medicinals see Table 9-11.

Table 9-11　Simple list of other blood-activating and stasis-resolving medicines

Name	Properties and Tastes	Meridian Entry	Effects	Application	Dosage
Yujin(Radix Curcumae)	Pungent, bitter and cold	Liver,heart, lung and gallbladder meridians	(1) Activate blood and relieve pain (2) Promote qi and disperse the stagnated qi (3) Clear heart and cool blood (4) Excrete bile and relieve jaundice	(1) Liver qi stagnation and blood stasis causing blockage (2) Mental confused by phlegm heat (3) Blood heat causing bleeding as haematemesis, epistaxis,hematuria and unsmooth menstruation (4) Dampness-heat jaundice and gallstone	3 - 10 g for decoction
Ruxiang (Olibanum)	Pungent, bitter and warm	Liver,heart and spleen meridians	(1) Activate blood and alleviate pain (2) Subside swelling and promote tissue regeneration	(1) Blood stasis causing pain (2) Trauma and sores and ulcers,abscess and swelling	3-5 g for decoction
Moyao(Myrrha)	Bitter and neutral	Heart,liver and spleen meridians	(1) Activate blood and alleviate pain (2) Subside swelling and promote tissue regeneration	(1) Blood stasis causing pain (2) Sores and ulcers after rupture	3-5 g for decoction

Continue to Table 9-11

Name	Properties and Tastes	Meridian Entry	Effects	Application	Dosage
Taoren(Semen Persicae)	Bitter, sweet and neutral	Heart, liver and large intestine meridians	(1) Promote blood circulation by removing blood stasis (2) Lubricate the bowels to relieve constipation	(1) Syndromes of blood stasis causing dysmenorrheal, amenorrhea, postpartum abdominal pain, pain in chest and hypochondrium, and trauma pain (2) Blood stasis of heat type causing pulmonary and intestine abscess (3) Constipation due to dry intestine	5 - 10 g for decoction
Honghua(Flos Carthami)	Pungent and warm	Heart and liver meridians	(1) Promote blood circulation by removing blood stasis (2) Regulate menstruation and relieve pain	(1) Blood stasis syndromes (2) Chest and hypochondriac pain and mass (3) Trauma pain and pains in joints (4) Stagnation of heat and blood stasis	3 - 10 g for decoction
Yimucao (Herba-Leonuri)	Pungent, bitter and slightly cold	Liver, pericardium and bladder meridians	(1) Activate blood and dispel stasis (2) Lnduce diuresis to alleviate edema	(1) Syndromes of blood stasis (2) Dysuria and edema	10 - 15 g for decoction
Wangbuliuxing (Semen Vaccariae)	Bitter and neutral	Liver and stomach meridians	(1) Activate blood circulation and stimulate meridians (2) Promote lactation and cure abscess (3) Induce diuresis to relieve stranguria	(1) Blood stasis causing amenorrhea, dysmenorrheal, dystocia (2) Postpartum, agalactia, breast abscess and swollen pain (3) Heat stranguria, blood stranguria and urolithic stranguria	5 - 10 g for decoction
Ezhu(Rhizoma Curcumae)	Pungent, bitter and warm	Liver and spleen meridians	(1) Break blood stasis and move qi (2) Eliminate stagnation and alleviate pain	(1) Stagnation of qi and blood stasis (2) Syndromes of food stagnancy and qi stagnation	6-9 g for decoction
Sanleng (Rhizoma Sparganii)	Pungent, bitter and neutral	Liver and spleen meridians	(1) Break blood stasis and move qi (2) Eliminate stagnation and alleviate pain	(1) Stagnation of qi and blood stasis (2) Stagnation of food with fullness and pain in epigastric abdomen	5 - 10 g for decoction

9.4.12 Phlegm-dispelling, cough-suppressing and panting-calming medicine

This group actually comprises two subgroups of medicines: phlegm-dispelling medicines and cough-suppressing and panting-calming medicines. The phlegm-dispelling medicines act principally to dissolve phlegm and eliminate sputum. Cough is usually accompanied by sputum and phlegm usually causes cough. In general, phlegm-dispelling medicines also can stop cough and relieve asthma and cough-stopping and asthma-relieving medicines also can dissolve phlegm. The two groups are therefore usually discussed together. Phlegm-dispelling medicines are mainly used to treat illnesses of phlegm causing much sputum and cough, cough with labored breathing or sputum that is difficult to expectorate. Cough-suppressing and panting-calming medicines are mainly used to treat cough and asthma due to either internal injury or exogenous pathogenic agent. Since both internal injury and exogenous illness can produce cough, asthma or much sputum, it is important to select these medicines on the basis of the cause and properties of the clinical condition being treated and to add appropriate supplemental medicines.

For cough with associated hemoptysis it is not appropriate to prescribe phlegm-dispelling medicines that are harsh and irritating, as these may aggravate the hemoptysis. For cough in the early stages of measles, the main medicines to use are in general those that clear and ventilate the lung rather than cough-stopping medicines. Cough-suppressing medicines that are warm or astringent are especially inappropriate as they may aggravate heat or affect the proper eruption of the measles rash.

Banxia(Pinellia Tuber, Pinelliae Rhizoma)

Properties and Tastes: pungent, warm and toxic.

Meridian Entry: spleen, stomach and lung meridians.

Effects: ①Dry dampness and eliminate phlegm. ②Direct qi downward to relieve vomiting. ③Relieve stuffiness and dissipate nodulation. ④Relieve swelling and pain for external use.

Application:

(1) Damp-phlegm syndromes

It's an important drug for clearing dampness to reduce phlegm. For failure of spleen to transport and transform water and obstruction by phlegm and dampness causing profuse sputum, cough and adverse rise of qi, it is usually combined with Chenpi and Fuling in Erchen Tang. For that accompanied with cold, profuse and clear sputum, Xixin and Ganjing are combined. For that with fever and thick and yellowish sputum, it is used together with Huangqin, Zhimu and Gualou. For dizziness due to damp-phlegm, it is combined with Baizhu and Tianma in Banxia Baizhu Tianma Tang.

(2) Adverse rise of stomach qi manifested as nausea and vomiting

For vomiting due to cold-fluid retention, it is usually combined with Shengjiang in Xiaobanxia Tang. For vomiting due to stomach deficiency, combined with Renshen and Baimi in Dabanxia Tang. For vomiting due to stomach heat, combined with Huanglian and Zhuru. For vomiting during pregnancy, combined with Zisugeng and Sharen. For vomiting due to stomach yin deficiency, combined with Shihu and Maidong.

(3) Chest and epigastric fullness and stuffiness, globus hystericus, goiter, subcutaneous nodule

For chest and epigastric fullness and stuffiness with vomiting due to mixed accumulation of phlegm and heat, it is combined with Huanglian and Gualou in Xiaoxianxiong Tang. For epigastric oppression due to phlegm and heat, it is usually combined with Ganjiang, Huanglian and Huangqin in Banxia Xiexin Tang. For globus hystericus without fever due to qi stagnation and phlegm accumulation, it is combined with Houpo, Zisuye and Fuling in Banxia Houpo Tang. For goiter and subcutaneous nodule, it is used together with Kunbu, Haizao and Zhebeimu.

(4)Large carbuncle, mammary sore, bite by poisonous snake

It can relieve swelling and pain by external use. It is ground into powder to apply on the affected parts.

In addition, it can dry dampness and harmonize stomach, so it is effective for disharmony of stomach and restlessness when combined with Shumi in Banxia Shumi Tang.

Usage and dosage: 3-9 g. It is made into powder and applied on the affected parts with appropriate amount. It is usually used after processing. For instance, Jiangbanxia is very effective for suppressing adverse rise of qi and stopping vomiting, and Fabanxia is usually used to dry dampness with mildly warm property.

Precautions: It is incompatible with Wutou. Since it is warm and dry, it is used with caution to treat dry cough due to yin deficiency, hemorrhagic diseases, dry-phlegm and heat-phlegm.

Chuanbeimu(Tendrilleaf Fritillary Bulb, Bulbus Fritillariae Cirrhosae)

Properties and Tastes: bitter, sweet and slightly cold.

Meridian Entry: lung and heart meridians.

Effects: ①Clear heat and resolve phlegm. ②Moisten lung and relieve cough. ③Dissipate mass and relieve swelling.

Application:

(1)Chronic cough due to lung deficiency, dry cough due to lung heat

It is slightly cold in nature and bitter in flavor and could relieve lung heat and resolve phlegm. Also, it is sweet and moist in flavor and could moisten the lung to relieve cough. Combined with Shashen and Maidong, it treats lung deficiency and yin deficiency causing chronic cough with phlegm. To treat lung heat resulting in dry cough, it is usually combined with Zhimu in Ermu San.

(2)Scrofula, carbuncle, mammary abscess, pulmonary abscess

It has the effect of clearing heat and congestion. For scrofula, it is usually combined with Xuanshen and Muli in Xiaoluo Wans. For carbuncle and mammary abscess, it is usually combined with Pugongying, Tianhuafen and Lianqiao. For pulmonary abscess, it is usually combined with Yuxingcao, Xianlugen and Yiyiren.

Usage and dosage: 3-10 g. It is ground into powder with 1-2 g each time.

Precautions: It is incompatible with Wutou.

Zhebeimu(Thunberg Fritillary Bulb, Bulbus Fritillariae Thunbergii)

Properties and Tastes: bitter and cold.

Meridian Entry: lung and heart meridians.

Effects: ①Clear heat and resolve phlegm. ②Remove stagnation and dissipate mass.

Application:

(1)Cough caused by wind-heat, dryness-heat and phlegm-heat

It is cold in flavor and has the effect of removing heat-phlegm and driving lung qi downward. For cough due to wind-heat, it is usually combined with Sangye, Niubangzi and Qianhu. For cough due to phlegm-heat accumulation in lung, it is usually combined with Gualou and Zhimu.

(2)Scrofula, goiter, carbuncle, pulmonary abscess

It has the effect of clearing heat and congestion. For scrofula, it is combined with Xuanshen and Muli in Xiaoluo Wan. For goiter, it is usually combined with Haizao and Kunbu. For carbuncle, it is often used together with Lianqiao and Pugongying. For pulmonary abscess, it is used together with Yuxingcao, Lugen and Taoren.

Usage and dosage: 5-10 g.

Precautions : It is incompatible with Wutou.

Kuxingren (Bitter Apricot Seed , Semen Armeniacae Amarum)

Properties and Tastes : bitter , slightly warm and mildly toxic.

Meridian Entry : lung and large intestine meridians.

Effects : ①Relieve cough and asthma. ②Moisten intestine and relax the bowels.

Application :

(1) Cough and asthma

It is an important drug to relieve cough and asthma. It treats cough due to wind-heat , combined with Sangye and Juhua , such as Sangju Tang. For cough due to wind-cold , combined with Mahuang and Gancao , such as Sanao Tang. It treats cough caused by dry-heat with Sangye , Chuanbeimu and Shashen , such as Sangxing Tang. In cases of cough and asthma resulting from lung-heat , it is usually combined with Mahuang and Shengshigao , such as Mahuang Xingren Gancao Shigao Tang.

(2) Intestinal dryness causing constipation

It is usually used together with Huomaren , Danggui and Zhiqiao , such as Runchang Wan ; and usually combined with Baiziren , Yuliren , Taoren and Songziren , such as Wuren Wan.

Usage and dosage : 5-10 g. The raw medicinal material is decocted later.

Precautions : It is mildly toxic , so it must be used within the amount listed. It must be used with caution when treating infants.

Simple list of other cough-suppressing and panting-calming medicinals see Table 9-12.

Table 9-12　Simple list of other cough-suppressing and panting-calming medicines

Name	Properties and Tastes	Meridian Entry	Effects	Application	Dosage
Xuanfuhua (Inula Flower)	Bitter , pungent , salty and slightly warm	Lung , spleen , stomach and large intestine meridians	(1) Direct qi downward to resolve phlegm (2) Direct qi downward to relieve vomiting	(1) It is used for phlegm-fluid congestion in lung causing cough and asthma with profuse sputum , phlegm and retained fluid causing oppressing in chest and diaphragm (2) It is used for belching , vomiting	3-9 g for decoction. Wrap-decoction
Gualou (Snakegourd Fruit)	Weet and cold	Lung , stomach and large intestine meridians	(1) Clear heat and resolve phlegm (2) Loosen chest to remove stasis (3) Moisten intestine and relieve constipation	(1) It is used for phlegm-heat causing cough and asthma (2) It is used for chest impediment , thoracic accumulation (3) It is used for pulmonary abscess , intestinal abscess , mammary abscess (4) It is used for intestinal dryness with constipation	9 - 15 g for decoction

Continue to Table 9-12

Name	Properties and Tastes	Meridian Entry	Effects	Application	Dosage
Zhuru(Bamboo Shavings)	Sweet and slightly cold	Lung, stomach and gallbladder meridians	(1) Clear heat and resolve phlegm (2) Alleviate restlessness and relieve vomiting	(1) It is used for phlegm-heat causing cough, inner disturbance by phlegm-fire causing restlessness and insomnia (2) It is used for stomach-heat causing vomiting	5 - 10 g for decoction
Jiegeng(Platyco-don Grandiflorus)	Bitter, pungent and neutral	Lung meridian	(1) Disperse lung qi and resolve phlegm (2) Relieve sore throat and eliminate abscess	(1) It is used for failure of lung qi in dispersion manifested as cough with profuse sputum, oppression in chest (2) It is used for sore throat and aphonia (3) It is used for pulmonary abscess	3 - 10 g for decoction
Zisuzi(Perilla Fruit)	Pungent and warm	Lung and large intestine meridians	(1) Send the adverse qi downward (2) Clear phlegm, relieve cough and asthma (3) Relax the bowels to relieve constipation	(1) It is used for phlegm accumulation, adverse rise of lung qi, cough and asthma (2) It is used for intestinal dryness with constipation	3 - 10 g for decoction
Baibu(Stemona Root)	Sweet, bitter and slightly warm	Lung meridian	(1) Moisten the lung and relieve cough (2) Kill worms and insects, including louse	(1) It is used for acute or prolonged cough, whooping cough, cough caused by pulmonary tuberculosis (2) It is used for enterobiasis, head louse, body louse, scabies	3-9 g for decoction
Ziwan(Tatarian Aster Root)	Pungent, bitter and warm	Lung meridian	(1) Nourish the lung to send the adverse qi downward (2) Relieve cough and asthma	(1) It treats external contraction by wind-cold manifested as cough with profuse sputum (2) It is used for lung deficiency causing prolonged cough with hemoptysis	5 - 10 g for decoction
Kuandonghua (Flos Farfarae)	Pungent, slightly bitter and warm	Lung meridian	(1) Moisten lung to send the adverse qi downward (2) Resolve phlegm and relieve cough	Cough and asthma	5-9 g for decoction

Continue to Table 9-12

Name	Properties and Tastes	Meridian Entry	Effects	Application	Dosage
Pipaye(Loquat Leaf)	Bitter and slightly cold	Lung and stomach meridians	(1) Clear lung and relieve cough (2) Suppress adverse rise of qi to stop vomiting	(1) It is used for lung heat causing cough (2) It is used for stomach heat manifested as thirst, vomiting	6 – 10 g for decoction
Sangbaipi (White Mulberry Root-bark)	Sweet and cold	Lung meridian	(1) Purge lung-heat to relieve asthma (2) Diuresis and eliminate edema	(1) It is used for lung heat causing cough and asthma (2) It is used for excess syndrome of fluid retention manifested as edema, difficult urination	6 – 12 g for decoction

9.4.13 Tranquillizing medicine

These are medicinals that have their principal action of tranquilliztion or calming the mind. Their principal application is the treatment of restlessness, agitation, palpitations of the heart, insomnia, excessive dreaming, as well as infantile convulsions, epilepsy and dementia.

Most medicinals in this category derive from minerals or the seeds of plants. In general, mineral medicinals are heavy and lowering in nature; hence many of them are sedating or tranquilizing. The seed medicinals are moistening and restorative in nature; hence many of them strengthen the heart and calm the mind.

When prescribing tranquillizing medicinal the physician must take full stock of the patient's illness; not only select an appropriate medicinal, but also supplement and complement it with appropriate other medicinals. For example, for yin deficiency and blood insufficiency, complement the mind-calming medicinals with medicinals that generate blood and augment yin. For abnormal ascent of liver-yang, complement with medicinals that calm the liver and suppress yang. For the blazing of heart-fire, complement with medicinals that cool the heart and clear fire. In such conditions as epilepsy and infantile convulsion, the approach is usually to use medicinals that dissolve phlegm and open orifices or those that calm the liver and extinguish wind as the main treatment. Tranquilizing medicinals are used only as supplement.

Mineral herbs when taken as pills or powders can easily injure the stomach and impair stomach qi. They must be complemented with herbs that nourish the stomach and strengthen the spleen. Some of them are quite toxic and must be used only with great care.

Zhusha(Cinnabar, Cinnabaris)

Properties and Tastes: sweet, slightly cold and toxic.

Meridian Entry: heart meridian.

Effects: ①Relieve palpitation and calm spirit. ②Clear heat and remove toxin.

Application:

(1) Irritability, palpitation, insomnia

For exuberance of heart fire causing irritability, restless fever in chest, palpitation and insomnia, it is combined with Huanglian and Gancao. For those accompanied by deficiency of heart blood, Danggui and Shengdihuang are added, such as Zhusha Anshen Wan. For palpitation due to fright or heart deficiency, it is put into a pig's heart and stewed for oral administration. For deficiency of yin and blood resulting in palpitation and insomnia, it is combined with Danggui, Baiziren and Suanzaoren.

(2)Convulsion and epilepsy

For high fever causing coma and convulsion, it is used with Niuhuang and Shexiang, such as Angong Niuhuang Wan. For infantile convulsion, it is combined with Niuhuang and Quanxie, such as Niuhuang San. For epilepsy, sudden coma and convulsion, it is combined with Cishi and Shenqu, such as Cizhu Wan.

(3)Carbuncle, sore throat and aphthae

To treat carbuncle, it is combined with Xionghuang and Daji, such as Zijin Troche. It treats sore throat and aphthae, with Bingpian and Pengsha in Bingpeng San for external application.

In addition, it is also used as coat of pills and boluses, strengthening the effect of calming spirit and preventing decaying.

Usage and dosage: 0. 1-0. 5 g is usually used in pill or powder form, not in decoction. It is used externally with appropriate dosage.

Precautions: Since it is toxic, it cannot be used in large amount or for a prolonged time. It contraindicates with abnormal function of liver and kidneys. It avoids being calcined, because mercury can be separated out, which is extremely toxic.

Suanzaoren(Spine Date Seed, Semen Ziziphi Spinosae)

Properties and Tastes: sweet, sour and neutral.

Meridian Entry: liver, gall bladder and heart meridians.

Effects: ①Nourish heart and benefit liver. ②Clam mind. ③Arrest sweating.

Application:

(1)Palpitation and insomnia

For blood deficiency of heart and liver resulting in palpitation and insomnia, it is combined with Danggui, Baishao and Heshouwu. For liver deficiency with heat causing vexation and insomnia, it is usually combined with Zhimu and Fuling, such as Suanzaoren Tang. For deficiency of heart and kidney and yin deficiency leading to hyperactive yang causing insomnia, palpitation, amnesia, it is combined with Shengdihuang, Xuanshen and Baiziren, such as Tianwang Buxin Wan.

(2)Weak constitution manifested as spontaneous sweating and night sweating

To treat spontaneous sweating and night sweating caused by weak constitution, it is usually combined with Dangshen, Wuweizi and Shanzhuyu.

Usage and dosage: 9-15 g. It is ground into powder for oral administration with 1. 5-3 g for each time.

Simple list of other tranquillizing medicinals see Table 9-13.

Table 9-13 Simple list of other tranquillizing medicines

Name	Properties and Tastes	Meridian Entry	Effects	Application	Dosage
Cishi(Magnetitum)	Salty and cold	Liver,heart and kidney meridians	(1)Induce sedation and calm mind (2)Calm liver and suppress yang (3)Improve auditory and visual acuity (4)Improve inspiration and relieve dyspnea	(1)Irritability,fright palpitation,insomnia and epilepsy (2)Liver yang hyperactivity manifested as dizziness and headache (3)Yin deficiency of liver and kidney causing tinnitus, deafness,blurred vision (4)Dyspnea of kidney deficiency type	9 – 30 g for decoction first
Longgu (Os Draconis)	Sweet, astringent and neutral	Heart,liver and kidney meridians	(1)Induce sedation and calm mind (2)Pacify liver and subdue hyperactive yang (3)Astringe and arrest discharge	(1)Restlessness,palpitation,insomnia,fright epilepsy and mania (2)Yin deficiency and yang hyperactivity manifested as irritability and dizziness (3)Loss and consumption syndromes	15 – 30 g for decoction
Baiziren(Semen Platycladi)	Sweet and neutral	Heart, kidney and large intestine meridians	(1)Nourish heart and calm mind (2)Moisten intestines to release bowels	(1)Palpitation,insomnia (2)Intestinal dryness with constipation	3 – 10 g for decoction
Yuanzhi(Radix Polygalae)	Bitter, pungent and warm	Heart, kidney and lung meridians	(1)Calm heart and tranquilize mind (2)Eliminate phlegm for resuscitation (3)Dissipate swelling and carbuncles	(1)Fright palpitation, insomnia and amnesia (2)Confusion of mind by phlegm causing epilepsy and mania (3)Cough with profuse sputum (4)Large carbuncle causing swelling pain	3 – 10 g for decoction
Hehuan pi(Cortex Albiziae)	Sweet and neutral	Heart,liver and lung meridians	(1)Calm mind and alleviate mental depression (2)Activate blood circulation and relieve swelling	(1)Emotional injury manifested as depression,insomnia and amnesia (2)Fracture caused by trauma,abscess of internal organs,carbuncle swelling	6 – 12 g for decoction

9.4.14　Tonifying and replenishing medicinal

These medicinals have their principal actions of replenishing the vital substances of the body and of strengthening its visceral organs. By doing so they enhance the body's resistance to illness and eliminate the deficiencies.

There are four types of deficiency: qi, blood, yin and yang. By their actions and applications restorative medicinals fall into four categories: those that augment qi, those that generate blood, those that restore yin and those that restore yang. Which medicinal to prescribe will depend upon the type of deficiency. Moreover, in conditions of deficiency or damage of qi, blood, yin and yang often interact and affect one another. Hence, medicinals from the different categories must often be prescribed together-restorative medicinals for qi and yang together and restorative medicinals for blood and yin together.

Tonifying and replenishing medicinals are inappropriate in strength illnesses due to exogenous pathogenic evils. Also, if they are used incorrectly, restoratives can do more harm than good. When prescribing them the physician must take proper care of the spleen and the stomach. To avoid impairing digestion and absorption, as well as to obtain the desired therapeutic effects, the physician must include appropriate medicinals that strengthen these organs.

Renshen(Ginseng, Radix Ginseng)

Properties and Tastes: sweet, slightly bitter and neutral.

Meridian Entry: lung, spleen and heart meridians.

Effects: ①Replenish the primordial qi. ②Reinforce the spleen and nourish the lung. ③Promote fluid production. ④Induce tranquilization and improve intelligence.

Application:

(1)Prostration syndrome of primordial qi

It is a vital life-saving medicinal and used to treat the crucial state due to prostration syndrome of primordial qi manifested as shortness of breath, listlessness, as well as a weak and faint pulse. It can be used alone such as in the Dushen Tang. For declination of yang qi manifested as cold extremities, it is used in combination with Fuzi, such as in the Shenfu Tang. For thirst due to deficiency of both qi and yin, it is used in combination with Maidong and Wuweizi, such as in the Shengmai San.

(2)Lung qi deficiency syndrome

For shortness of breath, dyspnea, reluctance to speak and a low voice due to deficient lung qi, it is usually used in combination with Huangqi and Wuweizi. For dyspnea due to deficiency of both the lung and kidney, it is used in combination with Gejie and Wuweizi, such as in the Renshen Gejie San.

(3)Spleen qi deficiency syndrome

For lassitude, lack of strength, anorexia and loose stools due to spleen qi deficiency, it is usually used in combination with Baizhu and Fuling, such as in the Sijunzi Tang. For various types of bleeding due to the failure of spleen to control blood, it is usually used in combination with Huangqi and Baizhu, such as in the Guipi Tang.

(4)Thirst due to qi deficiency and consumption of fluid in febrile diseases and diabetes

For febrile diseases with consumption of qi and body fluid manifested as thirst, large and feeble pulse, it is usually combined with Zhimu, Shigao, such as in Baihu Jia Renshen Tang. For Xiaoke(similar to diabetes), it is used in combination with Tianhuafen and Shengdihuang.

(5)Palpitation, insomnia and dreamful sleep

Due to its effect of replenishing heart qi, it is usually used in combination with Suanzaoren and Baiziren to treat heart qi deficiency syndrome manifested as palpitation, fearful throbbing, insomnia and dream-disturbed sleep.

In addition, it can replenish qi and strengthen yang and it is used to treat impotence. When combined with pathogen-expelling medicinal such as exterior-releasing medicinal, cathartic drugs, it has the efficacy to reinforce the healthy and dispel the pathogenic. It is used to treat excessive pathogens with healthy qi being deficient, such as in the case of qi deficiency with external contraction, or with heat accumulation of interior-excess.

Usage and dosage: 3-9 g. In case of prostration syndrome, the recommended dosage can be as much as 15-30 g. It should be simmered separately and later mixed with decoction of other medicinal herbs for oral administration. As to wild Renshen, it is ground into powder for swallows, 2 g each time, two times per day.

Precautions: It should not be used in combination with Lilu. Chronic administration of Renshen or Renshen preparations can cause diarrhea, rashes, insomnia, nervousness, increased blood pressure, melancholy, hypersexuality(or hyposexuality), headache or palpitations. Bleeding is indicative of acute poisoning of Renshen.

Huangqi(Milkvetch Root, Radix Astragali seu Hedysari)

Properties and Tastes: sweet and slightly warm.

Meridian Entry: spleen and lung meridians.

Effects: ①Tonify qi and raise yang. ②Strengthen the defensive and superficial. ③Induce diuresis to alleviate edema. ④Expel toxin and promote tissue regeneration.

Application:

(1)Spleen qi deficiency syndrome and syndrome of sinking of middle qi

It is an essential medicinal for invigorating the middle and replenishing qi. For lassitude, lack of strength, anorexia and loose stool, due to spleen qi deficiency, it is often used in combination with Dangshen and Baizhu. In cases of proctoptosis due to prolonged diarrhea, prolapse of internal organs, resulted from the sinking of middle qi, it is used with Renshen and Shengma, such as in the Buzhong Yiqi Tang. Furthermore, it functions to tonify qi and produce blood and treats blood deficiency syndrome in combination with Danggui, such as in the Danggui Buxue Tang. For loss of blood, which is due to the failure of spleen to control blood, it is combined with Renshen and Baizhu, such as in the Guipi Tang. To treat Xiaoke(similar to diabetes), which is due to the spleen failing to distribute fluid, it is usually combined with Tianhuafen and Gegen.

(2)Lung qi deficiency syndrome and spontaneous sweating due to qi deficiency

For chronic cough and dyspnea, shortness of breath, listlessness, which is due to lung qi deficiency, it is used in combination with Ziyuan, Kuandonghua. To treat spontaneous sweating due to exterior deficiency, it is used with Muli and Mahuanggen. For those with exterior deficiency syndrome presenting as spontaneous sweating, and vulnerability to pathogenic wind, it is combined with Baizhu and Fangfeng, such as in the Yupingfeng San.

(3)Edema due to qi deficiency

It is an essential medicine to treat edema due to qi deficiency. In this case, it is usually combined with Baizhu and Fuling.

(4)Deficiency syndrome of qi and blood, unruptured ulcers or unhealed ulcers after rupture. When the healthy qi is deficient and fails to expel interior toxins outwardly, there may appear even-shaped wide-rooted ulcers which fail to heal for a long period after rupturing. In this case, it is prescribed with Danggui and

Shengma, such as in the Tounong San. For that due to deficiency of qi and blood, it is combined with Danggui and Rougui, such as in the Shiquan Dabu Tang.

Furthermore, with the function of tonifying qi to promote blood circulation, it treats arthralgia syndrome and sequela of apoplexy.

Usage and dosage: 9–30 g. Honey-roasted, it is more effective for invigorating the middle and replenishing qi.

Danggui(Chinese Angelica, Radix Angelicae Sinensis)

Properties and Tastes: sweet, pungent and warm.

Meridian Entry: liver, heart and spleen meridians.

Effects: ①Tonify blood and activate blood. ②Regulate menstruation to relieve pain. ③Moisten the bowels to relieve constipation.

Application:

(1) Blood deficiency syndrome

It is the most essential medicinal for treating blood deficiency syndrome. In this case, it is usually combined with Huangqi, as in the Danggui Buxue Tang.

(2) Irregular menstruation, amenorrhea and menorrhagia

To treat irregular menstruation, amenorrhea and menorrhagia due to blood deficiency or blood stasis, it is usually combined with Shudihuang, Baishao and Chuanxiong, such as in the Siwu Tang. If it is accompanied by qi deficiency, it is combined with Renshen and Huangqi; if for accompanied by qi stagnation, it is used combined with Xiangfu and Yanhusuo; and if by blood heat, it is combined with Huangqin and Huanglian. For amenorrhea due to blood stasis, it is used in combination with Taoren and Honghua. For that due to blood deficiency and cold-stagnation, it is combined with Ejiao and Aiye.

(3) Abdominal pain due to deficiency cold, injuries from falls, carbuncles and ulcers and sores, arthralgia due to wind-cold

It treats abdominal pain due to blood deficiency, blood stasis or cold stagnation, it is used in combination with Guizhi, Shaoyao and Shengjiang, such as in the Danggui Jianzhong Tang. For injuries from falls marked by pains and ecchymoma, it is combined with Honghua and Taoren, such as in the Fuyuan Huoxue Tang. In the case of early stage of ulcers with redness, swelling and pain, it is combined with Jinyinhua, Chishao and Tianhuafen, such as in the Xianfang Huoming Tang. In the treatment of unhealed ulcers after rupture, it is combined with Huangqi, Renshen and Rougui, such as in the Shiquan Dabu Tang. It also treats arthralgia due to wind-cold, combined with Qianghuo, Fangfeng and Huangqi.

(4) Constipation due to blood deficiency with intestinal dryness

In this case, it is usually used in combination with Roucongrong and Niuxi.

Usage and dosage: 5–15 g.

Precautions: It is contraindicated in patients with excessive dampness with abdominal fullness and diarrhea.

Ejiao(Ass Hide Glue, Colla Corii Asini)

Properties and Tastes: sweet and neutral.

Meridian Entry: lung, liver and kidney meridians.

Effects: ①Tonify blood. ②Nourish yin. ③Moisten the dryness. ④Stop bleeding.

Application:

(1) Blood deficiency syndrome

It is an essential medicinal for treating blood deficiency. It is better at treating bleeding due to blood deficiency and usually prescribed with Shudihuang, Danggui and Shaoyao, such as in the Ejiao Siwu Tang. For palpitations, fearful throbbing, knotted and intermittent pulse, due to deficiency of qi and blood, it is usually prescribed with Guizhi and Gancao, such as the Zhigancao Tang.

(2) Hemorrhage

For bloody urine during pregnancy, it is baked by itself and ground into powder for oral administration. In cases of hematemesis and hemorrhage due to yin-deficiency with blood heat, it is combined with Puhuang and Shengdihuang. To treat hemoptysis, it is used together with Renshen and Tiandong. Also, for metrorrhagia and metrostaxis due to blood deficiency or blood cold, it is usually combined with Shudihuang and Danggui. To treat hemafecia or hematuria due to deficiency cold of spleen qi, it is combined with Baizhu and Zaoxintu in the Huangtu Tang.

(3) Yin deficiency with dry cough

For syndrome of lung heat with yin deficiency, manifested as dry cough with little phlegm, dry throat and bloody sputum, it is used in combination with Madouling, Niubangzi and Xingren. For syndromes of dryness injury to the lung manifesting as dry cough without sputum, dry nose and throat, it is combined together with Sangye, Xingren and Maidong.

(4) Dysphoria and insomnia, clonic convulsions of the four extremities

In combination with Huanglian and Baishao, such as in the Huanglian Ejiao Tang. It treats febrile disease with dysphoria and insomnia due to deficiency of kidney yin with exuberance of heart fire for clonic convulsions of the four extremities in the advanced stage of febrile disease encompassing exhaustion of true yin and yin deficiency stirring wind, it is combined with Guijia and Hen Egg Yolk, such as in the Dadingfengzhu Tang or Xiaodingfengzhu Tang.

Usage and dosage: 5-15 g, melted by heating for oral administration with water.

Precautions: It is sticky and greasy and may cause dyspepsia. Therefore, it should be administered cautiously for patient with weakness of spleen and stomach.

Maidong(Dwarf Lilyturf Tuber, Radix Ophiopogonis)

Properties and Tastes: sweet, bitter slightly and cold slightly.

Meridian Entry: stomach, lung and heart meridians.

Effects: ①Nourish Yin and moisten the lung. ②Tonify the stomach to promote the production of the body fluid. ③Dispell heat from the heart and relieve vexation.

Application:

(1) Stomach yin deficiency syndrome

In combination with Shengdihuang and Yuzhu, it treats deficiency of stomach yin due to heat, manifesting as dry mouth and tongue. For Xiaoke(similar to diabetes), it is combined with Tianhuafen and Wumei. It is combined with Banxia and Renshen to treat vomiting due to deficiency of stomach. To treat constipation due to pathogenic heat damaging fluid, it is prescribed with Shengdihuang and Xuanshen, such as in the Zengye Tang.

(2) Lung yin deficiency syndrome

Prescribed with Ejiao, Shigao and Sangye in Qingzao Jiufei Tang, it treats yin deficiency with dryness-heat in the lung, manifesting as dry nose and throat, dry cough with little phlegm, sore throat and hoarse voice.

(3) Heart yin deficiency syndrome

To treat deficiency of heart yin, manifested as dysphoria, insomnia, dream-disturbed sleep amnesia, palpitations and fearful throbbing. It is prescribed with Shengdihuang and Suanzaoren, such as in the Tianwang

Buxin Wan. To treat dysphoria and hyposomnia, due to heat invading heart-nutrient level it is used in combination with Huanglian and Shengdihuang.

Usage and dosage : 6-12 g.

Gouqizi(Lycii Fructus Barbary, Wolfberry Fruit)

Properties and Tastes : sweet and neutral.

Meridian Entry : liver and kidney meridians.

Effects : ①Nourish liver and kidney. ②Replenish essence and improve vision.

Application : Syndrome of liver-kidney yin deficiency.

It is indicated for dizziness, aching and limpness in the loins and knees, spermatorrhea, deafness, loosened teeth, early graying of hair, insomnia and dream-disturbed sleep, due to insufficiency of essence and blood, tidal fever, night sweating and Xiaoke(diabetes), due to yin deficiency of liver and kidney. To treat xerotic eyes, cataract and blurry vision, it is prescribed with Shudihuang, Shanzhuyu, Shanyao and Juhua, such as in the Qiju Dihuang Wan.

Usage and dosage : 6-12 g.

Simple list of other tonifying and replenishing medicinals see Table 9-14.

Table 9-14　Simple list of other tonifying and replenishing medicinals

Name	Properties and Tastes	Meridian Entry	Effects	Application	Dosage
Xiyang shen (Radix Panacis Quinquefolii)	Sweet, slightly bitter and cool	Lung, heart and kidney meridians	(1) Tonify qi and nourish yin (2) Clear heat and promote fluid production	(1) Syndrome of both qi and yin deficiency (2) Lung qi deficiency syndrome and lung yin deficiency syndrome (3) Thirst due to qi deficiency and consumption of fluid in febrile diseases and diabetes	3-6 g for decoction alone
Dangshen (Radix Codonopsis)	Sweet and neutral	Spleen and lung meridians	(1) Invigorate the middle energizer and replenish qi (2) Invigorate spleen and lung (3) Nourish blood and promote fluid production	(1) Insufficiency of middle qi (2) Lung qi deficiency syndrome (3) Qi and blood deficiency syndrome (4) Qi deficiency and fluid consumption syndrome	9-30 g for decoction
Taizishen (Radix Pseudostellariae)	Sweet, slightly bitter and neutral	Spleen and lung meridians	(1) Tonify spleen qi (2) Promote fluid production and nourish lung	(1) Spleen deficiency syndrome (2) Insufficiency of qi and yin after disease (3) Dry cough due to lung insufficiency	9-30 g for decoction

Continue to Table 9–14

Name	Properties and Tastes	Meridian Entry	Effects	Application	Dosage
Baizhu (Rhizoma Atractylodis Macrocephalae)	Sweet, bitter and warm	Spleen and stomach meridians	(1) Invigorate spleen and replenish qi (2) Dry dampness and induce diuresis (3) Stop sweating (4) Prevent abortion	(1) Spleen qi deficiency syndrome. (2) Edema, phlegm-fluid retention (3) Spontaneous sweating due to qi deficiency (4) Threatened abortion due to spleen deficiency	6 – 12 g for decoction
Shanyao(Rhizoma Atractylodis Macrocephalae)	Sweet and neutral	Spleen, lung and kidney meridians	(1) Nourish the spleen and stomach (2) Promote production of fluid and nourish lung (3) Tonify kidney and secure essence	(1) Spleen deficiency syndrome (2) Lung deficiency syndrome (3) Kidney deficiency syndrome (4) Xiaoke with deficiency of both qi and yin	15 – 30 g for decoction
Baibiandou (Semen Dalichoris Album)	Sweet and slightly warm	Spleen and stomach meridians	(1) Invigorate spleen and resolve dampness (2) Harmonize the middle and dispel summer-heat	(1) Spleen qi deficiency syndrome (2) Syndrome of summer-heat, vomiting and diarrhea	9 – 15 g for decoction
Gancao(Radix Glycyrrhizae)	Sweet and neutral	Heart, lung spleen and stomach meridians	(1) Tonify spleen and replenish qi (2) Dispel phlegm and arrest cough (3) Relive spasm and alleviate pain (4) Clear heat and relieve toxicity (5) Harmonize all medicinal	(1) Spleen qi deficiency syndrome (2) Heart qi insufficient syndrome (3) Cough and dyspnea (4) Spasm in the abdomen and extremities (5) Heat-toxin with ulcers, sore throat, medicinal or food poisoning (6) Moderating the properties of medicinal	2 – 10 g for decoction
Dazao(Fructus Jujubae)	Sweet and warm	Spleen and stomach meridians	(1) Tonify the middle and replenish qi (2) Nourish blood and induce tranquilization	(1) Spleen qi deficiency syndrome (2) Sallowness due to blood deficiency, and hysteria	6 – 15 g for decoction

Continue to Table 9-14

Name	Properties and Tastes	Meridian Entry	Effects	Application	Dosage
Lurong(Ccornu Cervi Pantotrichum)	Sweet, salty and warm	Kidney and liver meridians	(1)Tonify kidney yang (2)Replenish essence and blood (3)Strengthen tendons and bones (4)Regulate Chong (Thoroughfare) and Ren (Conception) vessels (5)Expel sores	(1) Kidney yang deficiency and essence blood deficiency (2) Kidney deficiency with bone weakness (3) Deficiency cold in thoroughfare and conception vessels (4) Unhealed chronic ulcers, deep-rooted yin abscess	1-2 g. It is ground into powder for swallows or used in pill for powder form
Yinyanghuo (Herba Epimedii)	Pungent, sweet and warm	Kidney and liver meridians	(1)Tonify kidney yang (2) Strengthen tendons and bones (3)Expel wind-damp	(1)Declination of kidney yang (2)Wind-cold-damp arthralgia, numbness in limbs	6 - 10 g for decoction
Bajitian(Radix Morindae Officinalis)	Pungent, sweet and slightly warm	Kidney and liver meridians	(1)Tonify kidney yang (2)Strengthen tendons and bones (3)Expel wind-damp	(1)Deficiency of kidney yang (2)Kidney deficiency limpness in the knees and lumbus, lumbago and impediment disease	3 - 10 g for decoction
Xianmao (Rhizoma Curculigins)	Pungent, hot and toxic	Kidney, liver and spleen meridians	(1)Tonify kidney yang (2) Strengthen tendons and bones (3)Expel wind-damp	(1)Deficiency of kidney yang (2)Pain and cold sensation in knees and lumbus, bone limpness, chronic impediment disease	3 - 10 g for decoction
Xuduan(Radix Dipsaci)	Bitter, pungent and slightly warm	Liver and kidney meridians	(1)Tonify kidney and liver (2)Strengthen tendons and bones (3)Heal bone fracture (4)Stop metrorrhagia and metrostaxis	(1)Impotence, spermatorrhea and enuresis (2) Soreness in knees and lumbus, arthralgia due to cold-dampness (3) Injuries from falls, soft tissue injuries and bone fracture (4)Metrorrhagia and metrostaxis, threatened abortion	9 - 15 g for decoction
Roucongrong (Herba Cistanches)	Sweet, salty and warm	Kidney and large intestine meridians	(1)Tonify kidney yang (2)Replenish essence and blood (3)Moisten bowels to relieve constipation	(1)Impotence, spermatorrhea, sterility (2)Constipation due to intestinal fluid consumption	6 - 10 g for decoction

Continue to Table 9-14

Name	Properties and Tastes	Meridian Entry	Effects	Application	Dosage
Tusizi(Semen Cuscutae)	Sweet and warm	Liver, kidney and spleen meridians	(1)Tonify kidney and replenish essence (2)Nourish liver to improve vision (3)Stop diarrhea and prevent abortion	(1)Kidney insufficiency with lumbago, impotence, spermatorrhea and frequent urination, sterility due to cold uterus (2)Insufficiency liver and kidney, dim and blurred vision (3)Deficiency of spleen and kidney yang, diarrhea (4)Kidney insufficiency with threatened abortion and habitual abortion	6-12 g for decoction
Hetaoren(Semen Juglandis)	Sweet and warm	Kidney, lung and large intestine meridians	(1)Tonify kidney and warm lung (2)Moisten bowels to relieve constipation	(1)Declination of kidney yang, lumbago and feet flaccidity, frequent urination (2)Deficiency of lung and kidney, cough and dyspnea due to deficiency cold (3)Constipation due to intestinal dryness	6-9 g for decoction
Shudihuang (Radix Rehmanniae Preparata)	Sweet and slightly warm	Liver and kidney meridians	(1)Nourishing yin and supplementing blood (2)Replenish essence and marrow	(1)Blood deficiency syndromes (2)Deficiency syndromes of liver-kidney yin	9-15 g for decoction
Baishao(Radix Paeoniae Alba)	Bitter, sour, slightly cold	Liver and spleen meridians	(1)Nourish blood and regulate menstruation (2)Suppress liver to relieve pain (3)Astringe yin to arrest sweating	(1)Irregular menstruation (2)Pain in the hypochondrium, stomach and abdomen, or spasm and pain in the extremities (3)Hyperactivity of liver yang with headache and vertigo (4)Sweating with aversion to wind, night sweating due to yin deficiency	6-15 g for decoction
Beishashen (Radix Glehniae)	Sweet, slightly bitter and slightly cold	Lung and stomach meridians	(1)Nourish yin and clear lung heat (2)Reinforce the stomach and promote fluid production	(1)Lung yin deficiency syndrome (2)Stomach yin deficiency syndrome	5-12 g for decoction

Continue to Table 9-14

Name	Properties and Tastes	Meridian Entry	Effects	Application	Dosage
Baihe(Bulbus Lilii)	Sweet and cold	Heart and lung meridians	(1)Nourish yin and moisten lung (2)Clear heart to induce tranquilization	(1)Lung yin deficiency syndrome (2)Insomnia,palpitations, lily disease	6-12 g for decoction
Tiandong(Radix Asparagi)	Sweet,bitter and cold	Lung and kidney meridians	(1)Nourish yin and moisten dryness (2)Clear lung and promote fluid production	(1)Lung yin deficiency syndrome (2)Kidney yin deficiency syndrome (3)Febrile disease with consumption of fluid, anorexia,thirst and constipation to intestinal dryness	6-12 g for decoction
Shihu(Herba Dendrobii)	Sweet,slightly cold	Stomach and kidney meridians	(1)Strengthen stomach and promote fluid production (2)Nourish yin and clear heat	(1)Stomach yin deficiency syndrome (2)Kidney yin deficiency syndrome	6-12 g for decoction
Yuzhu(Rhizoma Polygonati Odorati)	Sweet,slightly cold	Lung and stomach meridians	(1)Nourish yin and moisten dryness (2)Promote fluid production to relieve thirst	(1)Lung deficiency syndrome (2)Stomach yin deficiency syndrome	6-12 g for decoction
Huangjing (Rhizoma Polygonati)	Sweet and neutral	Spleen,lung and kidney meridians	(1)Tonify qi and nourish yin (2)Invigorate the spleen (3)Moisten the lung (4)Reinforce the kidney	(1)Ling yin deficiency syndrome (2)Spleen deficiency syndrome (3)Deficiency of kidney essence	9-15 g for decoction
Mohanlian(Herba Ecliptae)	Sweet,sour and cold	Liver and kidney meridians	(1)Nourish liver yin and kidney yin (2)Cool blood to stop bleeding	(1)Syndrome of liver-kidney yin deficiency (2)Hemorrhage due to yin deficiency with blood heat	6-12 g for decoction
Guijia(Carapax et Plastrum Testudinis)	Salty,sweet and slightly cold	Liver,kidney and heart meridians	(1)Nourish yin and suppress yang (2)Tonify kidney and strengthen bones (3)Nourish blood and replenish heart	(1)Syndrome liver-kidney yin deficiency (2)Kidney deficiency with flaccidity of the tendons and bones (3)Insufficiency of yin-blood with palpitations, insomnia and amnesia	9-24 g for decoction first

Continue to Table 9-14

Name	Properties and Tastes	Meridian Entry	Effects	Application	Dosage
Biejia(Carapax Trionycis)	Salty and cold	Liver and kidney meridians	(1)Nourish yin and suppress yang (2)Reduce bone-steaming fever (3)Soften hardness and dissipate nodulation	(1)Yin deficiency with internal heat,with wind stirring inside,with yang hyperactivity (2)Abdominal masses	9-24 g for decoction first

9.4.15 Astringent medicine

These are medicines that have their principal actions of astringing and stabilizing. Most of them are sour and astringent. Individual medicines have the ability to hold back sweat, stop diarrhea, hold back semen, reduce diuresis, curtail vaginal discharge, stop bleeding or stop cough. Hence they are suitable for use in a patient in whom the constitution has been weakened by chronic illness or genuine qi is infirm. Such a patient may show symptoms of unrestrained flow, such as spontaneous sweating, night sweat, chronic diarrhea, dysentery, spermatorrhea, premature ejaculation, enuresis, polyuria, chronic cough with labored breathing, persistent metrorrhagia and persistent vaginal discharge.

Astringent medicinals treat only the appearance, not the root. They can prevent exhaustion of genuine qi from the unrestrained and continual loss and avoid other complications. However, the fundamental cause of illnesses with such unrestrained loss is deficiency of genuine qi. Hence, complete treatment of both root and appearance requires the use of complementary restorative medicinals. For example, for spontaneous sweating due to qi deficiency or night sweat due to yin deficiency, add respectively medicines that augment qi or nourish yin. For chronic diarrhea, dysentery and persistent vaginal discharge due to insufficiency of the spleen and the kidney, add medicinals that nourish and strengthen the spleen and the kidney. For premature ejaculation, spermatorrhea, enuresis and polyuria due to kidney insufficiency, add medicinals that nourish and strengthen the kidney. For infirmity of the ren and chong meridians causing metrorrhagia, add medicinals that nourish the liver and the kidney and those that reinforce the ren and chong meridians. For chronic cough and labored breathing due to insufficiency of the lung and the kidney, add medicinals that nourish the lung and enhance the kidney's capacity to receive qi.

Astringent medicinal have the disadvantage of potentially retaining disease-causing evils. In general, if the exogenous pathogenic evil is still present in the exterior, if dampness has accumulated in the interior, or if interior heat has not been cleared, then it is inappropriate to prescribe these medicinals.

Mahuanggen(Ephedra Root,Radix Ephedrae)

Properties and Tastes: sweet, slightly astringent, and neutral.

Meridian Entry: lung meridian.

Effects: Strengthen superficies and stop sweating.

Application:

Spontaneous sweating and night sweating

For spontaneous sweating due to deficiency of qi, it can be used combined with Huangqi and Muli, such as in Muli San. In cases of night sweating due to yin deficiency, it is usually used together with Shudihuang and Danggui. To treat frequent perspiration after delivery due to asthenia, it can be used in combination with Danggui and Huangqi. Also, it can be used with Muli and prepared as powder for external application, for any sweating syndrome, due to asthenia.

Usage and dosage: 3-9 g is used for oral use. For external application, the amount should be appropriate.

Precautions: It is contraindicated in those patients who infected with exogenous pathogens.

Wuweizi(**Magnoliavine Fruit, Fructus Schisandrae Chinese**)

Properties and Tastes: sour, sweet and warm.

Meridian Entry: lung, heart and kidney meridians.

Effects: ①Astringe and strengthen. ②Benefit qi and promote the production of body fluid. ③Tonify the kidney and calm the mind.

Application:

(1)Chronic cough and dyspnea resulting from asthenia

It is used for chronic cough and dyspnea resulting from asthenia. It is the essential medicine for the treatment of this kind of syndrome in treating chronic cough due to deficiency of the lung. It is used in combination with Yingsuke such as in the formula Wuweizi Wan. To treat the syndrome of lung and kidney deficiency manifesting as heavy breathing, it is often used combined with Shanzhuyu and Shudihuang, such as in the formula Duqi Wan. In treating cough and asthma caused by lung cold, it should be used together with Mahuang and Xixin, such as in Xiaoqinglong Tang.

(2)Spontaneous perspiration and night sweating

It is used for spontaneous perspiration and night sweating, it is often used in combination with Mahuanggen and Muli.

(3)Emission and spermatorrhea

In treating spermatorrhea, it can be used with Sangpiaoxiao, Fuzi and Longgu. For treating emission while dreaming, it is often used together with Maidong and Shanzhuyu.

(4)Chronic diarrhea

It is indicated for chronic diarrhea, and it is often used together with Buguzhi, Roudoukou and Wuzhuyu, such as in the formula Sishen Wan.

(5)Thirst due to fluid loss and diabetes

To treat thirst of fluid loss resulting from thermal injury qi and yin, it is often used in combination with Renshen and Maidong, such as Shengmai powder. For polydipsia resulting from internal heat due to yin deficiency in diabetes, it is usually used in combination with Shanyao and Zhimu.

(6)Palpitation, insomnia and dreaminess

To treat deficiency of yin and blood, or heart-kidney imbalance manifesting as palpitation, insomnia and dreaminess, it is usually used in combination with Maidong, Danshen and Shengdihuang, such as Tianwang Buxin Wan.

Usage and dosage: 3-6 g is taken orally. It is ground into powder 1-3 g.

Precautions: It is not suitable for those with exterior pathogen factors which have not been eliminated and sthenic heat in the interior, manifesting as cough and measles in the initial stage.

Wumei(**Smoked Plum, Fructus Mume**)

Properties and Tastes: sour, astringent and neutral.

Meridian Entry: liver, spleen, lung, large intestine meridians.

Effects: ①Astringe the lung and relieve cough. ②Astringe the intestine and antidiarrheal. ③Promote the production of body fluid. ④Relieve ascaris colic.

Application:

(1) Prolonged cough due to deficiency of the lung

In treating prolonged cough with a small amount of sputum due to deficiency of the lung, or dry cough without sputum, it is often used together with Yingsuke and Kuxingren, such as in the formula Yifu San.

(2) Prolonged diarrhea or dysentery

For prolonged diarrhea or dysentery, it can be used together with Yingsuke and Hezi, such as in the formula Guchang Wan. In treating hygropyretic dysentery and purulent hematochezia, it can be combined with Huanglian, such as in the formula Wumei Wan.

(3) Xiaoke(diabetes) due to deficiency heat

Its single decoction is effective in treating Xiaoke(diabetes) due to heat of deficiency type, or used together with Tianhuafen, Maidong and Renshen, such as in the formula Yuquan San.

(4) Abdominal pain and vomiting caused by intestinal ascariasis

Ascaris becomes sedated when it meets a sour flavour, as this medicine is quite sour. It is a good medicine for ascariasis in treating abdominal pain, vomiting and cold extremities caused by intestinal ascariasis, it is often combined with Chuanjiao and Huanglian, such as in the formula Wumei Wan.

In addition, when carbonized it has the function of strengthening the thoroughfare vessel and stop metrostaxis, it can treat metrorrhagia and metrostaxis and hemafecia. Also, it is able to eliminate sores accompanied with toxins by external application, such as pterygium and head sore.

Usage and dosage: 3-10 g is taken orally, in a large dosage may be up to 30 g. For external application, the amount should be appropriate, and it can be pounded or carbonized and then ground into powder. In order to stop bleeding and diarrhea, the carbonized form is applicable.

Precautions: If taken orally, it is contraindicated for patients with exogenous factors or those with stagnation of sthenic heat.

Shanzhuyu(Asiatic Cornelian Cherry Fruit, Fructus Corni)

Properties and Tastes: sour, astringent and slightly warm.

Meridian Entry: liver and kidney meridians.

Effects: ①Tonify liver and kidney. ②Astringe essence and strengthen collapse.

Application:

(1) Soreness of waist and knees, dizziness, tinnitus, and impotence

It can be used for deficiency of the liver and kidney manifesting as dizziness, soreness of waist, tinnitus. It is often combined with Shudihuang, Shanyao, such as in the formula Liuwei Dihuang Wan. It can be used for weak fire of Mingmen manifesting as cold pain of waist and knees, dysuria, combined with Rougui and Fuzi, such as in the formula Shenqi Wan. For impotence due to insufficiency of kidney yang, it is combined with Lurong, Buguzhi and Bajitian.

(2) Emission, spermatorrhoea, enuresis, frequent urination

In treating emission, spermatorrhoea due to kidney deficiency leading to essence not being consolidated, it is often used together with Shudihuang and Shanyao. In treating enuresis and frequent urination with deficiency of kidney leading to bladder lost restriction, it is often used together with Fupenzi, Jinyingzi and Shayuanzi.

(3) Metrorrhagia and metrostaxis and menorrhagia

In treating metrorrhagia and metrostaxis and menorrhagia due to deficiency of liver and kidney, it is often used with Shudihuang and Baishao. In treating those due to deficiency of spleen, unconsolidation of thoroughfare and conception meridians, it is often used with Longgu and Huangqi.

（4）Profuse sweating and collapse due to weak constitution

For profuse sweating and collapse due to weak constitution, it is often used with Renshen, Fuzi, and Longgu.

In addition, it also can be used for Xiaoke(diabetes) , it is mostly combined with Shengdihuang and Tianhuafen.

Usage and dosage：3–10 g is used for oral use. Large dosage may be up to 20–30 g for emergency to strengthen collapse.

Precautions：It is not suitable for patients with dribbling and astringent pain during urination due to damp ness-heat in normal timer.

Simple list of other astringent medicinals see Table 9–15.

Table 9–15　Simple list of other astringent medicines

Name	Properties and Tastes	Meridian Entry	Effects	Application	Dosage
Fuxiaomai (Fructus Tritici Levis)	Sweet and cool	Heart meridian	（1）Strengthen superficies and arrest sweating （2）Tonify healthy qi and eliminate heat	（1）Spontaneous sweating and night sweating （2）Hectic fever and over-strain-fever	15–30 g for decoction
Wubeizi(Galla Chinensis)	Sour, astringent and cold	Lung, large intestine and kidney meridians	（1）Astringe lung and lower fire （2）Astringe intestines to stop diarrhea （3）Astringe perspiration and stop bleeding （4）Absorb dampness and heal sore	（1）Cough, emptysis （2）Prolonged diarrhea or dysentery （3）Spontaneous perspiration and night sweat （4）Metrorrhagia and metrostasis, hematochezia, hemorrhoids with bleeding （5）Damp sore, swollen sore with toxicity	3–6 g for decoction
Hezi(Fructus Chebulae)	Bitter, sour, astringent and neutral	Lung and large intestine meridians	（1）Astringe the intestines and lung （2）Drive fire downward and benefit the throat	（1）Prolonged diarrhea and dysentery （2）Prolonged cough, loss of voice	5–10 g for decoction
Roudoukou(Semen Myristicae)	Pungent and warm	Spleen, stomach and large intestine meridians	（1）Astringe the intestine to stop diarrhea （2）Warm the middle energizer to promote flow of qi	（1）Diarrhea of deficiency type and cold dysentery （2）Stomach cold leading to distending pain, poor appetite and vomiting	3–10 g for decoction
Chishizhi(Halloysitum Rubrum)	Sweet, sour, astringent and warm	Large intestine and stomach meridians	（1）Astringe the intestine to stop bleeding （2）Promote tissue regeneration and healing of wounds	（1）Chronic diarrhea and dysentery （2）Metrorragia and metrostaxis, bloody stool, leucorrhea （3）Unhealed chronic ulcer	9–12 g for decoction first

Continue to Table 9-15

Name	Properties and Tastes	Meridian Entry	Effects	Application	Dosage
Sangpiaoxiao (Oötheca Mantidis)	Sweet, salty and neutral	Liver and kidney meridians	(1) Benefit kidney and astringe essence (2) Reduce the frequency of urination to stop turbidity	(1) Impotence, emission, spermatorrhoea (2) Enuresis and frequent urination, white turbidity	5 – 10 g for decoction
Jingyingzi (Fructus Rosae Laevigatae)	Sour, sweet, astringent and neutral	Kidney, bladder, large intestine meridians	(1) Astringe essence (2) Reduce the frequency of urination (3) Astringe the intestine to relieve diarrhea	(1) Nocturnal emission, spermatorrhoea, enuresis, frequent micturition and excessive leucorrhea (2) Chronic diarrhea and dysentery	6 – 12 g for decoction
Haipiaoxiao(Os Sepiellae seu Sepiae)	Salty, astringent and warm	Spleen and kidney meridians	(1) Astringe to stop bleeding (2) Astringe essence and stop emission and leucorrhea (3) Control acid regurgitation (4) Promote sore healing	(1) Metrorrhagia and metrostasis, hematochezia, hemorrhoids with bleeding due to trauma (2) Nocturnal emission, spermatorrhoea, leucorrhea (3) Stomachache with acid regurgitation (4) Skin pyogenic infection, eczema, ulcer without being healed	5 – 10 g for decoction
Lianzi(Semen Nelumbinis)	Sweet, astringent and neutral	Spleen, kidney and heart meridians	(1) Invigorate the spleen and relieve diarrhea (2) Benefit the kidney to preserve the essence (3) Nourish the heart and tranquilize the mind	(1) Diarrhea due to deficiency of the spleen (2) Nocturnal emission, spermatorrhoea, leucorrhea (3) Palpitation, insomnia	6 – 15 g for decoction
Qianshi (Ssemen Euryales)	Sweet, astringent and neutral	Spleen and kidney meridians	(1) Benefit the kidney to preserve the essence (2) Invigorate the spleen and relieve diarrhea (3) Dispel dampness to relieve leucorrhea	(1) Nocturnal emission, spermatorrhoea (2) Prolonged diarrhea due to deficiency of the spleen (3) Leucorrhea	9 – 15 g for decoction

Sun Min, Zhai Fengting, Song Guanli, Zhang Zhinan

Chapter 10

Basic Knowledge of Prescription

Prescription, which is one of the important methods of TCM, is used for the prevention and treatment of diseases. Prescriptions are used under the guidance of TCM theory, upon syndrome differentiation and according to different diseases. The application of prescription involves the combination of medicinal, determination of dosage and preparation form, and the modification according to the syndrome development. This chapter starts with the basic theory of prescriptions and introduces the commonly used prescriptions in terms of main effect.

❯ Introduction

Prescriptions are formed with appropriate combination of selected Chinese medicinals according to the principle of prescription for the determination of dosage and preparation form of medicinals. As the important measure of TCM treatment, prescriptions are the specific expression of treatment upon syndrome differentiation. Prescriptions are composed of Chinese mdeicines, and comprehensive application of Chinese medicines form prescriptions.

10.1 Formation and modification of prescription

Prescription comes from combination of the Chinese medicinal. The efficacy and specific nature of each Chinese medicinal are different. Therefore, only by following the certain principle and reasonable collocation, to enhance the original efficacy of Chinese medicinal, harmonize the special aspects of their nature, restricting their toxicity, can the integrated use of various Chinese medicinal be fully utilized. At the same time, prescription has great flexibility. The ingredient, dosage and preparation form must be adjusted during the clinical practice.

10.1.1 Forming principles

The composition of each prescription must be confirmed by choosing appropriate combination and on the basis of syndrome differentiation and decision of therapeutic methods according to different conditions. The forming principles must be followed strictly during combination. In the prescription, different medicines play different roles with the help of special combination. According to the different roles and status of Chinese medicinal, this combination relationship can be described as sovereign(jun), minister(chen), assistant (zuo), and courier(shi) medicinals.

10.1.1.1 Sovereign medicine

Sovereign medicine is the essential component of the prescription and its pharmacological effect is stronger than others. Sovereign medicinal plays a primary curative role aiming at the main disease or syndrome.

10.1.1.2 Minister medicine

Minister medicinal plays a supporting role to sovereign medicinal and its pharmacological effects is second to the sovereign medicinal. There are two different conditions. In one condition, the minister medicinal helps sovereign medicinal to enhance the curative effect to main disease or syndrome. In another, minister medicinal plays a primary curative role aiming at the accompanying diseases or syndrome.

10.1.1.3 Assistant medicine

Assistant medicine can be used as three conditions.

Promotion assistant: it can help sovereign and minister medicinal to enhance the curative effect or treat secondary accompanying diseases or syndrome directly.

Restriction assistant: it is used to eliminate or slow the toxicity and potent nature of sovereign and minister medicine.

Counteracting assistant: in this condition, the pathogenic factors of disease are too serious to make patients refuse the medicinal. Thus, the medicinal that has opposite nature and flavor to those of sovereign medicinal but plays supplementing role in the treatment will be chosen.

10.1.1.4 Courier medicine

There are two conditions about the courier medicine. One is used as meridian ushering medicine, guiding the medicine of the prescription into the pathogenic location. The other is used as harmonizing medicinal, harmonizing all the medicine of the prescription.

In clinics, not all the prescription has the assistant medicinal and courier medicinal. In case of simple pathogenic condition, one or two ingredients of medicine can take effect. If there is not toxic or drastic in the sovereign and minister medicinal, it is not necessary to add assistant medicine. The meridian entry of the sovereign and minister medicinal can lead into the pathogenic location, and then courier medicinal as meridian ushering medicine is not also necessary. In a general way, the ingredients of sovereign medicinal should be fewer but with large dosage, while the minister medicine more than sovereign, and assistant medicine more than minister, and one or two courier medicinals. In a word, the quantity of medicinal ingredients and the application of sovereign, minister, assistant, and courier medicine should be based on the condition of disease state and the treatment method.

10.1.2　Modification of prescription

The composition of prescription has strict principle and also great flexibility. Forming prescription in clinical practice must be based on the specific condition and flexibility.

10.1.2.1 Modification of ingredients

Ingredient is the main factor that determines efficacy of prescription. So the increase or decrease of ingredients inevitably changes the efficacy of prescription. There are two cases of it. One is the increase or decrease of assistant medicine and courier medicinal, which is applied to the cases that the main disease is unchanged but accompanying syndrome different, and this will not lead to a fundamental change in the prescription. For example, Yinqiao San is the commonly used prescription for wind-heat exterior syndrome. If also accompanied by cough, it is lung qi failing to diffuse, so we can add Kuxingren to descend lung qi and relieve cough. The other is the increase or decrease of minister medicinals. Due to the forming relation changed of the prescription, it will make a fundamental change in the overall efficacy. For example, Mahuang Tang is a prescription for the treatment of wind-cold excess exterior syndrome. If the minister medicinal Guizhi is removed, which leads to the weakening of sweating power, the prescription will become a treatment for cough and asthma in cold syndrome. If Baizhu is added, with minister medicinal as Guizhi, the effects of prescription will increase resolving dampness effect based on promoting sweating to release the exterior, and the prescription becomes a treatment for wind-cold fixed impediment.

10. 1. 2. 2　Increase and decrease of dosage

The dosage is directly related to the pharmacological effects. Although the ingredients of prescription are the same, if one or more ingredients are changed, it will lead to the combination, effects and main indications different. For example, both Xiaochengqi Tang and Houpo Sanwu Tang contain same three kinds of herbs, Dahuang, Houpo, and Zhishi. Dahuang, the sovereign medicinal with great effect of purging heat accumulation, has been used with a big dosage in Xiaochenqi Tang in order to treat yangming fu-viscera excess syndrome; While Houpo, the sovereign medicinal with great effect of moving qi to resolve fullness, has been used with a big dosage in Houpo Sanwu Tang, for the treatment of constipation with qi stagnation syndrome.

10. 1. 2. 3　Modification of preparation forms

Prescription have a variety of preparation forms and different preparation form features. The same prescription with different preparation forms will lead to different strength and effect of the prescription, as well as the treatment of disease with its priorities. For example, Lizhong Wan and Renshen Tang, comprised of the same ingredients and dosages, but Lizhong Wan is a pill that grinds the above into a fine powder and makes it into the pill, which is for milds deficiency cold syndrome in middle energizer with gentle effect; while Renshen Tang is a decoction boiled by medicinals, with the features of fast absorption and taking effect quickly, which is the treatment of serious deficiency cold syndrome in upper and middle energizer.

10. 2　Preparation forms of prescription

Preparation form of prescription is a particular form, which can be made according to the needs and characteristics of medicinals after the combination of prescription, in order to make it easy to use or better for treatment of diseases. Traditional preparation forms of prescription include decoction, pill, powder, paste, pellet, wine preparation, soluble granule and syrup and so on. The commonly used preparation forms of prescription are introduced as follows.

10. 2. 1　Decoctions(tang)

Decoction is the most commonly used and most traditional preparation form of prescription. After completing the medicinals of prescription, the medicines are soaked with water or wine, or a mixture of 50 percent of wine and 50 percent of water for a period of time(often for half an hour), boiled to certain amount of water or boiled after a certain of time, remove the slag, then the decoction is obtained. Decoction is mostly orally used or for external wash. For example, Mahuang Tang and Guizhi Tang are made this way. The characteristics of decoction are fast absorption, rapid action and especially facilitate with modification of preparation form according to the disease. It is the most widely used in clinical practice, which is suitable for patients with severe or unstable conditions. The disadvantages of decoction are that some of the effective medicinals are not easy to be decocted, and the dosage is large, and inconvenient to carry.

10.2.2　Pills(wan)

Pills are a round solid fixed dosage form that grind the medicinals of the prescription into fine powder, and then add a proper amount of excipient. Pills have the advantages of slow absorption, lasting effect and more convenient to be taken and carried. It is suitable for chronic disease and debilitating diseases such as Liuwei Dihuang Wan and Lizhong Wan. There are also pills for first aids such as Angong Niuhuang Wan, which is made into pills, and thus can be easily stored for emergency use.

10.2.2.1　Honeyed pill

Honeyed pill is made by grinding medicinals into fine powder and adding honey as excipient. There are big honeyed pills and small honeyed pills with moderate and lasting effects.

10.2.2.2　Water-bindered pill

Water-bindered pill is made by grinding medicinals into fine powder and adding cooled boiled water or distilled water as excipient. Compared to honeyed pills, water-bindered pills are fast disintegrated and easy to be absorbed.

10.2.2.3　Starched pill

Starched pill is made by grinding medicinals into fine powder and adding paste such as rice paste, panada and leaven paste and so on as excipient. Starched pills are slowly disintegrated, which can prolong the effect of medicine and reduce adverse reactions when taken orally.

10.2.2.4　Condensed pill

Condensed pill is made by decocting medicinals into pastes, then mixed with other medicinal fine powders, and water or honey added, or decoction. It is easy to be accepted for its small in size and low dosage.

10.2.3　Powders(san)

Powders are made by the medicinals ground into fine powders and mixed evenly. There are two types of powders, for oral or external use. Oral use powders are divided into fine powder and coarser powder. Fine powders such as Qili San can be taken with water. Coarser powder such as Yinqiao San can be decocted and for oral use after subducting residue. Externally used powders such as Jinhuang San are generally used as external applications, which are applied to sore surface or to the wound. Others such as Bingpeng San are for throat sprinkle. The features of the powders are quick absorption, simple making, convenient for taking and caring, saving the medicinal materials.

10.2.4　Pastes(gao)

Pastes are made by medicinals decocted with water or plant oil and removing slag, for oral and external use. Oral use pastes such as Pipa Gao include three kinds, which are liquid pastes, semi-liquid pastes and decocted pastes, while externally used pastes include ointment such as Sanhuang ointment. Liquid pastes, semi-liquid pastes are used by blending with other prescriptions. Decocted pastes are semi-liquid pastes made by medicinals decocted with water and removing slag and added with honey or sugar. Decocted pastes are suitable for chronic diseases. The ointment made of fine powder and appropriate medicinal substrates with appropriate viscosity of semi-solid prescription for external use only, which is usually used for skins, mucosa or the surface of the wounds. Plaster also known as hard paste can be used for orthopedics and traumatology and impediment disease.

10.2.5   Pellets(dan)

There are two types of pellets. One is for oral used and the other is for external use. Oral pallets haven't fixed prescriptions like pills or powder. It is called "Dan" because the medicinals are precious, such as Zhibao Dan. Pellets are medicinals made of some mineral medicinals under the high temperature, which is often ground into powder and sprinkled on the surface of the wound. They are mainly for surgery use.

10.2.6   Wine preparation(jiu)

Wine preparation also known as medicinal liquor, is made of medicinals soaked in wine, removing slag, then taking the liquid for internal or external use. Wine has the characteristics of promoting blood circulation and promoting efficacy of the drug, which is suitable for impediment disease, weakness of nourishing and orthopedics and traumatology and so on, such as Duzhong Hugu Jiu. Wine for external use has the ability for activating blood, resolving edema and relieving pain, but not suitable for yin deficiency with excess fire syndrome.

10.2.7   Soluble granules(keli)

Soluble granules are granulated prescriptions made through the modern technology by extraction of active ingredients of medicinals, then being mixed with appropriate number of excipients such as starch or some of the medicinals fine powder. It is soluble in water, so it can be used by being dissolved in water. Soluble granules have the characteristic of storage, rapid effect, and convenience to take and so on. There are compound granules such as Ganmao granules(granules for cold) and single granules with one medicinal, and then combined into prescriptions.

10.2.8   Syrup(tangjiang)

Syrup is made by decocting medicinal, removing slag and concentrating and adding suitable sucrose in it. Syrup is characterized by sweet in taste and small in volume, especially suitable for children.

10.3   Classification and commonly used prescriptions

10.3.1   Exterior-releasing prescriptions

10.3.1.1   Concept

Those that are mainly composed of medicinals for relieving exterior syndrome, and can promote sweating, release the flesh and outthrust eruption, used for exterior syndrome, are known as exterior-releasing prescription.

10.3.1.2   Classification

Exterior syndrome generally includes two kinds of syndrome: wind-cold syndrome and wind-heat syndrome. Therefore, exterior-releasing prescription falls into two kinds as prescriptions for relieving the exterior syndrome with pungent-warm and those for relieving the exterior syndrome with pungent-cold accordingly. Prescriptions for relieving the exterior syndrome with pungent-warm are mainly formed with medicinals of pungent-warm, and have the effect of dispersing wind-cold, used for exterior syndrome of wind-cold. Contrarily, prescriptions for relieving the exterior syndrome with pungent-cold are mainly formed with medicinals of pungent-cold, and have the effect of dispersing wind-heat, used for exterior syndrome of wind-heat.

10.3.1.3　Notes

Exterior-releasing prescriptions should not be decocted too long; otherwise the pharmacological effects of the prescriptions would be lost greatly with dissipating drug property. That's because the medicinals for forming exterior-releasing prescriptions are those with light-textured property and pungent flavor, and are easy to dissipate with long decocted. What's more, the decoction of exterior-releasing prescriptions must be taken warm. Keeping warm should also be paid attention to after taking the decoction in order to eliminate the pathogenic factors out of the body with sweating slightly.

Mahuang Tang(Ephedra Decoction)

Ingredients:

Mahuang(Ephedrae Herba)9 g;Guizhi(Ramulus Cinnamomi)6 g;Kuxingren(Semen Armeniacae Amarum)6 g;Zhigancao(Radix Glycyrrhizae)3 g.

Administration:All medicinals above are decocted in water, for oral use.

Effects:Promote sweating to release the exterior and diffuse the lung to calm panting.

Application:This prescription is for the syndrome of wind-cold and exterior-excess caused by externally contracted wind-cold. The syndrome of wind-cold and exterior-excess is characterized by aversion to cold, fever, headache, generalized pain, no sweating, dyspnea, thin and white tongue coating, floating and tight pulse. It can be used for common cold, flu, acute bronchitis, bronchial dyspnea and other diseases main symptoms of which are aversion to cold without sweating, cough and dyspnea, and belonging to syndrome of wind-cold and exterior-excess.

Analysis:The syndrome treated by this prescription is caused by externally contracted wind-cold, block of defensive qi and yang, tight striae, failed diffusion of lung qi. This syndrome should be dealt with treatment methods as follows: diffuse the lung to calm panting, promote sweating to release the exterior.

(1)Sovereign medicinal:Mahuang

Promote sweating to release the exterior in order to dispel wind-cold and diffuse the lung to calm panting.

(2)Minister medicinal:Guizhi

Warm the meridian to dissipate cold and assist Mahuang to promote sweating to release the exterior.

(3)Assistant medicinal:Kuxingren

Diffuse and descend lung qi and assist Mahuang to calm panting.

(4)Courier medicinal:Zhigancao

Harmonize all the medicinals. Not only ease the middle, but also restrict the oversweating of Mahuang and Guizhi.

Modification:If complicated with dampness pathogen characterized by arthrosis pain and heavy limbs and trunk, add Baizhu to dispel dampness. If mainly showing cough and panting but slight aversion to cold, get rid of Guizhi to concentrate on diffuse the lung to calm panting. If with heavy aversion to cold, no sweating and generalized pain, complicated with interior heat and vexation, double Mahuang to enhance the sweating to dispel pathogen, then add Shigao to discharge interior heat.

Notes:Because this prescription is drastic in promoting sweating with pungent-warm and used to treat syndrome of wind-cold and exterior-excess, it is forbidden for exterior syndrome of wind-cold with sweating. It also should be caution for patient with serious yin deficiency, blood deficiency and interior heat.

Guizhi Tang(Cinnamon Twig Decoction)

Ingredients:Guizhi(Ramulus Cinnamomi)9 g;Baishao(Radix Alba Paeoniae)9 g;Shengjiang(Rhizoma Zingiberis Recens)9 g;Dazao(Fructus Jujubae)3 pcs;Zhigancao(Radix Glycyrrhizae)6 g.

Administration:All medicinals above are decocted in water,for oral use.

Effects:Release the flesh,harmonize nutrient qi and defensive qi to release exterior syndrome.

Application:This prescription is for the syndrome of wind-cold and exterior-deficiency,syndrome of nutrient-defense disharmony and yin-yang disharmony after cure or after delivery. These syndromes are characterized by headache,fever,sweating and aversion to wind,thin and white tongue fur,floating and relaxed pulse. It can be used for common cold,flu,lichen,pruritus cutanea,agnogenic low-grade fever,after-cure or after-delivery low-grade fever and other diseases belonging to syndrome of nutrient-defense disharmony and yin-yang disharmony.

Analysis:The syndrome treated by this prescription is caused by externally contracted wind-cold, weakness after cure or after delivery,disharmony of nutrient-defense and yin-yang. This syndrome should be dealt with treatment methods as follows:release the flesh and outthrust the exterior,harmonize the nutrient qi and defensive qi.

(1)Sovereign medicinal:Guizhi

Release the flesh and dissipate cold,warm the meridian to promote the yang qi and defensive qi.

(2)Minister medicinal:Baishao

Enrich yin and engender fluid,secure the nutrient qi to stop sweating. Guizhi and Baishao combine equally in this prescription,one for dissipating while the other securing,can lead to dissipating wind-cold exterior,securing nutrient interior,harmonization of nutrient and defense and yin and yang.

(3)Assistant medicinal:Shengjiang,Dazao

Shengjiang harmonizes the stomach and assists Guizhi to dissipate cold. Dazao tonifies the spleen and assists Baishao to enrich yin. These two midicinals not only strengthen the sovereign and minister to harmonize nutrient and defense,but also regulate the stomach and tonify the spleen to supplement the source of generation and transformation of nutrient and defense.

(4)Assistant and Courier medicinal:Zhigancao

On one hand,as assistant,this medicinal tonifies qi to harmonize the middle,combines with the sovereign in order to transform yang with pungent-sweet to release the flesh,combines with the minister in order to transform yin with sour-sweet to harmonize the nutrient. On the other hand,as courier,it harmonizes all the medicinals.

Modification:If complicated with painful stiff nape,add Gegen to release the flesh and exterior syndrome,engender fluid to relax sinews. If complicated with cough and panting,add Houpo and Kuxingren to direct qi downward to suppress cough and to calm panting.

Notes:Because this prescription is mild in promoting sweating,known as "release the flesh",it is unsuitable for exterior syndrome of wind-cold without sweating. After administration,the patient should have a bowl of warm congee and put on more clothes to promote sweating slightly.

10.3.2   Heat-cleaning Prescriptions

10.3.2.1   Concept

Those that are mainly composed of medicinals for heat-clearing,and can clear heat,purge fire,cool the blood aspect,detoxify and used for interior-heat syndrome,are known as heat-cleaning prescription.

10.3.2.2 Classification

There are differences in the interior-heat syndrome between qifen and blood aspect, between warm-heat and summerheat-heat, between excess heat and deficiency heat, between zang viscera and fu viscera. Therefore, heat-cleaning prescription can be divided into six categories: qifen heat-cleaning prescription, clean nutrient and cool blood prescription, heat-cleaning and detoxify prescription, zang-fu viscera heat-cleaning prescription, deficiency heat cleaning prescription and summerheat-heat cleaning prescription.

10.3.2.3 Notes

The nature and flavor of the medicinals which form heat-cleaning prescription are mainly cold and bitterness. Therefore, heat-cleaning prescription should not to be used for a long time in case that cold and bitterness property might decline the stomach qi, yin and yang. What is more, add some fortify the spleen and invigorate the stomach medicinals. It also should be cautious used for patient with weakness of spleen and stomach, torpid intake and sloppy stool. If interior-heat is flaming, the patient emesis immediately after taking heat cleaning prescription so call "reject-medicinals". In these cases, methods of counteracting assistant that administering warm or adding a few pungent-warm ginger juice would be taken to relieve or eliminate these situations.

Baihu Tang(White Tiger Decoction)

Ingredients: Shigao (Gypsum Fibrosum) 50 g; Zhimu (Rhizoma Anemarrhenae) 18 g; Jingmi (Semen Oryzae Nonglutionosae) 9 g; Zhigancao (Radix Glycyrrhizae) 6 g.

Administration: All medicinals above are decocted in water, for oral use.

Effects: Clear heat and generate fluid.

Application: This prescription is for the yangming meridian syndrome and exuberant heat in qifen. This syndrome is characterized by high fever, reddened complexion, vexation thirst, desire for cold drink, sweating and aversion to heat, yellow urine, hard bound stool, red tongue, and yellow fur, surging and large pulse or slippery and rapid pulse. It can be used for common cold, flu, lobar pneumonia, epidemic encephalitis B, songo fever, gingivitis and other diseases belonging to yangming meridian syndrome and exuberant heat in qifen. This syndrome would be recognized as four exuberant symptoms: exuberant heat, extreme thirst, excessive sweating, surging and large pulse.

Analysis: The syndrome treated by this prescription is caused by exuberant heat in yangming meridian or warm disease with qifen syndrome scorching body fluid. This syndrome should be dealt with treatment methods as cleaning heat and generating fluid.

(1) Sovereign medicinal: Shigao

This medicinal can clear heat and purge fire while protect fluid with the nature-flavor of pungent-sweet and extremely cold.

(2) Minister medicinal: Zhimu

The nature-flavor of this medicinal that is bitter-cold but smooth, assists the sovereign to clear heat and purge fire, and enriches yin to engender fluid.

(3) Assistant medicinal: Jingmi

Invigorate the stomach, protect the fluid, and also prevent the extremely cold of sovereign to harm stomach.

(4) Assistant and Courier medicinal: Zhigancao

On one hand, as assistant, this medicinal invigorates the stomach qi and protects the the damage of fluid cooperated with Jingmi. On the other hand, as courier, it harmonizes all the medicinals.

Modification: If exuberant heat damaging the body fluid, complicated with that drink does not quench thirst and week large pulse, add Renshen to enrich qi and engender. If warm diseases manifested as blazing of both qi and blood, complicated with mental confusion and delirious speech, macula on the body, add Dihuang, Shuiniujiao to clear heat and cool the blood. If extreme heat engendering wind, complicated with limbs twitch, add Lingyangjiao, Gouteng to extinguish wind to arrest convulsions. If interior-heat with dampness complication, or wind-dampness and heat arthralgia, add Cangzhu to dry dampness.

Notes: Because this prescription is used for yangming meridian syndrome and excess heat, it is unsuitable for deficiency heat syndrome characterized by surging and large pulse but weak, and pale tongue.

Huanglian Jiedu Tang(Decoction of Coptis for Detoxification)

Ingredients: Huanglian(Rhizoma Coptidis)9 g; Huangqin(Radix Scutellariae)6 g; Huangbai(Cortex Phellodendri)6 g; Zhizi(Fructus Gardeniae)9 g.

Administration: All medicinals above are decocted in water, for oral use.

Effects: Purge fire and detoxify.

Application: This prescription is for the syndrome of fire toxin and exuberant heat in triple energizer. This syndrome is characterized by high fever, vexation, thirst and desiring to drink, delirious speech, inability to sleep, or fever and diarrhea, or deep-rooted boil, red tongue, yellow fur, powerful rapid pulse. It can be used for epidemic encephalitis B, epidemic cerebrospinal meningitis, septicemia, septicopyemia, dysentery, pneumonia, urinary infection and other infection diseases belonging to syndrome of fire toxin and exuberant heat.

Analysis: The syndrome treated by this prescription is caused by exuberant heat binding in the triple energizer. This syndrome should be dealt with treatment methods as purging fire and detoxify with bitter-cold.

(1)Sovereign medicinal: Huanglian

Purge heart fire and middle energizer fire.

(2)Minister and assistant medicinals: Huangqin, Huangbai, Zhizi

Huangqin purges upper energizer fire, Huangbai purges lower energizer fire, Zhizi purges the whole triple energizer and directs medicinals downward.

All four medicinals purge fire toxin with their nature of bitter cold.

Modification: If complicated with constipation, add Dahuang to relax the bowels and purge fire and direct the heat toxin downward. If complicated with hematemesis, epistaxis, macula, add Dihuang, Xuanshen, and Mudanpi to clear heat and cool blood.

Notes: The medicinals of this prescription are all bitter cold one. These medicinals would damage the fluid and stomach, so this prescription just can be used in syndrome of exuberant heat-toxin. It needs to stop once it takes effect. It is forbidden for patients with fluid deficiency.

10.3.3　Purgative prescriptions

10.3.3.1　Concept

Those that are mainly composed of medicinals for purgating, with the effects that induce relaxing the bowels, purgating heat, removing accumulation, and expelling water, used for interior-excess syndrome, are known as purgative prescription.

10.3.3.2　Classification

Interior-excess syndrome would be different in heat accumulation, cold accumulation, dryness accumulation and dampness accumulation, and healthy qi of human would be different in deficiency and excess. Accordingly, purgative prescription can be divided into five categories: cold-purgative prescription, warm-purgative prescription, lubricant laxation prescription, expelling water prescription, and tonifying to relax bowels prescription.

10.3.3.3 Notes

Purgative prescription would be easy to damage middle, consume fluid, interrupt blood, and induced abortion. Thus, it must stop once it takes effects and can't be overused. It is caution or forbidden for patients who are worn with age, yin-blood deficiency, menstrual period or pregnancy.

Dachengqi Tang(Major Purgative Decoction)

Ingredients: Dahuang(Radix et Rhizoma Rhei)12 g; Houpo(Cortex Magnoliae Officinalis)12 g; Zhishi (Fructus Aurantii Immaturus)9 g; Mangxiao(Natrii Sulfas)9 g.

Administration: Decocte Houpo and Zhishi first, and Dahuang later. Decoction would be for oral use without medicine residues and dissolved with Mangxiao.

Effects: Drastically purge heat-accumulation.

Application: This prescription is for yangming fu viscera excess syndrome. This syndrome is characterized by constipation, abdominal pain with aversion to press, fever aggravated in the afternoon, thirst with great desire to drink, red tongue, yellow dry fur with prickly, or black, dry and cracked fur, sunken replete pulse. It can be used for acute simple intestinal obstruction, adhesive intestinal obstruction, acute cholecystitis, acute pancreatitis, and constipation in heat diseases that complicated with high fever, delirious speech, unconsciousness, eclampsia, even raving.

Analysis: The syndrome treated by this prescription is caused by heat-pathogen accumulation in the large intestine, stoppage of fu qi. This syndrome should be dealt with treatment methods as follows: purge heat accumulation and remove accumulation to relax the bowels.

(1)Sovereign medicinal: Dahuang

Purge heat and relax the bowels, remove accumulation of intestines and stomach.

(2)Minister medicinal: Mangxiao

Soften hardness and moisten dryness, assist the sovereign to purge heat and relax the bowels.

(3)Assistant medicinal: Houpo, Zhishi

Move qi to remove fullness, assist Dahuang and Mangxiao to remove and purge heat-accumulation.

Modification: If complicated with exuberant heat consuming qi, qi deficiency and overstrain, add Renshen to tonify qi and prevent qi desertion with drastic purgation. If complicated with heat-accumulation damaging yin, serious thirst with great desire to drink, red dry dongue, and less fur, add Xuanshen and Dihuang to tonify yin, generate fluid, and moisten dryness to relax the bowels.

Notes: It is caution for yangming fu viscera excess syndrome but without exuberant heat accumulation, or someone who has always dual deficiency of qi and yin, old age, weakness, and pregnancy.

Wenpi Tang(Warming Spleen Decoction)

Ingredients: Dahuang(Radix et Rhizoma Rhei)12 g; Fuzi(Radix Aconiti Lateralis Preparata)9 g; Ganjiang(Rhizoma Zingiberis)6 g; Renshen(Radix Ginseng)6 g; Gancao(Radix Glycyrrhizae)6 g.

Administration: All medicinals above are decocted in water, for oral use.

Effects: Purge cold accumulation, warm tonify the spleen yang.

Application: This prescription is for syndrome of yang deficiency and cold accumulation. This syndrome is characterized by constipation and abdominal pain, or chronic diarrhea with pus and blood, cold of the extremities, pale tongue, thin white fur, sunken string-like pulse. It can be used for acute simple intestinal obstruction, partial small-bowel obstruction, chronic dysentery, chronic appendicitis acute attack, and other diseases characterized by constipation and abdominal pain, spiritlessness and weakness, aversion to cold and prefer warm, which belonging to syndrome of yang deficiency and cold accumulation.

Analysis: The syndrome treated by this prescription is caused by deficiency of spleen yang, internal generation of cold, cold accumulation in the intestine. This syndrome should be dealt with treatment methods as follows: purge cold accumulation, warm tonify the spleen yang.

(1)Sovereign medicinal: Dahuang, Fuzi

Dahuang removes accumulation with purgation, and relaxes the bowels. Fuzi warm interior, support yang, and dispel cold. This combination can warm interior and dispel cold, removes cold accumulation.

(2)Minister medicinal: Ganjiang

Assist Fuzi to warm middle and dispel cold.

(3)Assistant medicinal: Renshen

Tonify qi and harmonize middle, combine Fuzi and Ganjiang to tonify qi, warm yang, and tonify spleen.

(4)Assistant and courier medicinals: Gancao

Tonify qi and harmonize middle, and harmonize all the medicinals.

Modification: If complicated with serious abdominal pain, add Rougui and Muxiang to strengthen the effect of warming yang and moving qi to check pain. If complicated with vomiting, add Banxia and Sharen to harmonize stomach and direct qi downward. If complicated with chronic diarrhea and dampness-heat, yellow slimy tongue fur, add Jinyinhua and Huangqin to clear intestine and relax the bowels.

Notes: Wenpi Tang is a kind of warming agent, it is not suitable for internal heat syndrome.

10.3.4   Wind-dispelling prescriptions

10.3.4.1   Concept

Those that are mainly composed of medicinals with pungent in flavor and disperse in nature and medicinals for extinguishing wind to arrest convulsions, used for wind diseases included internal wind syndrome and external wind syndrome, are known as wind-dispelling prescription.

10.3.4.2   Classification

Wind diseases are all those caused by wind pathogen. Wind pathogen can be divided into external wind and internal wind. Accordingly, wind-dispelling prescription would be divided into external wind-dispelling prescription and internal wind-extinguishing prescription.

10.3.4.3   Notes

When using wind-dispelling prescription, it is necessary to distinguish between external wind and internal wind, between cold, heat, deficiency, and excess. External wind would be dispersed while internal wind would be extinguished. If wind pathogen is complicated with cold, heat, dampness, and phlegm, combine with dispelling cold, cleaning heat, dispelling dampness, and resolving phlegm accordingly.

Chuanxiong Chatiao San(Ligusticum Powder)

Ingredients: Chuanxiong(Rhizoma Ligustici Chuanxiong)9 g; Qianghuo(Rhizoma et Radix Notopterygii)6 g; Baizhi(Radix Angelicae Dahuricae)6 g; Xixin(Herba Asari)3 g; Bohe(Herba Menthae)9 g; Jingjie(Herba Schizonepetae)12 g; Fangfeng(Radix Saposhnikoviae)6 g; Zhigancao(Radix Glycyrrhizae)6 g.

Administration: Grind the above medicinals into fine powder, take 6 g each time and twice daily with tea. Or all medicinals above are decocted in water, for oral use.

Effects: Dispel wind and relieve pain.

Application: This prescription is for headache with external contraction syndrome of wind pathogen.

This syndrome is characterized by headache, or migraine, or parietal headache, fever, aversion to cold, dizziness, stuffy nose, thin and white tongue couting, floating pulse. It can be used for migraine, vascular neuropathic headache, and headache in chronic rhinitis that are complicated with rhinobyon and floating pulse, caused by external contraction syndrome of wind pathogen.

Analysis: The syndrome treated by this prescription is caused by external contraction of wind pathogen. Wind pathogen upward to invade the head along meridian, and hamper lucid yang qi. This syndrome should be dealt with treatment methods as dispelling wind and relieving pain.

(1) Sovereign medicinal: Chuanxiong, Qianghuo, Baizhi

All these three medicinals can dispel wind and relieve pain. Chuanxiong is good at relieving pain, particularly relieving headache in shaoyang, jueyin meridian (vertex and tempus). Qianghuo is good at relieving headache in taiyang meridian (occiput). Baizhi is good at relieving headache in yangming meridian (forehead).

(2) Minister medicinal: Xixin, Bohe

Xixin can dispel cold and relieve pain, while Bohe dispels wind and refreshes the mind. Both assist the sovereigns to dispel wind pathogen.

(3) Assistant medicinal: Jingjie, Fangfeng

Jingjie and Fangfeng can dispel wind pathogen, enhancing the power of sovereign and minister.

(4) Courier medicinal: Zhuyexin

Harmonize all the medicinals.

Modification: If caused by external contraction of wind-cold, complicated with obvious aversion to cold, increase the dosage of Chuangxiong, add Zisuye and Shengjiang to enhance the effect of dispelling wind-cold. If caused by external contraction of wind-heat, complicated with obvious fever, dry mouth, and red tongue, subtract Qianghuo and Xixin and add Manjingzi, and Juhua to dispel wind-heat. In case of long treatment of headache, add Quanxie, Jiangcan, and Taoren to seek wind, activate blood, and relieve pain.

Notes: It is forbidden for headache caused by deficiency of qi and blood, or stirring wind due to hyperactivity of yang.

Duhuo Jisheng Tang (Pubescent Angelica and Taxillus Decoction)

Ingredients: Duhuo (Rhizoma Ligustici Chuanxiong) 9 g; Qinjiao (Radix Gentianae Macrophyllae) 9 g; Fangfeng (Radix Saposhnikoviae) 9 g; Rougui (Cortex Cinnamomi) 6 g; Xixin (Herba Asari) 3 g; Sangjisheng (Herba Taxilli) 15 g; Duzhong (Cortex Eucommiae) 9 g; Niuxi (Radix Achyranthis Bidentatae) 9 g; Renshen (Radix Ginseng) 6 g; Fuling (Poria) 9 g; Danggui (Radix Angelicae Sinensis) 9 g; Chuanxion (Rhizoma Ligustici Chuanxiong) 6 g; Dihuang (Radix Rehmanniae) 9 g; Baishao (Radix Paeoniae Alba) 9 g; Gancao (Radix Glycyrrhizae) 6 g.

Administration: All medicinals above are decocted in water, for oral use.

Effects: Dispel wind-dampness, relieve impediment-pain, benefit liver and kidney, and tonify qi and blood.

Application: This prescription is for syndrome of wind-cold-dampness obstructing arthralgia. This syndrome is characterized by arthralgia in long treatment, depletion of liver and kidney, deficiency of qi and blood, cold pain and flaccid in waist and knee, unsmooth bend and stretch of limbs, or numbness, aversion to cold, flavor warm, pale tongue, white fur, fine and week pulse. It can be used for chronic arthritis, rheumatoid arthritis, ischialgia, lumbar muscle degeneration, osteoproliferation, poliomyelitis, and other diseases belonging to syndrome of wind-cold-dampness obstructing arthralgia.

Analysis: The syndrome treated by this prescription is caused by arthralgia in long treatment, consumption of liver, kidney, qi, and blood, pathogen retaining in the arthrosis. So this syndrome is manifested as cooccurrences of agonizing-fixed arthralgia and depletion of liver and kidney.

(1) Sovereign medicinal: Duhuo

Dispel wind-cold-dampness pathogen in lower body, dredge arthralgia and relieve pain.

(2) Minister medicinal: Qinjiao, Fangfeng, Rougui, Xixin

Qinjiao and Fangfeng dispel wind and dampness. Rougui dispells cold and relieves pain, warm through blood vessels. Xixin dispels cold and relieves pain with its pungent-warm nature.

(3) Assistant medicinal: Sangjisheng, Duzhong, Niuxi, Renshen, Fuling, Danggui, Chuanxion, Dihuang, Baishao

Sangjisheng, Duzhong, and Niuxi tonify liver and kidney, and strengthen the sinews and bones. Danggui, Chuanqiong, Dihuang, and Baishao nourish blood, and activate blood. Renshen and Fuling tonify qi to fortify the spleen and strengthen health qi.

(4) Assistant and courier medicinals: Gancao

As assistant, it strengthen health qi. As courier, it harmonize all the medicinals.

Modification: If complicated with serious arthralgia pain, add Zhichuanwu, Zhicaowu, Baihuashe and Dilong and Honghua to seek and dispel wind pathogen to free collateral vessels, activate blood and relieve pain. If complicated with serious cold pathogen, add Fuzi and Ganjiang to warm yang qi and dispel cold. If complicated with serious dampness pathogen, subtract Dihuang, and add Fangji and Yiyiren to drain dampness to alleviate edema.

Notes: Arthralgia syndrome belongs to those with dampheat evidence and should not be used.

10.3.5 Dampness-draining prescriptions

10.3.5.1 Concept

Those that are mainly composed of medicinals of clearing dampness, and with the effect of induce diuresis to drain dampness and free strangury, used for diseases caused by dampness pathogen, are known as dampness-draining prescription.

10.3.5.2 Classification

About dampness pathogen, the generation would include external contraction and internal generation; the location would be different in exterior, interior, upper, and lower; the nature also would be cold or heat. Therefore, dampness-draining prescription would be divided into five categories: dry dampness to harmonize stomach prescription, clear heat and dispel dampness prescription, induce diuresis to drain dampness prescription, warm-dispel dampness prescription, and dispel wind and drain dampness prescription.

10.3.5.3 Notes

The prescription would damage the yin fluid with the medicinals of aroma dry-warm or sweet-tasteless draining. Thus, it is unsuitable for those who always have deficiency of yin fluid, weakness, or for pregnant women.

Huoxiang Zhengqi San(Patchouli Qi-restoring powder)

Ingredients: Huoxiang(Herba Pogostemonis)9 g; Zisuye(Folium Perillae)6 g; Baizhi(Radix Angelicae Dahuricae)6 g; Banxia(Rhizoma Pinelliae)9 g; Houpo(Cortex Magnoliae Officinalis)6 g; Chenpi(Pericarpium Citri Reticulatae)6 g; Dafupi(Pericarpium Arecae)9 g; Baizhu(Rhizoma Atractylodis Macrocephalae)9 g; Fuling(Poria)9 g; Jiegeng(Radix Platycodonis)9 g; Zhigancao(Radix Glycyrrhizae)6 g.

Administration: Grind the above medicinals into fine powder, take 6-9 g each time, add Shengjiang 3 slices, Dazao 1 piece, decocted in water, for oral use.

Effects : Release the exterior with resolve dampness, regulate qi and harmonize the middle.

Application : This prescription is for external contraction of wind-cold combine internal damaging of dampness syndrome. These syndromes are characterized by aversion to cold, fever, headache, stomach and abdominal pain, vomiting, diarrhea, white slimy tongue fur, floating or soggy pulse. It can be used for acute gastroenteritis, gastrointestinal influenza, and other diseases that characterized by exterior-cold and interior-dampness.

Analysis : The syndrome treated by this prescription is caused by externally contracted wind-cold, stagnant defensive qi, internal obstruction of dampness-turbidity, unharmonization of spleen-stomach, abnormal of upward and downward. This syndrome should be dealt with treatment methods as follows: release the exterior with resolve dampness, regulate qi and harmonize the middle.

(1) Sovereign medicinal: Huoxiang

Dispel wind-cold, resolve dampness-turbidity, harmonize the middle and check vomiting.

(2) Minister medicinal: Zisuye, Baizhi

Assist the sovereign to dispel wind-cold and resolve dampness with the nature of pungent-aroma.

(3) Assistant medicinal: Fuling, Baizhu, Banxia, Chenpi, Houpo, Dafupi, Jiegeng

Fuling and Baizhu fortify spleen to transport dampness, and harmonize middle jiao to stop diarrhea. Banxia and Chenpi dry dampness and harmonize stomach, and direct the qi downward to check vomiting. Houpo and Dafupi move qi to resolve dampness. Jiegeng diffuses the lung to relieve the exterior and resolves the dampness.

(4) Courier medicinal: Zhigancao

Harmonize all the medicinals.

Modification : If exterior syndrome is serious, complicated aversion to cold and no sweating, add Xiangru to support the effect of relieving exterior. If complicated with qi stagnation and serious distending pain in stomach and abdominal, add Muxiang and Yanhusuo to move qi and check pain.

Notes : Because the aroma and pungent-dispelling are nature, the medicinals of this prescription would not be decocted too long.

Yinchenhao Tang(Oriental Wormwood Decoction)

Ingredients : Yinchen(Herba Artemisiae Scopariae)19 g; Zhizi(Fructus Gardeniae)9 g; Dahuang(Radix et Rhizoma Rhei)6 g.

Administration : All medicinals above are decocted in water, for oral use.

Effects : Clear heat and drain dampness to resolve jaundice.

Application : This prescription is for jaundice with dampness-heat syndrome. These syndromes are characterized by bright yellow on whole body, face, and eyes, slight abdominal fullness, thirst, inhibited urination, yellow slimy tongue fur, sunken rapid pulse. It can be used for acute icterohepatitis, cholecystitis, cholelithiasis, leptospirosis and other diseases that characterized by jaundice with bright yellow, yellow slimy tongue fur, internal dampness-heat syndrome.

Analysis : The syndrome treated by this prescription is caused by internal stagnation with dampness-heat and stasis-heat, heat without outthrust, dampness without purgation. This syndrome should be dealt with treatment methods as follows: clear heat and drain dampness to resolve jaundice.

(1) Sovereign medicinal: Yinchen

The important medicinal for resolving jaundice, cleaning heat and draining dampness.

(2) Minister medicinal: Zhizi

Clear heat and purge fire, drain through triple energizer, and direct the dampness-heat expelling with urinate.

(3) Assistant medicinal: Dahuang

Expel stasis and purge heat, and direct the stasis-heat purging with stool.

All three medicinals combine to expel dampness-heat out with urinate and stool separately. As a result, jaundice would be resolved follow clearing of dampness-heat and purgation of stasis-heat.

Modification: If complicated with serious dampness syndrome, add Fuling and Zexie to induce diuresis to drain dampness. If complicated with serious heat syndrome, add Huangbai and Longdancao to clear heat and resolve dampness. If complicated with hypochondriac pain, add Chaihu and Chuanlianzi to soothe the liver and regulate qi.

Notes: It is unsuitable for yin jaundice syndrome.

10.3.6 Digestant prescriptions

10.3.6.1 Concept

Those that are mainly composed of medicinals for improving appetite and digestion, with the effect of promoting digestion and removing food stagnation, fortifying spleen and harmonizing stomach, used for indigestion with food stagnation, are known as digestant prescription.

10.3.6.2 Classification

The cause of retained food is always due to overeating and spleen-stomach failing in transportation. Therefore, digestant prescription can be divided into two categories: promote digestion and remove food stagnation prescription and fortify spleen to promote digestion prescription.

10.3.6.3 Notes

Internal stagnation of retained food can induce inhibited qi movement, and easily generate dampness and heat. Therefore, the degree of food, qi, heat, and dampness stagnation will be distinguished when forming the prescription. Meanwhile, appropriate medicinals will be added necessarily in different conditions. If accumulation formed with retained food and dampness-heat, induced abdominal pain, constipation, and diarrhea, medicinals for purgating will be used in order to remove food stagnation and purge accumulation.

Baohe Wan(Harmony-preserving Pill)

Ingredients: Shanzha(Fructus Crataegi)18 g; Shenqu(Massa Medicata Fermentata)6 g; Laifuzi(Semen Raphani)6 g; Banxia(Rhizoma Pinelliae)9 g; Chenpi(Pericarpium Citri Reticulatae)9 g; Fuling(Poria)9 g; Lianqiao(Fructus Forsythiae)6 g.

Administration: For pills, take 6–9 g each time and twice or thrice daily. Or all medicinals above are decocted in water, for oral use.

Effects: Promote digestion and harmonize stomach.

Application: This prescription is for food accumulation syndrome. This syndrome is characterized by stuffiness and fullness and distending pain in the stomach and abdominal, belching, acid regurgitation, anorexia, and vomiting, or diarrhea, thick slimy tongue coating, slippery pulse. It can be used for acute gastritis, chronic gastritis, acute enteritis, chronic enteritis, dyspepsia, infantile diarrhea and other diseases belonging to food accumulation syndrome.

Analysis: The syndrome treated by this prescription is caused by dietary irregularities, overeat, food stagnation, inhibited qi movement, spleen-stomach disharmony, generating dampness-heat. This syndrome should be dealt with treatment methods as follows:promote digestion and harmonize stomach.

(1)Sovereign medicinal:Shanzha

Shanzha can digest every food accumulation,even meat and greasy food.

(2)Minister medicinal:Shenqu,Laifuzi

Shenqu promotes digestion and fortifies stomach,good at digesting wine and stained food. Laifuzi directs qi downward to promote digestion,good at digesting grain food.

The combination of sovereign and minister can digest every stained food.

(3)Assistant medicinal:Banxia,Chenpi,Fuling,Lianqiao

Banxia and Chenpi move qi to dispel accumulation,and harmonize stomach to check vomiting. Fuling drains dampness,fortifies spleen,and harmonizes middle jiao to stop diarrhea. Lianqiao clears heat and dispels accumulation.

Modification:If complicated with serious food accumulation,add Zhishi and Binglang(Arecae Semen) to strengthen the effect of promoting digestion and removing food stagnation. If complicated with exuberant heat,add Huangqin and Huanglian to clear heat. If complicated with spleen deficiency and solppy diarrhea, add Baizhu to fortify spleen and promote transportation.

Notes:The power of this prescription is slight with the effect of promoting digestion and harmonizing stomach. It is unsuitable for constipation with abdominal distending pain.

10.3.7　Phlegm-dispelling and cough-suppressing prescriptions

10.3.7.1　Concept

Those that are mainly composed of medicinals for treating phlegm,cough,and asthma,with the effect of dispelling phlegm-retained fluid,relieving cough and asthma,used for kinds of phlegm and cough diseases, are known as phlegm-dispelling and cough-suppressing prescription.

10.3.7.2　Classification

Phlegm diseases would be different in dampness phlegm,heat phlegm,dry phlegm,and cold phlegm, according to disease cause. Therefore,phlegm-dispelling and cough-suppressing prescription can be divided into five categories:dry dampness to resolve phlegm prescription,clear heat to resolve phlegm prescription, moisten dryness to resolve phlegm prescription,warm cold to resolve phlegm prescription,and relieving cough and dyspnea prescription.

10.3.7.3　Notes

The phlegm generated from dampness accumulation,and spleen moving and transforming dampness. Therefore,spleen is known as the source of the phlegm generation. What is more,as a tangible pathogen, phlegm is easy to block qi movement. Phlegm-dispelling prescription is always used combining medicinals for fortifying spleen to treat the source of phlegm generation,combining medicinals for regulating qi to move qi and dispel phlegm. The medicinals for drying dampness to dispel phlegm are always warm dryness of their nature,easy to interrupt blood,so it is caution for hemoptysis tendency.

Erchen Tang(Two Old Ingredients Decoction)

Ingredients:Banxia(Rhizoma Pinelliae)15 g;Juhong(Exocarpium Citri rubrum)15 g;Fuling(Poria) 9 g;Zhigancao(Radix Glycyrrhizae)5 g.

Administration:Add Shengjiang 7 slices,Wumei 1 pcs,decocted all in water,for oral use.

Effects:Dry dampness to dispel phlegm and regulate qi to harmonize middle.

Application:This prescription is for cough or vomiting with dampness-phlegm syndrome. This syndrome is characterized by cough with much phlegm which is white and easily expectorated, stuffiness in the chest, nausea and vomiting, lack of strength, or dizziness and palpitations, white slimy tongue coating, slippery pulse. It can be used for chronic bronchitis, pulmonary emphysema, chronic gastritis, vomitus gravidarum, nervous vomiting, and other diseases belonging to dampness-phlegm syndrome with much white phlegm.

Analysis: The syndrome treated by this prescription is caused by spleen failing in transportation, dampness pathogen retention, dampness accumulation forming phlegm, and inhibited qi movement. This syndrome should be dealt with treatment methods as follows: dry dampness to dispel phlegm and regulate qi to harmonize middle.

(1) Sovereign medicinal: Banxia

Banxia can dry dampness to dispel phlegm and check cough, lower adverse qi and harmonize stomach to check vomiting, with pungent-warm and dryness in flavor nature.

(2) Minister medicinal: Juhong

Assist the sovereign to strengthen the effect of dispelling phlegm and harmonize stomach. What is more, move qi to smoothen the phlegm expectoration.

(3) Assistant medicinal: Fuling

Fortify spleen to drain dampness and treat the source of phlegm generation. Combine with the sovereign and minister to treat both symptoms and root causes.

(4) Courier medicinal: Zhigancao

Harmonize middle and fortify spleen, and harmonize all the medicinals.

When decocted, add Shengjiang to assist sovereign and minister, strengthening the effect of moving qi to dispel phlegm, harmonizing stomach to check vomiting, restrict the toxicity of Banxia in the meantime. Combine 1 pcs of Wumei to astringe lung qi and avoid damaging the healthy qi. It is the basic method for phlegm-dispelling. Therefore, this prescription is known as commonly used phlegm-dispelling prescription.

Modification: This prescription is the basic prescription for dispelling phlegm, which can be used combining relevant medicinals for kinds of phlegm diseases. If complicated with heat phlegm, add Huangqin and Dannanxing to clear heat and dispel phlegm. If complicated with cold phlegm, add Ganjiang and Xixin to warm-dispel cold-phlegm. If complicated with wind phlegm, add Tiannanxing and Zhuli to extinguish wind and dispel phlegm. If complicated with food phlegm, add Laifuzi and Shenqu to digest food stagnation and dispel phlegm.

Notes: Because the warm dryness nature, it is forbidden for the patients with yin deficiency and lung dryness syndrome.

Suzi Jiangqi Tang(Perilla Fruit Decoction for Directing Qi Downward)

Ingredients: Zisuzi(Fructus Perillae)15 g; Banxia(Rhizoma Pinelliae)15 g; Houpo(Cortex Magnoliae Officinalis)6 g; Qianhu(Radix Peucedani)6 g; Rougui(Cortex Cinnamomi)9 g; Danggui(Radix Angelicae Sinensis)9 g; Zhigancao(Radix Glycyrrhizae)12 g.

Administration: Add 2 slices Shengjiang, 1 pcs Dazao, and Zisuye 3 g, all medicinals above are decocted in water, for oral use.

Effects: Direct qi downward to calm dyspnea and dispel phlegm to check cough.

Application: This prescription is for cough-dyspnea syndrome due to upper excess and lower deficiency. This syndrome is characterized by cough, dyspnea, with much white phlegm, stuffiness in the chest, pain and flaccid in waist and knee, or limbs edema, white slimy or slippery coating, slippery and wiry-like pulse. It can be used for chronic bronchitis, pulmonary emphysema, bronchial asthma and other diseases belonging to chest stuffiness, much white phlegm with white slimy or slippery coating.

Analysis: The syndrome treated by this prescription is caused by that phlegm accumulation in the lung, lung failing to diffuse and depurate, complicated with kidney yang deficiency, failing to receive qi. Thus, this syndrome is called as upper excess and lower deficiency syndrome. According to principle of treating symptoms when an acute attack occurs, this syndrome should be dealt with treatment methods as follows: direct qi downward to calm dyspnea and dispel phlegm to check cough.

(1) Sovereign medicinal: Zisuzi

Direct qi downward and dispel phlegm, relieve cough and calm dyspnea.

(2) Minister medicinal: Banxia, Houpo, Qianhu

Banxia drains dampness to dispel phlegm and directs qi downward. Houpo directs qi downward to calm dyspnea. Qianhu diffuses lung to dispel phlegm and relieve cough. All these three medicinals assist sovereign to direct qi downward, dispel phlegm and calm dyspnea.

Sovereign combine minister to treat upper excess syndrome.

(3) Assistant medicinal: Rougui, Danggui

Rougui warms tonify kidney qi, receives qi to calm dyspnea. Danggui nourishs blood and moistens the dryness.

The combination of assistant treats the lower deficiency syndrome.

(4) Courier medicinal: Zhigancao

Harmonize all the medicinals.

Modification: If cough and dyspnea complicated with inability to lie on back, add Chenxiang to strengthen the effect of directing qi downward to calm dyspnea. If complicated with exterior syndrome, aversion to cold and fever, add Mahuang and Kuxingren to diffuse lung and calm dyspnea. If complicated with qi deficiency, add Renshen and Wuweizi to tonify lung qi. If without lower deficiency, subduct Rougui and Danggui.

Notes: Because of the warm dryness nature, it is forbidden for the patients with yin deficiency of lung and kidney, or lung heat and phlegm-dyspnea.

10.3.8　Interior-warming prescriptions

10.3.8.1　Concept

Those that are mainly composed of medicinals for warming the interior, with the effect of warming the interior and tonifying yang, dissipating cold and freeing collateral vessels, used for interior cold syndrome are known as interior-warming prescription.

10.3.8.2　Classification

Regarding interior cold syndrome, the location would be different in zang-fu viscera and meridian. Therefore, interior-warming prescriptions can be devided into three categories: prescriptions of warming middle jiao to dissipate cold, prescriptions of restoring yang from collapse, and prescriptions of warming the meridian to dissipate cold.

10.3.8.3　Notes

The pungent-warm and dryness-heat nature of interior-warming prescription are easy to damage yin, assist heat, and interrupt blood, therefore, it is caution for those who are always yin deficiency with interior heat, and on menstrual period.

Lizhong Wan(Middle-regulating Pill)

Ingredients: Ganjiang(Rhizoma Zingiberis)9 g; Renshen(Radix Ginseng)9 g; Baizhu(Rhizoma Atractylodis Macrocephalae)9 g;Zhigancao(Radix Glycyrrhizae)9 g.

Administration:For pills with honey,take 6 g each time and thrice one day with warm water. Or all medicinals above are decocted in water,for oral use.

Effects:Warm the middle to dissipate cold,tonify qi and fortify the spleen.

Application:This prescription is for deficiency cold syndrome of spleen-stomach. This syndrome is characterized by stomach and abdominal pain with preferring warm and pressure,aversion to cold,limb cold,inappetence,vomiting and diarrhea,or bleeding due to yang deficiency with little dark blood,pale tongue,white coating,sunken fine pulse. It can be used for acute gastroenteritis,chronic gastroenteritis, stomach and duodenal ulcer,chronic colitis,and other diseases main symptoms of which are shown as vomiting,diarrhea,cold,and pain,belonging to deficiency cold syndrome of spleen-stomach.

Analysis:The syndrome treated by this prescription is caused by deficiency of middle yang,deficiency cold of spleen and stomach,and failing in transportation and transformation. This syndrome should be dealt with treatment methods as follow:warm the middle to dissipate cold,tonify qi and fortify the spleen.

(1)Sovereign medicinal:Ganjiang

Warm middle,promote yang qi,and dissipate cold.

(2)Minister medicinal:Renshen

Tonify qi,fortify spleen,and promote the transportation.

(3)Assistant medicinal:Baizhu

Tonify qi,fortify spleen,and drain dampness. On one hand,it combines sovereign to warn-transport spleen yang. On the other hand,it combines minister to tonify qi and fortify spleen.

(4)Assistant and courier medicinals:Zhigancao

As assistant,it tonifies middle with pungent-warm nature,assisting above three medicinals to warm and tonify the spleen. As courier,harmonize all the medicinals.

Modification:If complicated with serious cold,use heavy dosage of Ganjiang or add Fuzi to promote the effect of warming middle and assisting yang. If used for yang deficiency bleeding syndrome,change Ganjiang to Paojiang. If complicated with serious deficiency,use heavy dosage of Renshen,to strengthen the effect of tonifying qi and fortifying spleen. If complicated with serious diarrhea,use heavy dosage of Baizhu to fortify spleen and promote transport to check diarrhea. If complicated with serious vomitting,add Wuzhuyu and Shengjiang to warm stomach and check vomiting. If complicated with dampness phlegm,add Banxia and Fuling to warm-dispel phlegm.

Notes:Avoid seaweed,cabbage,peach,plum,and bird meat.

Sini Tang(Resuscitation Decoction)

Ingredients:Fuzi(Radix Aconiti Lateralis Preparata)15 g;Ganjiang(Rhizoma Zingiberis)9 g;Zhigancao(Radix Glycyrrhizae)9 g.

Administration:All medicinals above are decocted in water,for oral use.

Effects:Restore yang to save from collapse.

Application:This prescription is for the syndrome of yin exuberance with yang debilitation. This syndrome is characterized by reversal cold of the extremities,aversion to cold with cowered in bed,vomiting with no sweating,abdominal pain,diarrhea,lassitude of spirit,somnolence,white slippery tongue coating, faint fine pulse. It can be used for myocardial infarction,acute heart failure,acute or chronic gastroenteritis with over exhaling,or shock due to over sweating disease belonging to syndrome of yin exuberance with yang debilitation,even yang collapse.

Analysis:The syndrome treated by this prescription is caused by yin exuberance with heart and kidney yang debilitation. This syndrome should be dealt with treatment methods as restoring yang to save from collapse.

(1)Sovereign medicinal:Fuzi

Warm interior to dissipate cold and restore yang to save from collapse with great pungent-heat.

(2)Minister medicinal:Ganjiang

Warm middle to dispel cold, combine Fuzi to strengthen the effect of restoring yang and dissipating cold. That is called as Fuzi do not heat without Ganjiang.

(3)Assistant and courier medicinals:Zhigancao

As assistant, it assists the sovereign and minister with tonifying qi to warm middle, and relieves the toxic substances and dryness nature of Fuzi and Ganjiang. As courier, it harmonizes all the medicinals.

Modification:If complicated with exuberant yin repelling yang, reddened complexion, which is known as true cold with false heat, use heavy dosage of Fuzi and Ganjiang to strengthen the effect of restoring yang to save from collapse. If complicated with water internal retention due to yang deficiency, limb edema, add Dangshen, Zexie, and Fuling to fortify spleen, drain dampness, and alleviate edema.

Notes:Syndrome of deficiency cold of spleen-stomach is always shown as true cold with false heat with exuberant yin repelling yang or upcast yang syndrome. In this case, do not misuse the heat cleaning prescription. Emesis immediately after taking this prescription is called as "rejecting-medicinals". In these cases, method of counteracting assistant like adding a few cold midicinals into the prescription would be taken to relieve or eliminate these situations.

10.3.9　Qi-regulating prescriptions

10.3.9.1　Concept

Those that are mainly composed of medicinals for regulating qi, with the effect of regulating qi movement, used for disordered qi movement syndrome known as qi-regulating prescription.

10.3.9.2　Classification

Disordered qi movement syndrome includes qi stagnation and qi counterflow in a general way. Accordingly, qi-regulating prescription can be devided into two categories:qi-moving prescription and directing qi downward prescription. Qi-moving prescription can be used for qi stagnation in liver and spleen syndrome and qi stagnation in liver syndrome with the effect of moving qi to resolve stagnation, and dispersing stuffiness and removing fullness. Directing qi downward prescription can be used for lung qi counterflow syndrome and stomach qi counterflow syndrome with the effect of directing qi downward, and calm dyspnea and check vomiting. The directing qi downward prescription for treating lung qi counterflow is described in the section of phlegm-dispelling and cough-suppressing prescription.

10.3.9.3　Notes

The nature and flavor of the medicinals which form qi-regulating prescription, are mainly pungent-warm and dryness. Therefore, qi-regulating prescription should not to be used for a long time in case the property might damage fluid and consume qi. It is also caution for senile people, pregnant woman, and someone with syndrome of yin deficiency with effulgent fire.

Yueju Wan(Relieving Stagnation Pill)

Ingredients:Xiangfu(Rhizoma Cyperi)9 g;Chuanxiong(Rhizoma Ligustici Chuanxiong)9 g;Cangzhu(Rhizoma Atractylodis)9 g;Zhizi(Fructus Gardeniae)9 g;Shenqu(Massa Medicata Fermentata)9 g.

Administration:For pills, take 6−9 g each time and twice one day with warm water. Or all medicinals above are decocted in water, for oral use.

Effects: Move qi to resolve stagnation.

Application: This prescription is for six stagnations syndrome such as qi, blood, phlegm, fire, damp-ness, and food stagnation. This syndrome is characterized by stuffiness in the chest and diaphragm, disten-ding pain in stomach and abdominal, acid regurgitation and vomiting, and food accumulation. It can be used for gastroneurosis, chronic gastritis, stomach and duodenal ulcer, cholelithiasis, cholecystitis, hepatitis, inter-costal neuralgia, dysmenorrhea, irregular menstruation, and other diseases belonging to six stagnations syn-drome.

Analysis: The syndrome treated by this prescription is caused by qi stagnation in liver and spleen. Qi stagnation in the liver or constrained liver qi for long, lead to liver qi invading the spleen, spleen failing to transport, dampness accumulation generating phlegm, food accumulation not digested, or blood flow being not smooth, stagnation transforming into fire, result in qi, blood, phlegm, fire, food, and dampness stagnation appearing at the same time. Because qi stagnation appearing first in the six stagnations, this syndrome will be dealt with treatment methods mainly as moving qi to resolve stagnation.

(1) Sovereign medicinal: Xiangfu

Moving qi to resolve stagnation, in order to treat qi stagnation.

(2) Minister and assistant medicinals: Chuanxiong, Cangzhu, Zhizi, Shenqu

Chuanxiong promotes blood circulation for removing blood stasis in order to treat blood stagnation, and also assists Xiangfu to move qi to resolve stagnation. Zhizi clears heat and purges fire, in order to treat fire stagnation. Cangzhu dries dampness to fortify spleen, in order to treat dampness stagnation. Shenqu digests food to treat food stagnation. Phlegm stagnation is always due to spleen-dampness, and is related to qi, fire, and food stagnation. Thus, phlegm stagnation will be resolved with the other stagnation gone.

Modification: If complicated with obvious qi stagnation syndrome, use heavy dosage of Xiangfu, add Muxiang and Zhike to strengthen moving qi. If complicated with obvious blood stagnation syndrome, use heavy dosage of Chuanxiong, add Taoren and Honghua to promote blood circulation. If complicated with ob-vious dampness stagnation syndrome, use heavy dosage of Cangzhu, add Fuling and Zexie to drain damp-ness. If complicated with obvious food stagnation syndrome, use heavy dosage of Shenqu, add Shanzha and Maiya to promote digestion. If complicated with obvious fire stagnation syndrome, use heavy dosage of Zhizi, add Huangqin and Huanglian to purge fire. If complicated with obvious phlegm stagnation syndrome, add Banxia and Gualouzi to dispel phlegm.

Notes: Although this prescription can treat all the six stagnations, it just shows the basic method for treating the stagnation syndrome. In the clinical practice, modification will be taken flexibly in accordance with the syndrome.

Chaihu Shugan San(Bupleurum Soothing Liver Powder)

Ingredients: Chaihu(Radix Bupleuri) 6 g; Chuanxiong(Rhizoma Ligustici Chuanxiong) 5 g; Xiangfu (Rhizoma Cyperi) 5 g; Zhike(Fructus Aurantii) 5 g; Juhong(Exocarpium Citri rubrum) 6 g; Baishao(Radix Paeoniae Alba) 5 g; Gancao(Radix Glycyrrhizae) 3 g.

Administration: All medicinals above are decocted in water, for oral use.

Effects: Soothe liver to resolve stagnation and move qi to check pain.

Application: This prescription is for liver qi stagnation syndrome. This syndrome is characterized by distending pain in lateral thorax, stomach, and abdominal, belching and sighing, wiry-like pulse. It can be used for hepatitis, chronic gastritis, intercostal neuralgia, and other diseases belonging to liver qi stagnation syndrome.

Analysis:The syndrome treated by this prescription is caused by emotion depression, liver failing to free flow and rise of qi, qi stagnation in liver. This syndrome will be dealt with treatment methods mainly as soothing liver to resolve stagnation and moving qi to check pain.

(1)Sovereign medicinal:Chaihu

Soothe liver to resolve stagnation.

(2)Minister medicinal:Chuanxiong, Xiangfu

Chuanxiong moves qi and promotes blood circulation. Xiangfu regulates qi to soothe liver. This combination supports sovereign to resolve stagnation and check pain.

(3)Assistant medicinal:Zhike, Juhong, Baishao

Zhike and Juhong regulate qi and move stagnation. Baisho nourishes blood to soothe liver and check pain.

(4)Assistant and courier medicinals:Gancao

As assistant, combine Baishao to nourish blood and soothe liver. As courier, harmonize all the medicinals.

Modification:If complicated with serious pain, add Danggui and Yujin to strengthen the moving qi, activating blood, and checking pain effect. If liver stagnation transform to fire, with dryness of mouth and red tongue, add Zhizi and Chuanlianzi to clear liver and purge fire.

Notes:Qi deficiency syndrome, liver and kidney yin deficienly syndrome, cold cyndrome, etc. , should not be used.

10.3.10　Blood-regulating prescriptions

10.3.10.1　Concept

Those that are mainly composed of medicinals for regulating blood, with the effect of promoting blood circulation or stopping bleeding, used for blood stasis syndrome and bleed syndrome, are known as blood-regulating prescription.

10.3.10.2　Classification

In a general way, blood-disorder syndrome includes blood stasis and bleed. Blood stasis syndrome comes from blood flow being suffocated, then blood stagnation transforms into stasis. Bleed syndrome is caused by blood going out from the vessels. Accordingly, blood-regulating prescription can be devided into two categories:activate blood and resolve stasis prescription and stop bleeding prescription.

10.3.10.3　Notes

The nature of the medicinals which form blood-regulating prescription, are mainly drastic and purgative. These prescriptions are easy to consume blood and damage healthy qi, and liable to disturb blood circulation and fetus. The dosage of the prescription will not be too heavy in case it might damage healthy qi, or add some medicinals for tonifying. It is also caution for hypermenorrhea patient and pregnant woman. Because the astringent nature of stop bleeding prescription, the medicinals for promoting blood circulation will be combined to prevent stasis retention. What is more, whether the blood stasis syndrome or bleed syndrome, the pathogenesis will be different in cold and heat, excess and deficiency. Therefore, the incidental and fundamental or primary and secondary, are necessary to be distinguished in clinical.

Xuefu Zhuyu Tang(Expelling Chest Stasis Decoction)

Ingredients:Taoren(Semen Persicae)12 g; Honghua (Flos Carthami)9 g; Chishao (Radix Paeoniae Rubra)6 g; Chuanxiong(Rhizoma Ligustici Chuanxiong)6 g; Niuxi(Radix Achyranthis Bidentatae)9 g; Dihuang(Radix Rehmanniae)9 g; Danggui(Radix Angelicae Sinensis)9 g; Chaihu(Radix Bupleuri)3 g; Jiegeng(Radix Platycodonis)6 g; Zhike(Fructus Aurantii)6 g; Gancao(Radix Glycyrrhizae)3 g.

Administration: All medicinals above are decocted in water, for oral use.

Effects: Activate blood to expel stasis, move qi to relieve pain.

Application: This prescription is for the syndrome of blood stasis in the chest. This syndrome is characterized by prolonged chest pain and headache, pain like being pricked at fixed location, or hiccup in chronic process, or internal heat with vexation, or palpitation and inability to sleep, impatience and be fractious, tidal fever at night, dark lip, deep red tongue even with ecchymosis, rough or tight-string like pulse. It can be used for stenocardia of coronary heart disease, rheumatic heart disease, chest pain of chest trauma and costal chondritis, headache, dizzy, and depression of concussion sequela, and other diseases belonging to syndrome of blood stasis and qi stagnation of upper location.

Analysis: The syndrome treated by this prescription is caused by blood stasis obstructing in the chest and qi movement stagnation. This syndrome should be dealt with treatment methods as activating blood to expel stasis, moving qi to relieve pain.

(1)Sovereign medicinal: Taoren, Honghua

Taoren and Honghua are both importance medicinals for activating blood to expel stasis. This combination bring out the best in each other with the effect of activating blood to expel stasis.

(2)Minister medicinal: Chishao, Chuanxiong, Niuxi

Chishao activates blood to expel stasis. Chuanxiong moves qi to activate blood. Niuxi directs blood stasis downward. This combination strengthens the effect of activating blood to expel stasis.

(3)Assistant medicinal: Zhike, Jiegeng, Chaihu

Zhike and Jiegeng move qi to soothe the chest, Chaihu soothes the liver to resolve stagnation. This combination regulates the qi movement, moving qi to promote blood circulation and expel the stasis. Dihuang and Danggui nourish blood and tonify yin, and clear heat of the blood.

(4)Courier medicinal: Gancao

Harmonize all the medicinals.

Modification: If complicated with mass and nodules in coastal region, add Yujin and Danshen to activate blood to expel stasis and disperse mass and nodules.

Notes: Avoid use for pregnant women, use with caution for women during menstrual period, use with caution for those who are weak.

Buyang Huanwu Tang(Tonifying Yang and Returning Five Decoction)

Ingredients: Huangqi(Radix Astragali seu Hedysari)120 g; Danggui(Radix Angelicae Sinensis)6 g; Chishao(Radix Paeoniae Rubra)6 g; Chuanxiong(Rhizoma Ligustici Chuanxiong)3 g; Taoren(Semen Persicae)3 g; Honghua(Flos Carthami)3 g; Dilong(Lumbricus)5 g.

Administration: All medicinals above are decocted in water, for oral use.

Effects: Tonify qi, activate blood, and regulate the collateral vessels.

Application: This prescription is for sequela of stroke with syndrome of qi deficiency and blood-stasis. This disease is characterized by hemiplegia, deviation of eyes and mouth, salivation, frequent micturition or incontinence of urinary, dark pale tongue, thin white coating, and moderate pulse. Hemiplegic paralysis, paraplegia, flaccidity syndrome of upper or lower limbs, and other diseases due to sequela of stroke belonging to syndrome of qi deficiency and blood-stasis, can be treated by this prescription.

Analysis: The syndrome treated by this prescription is caused by qi deficiency cannot move blood, induce to stasis stagnation in the vessels, tendons and muscle failing to be nourished. This syndrome should be dealt with treatment methods as tonifying qi, activating blood, freeing the collateral vessels.

(1) Sovereign medicinal: Huangqi

Use heavy dosage of Huangqi to greatly tonify original qi, for qi being exuberant to move blood.

(2) Minister medicinal: Danggui

Activate blood to expel stasis, for freeing the collateral vessels.

(3) Assistant medicinal: Chishao, Chuanxiong, Taoren, Honghua, Dilong

The combination of Chishao, Chuanxiong, Taoren, and Honghua assists Danggui to activate blood to expel stasis. Dilong unblocks the meridian and activate collateral, for expelling the stasis in the vessels.

Modification: If complicated with much phlegm, add Banxia, and Tianzhuhuan to resolve phlegm. If complicated with unsmooth speech, add Shichangpu, Yuanzhi and Yujin to open the orifices and free the collateral vessels. If complicated with yang deficiency, aversion to cold and cold limbs, add Fuzi to warm yang to dispel cold. If complicated with serious lower limbs flaccidity syndrome, add Duzhong and Niuxi to tonify liver-kidney, strong the tendons and bones.

Notes: In this prescription, the dosage of Huangqi are generally starting from 30–60 g, and will be increasing little by little when it did not work. What is more, it will be taken for a while after cure, for consolidating curative effect.

10.3.11　Tranquilizing prescriptions

10.3.11.1　Concept

Those that are mainly composed of medicinals for mental disease, with the effect of tranquilizing and settling will, used for mind disturbed and metal disorder diseases, are known as tranquilizing prescription.

10.3.11.2　Classification

Mind disturbed diseases are characterized by restless syndrome of heart spirit such as palpitation, inability to sleep, dysphoria, and manic psychosis. The basic mechanisms of these diseases are that heat damaging heart spirit and heart blood deficiency. Accordingly, tranquilizing prescription can be devided into two categories: tranquilize by heavy settling prescription and nourish the heart to tranquilize prescription.

10.3.11.3　Notes

The tranquilization and mental controlling prescription should not be administered for long time because mineral medicinals are used, which would damage stomach qi if taken too much.

Suanzaoren Tang(Wild Jujube Seed Decoction)

Ingredients: Suanzaoren(Semen Ziziphi Spinosae)15 g; Fuling(Poria)9 g; Zhimu(Rhizoma Anemarrhenae)9 g; Chuanxiong(Rhizoma Ligustici Chuanxiong)6 g; Gancao(Radix Glycyrrhizae)6 g.

Administration: All medicinals above are decocted in water, for oral use.

Effects: Nourish the blood to tranquilize, clear heat to relieve vexation.

Application: This prescription is for deficiency vexation syndrome with inability to sleep. This syndrome is characterized by inability to sleep, palpitation, restlessness in heart, dizziness, dryness of mouth and throat, red tongue, fine and string-like pulse. It can be used for neurasthenia, cardiac neurosis, climacteric syndrome, and other diseases belonging to deficiency restlessness syndrome with inability to sleep.

Analysis: The syndrome treated by this prescription is caused by liver-blood deficiency, deficiency heat disturbing interior, and restlessness of heart spirit. This syndrome should be dealt with treatment methods as follow: nourish the blood to tranquilize and clear heat to relieve vexation.

(1)Sovereign medicinal:Suanzaoren

Tonify the liver to nourish blood and calm heart to tranquilize.

(2)Minister medicinal:Fuling,Zhimu

Fuling calms heart to tranquilize. Zhimu nourishes yin to clear heat. This combination strengthens the relieving vexation and tranquilization effect of the sovereign.

(3)Assistant medicinal:Chuanxiong

Regulate the qi movement and soothe liver qi. Chuanxiong soothes liver qi while Suanzaoren nourishes liver blood. Chuanxiong combines Suanzaoren,meaning opposite and supplementary to each other.

(4)Courier medicinal:Gancao

Gancao clears heat and regulates middle energizer,and harmonizes all medicinals.

Modification:If complicated with fire deficiency syndrome, heat vexation, inability to sleep with dreaminess,subduct Chuanxiong,add Dihuang,Baishao,and Huanglian to nourish yin,clear heat,and remove vexation. If complicated with serious night sweating,add Muli and Fuxiaomai to astringe yin and calm heart. If complicated with frequent fright waking-up,palpitation with dreaminess,pale tongue,fine and wiry-like pules,which are the symptoms of the qi deficiency of heart and gallbladder,add Dangshen and Zhenzhumu to tonify qi and settle fright.

Notes:It is unsuitable for serious liver fire syndrome manifested as vexation and inability to sleep, headache with reddened complexion,bitter taste in the mouth,dry throat,and strong string-like and rapid pules.

10.3.12   Tonifying and replenishing prescriptions

10.3.12.1   Concept

Those that are mainly composed of medicinals for tonifying deficiency,with the effect of tonifying and nourishing qi,blood,yin,and yang,used for kinds of deficiency syndromes,are known as tonifying and replenishing prescription.

10.3.12.2   Classification

In a general way,deficiency syndromes include qi deficiency syndrome,blood deficiency syndrome,yin deficiency syndrome,and yang deficiency syndrome. Accordingly, tonifying and replenishing prescriptions can be devided into four categories:tonifying qi prescription,tonifying blood prescription,tonifying yin prescription,and tonifying yang prescription.

10.3.12.3   Notes

Tonifying and replenishing prescriptions should not be administered for long because of the thick and greasy flavor damaging the spleen-stomach and not easy to be digested. It is also cautions for patients always with spleen-stomach deficiency, eating less and sloppy stool. For preventing that, medicinals for tonifying and replenishing spleen-stomach and regulating qi to promote transportation should be added when using tonifying and replenishing prescription. For patients with deficiency syndrome and intolerance of tonifying and nourishing,spleen-stomach must be regulated first. What is more, tonifying and replenishing prescriptions should be decocted slowly with mild fire,administrated before the meal for promoting the absorption and digestion.

Sijunzi Tang(Four Gentlemen Decoction)

Ingredients:Renshen(Radix Ginseng)9 g;Baizhu(Rhizoma Atractylodis Macrocephalae)9 g;Fuling (Poria)9 g;Zhigancao(Radix Glycyrrhizae)6 g.

Administration: All medicinals above are decocted in water, for oral use.

Effects: Tonify qi and fortify the spleen.

Application: This prescription is for the spleen-stomach qi deficiency syndrome. This syndrome is characterized by sallow white complexion, speaking in a low and week voice, qi shortage and lack of strength, torpid intake and sloppy stool, pale tongue, white coating, find and week pule. It can be used for chronic gastritis, stomach and duodenal ulcer, and other diseases belonging to spleen-stomach qi deficiency syndrome with mainly symptoms shown as above.

Analysis: The syndrome treated by this prescription is caused by qi deficiency of spleen-stomach, lack of strength for transportation. This syndrome should be dealt with treatment methods as tonifying qi and fortifying the spleen.

(1) Sovereign medicinal: Renshen

Tonify qi to fortify spleen and nourish stomach.

(2) Minister medicinal: Baizhu

Tonify qi to fortify spleen and drain dampness.

(3) Assistant medicinal: Fuling

Drain dampness and fortify spleen for promoting transportation.

(4) Courier medicinal: Zhigancao

On one hand, tonify qi with nourishing the middle. On the other hand, harmonize all the medicinals.

All four medicinals combine, tonifying but not accumulating, warm but not dry, to form a neutral supplementation prescription for spleen-stomach.

Modification: If complicated with qi stagnation, stuffiness and fullness in the chest, add Chenpi to move qi and resolve stagnation. If complicated with phlegm-dampness obstructing the lung, cough with much phlegm, add Chenpi and Banxia to drain dampness and resolve phlegm, namely Liujunzi Tang (Six Gentlemen Decoction). If complicated with dampness syndrome, with symptoms shown as limbs lack of strength, emaciation, food accumulation, vomiting or diarrhea, stuffiness and fullness in the stomach and abdominal, sallow complexion, pale tongue, white slimy coating, vacuous and moderate pulse, add Lianzi, Yiyiren, Sharen, Jiegeng, Baibiandou, and Shanyao to tonify qi and fortify spleen, drain dampness and check diarrhea, namely Shenling Baizhu San (Ginseng, Poria, and Bighead Atractylodes Powder).

Siwu Tang (Four Ingreddients Decoction)

Ingredients: Shudihuang (Radix Rehmanniae Praeparata) 12 g; Danggui (Radix Angelicae Sinensis) 9 g; Baishao (Radix Paeoniae Alba) 9 g; Chuanxiong (Rhizoma Ligustici Chuanxiong) 6 g.

Administration: All medicinals above are decocted in water, for oral use.

Effects: Nourish and harmonize the blood.

Application: This prescription is for the deficiency and stagnation of nutrient blood syndrome. This syndrome is characterized by palpitation and inability to sleep, dizzies, pale complexion, or irregular menstruation, scanty menstruation or amenorrhea, dull pain in abdominal, pale tongue, and fine pulse. It can be used for irregular menstruation, chronic skin diseases like chronic eczema and lichen, orthopedics diseases, anaphylactoid purpura, nerve headache, and other diseases belonging to deficiency and stagnation of nutrient blood syndrome.

Analysis: The syndrome treated by this prescription is caused by deficiency of nutrient blood and blood moving unsmooth. This syndrome should be dealt with treatment methods as nourishing and harmonizing the blood.

(1)Sovereign medicinal:Shudihuang

Nourish the yin and blood.

(2)Minister medicinal:Danggui

Tonify blood and nourish the liver,harmonize the blood and regulate the vessels.

(3)Assistant medicinal:Baishao,Chuanxiong

Baishao nourishes blood,soothes the liver,and harmonizes the nutrient. Chuanxiong activates blood and moves qi,preventing nourishing from stagnation.

In this prescription,the sovereign and the minister focus on nourishing nutrient blood,while the assistants on nourishing with moving the blood and qi. All combine,on one hand,nourish the blood but not stagnation. On the other hand,move blood but not damage the blood.

Modification:If complicated with qi deficiency,lassitude of spirit,shortage of qi,add Renshen and Huangqi to tonify qi for nourishing blood. If complicated with obvious stasis,dysmenorrhea,change Baishao to Chishao,add Taoren and Honghua to strengthen the activating blood and relieving stasis effect,namely Taohong Siwu Tang. If complicated with cold syndrome,abdominal pain and desire for warm,add Rougui, Paojiang,and Wuzhuyu to warm and free the meridian. If complicated with heat syndrome,dryness of mouth and throat,change Shudihuang to Dihuang,add Huangqin and Mudanpi to clear heat and cool the blood.

Notes:It is forbidden for irregular menstruation with serious stasis,stabbing pain in abdominal,or collapse of blood and qi.

Liuwei Dihuang Wan(Six Ingreddients with Rehmanniae Pill)

Ingredients:Shudihuang(Radix Rehmanniae Praeparata)24 g;Shanzhuyu(Fructus Corni)12 g;Shanyao(Rhizoma Dioscoreae)12 g;Zexie(Rhizoma Alismatis)9 g;Fuling(Poria)9 g;Mudanpi(Cortex Moutan Radicis)9 g.

Administration:For pills with honey,take 6-9 g each time and thrice one day with warm water or light salt brine. Or all medicinals above are decocted in water,for oral use.

Effects:Nourish yin and tonify kidney.

Application:This prescription is for the kidney yin deficiency syndrome. This syndrome is characterized by soreness and weakness of waist and knees,dizziness,tinnitus or deafness,night sweating,emission, wasting-thirst,bone steaming and tidal fever,feverishness in palms and soles,tongue dryness and throat pain,gomphiasis,heel pain,dribbling urination,infants fontanel not closed,red tongue,little coating,fine and rapid pulse. It can be used for chronic nephritis,hypertension,diabetes,tuberculosis,nephrotuberculosis,hyperthyroidism,anovulia functional uterine bleeding,climacteric syndrome,and other diseases belonging to kidney yin deficiency syndrome.

Analysis:The syndrome treated by this prescription is caused by deficiency of kidney yin,deficiency fire flaming upward. This syndrome should be dealt with treatment methods as nourishing yin and tonifying kidney.

(1)Sovereign medicinal:Shudihuang

Nourish the yin and tonify kidney,strengthen and nourish marrow and essence.

(2)Minister medicinal:Shanzhuyu,Shanyao

Shanzhuyu tonifies liver and kidney and astringes essence. Shanyao tonifies spleen and kidney,and secures essence.

(3)Assistant medicinal:Zexie,Mudanpi,Fuling

Zexie drains dampness and purges turbidity,preventing Shudihuang from greasy. Mudanpi clears liver and purges fire,countering the warm nature of Shanzhuyu. Fuling drains spleen dampness,assisting Shanyao to promote transportation.

In this prescription, three tonics combine three purgation to be a treatment method as nourishing and tonifying yin with purging fire. Spleen, liver, and kidney would be tonified at the same time, but mostly the kidney yin.

Modification : If yin deficiency complicated with flame fire, add Zhimu and Huangbai to strengthen the cleaning heat and purge fire effect, namely Zhibai Dihuang Wan. If complicated with liver-yin deficiency, blurred vision, add Gouqizi and Juhua to nourish liver and clear eyes, namely Qiju Dihuang Wan. If complicated with lung yin deficiency, cough and dyspnea, add Maidong and Wuweizi to nourish yin and astringe lung qi, namely Maiwei Dihuang Wan.

Shenqi Wan(Kidney Qi Pill)

Ingredients : Fuzi(Radix Aconiti Lateralis Preparata)3 g; Guizhi(Ramulus Cinnamomi)3 g; Shudihuang(Radix Rehmanniae Praeparata)24 g; Shanzhuyu(Fructus Corni)12 g; Shanyao(Rhizoma Dioscoreae)12 g; Zexie(Rhizoma Alismatis)9 g; Fuling(Poria)9 g; Mudanpi(Cortex Moutan Radicis)9 g.

Administration : For pills with honey, take 6−9 g each time and twice one day with warm water or light salt brine. Or all medicinals above are decocted in water, for oral use.

Effects : Nourish yang and tonify kidney.

Application : This prescription is for the kidney yang deficiency syndrome. This syndrome is characterized by soreness and weakness of waist and knees, sense of coldness in lower body, lower abdominal contracture, inhibited urination, or spontaneous urination, pale and enlarged tongue, weak pulse with sunken and fine in chi. Phlegm fluid, edema, wasting-thirst, dermatophytosis, and shifted bladder can be seen in this syndrome. This prescription can be used for chronic nephritis, renal edema, diabetes, hypothyroidism, neurasthenia, hypoadrenocorticism, repeated attack of bronchial asthma, climacteric syndrome and other diseases belonging to kidney yang deficiency syndrome.

Analysis : The syndrome treated by this prescription is caused by deficiency of kidney yang, failing to transform qi to move water. This syndrome should be dealt with treatment methods as nourishing the kidney yang.

(1) Sovereign medicinal : Fuzi, Guizhi

Warm tonify kidney yang.

(2) Minister medicinal : Shudihuang, Shanzhuyu, Shanyao

Nourish kidney yin. The combination of sovereign and minister, is aimed at persuiting yang from yin, for strengthening the tonifying yang effect. Less medicinals for tonifying yang with more medicinals for nourishing yin, meaning that generating fire slightly to encourage the kidney qi.

(3) Assistant medicinal : Zexie, Mudanpi, Fuling

The assistant combination induce diuresis to drain dampness and promote blood circulation, prevent tonic from greasy.

All medicinals combine, warm but not dryness, nourishing but not greasy, for encouraging kidney yang, recovering qi transformation, and then all syndromes gone.

Modification : In this prescription, Guizhi and changed to Rougui, for strengthening the warm yang effect. If complicated obvious edema, add Cheqianzi and Niuxi to induce diuresis to alleviate edema. If complicated with impotence, add Yinyanghuo, Buguzhi, and Bajitian to invigorate yang and raise impotence.

Notes : It is forbidden for patients who with dryness of mouth and throat, red tongue, and little coating.

10.3.13   Astringent prescriptions

10.3.13.1   Concept

Those that are mainly composed of astringent medicinals, with the effect of securing and astringing, used for consumption and prostration syndrome of qi, blood, essence, fluid, and liquid, are known as astringent prescription.

10.3.13.2   Classification

Kinds of consumption and prostration syndromes of qi, blood, essence, fluid, and liquid are different in pathogenic factor and location, even the clinical manifestation. Accordingly, astringent prescription can be devided into four categories: securing the exterior to check sweating prescription, astringing the intestines and check diarrhea prescription, securing essence to check emission prescription, and securing the chong vessel and stanching vaginal discharge prescription.

10.3.13.3   Notes

It is caution that pathogenic factor would be astringed when using astringent prescription. This kind of prescription is forbidden for prostration syndrome, such as sweating with heat diseases, diarrhea with food accumulation, emission with fire interruption, and metrorrhagia with blood heat. In case of deficiency complicated by excess, it is necessary to combine medicinals for expelling pathogenic factor, do not use medicinals for astringing only.

Muli San(Oyster Shell powder)

Ingredients: Duanmuli(Calcined Concha Ostreae)30 g; Huangqi(Radix Astragali seu Hedysari)30 g; Mahuanggen(Radix Ephedrae)30 g.

Administration: Grind the above medicinals into fine powder, decoct 9 g each time and twice one day with Xiaomai 30 g, for oral use in warm without residue.

Effects: Enrich qi to secure the exterior and astringent yin to arrest sweating.

Application: This prescription is for qi deficiency and exterior insecurity syndrome of spontaneous sweating and night sweating. This syndrome is characterized by always sweating, worsen in sleeping, palpitation and feeling apprehensive, lack of strength, vexation, pale red tongue, fine and week pules. It can be used for spontaneous sweating and night sweating caused by weakness after the illness, operation, and childbirth.

Analysis: The syndrome treated by this prescription is caused by qi deficiency and defense-exterior insecurity, leakage of yin fluid, heart yang damaging heart yin. This syndrome should be dealt with treatment methods as follow: enrich qi to secure the exterior and astringent yin to arrest sweating.

(1)Sovereign medicinal: Duanmuli

Astringe yin to arrest sweating, and suppress yang.

(2)Minister medicinal: Huangqi

Enrich qi to secure the exterior, for arresting sweating.

(3)Assistant medicinal: Mahuanggen, Xiaomai

Mahuanggen is specialized in astringing to check sweating. Xiaomai nourish heart to remove vexation.

Modification: If complicated with limbs cold, aversion to cold and desiring for warm, add Fuzi to enrich yang to expel cold. If complicated with lack of strength, worsening after movement, use heavy dosage of Huangqi, add Renshen and Baizhu to enrich qi and tonify deficiency. If complicated with serious yin deficiency, dryness of mouth, red tongue, add Dihuang and Baishao to nourish yin and astringe fluid.

Notes：Because of the astringing nature, it is caution for patients who with interior heat or phlegm dampness.

10.3.14 Harmonizing prescriptions

10.3.14.1 Concept

Those that are with the effect of harmonizing and regulating, used for cold damage disease in shaoyang meridian, un-harmonization of liver and spleen, cold-heat complex, and dual disease of the exterior and interior, are known as harmonizing prescription.

10.3.14.2 Classification

According to pathogen location, the harmonizing prescription can be divided into four categories：harmonizing shaoyang prescription, regulating liver and spleen prescription, regulating cold and heat prescription, and dually releasing exterior-interior prescription.

10.3.14.3 Notes

When using the harmonizing prescription, the dosage of medicinal is going to be weighed based on distinguishing of primary and secondary syndrome between zang and fu, exterior and interior.

Xiaochaihu Tang(Minor Bupleurum Decoction)

Ingredients：Chaihu(Radix Bupleuri)9 g；Huangqin(Radix Scutellariae)6 g；Banxia(Rhizoma Pinelliae)6 g；Shengjiang(Rhizoma Zingiberis Recens)6 g；Renshen(Radix Ginseng)6 g；Zhigancao(Radix Glycyrrhizae)3 g；Dazao(Fructus Jujubae)4 pcs.

Administration：All medicinals above are decocted in water, for oral use.

Effects：Harmonize and regulate shaoyang.

Application：This prescription is for cold damage disease with shaoyang syndrome. This syndrome is characterized by alternating chills and fever, fullness and discomfort in chest and hypochondrium, vexation in heart, vomiting, bitter taste in mouth, dryness in throat, thin and white tongue coating, string-like pulse. It can be used for common cold, flu, chronic hepatitis, acute and chronic cholecystitis, pleuritis, nephropyelitis, gastric ulcer, postpartum infection, and other diseases belonging to shaoyang syndrome.

Analysis：The syndrome treated by this prescription is caused by pathogenic factor in the shaoyang meridian, heathly qi and pathogenic qi conflicting in half-exterior and half-interior. This syndrome should be dealt with treatment methods as harmonizing and regulating shaoyang.

(1)Sovereign medicinal：Chaihu

Expel the pathogenic factor of half exterior, regulate and free the qi stagnation of shaoyang.

(2)Minister medicinal：Huangqin

Clear and purge the heat of half interior. The combination of Chaihu and Huangqin, is expelling and the other cleaning, reliving the pathogenic factor of shaoyang together, known as the important combination of harmonizing and regulating shaoyang.

(3)Assistant medicinal：Banxia, Shengjiang, Renshen, Dazao

Banxia and Shengjiang harmonize the stomach to check vomiting. Renshen and Dazao tonify qi to support the health qi, enriching interior to prevent pathogen entering the interior.

(4)Assistant and Courier medicinal：Zhigancao

On one hand, tonify qi to assist the Renshen and Dazao. On the other hand, harmonize all the medicinals.

Modification：If complicated with vexation but not vomiting, that is heat stagnation in the chest, subduct Banxia and Renshen, add Gualou to clear heat and regulate qi movement to free chest. If heat damaging fluid, complicated thirst, subduct Banxia and add Tianhuafen to generate fluid to check thirst. If liver qi invading the spleen, complicated with abdominal pain, subduct Huangqin and add Baishao to emolliate the liver and check pain.

Notes: It is caution for shaoyang syndrome with deficiency of yin and blood because Chaihu dispelling while Huangqin and Banxia drying.

Xiaoyao San(Ease Powder)

Ingredients: Chaihu(Radix Bupleuri)9 g; Baishao(Radix Paeoniae Alba)9 g; Danggui(Radix Angelicae Sinensis)9 g; Baizhu(Rhizoma Atractylodis Macrocephalae)9 g; Fuling(Poria)9 g; Zhigancao(Radix Glycyrrhizae)6 g.

Administration: Grind the above medicinals into fine powder, taken 9 g each time and twice a day with decoction of little Weishengjiang and Bohe for oral use. Or all medicinals above are decocted in water, for oral use.

Effects: Soothe liver to relive stagnation and nourish blood to fortify spleen.

Application: This prescription is for liver depression and deficiency of spleen and blood syndrome. This syndrome is characterized by hypochondrium pain, headache and dizziness, dryness of mouth and throat, lassitude of spirit, or alternating chills and fever, or irregular menstruation, distending pain in the breast, pale red tongue, fine and string-like pulse. It can be used for chronic hepatitis, cholelithiasis, stomach and duodenal ulcer, chronic gastritis, gastrointestinal neurosis, premenstrual tension, lobules of mammary gland, climacteric syndrome, chronic pelvic inflammatory disease, and other diseases belonging to liver depression and deficiency of spleen and blood syndrome.

Analysis: The syndrome treated by this prescription is caused by liver stagnation for long, consumption of yin blood, liver stagnation invading the spleen, and spleen failing to transport. This syndrome should be dealt with treatment methods as soothing liver to relive stagnation and nourishing blood to fortify spleen.

(1)Sovereign medicinal: Chaihu

Soothe liver to relive stagnation.

(2)Minister medicinal: Baishao, Danggui

Nourish blood and astringent yin, soothe liver and relive urgency.

(3)Assistant medicinal: Fuling, Baizhu

Enrich qi to tonify the middle, fortify spleen to support transportation, enrich spleen to prevent liver invading, for nourishing the generating source of qi and blood.

(4)Assistant and Courier medicinal: Zhigancao

As assistant, tonify qi to support the assistant. As courier, harmonize all the medicinals.

Modification: If liver stagnation transformed to fire, complicated with bitter taste and dryness in mouth, add Mudanpi and Zhizi to purge liver fire, namely Jiawei Xiaoyao San. If complicated with serious deficiency of blood, pale complexion, dizziness and pale tongue, add Shudihuang to nourish yin and blood, namely Heixiaoyao San.

Banxia Xiexin Tang(Pinellia Heart-draining Decoction)

Ingredients: Banxia(Rhizoma Pinelliae)12 g; Ganjiang(Rhizoma Zingiberis)9 g; Huanglian(Rhizoma Coptidis)3 g; Huangqin(Radix Scutellariae)9 g; Renshen(Radix Ginseng)9 g; Dazao(Fructus Jujubae)4 pcs; Zhigancao(Radix Glycyrrhizae)9 g.

Administration: All medicinals above are decocted in water, for oral use.

Effects: Mildly regulate cold and heat, relieve stuffiness and masses.

Application:This prescription is for stuffiness syndrome of cold and heat inter-stagnation. This syndrome is characterized by stuffiness and fullness but no pain in the upper abdomine,retching or vomiting, borborygmus and diarrhea,thin yellow and slimy tongue coating,rapid and string-like pulse. It can be used for acute and chronic gastroenteritis,chronic colitis,nervous gastritis,chronic hepatitis,chronic cholecystitis,and other diseases belonging to excess-deficiency and cold-heat complex,manifested as stuffiness,vomiting,and diarrhea.

Analysis:The syndrome treated by this prescription is caused by deficiency of middle yang,inter-stagnation of cold and heat,disorder of upward and downward qi movement. This syndrome should be dealt with treatment methods as mildly regulating cold and heat,relieving stuffiness and masses.

(1)Sovereign medicinal:Banxia

Relieve stuffiness and masses,harmonize stomach and descend adverse qi.

(2)Minister medicinal:Ganjiang,Huanglian,Huangqin

Ganjiang combining Banxia to relive stuffiness, harmonize middle and dispel cold. Huanglian and Huangqin purge and clear heat.

(3)Assistant medicinal:Renshen,Dazao

Renshen and Dazao tonify qi to support the health qi,combining Ganjiang to warm middle and tonify deficiency,fortify spleen and nourish stomach.

(4)Assistant and Courier medicinal:Zhigancao

On one hand,tonify qi to assist the Renshen and Dazao. On the other hand,harmonize all the medicinals.

The medicinals in this prescription include the functions of warming and clearing,and the effects of tonify and reduction. Pungent medicinals can dispel while bitter ones can descend,then cold-heat will be driven out and qi's up-downward movement recovered. Finally,stuffiness and fullness will be resolved,vomiting and diarrhea treated.

Modification:If stuffiness with vomiting,while the deficiency syndrome is not so serious,subduct Renshen and Dazao,add Zhishi and Shengjiang to regulate qi and harmonize stomach to stop vomiting.

Notes:It is forbidden for stomach stuffiness and fullness due to qi stagnation or food accumulation.

10.3.15　Resuscitative prescriptions

10.3.15.1　Concept

Those that are mainly composed of medicinals for causing resuscitation with aromatics,with the effect of opening the orifices and resuscitating,used for syndrome of orifices block with unconsciousness, are known as resuscitative prescription.

10.3.15.2　Classification

In a general way,syndrome of orifices block with unconsciousness include two kinds such as heat block and cold block. Accordingly,resuscitative prescription can be devided into two categories:cold resuscitative prescription and warm resuscitative prescription.

10.3.15.3　Notes

Orifices block syndrome is mainly caused by pathogenic factors such as warm-heat,phlegm-heat,qi stagnation,and turbid phlegm,blocking the heart orifices. Unconsciousness characterizes orifices block syndrome,but it is not all caused by heart orifices block. Therefore,when using the resuscitative prescription, unconsciousness due to collapse syndrome or heat accumulation in yangming must be excluded. What is more, aromatics medicinals cannot be decocted to prevent the volatilizing of active ingredients and declining of curative effect. So resuscitative prescription is always made into power and pills. Finally, the pungent nature of the prescription is easy to damage original qi and fetus qi. For this reason, resuscitative prescription is mainly used as first aid, and will be stopped immediately when it takes effect. It will not be taken for long, also caution for pregnant women.

Angong Niuhuang Wan(Peaceful Palace Bezoar Pill)

Ingredients: Niuhuang(Calculus Bovis) 30 g; Shexiang(Moschus)7. 5 g; Shuiniujiao(Cornu Bubali) 30 g; Huanglian(Rhizoma Coptidis)30 g; Huangqin(Radix Scutellariae)30 g; Zhizi(Fructus Gardeniae) 30 g; Bingpian(Borneolum Syntheticum)7. 5 g; Yujin(Radix Curcumae)30 g; Zhenzhu(Margarita)15 g; Zhusha(Cinnabaris)30 g; Xionghuang(Realgar)30 g.

Administration: Grind the above medicinals into fine powder made into pills with honey, weighing 3 g each. Take 1 pill each time and once or twice one day.

Effects: Clear heat and open orifices, sweep phlegm and detoxify.

Application: This prescription is for heat pathogen inward invading into pericardium syndrome. This syndrome is characterized by high fever, agitation, unconsciousness with delirious speech, dryness of mouth and tongue, exuberant phlegm accumulation, red or crimson tongue and rapid pulse. It is involved in stroke, epidemic encephalitis B, epidemic cerebrospinal meningitis, toxic dysentery, uremia, hepatic coma, and other diseases belonging to heat pathogen inward invading into pericardium syndrome.

Analysis: The syndrome treated by this prescription is caused by warm-heat pathogen inward invading into pericardium, orifices confused by phlegm-heat. This syndrome should be dealt with treatment methods as cleaning heat and opening orifices, sweeping phlegm and detoxifying.

(1) Sovereign medicinal: Niuhuang, Shexiang

Niuhuang clears heart and detoxify, extinguishes wind to tranquilize fright, sweeps phlegm and opens orifices. Shexiang frees the twelve meridians, opens orifices and induces resuscitation. This combination aim at cleaning heart and opening orifices.

(2) Minister medicinal: Shuiniujiao, Huanglian, Huangqin, Zhizi, Bingpian, Yujin

Shuiniujiao, Huanglian, Huangqin, and Zhizi clear heat, purge fire, and detoxify, supporting the Niuhuang to clear pericardium heat. Bingpian and Yujin repel foulness and open the block, supporting Shexiang to open orifices and induce resuscitation.

(3) Assistant medicinal: Zhusha, Zhenzhu, Xionghuang

Zhusha and Zhenzhu settle the heart to tranquilize, for reliving vexation. Xionghuang assist the Niuhuang to sweep phlegm and detoxify.

(4) Courier medicinal: honey

For pills with honey, harmonize the stomach and regulate the middle.

Modification: If complicated with replete and strong pulse, take it with decoction of Jinyinhua and Bohe for strengthening the effect of cleaning heat and expelling the pathogenic factor. If complicated with week pulse, take it with decoction of Renshen for strengthening the effect of supporting healthy qi to expel pathogenic factor. If complicated with yangming fu viscera excess syndrome, unconsciousness, and constipation, dissolve 2 pills and taken with powder of Dahuang 9 g, namely Niuhuang Chengqi Tang.

Zhu Mingmin

Chapter 11

Basic Knowledge of Acupuncture and Moxibustion

Acupuncture and moxibustion discipline is a subject using meridian theory and techiques of acupuncture and moxibustion to prevent and cure diseases, which is guided by the theory of traditional Chinese medi-cine traditional Chinese medicine. As an important component of TCM, after a long process of development, acupuncture and moxibustion discipline has gradually become an independent subject with rich theoretical contents and high clinical application value.

Acupuncture and moxibustion have the following characteristics. Firstly, they are widely used in various clinical diseases and have significant curative effect. Secondly, adverse reactions happen infrequently if standardized manipulations of acupuncture and moxibustion are strictly followed. Thirdly, necessary instruments such as needles, moxa and disinfection materials are small in size and convenient for the doctor to carry. So acupuncture and moxibustion are suitable for emergency treatment especially. Acupuncture and moxibustion originated in China. They not only play an important role in reproduction and prosperity of the Chinese nation, but also make a great contribution to the development of the world medicine. Today, acupuncture and moxibustion are applied in more and more countries and regions.

11.1　General introduction to meridians and collaterals

11.1.1　The basic concepts of meridians and collaterals

Meridians and collaterals are pathways that transport qi and blood, and connect the zang-fu viscera with the surface and other parts of the body. Meridians mean main paths or straight lines. Collaterals refer to branches that separate from the meridians and distribute throughout the body like a net.

The meridian and collateral system consists of the twelve meridians, the eight extra meridians, the fifteen collaterals, the twelve divergent meridians, tendons along the twelve meridians, and the twelve skin regions as listed in Figure 11-1.

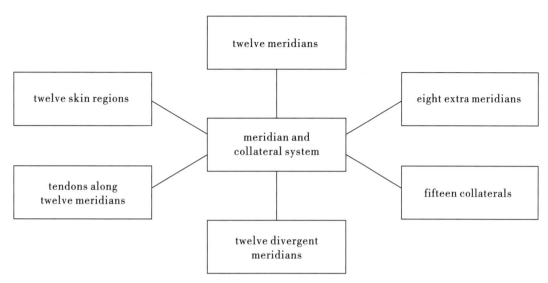

Figure 11-1   The meridian and collateral system

11.1.2   The twelve meridians

11.1.2.1   The nomenclature of the twelve meridians

The nomenclature of the twelve meridians comprises three elements: hand and foot, yin and yang, and viscera. Hand and foot refers to the external distribution and origin or termination of a meridian on upper or lower limb. Yin and yang designates the nature of the meridian. There are three hand and foot pairs of yin and three hand and foot pairs of yang meridians. Those with the most abundant yin are called taiyin; those with a lesser amount are called shaoyin; those with the least are called jueyin. Similarly those with the most abundant yang are called yangming; those with a lesser amout are called taiyang; those with the least are called shaoyang. Each yin meridian is also paired with its corresponding yang meridian to form six interior and exteriorly related pairs: hand taiyin and hand yangming; foot yangming and foot taiyin; hand shaoyin and hand taiyang; foot taiyang and foot shaoyin; hand jueyin and hand shaoyang; foot shaoyang and foot jueyin.

In the twelve meridians, qi circulates cyclically. Beginning with the lung meridian of hand taiyin, it moves through the meridians one by one. After the twelfth, the liver meridian of foot jueyin, it reenters the lung meridian to circulate again.

11.1.2.2   The distribution regularities of the twelve meridians

(1) Exterior distribution

1) The four limbs

The three yin meridians of hand run sequentially on the medial or palmar aspect of the upper limb; from anterior to posterior the order is hand taiyin, hand jueyin, and hand shaoyin. The three yang meridians of hand run sequentially on the lateral or dorsal aspect of the upper limb; from anterior to posterior the order is hand yangming, hand shaoyang, and hand taiyang. The three yin and three yang meridians of foot are similarly distributed on the lower limb, with the three yin meridians of foot ordered on the medial portion from anterior to posterior and the three yang meridians of foot on the lateral aspect from anterior to posterior. In an exception to this arrangement, the liver meridian of foot jueyin runs anterior to the spleen meridian of foot taiyin until the two meridians intersect eight cun above the medial malleolus where the liver meridian of foot jueyin returns to its regular position between the spleen meridian of foot taiyin and the kidney meridian of foot shaoyin.

2)The head,face and trunk

The three yin meridians of hand run from the chest to the medial or palmar aspect of the hand. The three yin meridians of foot begin at the foot and end at the abdomen and the chest region. All the yang meridians either begin or end at the head and face region;as the saying goes,"the head is the convergence of all yang meridians". The three yang meridians of hand are not externally distributed on the trunk. They begin at the lateral aspect of the hand and end at the head or face. The three yang meridians of foot travel from head to the foot and are the longest of the twelve meridians. The stomach meridian of foot yangming travels on the anterior aspect of the body;the gallbladder meridian of foot shaoyang,on the lateral aspect;the bladder meridian of foot taiyang,on the posterior aspect.

(2)Interior distribution

Interior distribution of the twelve meridians refers to the portion of each meridian that enters the chest and abdomen internally to connect with the related zang-fu viscera and tissues. Each of the twelve meridians belongs to its respective zang-fu viscera. As zang viscus belong to yin and fu viscera belong to yang, the three yin meridians of hand connect with the chest and belong respectively to the lung,the pericardium and the heart. The three yin meridians of foot connect with the abdomen and belong to the spleen,the liver and the kidney. The three yang meridians of foot belong to the stomach,the gallbladder and the urinary bladder. The three yang meridians of hand belong to the large intestine,the triple energizer and the small intestine.

(3)Exterior-Interior relationships of the twelve meridians

The zang and fu viscera have exterior-interior relationships with each other. Because the twelve meridians belong to the zang-fu viscera internally,each shares an exterior-interior relationship with its corresponding zang or fu viscera. The yin meridians belong to the interior and to zang viscera;the yang meridians,to the exterior and to fu viscera. The exterior and interior relationship of yin and yang meridians share pertaining and connecting relationships within the body. Each yin meridian pertains to a zang viscus and connects to a fu viscera,each yang meridian pertains to a fu viscera and connects to a zang viscera. For example,the lung meridian of hand taiyin pertains to the lung and connects to the large intestine,the exterior-interior related viscera of the lung;conversely,the large intestine meridian of hand yangming pertains to the large intestine and connects to the lung. According to these exterior-interior,pertaining and connecting relationships,the twelve meridians are divided into six pairs:lung meridian of hand taiyin and large intestine mendian of hand yangming,heart meridian of hand shaoyin and small intestine meridian of hand taiyang,interior meridian(yin meridian) and exterior meridian(yang meridian),lung meridian of hand taiyin and large intestine meridian of hand yangming,heart meridian of hand shaoyin and small intestine meridian of hand taiyang,pericardium meridian of hand jueyin and triple energizer meridian of hand shaoyang,spleen meridian of foot taiyin and stomach meridian of foot yangming,kidney meridian of foot shaoyin and bladder meridian of foot taiyang,liver meridian of foot jueyin and gallbladder meridian of foot shaoyang.

The exterior-interior relationships of the twelve meridians are also strengthened by the divergent meridians and collaterals,which facilitate communication and strengthen the connections between the exterior-interior related viscera and the relevant parts and regions of the body.

11. 1. 2. 3　Flow and entry of qi and blood into the twelve meridians

Movement of qi and blood inside a meridian is known as "flow";influx of qi and blood from one meridian to another is known as "entry". The general rule is that the three yin meridians of hand travel from chest to hands;the three yang meridians of hand,from hands to head;the three yang meridians of foot,from head to feet;the three yin meridians of foot,from feet to abdomen or chest. The connections between the twelve meridians also follow a pattern: ①The exterior-interiorly related meridians connect at the extremities; e. g. ,the lung meridian of hand taiyin and the large intestine meridian of hand yangming connect at the tip of the radial side of the index finger. ②Yang meridians with the same nomenclature connect at the head and facial region; e. g. ,the hand and foot yangming meridians connect next to the nose. ③Yin meridians connect inside the chest; e. g. ,the spleen meridian of foot taiyin connects with the heart meridian of hand shaoyin inside the heart.

Based on their distribution and conjunction, the twelve meridians connect with each other to form a closed system.

The lung meridian of hand taiyin starts from the lung and ends at the index finger. The large intestine meridian hand yangming starts from the index finger and ends at the lateral side of the nose. The stomach meidian of foot yangming starts from the lateral side of the nose and ends at the big toe. The spleen meridian of foot taiyin starts from the big toe and ends at the heart. The heart meridian of hand shaoyin starts from the heart and ends at the little finger. The small intestine meridian of hand taiyang starts from the little finger and ends at the inner corner of the eye. The bladder meridian of foot taiyang starts from the inner corner of the eye and ends at the little toe. The kidney meridian of foot shaoyin starts from the little toe and ends at the chest. The pericardium meridian of hand jueyin starts from the chest and ends at the ring finger. The triple energizer meridian of hand shaoyang starts from the ring finger and ends at the outer corner of the eye. The gallbladder meridian of foot shaoyang starts from the outer corner of the eye and ends at the big toe. The liver meridian of foot jueyin starts from the big toe and ends at the lung.

Qi and blood flows continuously inside the closed loop formed by the connection of the twelve meridians in a circulation affected by the patterns of nature. For example, the day may be divided into twelve two-hour intervals: the flow of qi and blood in each meridian correlates to one interval, after which it moves to the next meridian following the natural cycle of the earth's movement around the sun. This concept is the foundation of stem-branch acupuncture. In the eight extra meridians, the conception vessel and the governor vessel were later incorporated into the loop system to form the circulation of the fourteen meridians.

11.1.3   The eight extra meridians

The eight extra meridians, governor vessel, conception vessel, thoroughfare vessel, belt vessel, yang heel vessel, yin heel vessel, yang link vessel and yin link vessel, have unique functions, including governing, connecting, and regulating qi and blood within the meridians. They differ from the twelve meridians in that they do not belong directly to zang-fu viscera and have no exterior-interior relationships. However, they are closely related to extraordinary fu-viscera such as the uterus, the brain and the marrow, and they intersect the twelve meridians. Governor vessel runs along the posterior midline; conception vessel travels the anterior midline. Like the twelve meridians, the governor vessel and conception vessel have points of their own. Thus they are often grouped with the twelve meridians into the arrangement known as the fourteen meridians. With no points of their own, the remaining six meridians connect with the twelve meridians at various points throughout the body. Thoroughfare vessel runs along the first lateral line on the abdomen, where it connects with the kidney meridian of foot shaoyin. The conception vessel, governor vessel and thoroughfare vessel all originate in the uterus(uterus in females; essence chamber in males). These three meridians emerge at the perineum and separate thereafter; hence the saying, "one origin and three divisions". The belt vessel encircles the waist and abdomen like a belt and intersects points on the gallbladder meridian of foot shaoyang. Yang heel vessel runs laterally on the lower limbs and ascends to the shoulder and head; it intersects points on meridians such as the bladder meridian of foot taiyang. Yin heel vessel travels on the medial aspect of the lower limbs and ascends to the head, face and eye; it intersects the kidney meridian of foot shaoyin. Yang link vessel travels laterally on the lower limbs and ascends to the shoulder, head, and nape of of the neck; it intersects points on meridians such as the bladder meridian of foot taiyang and the governor vessel. Yin link vessel travels on the medial aspect of the lower limbs and along the third lateral line of the abdomen to the neck; it intersects points on meridians such as the kidney meridian of foot shaoyin and the conception vessel.

11.1.4　The fifteen collaterals

The fifteen collaterals consist of the twelve collaterals which branch out from the twelve meridians on the limbs; one collateral for the conception vessel on the front, one collateral for the governor vessel on the back, and the major collateral of the spleen on the lateral side of the trunk. The twelve collaterals strengthen qi and blood communication between exterior-interior related meridians. The twelve collaterals start from the connecting points on the twelve meridians and go towards their exterior-interiorly paired meridians. The three collaterals on the trunk infuse qi and blood to the anterior, posterior and the lateral side of the body.

11.1.5　The twelve divergent meridians

The twelve divergent meridians are the divergent passages of the twelve meridians which travel deep inside the body in order to strengthen connection between exterior-interior related meridians. Their traveling characteristics can be summarized as "leaving", "entering", "exiting" and "merging". They "leave" from the twelve meridians in the areas above elbow or knee, "enter" thoracic and abdominal cavities, connect with their pertaining and connecting zang-fu viscera, "exit" at the neck or the face, then the yang divergent meridians "merge" with the yang meridians they leave from, while yin divergent meridians "merge" with their exterior-interior related yang meridians. For example, divergent meridian of foot taiyang and divergent meridian of foot shaoyin branch out from bladder meridian and kidney meridian at the popliteal fossa. They enter the body and connect with the kidney and the bladder, exit at the nape and merge with the bladder meridian.

11.1.6　Tendons along twelve meridians

Tendons along twelve meridians refer to the corresponding muscles and tendons around the twelve meridians. Each bundle of tendons corresponds to a meridian and is nourished by the meridian. All tendons along twelve meridians start from the tips of the fingers or toes, accumulate at joints, travel along the superficial part of the body, and finally reach the trunk or head. They do not connect the internal viscera. The tendons along three yang meridians of foot start from the tips of the toes and arrive at the face. The tendons along three yin meridians of foot start from the tips of the toes and reach the external genitalia. The tendons along three yang meridians of hand start from the tips of the fingers and reach the head. The tendons along three yin meridians of hand start from the tips of the fingers and end at the chest. The twelve meridians distribute, retain, and accumulate qi and blood in their respective tendon area.

11.1.7　Twelve skin regions

Twelve skin regions are the regions of the skin reflecting the functional condition of the twelve meridians. One skin region reflects the functional condition of one meridian. Like tendons along twelve meridians, the twelve skin regions also need the nourishment of qi and blood from the corresponding meridians.

11.1.8   Effects of meridians and collaterals

11.1.8.1   Linking the interior with the exterior throughout the body

The tissues and viscera in the human body, including the zang-fu viscera and extraordinary fu-viscera, five sensory viscera, nine orifices, skin, muscles, tendons and bones, have individual physiological functions. Nevertheless, they are interconnected and coordinated via the meridian system. The twelve meridians form the main body; the twelve divergent meridians and the fifteen collaterals are the large branches; the twelve skin regions and tendons along twelve meridians correspond to the twelve meridians on the skin, muscles and tendons. The eight extra meridians traverse, intersect, and connect the twelve meridians. The meridians and collaterals are independent from each other, but they interconnect and converge to form a network that integrates the whole body into a complete organism.

The twelve meridians connect the body surface with the internal viscera and strengthen communication among the zang-fu viscera. The twelve divergent meridians strengthen connection between yin and yang meridians and connection among meridians, zang-fu viscera, and the head and facial region. The fifteen collaterals strengthen the relationship between the surface and the meridians. The eight extra meridians strengthen the relationship among the twelve meridians.

11.1.8.2   Circulating qi and blood, coordinating yin and yang

The *Miraculous Pivot* says, "The meridians move qi and blood, nourish yin and yang, and lubricate the joints and tendons". Qi and blood are the material foundation of all activities in the human body. The yang fu viscera and tissues conduct their normal physiological functions relying on the nourishment provided by qi and blood, which are transported by the meridians and collaterals throughout the body. Yin and yang differ throughout the human body. Meridians and collaterals connect the whole body to facilitate yin-yang balance, harmony, and normal physiological functions.

11.1.8.3   Resisting pathogenic qi, reflecting signs and symptoms of disorders

External pathogens usually attack the body through the meridians and collaterals, penetrating from the exterior to the interior via collaterals, meridians, fu viscera and zang viscera. If meridian qi is robust, it can defend the body and prevent pathogenic qi from penetrating deeply into the body. If it is weak, it cannot withstand the attack, and pathogenic qi remains, lingering at different levels of the meridian and collateral system and ultimately penetrating the zang-fu viscera.

Because meridians and collaterals communicate with the interior and exterior of the body, pathological changes within the zang-fu viscera can be reflected on the body's surface through the meridians and collaterals. Internal disorders can manifest as tenderness, nodules, depressions, and saturated blood vessels on the body surface. Such signs and symptoms serve as important evidence for diagnosing internal disorders.

11.1.8.4   Transmitting sensation, regulating deficiency and excess

Meridians and collaterals play an important role during treatment, as they react to acupuncture, moxibustion and tuina. The transmission of the needling sensation along the meridians is shown in such phenomena as the arrival, movement and spreading of qi to affected areas. Needling sensation is the key to therapeutic efficacy in acupuncture; it is conducted through the meridians to diseased areas to regulate deficiencies and excesses. Notably, acupuncture's regulating effects are optimizing: stimulating a point using the same method under different conditions can produce opposite therapeutic effects, but acupuncture always moves the body towards homeostasis and almost never has effects on healthy individuals. Hence needling Neiguan(PC 6) increases the heart rate in bradycardia and reduces it in tachycardia, and needling Tianshu

(ST 25)can relieve constipation as well as diarrhea.

11.2 General introduction on acupoints

11.2.1 Nomenclature of acupoints

The name of an acupoint usually has its specific meaning. Ancient scholars assigned names based on variety of subjects ranging from astronomy, geography, daily life, natural objects and anatomy to distribution characteristics, functions and indications of acupoint. Nomenclature of acupoint is summarized below.

11.2.1.1 Nomenclature based on astronomy and geography

Acupoints named for the sun, moon or stars: Riyue(GB 24)refers to the sun and the moon. Shangxing (GV 23), Xuanji(CV 20), Taiyi(ST 23)and Taibai(SP 3)are all names of stars.

Acupoints named for the mountains, hills or valleys: Chengshan (BL 57) means supporting the mountains. Daling(PC 7)means a large mound. Liangqiu(ST 34)refers to a ridge in the hill. Hegu(LI 4) means the junction of valleys.

Acupoints named for seas, rivers, streams or ponds: Shaohai(HT 3)means the smaller sea. Sidu(SJ 9) is the four rivers. Houxi(SI 3)means the back stream. Quchi(LI 11)refers to a crooked pond.

Acupoints named for roads, paths or passes: Qichong(ST 30)means the pathway of qi. Shuidao(ST 28)means the pathway of water. Neiguan(PC 6)is an internal pass.

11.2.1.2 Nomenclature based on activities of human beings and objects

Acupoints named for animals and plants: Jiuwei(CV 15)is the tail of a turtledove. Futu(ST 32)means a crouching rabbit. Cuanzhu(BL 2)means a clump of bamboo.

Acupoints named for buildings: Kufang(ST 14)is a warehouse. Tianchuang(SI 16)is a skylight. Zigong (CV 19)means royal palace.

Acupoints named for commonly used tools: Xuanzhong(GB 39)refers to a suspended bell. Dazhu(BL 11)is a large shuttle. Quepen(ST 12)is a basin.

Acupoints named for human affairs: Guilai(ST 29)means returning to the original place. Yanglao(SI 6)means providing for the aged.

11.2.1.3 Nomenclature based on acupoint location and function

Acupoints named for their anatomical locations: Dazhui(GV 14)is a large vertebra. Wangu(SI 4)is the carpus. Rangu(KI 2)is the navicular bone.

Acupoints named for the functions of zang-fu viscera: Shentang(BL 44)means the palace of mind. Po-hu(BL 42)means the door of the corporeal soul. Hunmen(BL 47)is the door of the soul. Yishe(BL 49)is the house of thought. Zhishi(BL 52)is the room of will.

Acupoints named for meridians, collaterals, and yin-yang: Sanyinjiao(SP 6)is the intersection of the three yin meridians of foot. Sanyangluo(TE 8)is the junction of three yang meridians of hand.

Acupoints named according to the functions of acupoint: Guangming(GB 37)is for clear vision. Ying-xiang(LI 20)is for sense of smell. Tinggong(SI 19)and Tinghui(GB 2)are for hearing.

11.2.2 Classification of acupoints

Acupoints are classified as meridian points, extra points and ashi points.

11.2.2.1   Meridian points

The acupoints distributed along the course of the fourteen meridians(twelve regular meridians plus the-governor vessel and the conception vessel)are called "acupoints of the fourteen meridians", or "meridian points" for short. A meridian point has its definite name, fixed location and specific indication. The *Source of Acupuncture and Moxibustion*, compiled in 1871 A. D. , recorded 361 acupoints, which is the number of meridian points still used today.

11.2.2.2   Extra points

The acupoints that have fixed locations but do not belong to the fourteen meridians are called "extra points". They have specific names and indications, and most of them are used for specific disorders. For example, Dingchuan(EX–B 1)is used for asthma; Yaotongdian(EX–UE 7)are used for acute lumbar muscle sprain; Dannang(EX–LE 6)is effective for acute cholecystitis.

11.2.2.3   Ashi points

Ashi points refer to tender points or other sensitive spots due to diseases. They have neither definite names nor fixed locations. Most of them are located near the affected part, but some are distal to the affected part.

11.2.3   Rules for the effects and indications of acupoints

11.2.3.1   Rules for the effects of acupoints

Acupoints are reaction points of diseases. They receive various stimulation including acupuncture and moxibustion. They prevent and treat diseases and are sites where qi and blood are transported and pathogenic qi invades. Acupoints are stimulated by acupuncture and moxibustion in order to strengthen healthy qi and remove pathogenic qi through dredging the meridians, regulating the flow of qi and blood, harmonizing yin and yang with each other and harmonizing zang-fu viscera functions. The rules for the effects of acupoints are classified as follows.

(1)Local therapeutic effects

Local therapeutic effect is a characteristic of all acupoints, including meridian points, extra points an-dashi points. All points can treat disorders of their adjacent locations. For example, Quchi(LI 11)located near the elbow is used to treat pain of the elbow. Zusanli(ST 36)and Yanglingquan(GB 34)located on the leg, are effective for pain and paralysis of the lower limbs.

(2)Remote therapeutic effects

Remote therapeutic effects is a characteristic of meridian points, especially those of the twelve meridi-ans located blow the elbow and the knee. They are effective not only for local disorders but also for disorders of remote locations on the course of their pertaining meridians. This is what the saying "the indications of the acupoints extend to where their pertaining meridians reach" means. For example, Zusanli (ST 36)is used to treat gastro-intestinal disorders according to the course of the stomach meridian of foot yangming.

(3)Special therapeutic effects

In addition to local and remote therapeutic effects, some acupoints have special therapeutic effects such as bidirectional regulation, general regulation, and other specific effects. Many acupoints have the effects of bidirectional regulation. For instance, Tianshu(ST 25)and Zusanli(ST 36)relieves diarrhea or constipation. Neiguan(PC 6)decreases heart rate in patients with tachycardia but increases it in bradycardia. Some acu-points, especially in yangming meridians, governor vessel and conception vessel, have effects of general reg-ulation. For example, Hegu(LI 4),Quchi(LI 11)and Dazhui(GV 14)are used to treat fever caused by external pathogenic qi. Guanyuan(CV 4) and Zusanli(ST 36) have the effects of tonification and preserving health. Some acupoints have relatively specific effects, for example, Shaoze(SI 1) treats mastitis, and Zhiyin (BL 67) corrects malpresentation.

11.2.3.2 Rules for indications of acupoints

Each acupoint has wide range of indications directly related to its location and meridian. Acupoints from different meridians have some common indications in addition to their own characteristics. Acupoints located in the same region also have some common indications. The rules for acupoint indications in different meridians are summarized in Table 11-1.

Table 11-1　Indications for acupoints of the fourteen meridians

Meridians	Indications of the meridian	Common indications	
Lung meridian of hand taiyin	Disorders of the lung and throat		Disorders of the chest
Pericardium meridian of hand jueyin	Disorders of the heart and stomach	Disorders of the mind	
Heart meridian of hand shaoyin	Disorders of the heart		
Large intestine meridian of hand yangming	Disorders of the forehead, nose, mouth and teeth		Disorders of the eyes and throat, fever
Triple energizers meridian of hand shaoyang	Disorders of the temporal region and hypochondrium	Disorders of the ears	
Small intestine meridian of hand taiyang	Disorder of the occipital region, scapula and mind		
Stomach meridian of foot yangming	Disorders of the forehead, mouth, teeth, throat, stomach and intestine		Disorders of the mind, fever
Gallbladder meridian of foot shaoyang	Disorders of the temporal region, ear, neck, gallbladder and hypochondrium	Disorders of the eyes	
Bladder meridian of foot taiyang	Disorders of the occipital region, neck and back, anorectal disorders and zang-fu viscera disorders		
Spleen meridian of foot taiyin	Disorders of the spleen and stomach		Disorders in the abdomen, gynecological disorders
Liver meridian of foot jueyin	Disorders of the liver	Disorders of the externalia	
Kidney meridian of foot shaoyin	Disorders of the kidney, lung and throat		
Governor vessel	Fever, disorders of the head	Stroke, disorders of the mind and zang-fu viscera	
Conception vessel	Deficiency cold syndrome, disorders of lower energizer		

Acupoints located in fo forehead and temporal region have indication for disorders of the eyes and nose.

Acupoints located in occipital region have indication for disorders of the head and mind.

Acupoints located at nape have indication for disorders of the mind, throat, eyes, head and nape.

Acupoints located at eyes have indication for disorders of the eyes.

Acupoints located at nose have indication for disorders of the nose.

Acupoints located at neck have indication for disorders of the tongue, throat, trachea and neck.

Acupoints located at chest and upper back have indication for disorders of the lung and heart (upper energizer).

Acupoints located at hypochondrium and upper abdomen and lower back have indication for disorders of the liver, gallbladder, spleen and stomach (middle energizer).

Acupoints located at lower abdomen and lumbosacral region have indication for disorders of the externalia and anus, kidney, intestine and bladder (lower energizer).

11.2.4 Specific points

Specific points refer to those acupoints of the fourteen meridians that have special therapeutic effects and are classified as specific categories. Specific points make up a considerable proportion of the acupoints of the fourteen meridians and play an important role in the basic theory and clinical application of acupuncture and moxibustion.

11.2.4.1 Five transport points

Five transport points refer to five groups of points distal to elbow or knee, namely well, spring, stream, river and sea points. The ancient doctors described qi flowing in the meridians as water flowing from a spring to the sea, from shallow to deep. The qi of meridians flows from the distal extremities to the elbows or knees, from well point, to spring, stream, river and sea point in sequence. Most well points are located at the tips of the fingers or toes where the meridian qi starts to bubble like water coming out of a well. The spring points are distal to metacarpal-phalangeal or metatarso-phalangeal joints where meridian qi starts to rush like a spring. The stream points are proximal to the metacarpal-phalangeal or metatarso-phalangeal joints where meridian qi flows like a stream. The river points are proximal to the wrist or ankle where meridian qi pours abundantly like a river. Finally, sea points are near the elbows and knees where meridian qi enters the body and gathers in the zang-fu viscera like rivers converging to the sea.

Five transport points are widely applied clinically corresponding to the five elements. The details of the five transport points and their attributes of five elements are listed in Table 11-2 and Table 11-3.

Table 11-2   Five transport points of the six yin meridians

Six yin meridians		Well points (wood)	Spring points (fire)	Stream points (earth)	River points (metal)	Sea points (water)
Three yin meridians of hand	Lung (metal)	Shaoshang (LU 11)	Yuji (LU 10)	Taiyuan (LU 9)	Jingqu (LU 8)	Chize (LU 5)
	Pericardium (ministerial fire)	Zhongchong (PC 9)	Laogong (PC 8)	Daling (PC 7)	Jianshi (PC 5)	Quze (PC 3)
	Heart (fire)	Shaochong (HT 9)	Sha fu (HT 8)	Shenmen (HT 7)	Lingdao (HT 4)	Shaohai (HT 3)

Continue to Table 11-2

Six yin meridians		Well points (wood)	Spring points (fire)	Stream points (earth)	River points (metal)	Sea points (water)
Three yin meridians of foot	Spleen(earth)	Yinbai (SP 1)	Dadu (SP 2)	Taibai (SP 3)	Shangqiu (SP 5)	Yinlingquan (SP 9)
	Liver(wood)	Dadun (LR 1)	Xingjian (LR 2)	Taichong (LR 3)	Zhongfeng(LR 4)	Ququan (LR 8)
	Kidney(water)	Yongquan (KI 1)	Rangu (KI 2)	Taixi (KI 3)	Fuliu (KI 7)	Yingu (KI 10)

Table 11-3   Five transport points of the six yang meridians

Six yang meridians		Well points (metal)	Spring points (water)	Stream points (wood)	River points (fire)	Sea points (earth)
Three yang meridians of hand	Large intestine (metal)	Shangyang (LI 1)	Erjian (LI 2)	Sanjian (LI 3)	Yangxi (LI 5)	Quchi (LI 11)
	Triple energizer (ministerial fire)	Guanchong (TE 1)	Yemen (TE 2)	Zhongzhu (TE 3)	Zhigou (TE 6)	Tianjing (TE 10)
	Small intestine (fire)	Shaoze (SI 1)	Qiangu (SI 2)	Houxi (SI 3)	Yanggu (SI 5)	Xiaohai (SI 8)
Three yang meridians of foot	Stomach(earth)	Lidui (ST 45)	Neiting (ST 44)	Xiangu (ST 43)	Jiexi (ST 41)	Zusanli (ST 36)
	Gallbladder(wood)	Zuqiaoyin (GB 44)	Xiaxi (GB 43)	Zulingqi (GB 41)	Yangfu (GB 38)	Yanglingquan (GB 34)
	Bladder(water)	Zhiyin (BL 67)	Zutonggu (BL 66)	Shugu (BL 65)	Kunlun (BL 60)	Weizhong (BL 40)

Based on ancient documents and contemporary clinical practice, the five transport points are applied as follows.

(1)Selecting the five transport points according to their characteristics

The indications of the five transport points are various in ancient documents. As stated in *Miraculous Pivot*, "well points are selected for diseases of zang viscera, spring points for diseases with changes in colors, stream points for intermittent conditions, river points for abnormality in voice, and sea points for stomach disorders caused by irregular diet". *Classic of Difficult Issues* states, "well points are indicated for epigastric fullness, spring points for fever, stream points for heaviness of the body and pain of the joints, river points for asthma, cough, chill and fever, and sea points for reversed flow of qi and diarrhea." This statement mainly focuses on therapeutic effects of the five transport points from the perspective of relation between the attributes of the five transport points of yin meridians and attributes of their internally related zang viscera.

(2)Selecting the five transport points according to mutual relations of generation and restraint

The five transport points follow the law of five element theory. According to the principle for reinforcing and reducing established by *Classic of Difficult Issues*："Reinforce the mother when the son is deficient and reduce the son when the mother is excessive",the mother or son point from the five transport points on the diseased meridian are selected. For instance,the lung corresponds to metal,whose son is water and mother is earth. When the lung is excessive,Chize(LU 5),the sea point of the lung meridian corresponding to water,is reduced. When the lung is deficient,Taiyuan(LU 9),the stream point of the lung meridian corresponding to earth,is reinforced. These are typical examples of application of the mother or son point on diseased meridian.

In addition,the mother point from the mother meridian and the son point from the son meridian are also applied clinically. For example,when the lung is excessive,Yingu(KI 10),the sea point corresponding to water from the kidney meridian corresponding to water too,is reduced. When the lung is deficient,Taibai (SP 3),the stream point corresponding to earth from the spleen meridian corresponding to earth too,is reinforced.

11.2.4.2　Back transport points and alarm points

Back transport points are the points on the back where the qi of the respective zang-fu viscera is infused. Alarm points are the points on the chest or abdomen where the qi of the respective zang-fu viscera infuses and converges.

All back transport points are located on the first lateral line of the bladder meridian of foot taiyang. All alarm points are located close to their corresponding zang-fu viscera. Each of the six zang and six fu viscera has one alarm point and one back transport point on each side of the spine(Table 11-4).

Table 11-4　Back transport and alarm points of the zang-fu viscera

Zang-fu viscera	Back transport points	Alarm points
Lung	Feishu(BL 13)	Zhongfu(LU 1)
Pericardium	Jueyinshu(BL 14)	Danzhong(CV 17)
Heart	Xinshu(BL 15)	Juque(CV 14)
Liver	Ganshu(BL 18)	Qimen(LR 14)
Gallbladder	Danshu(BL 19)	Riyue(GB 24)
Spleen	Pishu(BL 20)	Zhangmen(LR 13)
Stomach	Weishu(BL 21)	Zhongwan(CV 12)
Triple energizer	Sanjiaoshu(BL 22)	Shimen(CV 5)
Kidney	Shenshu(BL 23)	Jingmen GB 25)
Large intestine	Dachangshu(BL 25)	Tianshu(ST 25)
Small intestine	Xiaochangshu(BL 27)	Guanyuan(CV 4)
Bladder	Pangguangshu(BL 28)	Zhongji(CV 3)

In general,back transport points are more often used for yin diseases including disorders of zang viscera,cold or deficiency syndrome. Alarm points are more often used for yang diseases including disorders of fu-viscera,heat or excess syndrome. For example,Shenshu(BL 23),the back transport point of kidney,is indicated for kidney deficiency syndrome. Tianshu(ST 25),the alarm point of large intestine,is used to treat disorders of intestines,such as abdominal distension or pain,diarrhea,constipation and so on.

Back transport points and alarm points can be used either alone or in combination. The latter is called "back transport and alarm point combination method". For example, Danshu(BL 19) and Riyue(GB 24) are both selected to treat gallbladder diseases.

11.2.4.3 Source points and connecting points

Source points are a group of twelve meridian points located near the wrist or ankle where the original qi of zang-fu viscera and meridians passes and gathers. Source point of a yin meridian is identical to its stream point, whereas source point of a yang meridian is independent from its stream point.

Connecting points are locations where the fifteen collaterals branch out from the meridians. There is one-connecting point on each of the twelve meridians, the governor vessel, the conception vessel, and the major collateral of the spleen. Therefore, they are called "fifteen connecting points"(Table 11-5).

Table 11-5   Source points and connecting points of the meridians

Meridians	Source points	Connecting points
Lung meridian	Taiyuan(LU 9)	Lieque(LU 7)
Pericardium meridian	Daling(PC 7)	Neiguan(PC 6)
Heart meridian	Shenmen(HT 7)	Tongli(HT 5)
Spleen meridian	Taibai(SP 3)	Gongsun(SP 4)
Liver meridian	Taichong(LR 3)	Ligou(LR 5)
Kidney meridian	Taixi(KI 3)	Dazhong(KI 4)
Large intestine meridian	Hegu(LI 4)	Pianli(LI 6)
Triple energizer meridian	Yangchi(TE 4)	Waiguan(TE 5)
Small intestine meridian	Wangu(SI 4)	Zhizheng(SI 7)
Stomach meridian	Chongyang(ST 42)	Fenglong(ST 40)
Gallbladder meridian	Qiuxu(GB 40)	Guangming(GB 37)
Bladder meridian	Jinggu(BL 64)	Feiyang(BL 58)
Governor vessel		Changqiang(GV 1)
Conception vessel		Jiuwei(CV 15)
Major collateral of the spleen		Dabao(SP 21)

Source points and connecting points can be used either alone or in combination. When a source point of a primary diseased meridian is combined with connecting point of the interior-exterior related meridian which is affected subsequently, it is called "source-connecting points combination" or "host-guest points combination". For example, when the liver meridian is diseased first and the gallbladder meridian is affected subsequently, Taichong(LR 3) which is the source point of the liver meridian, and Guangming(GB 37) which is the connecting point of the gallbladder, are used in combination.

11.2.4.4 Confluence points of the eight extra meridians

The confluence points of the eight extra meridians are the eight points on the four limbs where the twelve meridians communicate with the eight extra meridians(Table 11-6).

Table 11-6   Confluence points of the eight extra meridians

Eight confluence points and their related extrao meridians	Indications
Gongsun(SP 4)(thoroughfare vessel) Neiguan(PC 6)(yin link vessel)	Problems of the stomach, heart and chest
Houxi(SI 3)(governor vessel) Shenmai(BL 62)(yang heel vessel)	Problems of the inner canthus, nape, ear and shoulder
Zulinqi(GB 41)(belt vessel) Waiguan(TE 5)(yang link vessel)	Problems of the outer canthus, cheek, neck, the posterior of the ear, and shoulder
Lieque(LU 7)(conception vessel) Zhaohai(KI 6)(yin heel vessel)	Problems of the chest, lung, diaphragm and throat

In clinical practice, each confluence point is effective for diseases of its related extra meridian. For instance, Houxi(SI 3), a confluence point communicating with the governor vessel, is applicable for diseases of the governor vessel such as stiffness or pain of the spine.

The eight confluence points are usually used in pairs according to the relationship of the eight extra meridians and areas where two extra meridians meet. For example, Gongsun(SP 4) and Neiguan(PC 6) are the confluence points of the thoroughfare vessel and yin link vessel respectively; they are used in combination to treat diseases of the heart, chest and stomach, where the two meridians both distribute.

11.2.4.5   The eight meeting points

The eight meeting points are eight points corresponding respectively to eight kinds of viscera and tissues, including zang viscera, fu viscera, qi, blood, sinew, vessels, bones and marrow. Each of points treats diseases of its corresponding viscera or tissue. For example, Danzhong(CV 17), the meeting point of qi, is applicable for qi disorders. Yanglingquan(GB 34), the meeting point of sinew, treats sinew disorders(Table 11-7).

Table 11-7   The eight meeting points

Eight meeting points	Viscera or tissues
Zhangmen(LR 13)	zang viscera
Zhongwan(CV 12)	fu viscera
Danzhong(CV 17)	qi
Geshu(BL 17)	blood
Yanglingquan(GB 34)	tendons
Taiyuan(LU 9)	vessels
Dazhu(BL 11)	bones
Xuanzhong(GB 39)	marrow

11.2.4.6   Cleft points

Cleft points are locations where the meridian qi is deeply converged and accumulated in the limbs. Most cleft points are situated distal to elbow or knee. Each of the twelve meridians and the four extra vessels, yin and yang link vessel, yin and yang heel vessel, has one cleft points. There are sixteen cleft points in all(Table 11-8).

Table 11-8 Cleft points of the meridians

Yin meridians	Cleft points	Yang meridians	Cleft points
Lung meridian	Kongzui(LU 6)	Large intestine meridian	Wenliu(LI 7)
Spleen meridian	Diji(SP 8)	Stomach meridian	Liangqiu(ST 34)
Heart meridian	Yinxi(HT 6)	Small intestine meridian	Yanglao(SI 6)
Kidney meridian	Shuiquan(KI 5)	Bladder meridian	Jinmen(BL 63)
Pericardium meridian	Ximen(PC 4)	Triple energizer meridian	Huizong(TE 7)
Liver meridian	Zhongdu(LR 6)	Gallbladder meridian	Waiqiu(GB 36)
Yin link vessel	Zhubin(KI 9)	Yang link vessel	Yangjiao(GB 35)
Yin heel vessel	Jiaoxin(KI 8)	Yang heel vessel	Fuyang(BL 59)

Cleft points are frequently used for acute diseases of their respective meridians and their internally connected zang-fu viscera. Specifically, cleft points of yin meridians are effective for bleeding, while those of yang meridians are more frequently used for acute pain. For example, Kongzui(LU 6), the cleft point of the lung meridian, is applicable for hemoptysis. Liangqiu(ST 34), the cleft point of the stomach meridian, is effective for stomachache. In addition, cleft points are often used in combination with the eight meeting points, hence the name "cleft-confluent points combination". For instance, Geshu(BL 17), the meeting point of blood, is combined with Kongzui(LU 6)to treat hemoptysis. Zhongwan(CV 12), the meeting point of fu viscera, is used in combination with Liangqiu(ST 34)for stomachache.

11.2.4.7 Lower sea points

The lower sea points, also called lower sea points of the six fu viscera, are the six points where the qi of the six fu viscera flows down towards the three yang meridians of foot. The lower sea points of the stomach, gallbladder and bladder are identical to sea points of respective meridian, while the lower sea points of the large intestine, small intestine and triple energizer are independent of sea points in respective meridian(Table 11-9).

Table 11-9 Lower Sea points of six fu viscera

The six fu viscera	Lower sea points
Stomach	Zusanli(ST 36)
Large intestine	Shangjuxu(ST 37)
Small intestine	Xiajuxu(ST 39)
Triple energizer	Weiyang(BL 39)
Bladder	Weizhong(BL 40)
Gallbladder	Yanglingquan(GB 34)

As stated in Miraculous Pivot, "the lower sea points treat diseases of the fu-viscera". For example, Zusanli(ST 36), the lower sea point of stomach, is the main point to treat vomiting, stomach bloating and pain. Weizhong(ST 40), the lower sea point of bladder, is effective for uroschesis and enuresis.

11.2.4.8 Crossing points

Crossing points are those at which two or more meridians intersect. Most crossing points are distributed on the head, face and trunk.

A crossing point is indicated for diseases of its pertaining meridian and the meridians that intersect at the point. For instance, Sanyinjiao(SP 6), a crossing point where three yin meridians of foot cross, is used not only for diseases of the spleen meridian, but also for diseases of the liver meridian and the kidney meridian. Chengjiang(CV 24), the crossing point of the conception vessel, the governor vessel, the large intestine meridian and the stomach meridian, treats diseases of these four meridians.

11.2.5 Methods for locating acupoints

In general, commonly used methods for locating acupoints include anatomical landmarks measurement, proportional bone measurement, finger cun measurement and simplified measurement.

11.2.5.1 Location of acupoints according to anatomical landmarks on body surface

The anatomical landmarks used to locate acupoints are divided into fixed landmarks and moving landmarks.

(1) Fixed anatomical landmarks

Fixed anatomical landmarks refer to prominences and depressions formed by the joints and muscles, contours of the eyes, ears, nose and mouth, fingernails and toenails, the nipples, the umbilicus and so on. For example, Cuanzhu(BL 2) is in the depression at the medial end of the eyebrow. Danzhong(CV 17) is between the nipples. Chengshan(BL 57) is on the posterior aspect of the leg where the calcaneal tendon connects with the two muscle bellies of the gastrocnemius. Yanglingquan(GB 34) is in the depression anterior and distal to the head of the fibula.

Commonly used anatomical landmarks on the back for locating acupoints are listed in Table 11-10.

Table 11-10   Commonly used anatomical landmarks on the back

Anatomical landmarks	Notes
The sternal angle	At the same level as the second rib
The nipples in males	At the same level as the fourth intercostal space
The spinous process of the seventh cervical vertebra	The most prominent spinous process on the posterior median line of the neck
The medial ends of the two spines of the scapula	At the same level as the spinous process of the third thoracic vertebra
The inferior angles of the scapula	At the same level as the spinous process of the seventh thoracic vertebra
The spinous process of the twelfth thoracic vertebra	At the same level as the midpoint of the line connecting the inferior angle of the scapula with the highest point of the iliac crest
The highest points of the iliac crests	At the same level as the spinous process of the fourth lumbar vertebra

(2) Moving landmarks

Moving landmarks refer to the depressions and folds on the joints, muscles and skin with reference to specific body movements. For instance, Ermen(TE 21), Tinggong(SI 19) and Tinghui(GB 2) are located with the mouth open. Xiaguan(ST 7) is located when the mouth closed. Jiache(ST 6) is at the prominence of the masseter muscle when teeth are clenched.

11.2.5.2 Location of acupoints by bone proportional cun

Location of acupoints by bone proportional cun refers to a method that using bones and joints as landmarkers to measure the length and width of various parts of the body and then convert them into proportional units for locating points. This method is based on the patient's own body: the length of a given bone or the distance between two joints is divided into equal units, and each unit is considered as one cun. This method of measurement is applicable for locating points on patients of different sexes, ages and body types. There are 4 proportional bone measurements at head and face. With longitudinal measurement, the distance is 12 cun from the midpoint of the anterior hairline to the midpoint of the posterior hairline and 3 cun from the glabella to the midpoint of the anterior hairline. If the anterior and posterior hairlines are indistinguishable, the distance from the glabella to Dazhui(GV 14) is measured as 18 cun. The distance from Dazhui(GV 14) to the posterior hairline is 3 cun. With transverse measurement, the distance is 9 cun between the bilateral corners of the anterior hairline on the forehead and 9 cun Between the bilateral mastoid processes.

There are 5 proportional bone measurements at chest and abdomen. With longitudinal measurement, the distance is 9 cun from the suprasternal fossa to the midpoint of the xiphisternal symphysis, 8 cun from the midpoint of the xiphisternal symphysis to the center of the umbilicus and 5 cun from the center of the umbilicus to the superior border of the pubic symphysis. With transverse measurement, the distance is 12 cun between the bilateral medial borders of the coracoid and 8 cun between the two nipples. For female, the distance between the two nipples may be substituted by the two mid-clavicular lines. There are 1 proportional bone measurements at back. With transverse measurement, the distance is 3 cun from the medial border of the scapula to the posterior midline. There are 2 proportional bone measurements at upper limbs. With longitudinal measurement, the distance is 9 cun from the anterior or posterior axillary fold to the cubital crease and 12 cum from the cubital crease to the wrist crease. There are 8 proportional bone measurements at lower limbs. With longitudinal measurement, the distance is 18 cun from the superior border of the pubic symphysis to the base of patella, 2 cun from the base of the patella to the apex of the patella, 15 cun from the apex of the patella(the center of the popliteal fossa) to the prominence of the medial malleolus, 13 cun from the inferior border of medial condyle of the tibia to the prominence of the medial malleolus, 19 cun from the prominence of the greater trochanter of femur to the popliteal crease, 14 cun from the gluteal fold to the popliteal crease, 16 cun from the popliteal crease to the prominence of the lateral malleolus and 3 cun from the prominence of medial malleolus to the sole.

11.2.5.3 Location of acupoints by cun measurement

Finger cun measurement refers to a method using the length or width of the patient's fingers for locating acupoints. Commonly used finger cun measurement methods include middle finger cun, thumb cun and finger-breadth cun.

(1)Middle finger cun: The distance between the ends of the two radial creases of the interphalangeal joints of the middle finger is taken as one cun when the middle finger is bent.

(2)Thumb body cun: The width of the interphalangeal joint of the thumb is taken as one cun.

(3)Finger-breadth cun: When the patient's four fingers(the index, middle, ring and little finger) are extended and closed together, the width of the four fingers at the level of the crease of the proximal interphalangeal joint of the middle finger is taken as three cun. This method is also called "four-finger measurement".

11.2.5.4 Simplified measurement

Simplified measurement is a simple method to locate acupoints. For example, when the index fingers and thumbs of both hands are crossed with one index finger in extending position, Lieque(LU 7) is under the tip of the index finger. When a loose fist is made, Laogong(PC 8) is just under the tip of the middle finger. Baihui(GV 20) is located at the center of the line between the ear apexes. Simplified measurement is usually applied as an auxiliary to other methods of point locating.

11.3   Meridians and acupoints

11.3.1   Frequently used acupoints on the twelve meridians

11.3.1.1   Frequently used acupoints on lung meridian of hand taiyin

Lung meridian of hand taiyin originates from the middle energizer, and descends to connect with the large intestine. It then returns to connect the lung and exits transversely from lung system where the lung communicates with the throat. It descends along the anterior side of forearm and the upper arm and enters the cun kou. It then passes through the major thenar eminence, goes out to terminate at the medial side of the tip of the thumb. A branch of this meridian splits from the styloid process of the wrist and runs to the radial side of the tip of the index finger(Figure 11-2).

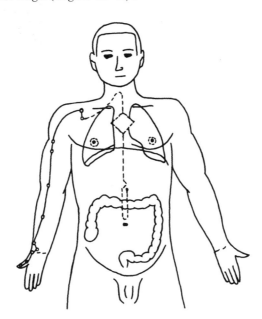

Figure 11-2   The course of lung merdian of hand taiyin

(1)Zhongfu(LU 1)alarm point of the lung

Location: On the upper lateral chest, 6 cun lateral to the anterior midline and at the same level of the first intercostal space(Figure 11-3).

Indications: ①Cough, asthma, fullness in the chest, chest pain. ②Upper back pain.

Manipulation: Insert the needle obliquely into the lateral side of the chest, 0.5-0.8 cun deep. Deep perpendicular insertion toward the medial aspect is prohibited in order to avoid puncturing the lung and causing pneumothorax.

(2)Chize(LU 5)sea point

Location: On the transverse crease of the elbow, in the radial depression of the tendon of the biceps muscle(Figure 11-4).

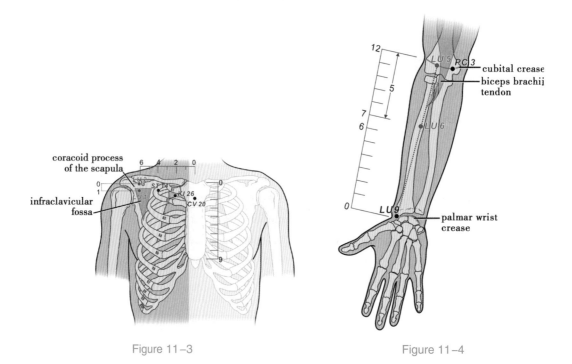

Figure 11-3　　　　　　　　　　　　　　Figure 11-4

Indications：①Cough，asthma，coughing up blood，sore throat，tidal fever. ②Spasm and pain in the upper arm. ③Acute vomiting and diarrhea. ④Infantile convulsion.

Manipulation：Insert the needle perpendicularly by 0.5-0.8 cun deep or prick to allow bleeding.

(3)Kongzui(LU 6)cleft point

Location：On the medial side of the forearm，along the line linking Taiyuan(LU 9)and Chize(LU 5)，7 cun above the transverse crease of the wrist(Figure 11-5).

Indications：①Cough，coughing up blood，asthma，nosebleed，sore throat. ②Spasm and pain in the arm.

Manipulation：Insert the needle perpendicularly by 0.5-1.0 cun deep.

(4)Lieque(LU 7)connecting point；one of the eight confluence points associating with the conception vessel

Location：On the radial aspect of the forearm beween the extensor pollicis brevis tendon and the abductor pollicis longus tendon in the groove of the abductor pollicis longus tendon，1.5 cun superior to the palmar wrist crease(Figure 11-5).

Indications：①Lung system diseases like cough，asthma，sore throat，etc. ②Craniofacial diseases like rigidity of nape with headache，deviated mouth and eyes，toothache，etc. ③Pain in the wrist.

Manipulation：Insert the needle obliquely upward by 0.3-0.8 cun deep.

(5)Taiyuan(LU 9)stream point，source point，one of the eight meeting points(vessels convergence)

Location：Between the radial styloid process and the scaphoid，in the depression ulnar to the abductor pollicis longus tendon，on the radial side of the transverse crease of the wrist where radial artery pluses(Figure 11-6).

Indications：①Cough，asthma，coughing blood，chest pain，sore throat. ②Acrotism. ③Pain in the wrist.

Manipulation：Keep away from artery and insert the needle perpendicularly by 0.2-0.3 cun deep.

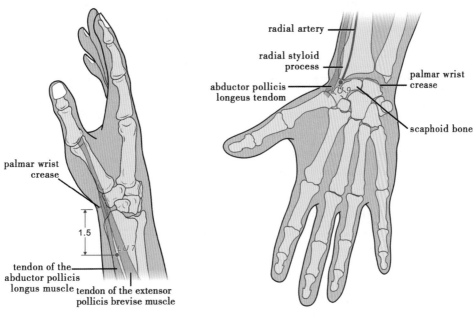

Figure 11-5   Figure 11-6

(6) Yuji(LU 10) spring point

Location: On the midpoint of the 1st metacarpal bone, on the junction of the red and white skin (Figure 11-7).

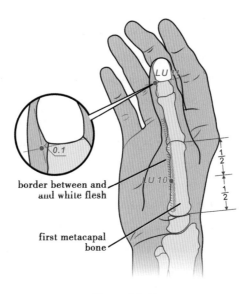

Figure 11-7

Indications: ①Cough, asthma, coughing up blood, sore throat, sudden loss of voice. ②Palm hot. ③Infantile malnutrition.

Manipulation: Insert the needle perpendicularly by 0.5-0.8 cun deep. Subcutaneous tissue resection therapy to treat infantile malnutrition is available.

(7) Shaoshang(LU 11) well point

Location: On the radial side of the thumb, about 0.1 cun from the corner of the fingernail.

Indications: ①Swollen and sore throat, cough, nosebleed, high fever, unconsciousness. ②Psychosis.

Manipulation: Insert the needle superficially by 0. 1 cun, or prick to allow bleeding.

Other points on lung meridian of hand taiyin see Table 11-11.

Table 11-11　Other points on lung meridian of hand taiyin

Points	Code	Location	Indication
Yunmen	LU 2	On the upper lateral chest, superior to the coracoid process of the scapula, in the depression of the infraclavicular fossa, 6 cun lateral to the anterior midline	①Cough, asthma, pain in the chest. ②Shoulder and upper back pain
Tianfu	LU 3	On the radial border of the biceps muscle, 3 cun below the front end of the axillary fold	①Cough, asthma, nosebleed, goiter. ②Pain in the upper arm
Xiabai	LU 4	On the radial side of the tendon of the biceps muscle, 4 cun below the front end of the axillary fold	①Cough, asthma, nausea. ②Pain in the upper arm
Jiingqu (river point)	LU 8	In the depression between the styloid process of the radius and the radial side, 1 cun above the transverse crease of the wrist	①Cough, asthma, chest pain. ②Swelling and pain in the throat. ③Pain in the wrist

11.3.1.2　Frequently used acupoints on large intestine meridian of hand yangming

Large intestine meridian of hand yangming starts from the tip of the index finger, proceeding upward along the radial side of the index finger, then goes upwards along the anterior aspect of the forearm and the lateral anterior aspect of the upper arm and reaches the anterior upper aspect of the shoulder joint. It then goes backward crossing Dazhui(GV 14) and descents to the supraclavicular fossa and enters into chest to connect with the lung, and then it goes downwards to connect the pertaining large intestine. Its branch splits from the supraclavicular fossa and runs upwards to the head.

It splits from the supraclavicular fossa and runs upwards along the neck, passes through the cheek and enters the gingiva of the lower teeth. It then curves around the corner of the mouth and intersects at the philtrum with the opposite side of the same meridian, with this intersection the meridian on the right hand proceeds to the left while the left to right. It finally terminates on the lateral side of the nose(Figure 11-8).

(1)Shangyang(LI 1)well point

Location: 0. 1 cun lateral to the radial nail corner of the index finger(Figure 11-9).

Indications: ①Swollen and sore throat, toothache. ②Loss of consciousness, sunstroke. ③Febrile diseases.

Manipulation: Insert the needle superficially by 0. 1 cun deep, or prick to induce bleeding.

(2)Hegu(LI 4)source point

Location: Between the 1st and 2nd metacapal bones, approximately in the middle of the 2nd metacarpal bone on the radial side(Figure 11-10).

Indications: ①Headache, deviated mouth and eye, toothache, conjunctival congestion, nosebleed, deafness. ②Fever, aversion to cold, with or without sweating. ③Amenorrhea, delayed labour. ④Paralysis of the forearm, unable to move voluntarily, painful wrist and forearm.

Manipulation : Insert the needle perpendicularly by 0. 5–1. 0 cun deep. It is contraindicated for pregnant women.

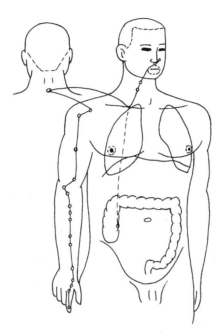

Figure 11–8　The course of large intestine meridian of hand yangming

(3) Yangxi(LI 5) river point

Location : At the radial side of the dorsal wrist crease, distal to the radial styloid process in the depression of the anatomical snuffbox, between the tendons of the extensor pollicis longus and extensor pollicis brevis(Figure 11–10).

Indications : ①Headache, toothache, sore throat. ②Pain in the wrist.

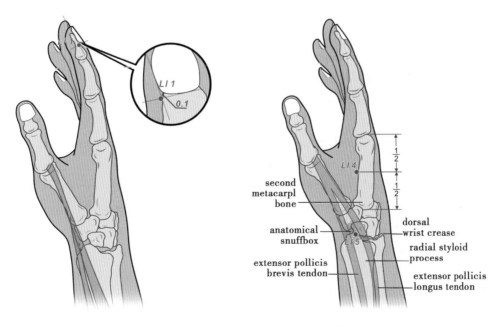

Figure 11–9　　　　　　　　　　　　　　　　Figure 11–10

Manipulation:Insert the needle perpendicularly by 0.3–0.5 cun deep.

(4)Pianli(LI 6)connecting point

Location:With the elbow slightly flexed,on the radial side of the dorsal surface of the forearm and on the line connecting Yangxi(LI 5)and Quchi(LI 11),3 cun above the crease of the wrist(Figure 11–11).

Indications:①Nosebleed,tinnitus,deafness. ②Pain in the forearm. ③Abdominal distending pain. ④Edema.

Manipulation:Insert the needle perpendicularly by 0.3–0.5 cun deep.

(5)Shousanli(LI 10)

Location:On the line linking the Yangxi(LI 5)and Quchi(LI 11)points,2 cun below Quchi(LI 11) (Figure 11–12).

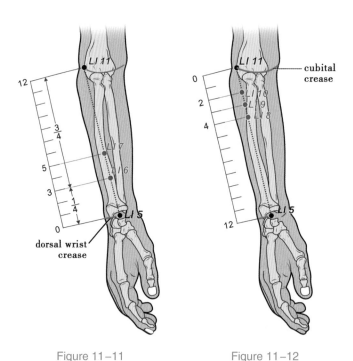

Figure 11–11   Figure 11–12

Indications:①Paralysis of the forearm,pain and numbness in the elbow and arm. ②Toothache,swollen cheek. ③Abdominal pain,diarrhea.

Manipulation:Insert the needle perpendicularly by 0.8–1.2 cun deep.

(6)Quchi(LI 11)sea point

Location:With the elbow flexed,at the lateral end of the transverse cubital crease,midway between Chize(LU 5)and the lateral epicondyle of the humerus(Figure 11–13).

Indications:①Swollen and sore throat,toothache,redness and pain in the eyes. ②Febrile diseases. ③Rubella,eczema. ④Hypertension. Paralysis of the arm,pain and weakness in the elbow. ⑤Psychosis. ⑥Abdominal pain,diarrhea.

Manipulation:Insert the needle perpendicularly by 0.8–1.5 cun deep.

(7)Binao(LI 14)

Location:On the lateral side of the arm anterior to the border of the deltoid muscle,7 cun superior to Quchi(LI 11)(Figure 11–14).

Indications:①Painful upper arm and shoulder,impaired arm movement. ②Eye diseases. ③Scrofula.

Manipulation:Insert the needle perpendicularly or obliquely upward by 0.8–1.5 cun deep.

(8) Jianyu(LI 15)

Location: On the shoulder girdle in the depression between the anterior end of the lateral border of the acromion and the greater tubercle of the humerus(Figure 11−14).

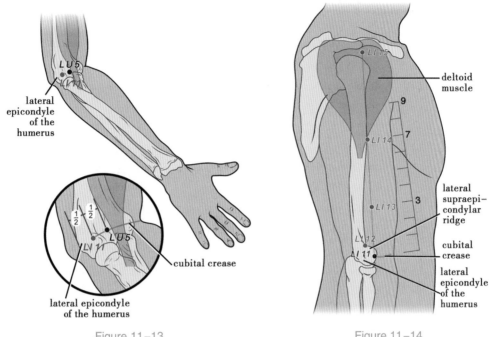

Figure 11−13   Figure 11−14

Indications: ①Pain and numbness in the upper arm and shoulder, impaired movement of arm. ②Scrofula.

Manipulation: Insert the needle perpendicularly or obliquely downward by 0.8−1.5 cun deep.

(9) Yingxiang(LI 20)

Location: 0.5 cun beside the lateral border of the nasal ala, in the nasolabial groove(Figure 11−15).

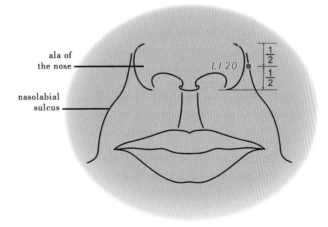

Figure 11−15

Indications: ①Nasal obstruction, nosebleed, sinusitis. ②Facial paralysis, facial itchiness. ③Ascariasis of the biliary tract.

Manipulation: 0.2−0.5 cun deep perpendicular or oblique insertion.

Other points on large intestine meridian of hand yangming see Table 11-12.

Table 11-12 **Other points on large intestine meridian of hand yangming**

Points	Code	Location	Indication
Erjian(spring point)	LI 2	In the depression of the radial side, distal to the 2nd metacarpopbalangeal joint when a loose fiat is made	①Nosebleed, toothache, red and swollen eyes, deviated mouth and eye. ②Febrile disease
Sanjian(stream point)	LI 3	In the depression of the radial side and proximal to the 2nd metacarpophalangeal joint	①Toothache, nosebleed, sore throat. ②Fever
Wenliu(cleft point)	LI 7	With the elbow flexed, on the line linking theYangxi(LI 5) and Quchi(LI 11) points, 5 cun above the wrist crease	① Headache, swollen of the face, sore throat. ② Aching shoulders and back. ③Abdominal pain, borborygmus
Xialian	LI 8	On the line connecting Yangxi(LI 5) and Quchi(LI 11), 4 cun below the cubital crease	①Headache, vertigo and pain in the elbow. ② Abdominal distention, abdominal pain, pain in the elbow and arm
Shanglian	LI 9	On the line connecting Yangxi(LI 5) and Quchi(LI 11), 3 cun below the cubital crease	①Pain and numbness in the elbow and arm, paralysis of the forearm, headache. ②Borborygmus, abdominal pain
Zhouliao	LI 12	With the elbow flexed, 1 cun above the Quchi(LI 11) point, on the border of the humerus	Aching, numbness and spasm of the elbow and arm
Shouwuli	LI 13	On the line connecting Quchi(LI 11) and Jianyu(LI 15), 3 cun above Quchi(LI 11)	①Spasm and pain in the elbow and arm. ②Scrofula
Jugu	LI 16	In the upper portion of the shoulder, in the depression between the acromial extremity of the clavicle and the scapular spine	①Pain of the shoulder and upper back. ②Scrofula, goiter
Tianding	LI 17	On the lateral side of the neck, on the posterior border of sternocleidomastoid muscle, at the midpoint of the line linking the Futu(LI 18) and Quepen(ST 12) points	①Sore throat, sudden loss of voice. ②Scrofula, goiter
Futu	LI 18	3 cun lateral to the tip of the Adam's apple, between the sternal head and clavicular head of musculus sternocleidomatoideus	①Sore throat, sudden loss of voice. ②Scrofula, goiter. ③Cough and asthma
Kouheliao	LI 19	On the upper lip, directly below the lateral border of the nostril, on the level of Shuigou (GV 26)	Nosebleed, nasal obstruction, deviated face, trismus

11.3.1.3 Frequently used acupoints on stomach meridian of foot yangming

The stomach meridian of foot yangming starts from the lateral side of the nose. It travels upward to the root of the nose where it meets the foot taiyang meridian. Turning downward along the lateral side of the nose, it enters the upper gingiva. Curving around the lips, it meets Chengjiang(CV 24) in the mentolabial groove. It then travels to the posterior aspect of the mandible passing through the facial artery, ascending in front of the ear and following the anterior hairline, it reaches the forehead at last.

Cheek Branch: Its cheek branch splits from the front of the Daying(ST 5) and passes through the carotid artery. Passing along the throat, it enters the supraclavicular fossa. It further descends and passes through the diaphragm, and then enters its pertaining organ, the stomach, and connects to the spleen, the related organ.

The stomach meridian descends from face to throat and enters the supraclavicular fossa then enters its pertaining organ, the stomach, and connects to the spleen, the related organ. The straight branch of the meridian emerges from the supraclavicular fossa, which passes through the nipple descends along the lateral side of umbilicus and enters Qichong(ST 30) which is located in the lower abdomen.

The branch starts from the lower orifice of the stomach, and descends inside of the abdomen, reaching Qichong(ST 30). From here, it further descends to Biguan(ST 31) and goes downward to the knee. From the knee, it continues further down along the anterior border of the lateral aspect of the tieba to the dorsum of the foot and reaches the lateral side of the tip of the second toe.

The tibial branch of the meridian splits from the place 3 cun below the knee and runs downward and ends at the lateral side of the middle toe. Another branch on the foot emerges from the dorsum of the foot to enter the medial side of the tip of big toe(Figure 11-16).

(1)Chengqi(ST 1)

Location: On the face, directly below the pupil with the eyes looking straight forward, between the eyeball and the infraorbital ridge(Figure 11-17).

Indications: ①Trembling eyelids, red and swollen eyes, night blindness, lacrimation upon exposure to wind. ②Deviation of the mouth and eyes, prosopospasm.

Manipulation: With the eyes closed, push the eyeball upward slightly with the left thumb and puncture perpendicularly and slowly by 0.5-1.0 cun along the infraorbitalridge. It is not advisable to manipulate the needle with a large amplitude, compress the needling hole after withdrawing the needle.

(2)Sibai(ST 2)

Location: On the face, directly below the pupil with the eyes looking straight forward, in the depression of the infraorbital foramen(Figure 11-17).

Indications: ①Red and painful eyes, lacrimation upon exposure to wind, superficial visual obstruction, blurred vision. ②Deviation of the mouth and eye, twitching of the eyelids, facial pain and itchiness. ③Vertigo.

Manipulation: 0.3-0.5 cun deep perpendicular insertion. It is not advisable to manipulate the needle with large amplitude.

(3)Dicang(ST 4)

Location: On the face, 0.4 cun beside the corner of the mouth(Figure 11-18).

Indications: Deviation of the mouth and eyes, trembling lips, lacrimation.

Manipulation: 0.5-0.8 cun horizontal insertion toward Jiache(ST 6).

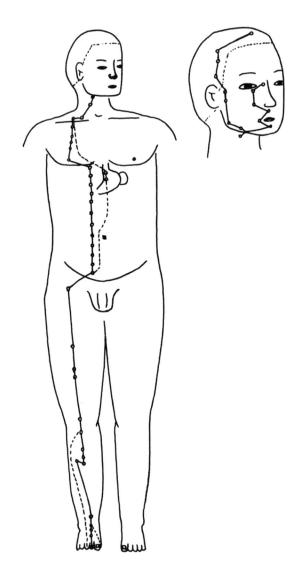

Figure 11–16   The course of stomach meridian of foot yangming

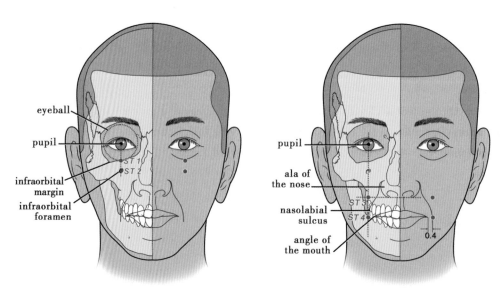

Figure 11–17

Figure 11–18

(4) Jiache(ST 6)

Location: On the cheek, one finger width anterior and superior to the mandibular angle, in the depression where the masseter muscle is prominent(Figure 11-19).

Indications: Deviation of the mouth and eyes, swollen cheeks, toothache, locked jaw, spasm of facial muscles.

Manipulation: 0. 3-0. 5 cun deep perpendicular insertion or 1. 3-1. 5 cun oblique insertion toward Dicang(ST 4).

(5) Xiaguan(ST 7)

Location: On the face, anterior to the ear, in the depression between the zygomatic arch and mandibular notch(Figure 11-20).

Indications: ①Lower mandible pain, locked jaw, deviated mouth and eyes, toothache, swollen cheek, facial pain. ②Deafness, tinnitus, ear infection.

Manipulation: 0. 5-1. 0 cun deep perpendicular insertions. It is not advisable to open mouth when retaining the needle so as to avoid curving or breaking the needle.

(6) Touwei(ST 8)

Location: On the lateral side of the head, 0. 5 cun above the anterior hairline, and 4. 5 cun lateral to the anterior midline of the forehead(Figure 11-20).

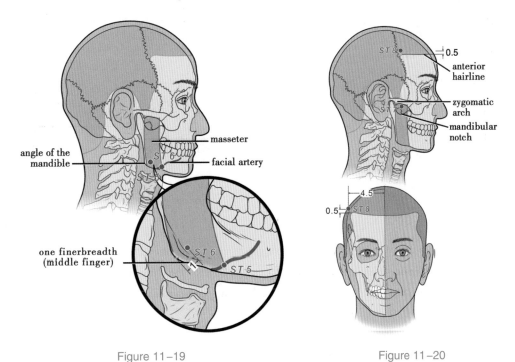

Figure 11-19　　　　　　　　　　　　Figure 11-20

Indications: Headache, vertigo, lacrimation upon exposure to wind, eyes pain.

Manipulation: 0. 5-1. 0 cun horizontal insertions backward.

(7) Liangmen(ST 21)

Location: On the upper abdomen, 4 cun above the center of the umbilicus, 2 cun lateral to the anterior midline of the abdomen(Figure 11-21).

Indications: Stomachache, vomiting, poor appetite, and abdominal distension.

Manipulation: 0. 8-1. 2 cun perpendicularly insertion. Needling is not advisable for people with hepatomegaly or who have recently had a great feed. It is not advisable to manipulate the needle with large amplitude.

(8) Tianshu(ST 25) alarm point of the large intestine

Location: 2 cun lateral to the center of the umbilicus(Figure 11-21).

Indications: ①Abdominal pain, abdominal distension, borborygmus, diarrhea, dysentery, constipation, intestinal abscess. ②Irregular menstruation, dysmenorrhea.

Manipulation: 1.0-1.5 cun perpendicular insertion.

(9) Guilai(ST 29)

Location: 4 cun below the umbilicus, 2 cun lateral to the anterior midline of the abdomen(Figure 11-22).

Indications: ① Amenia, prolapse of the uterus, dysmenorrheal, leucorrhea, irregular menstruation. ②Lower abdominal pain, hernia.

Manipulation: 0.8-1.2 cun perpendicular insertion.

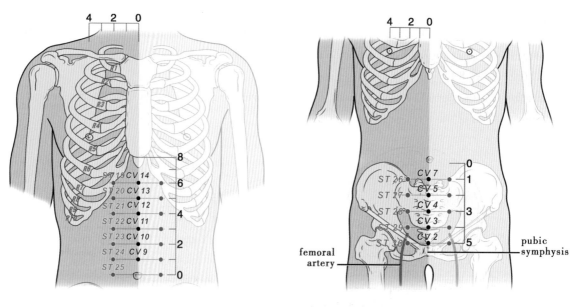

Figure 11-21   Figure 11-22

(10) Futu(ST 32)

Location: On the anterolateral aspect of the thigh on the line connecting the lateral end of the base of the patella with the anterior superior iliac spine, 6 cun superior to the base of the patella(Figure 11-23).

Indications: ①Pain and paralysis of the legs. ②Hernia. ③Abdominal distention.

Manipulation: 1.0-2.0 cun perpendicular insertion.

(11) Liangqiu(ST 34) cleft point

Location: On the anterolateral aspect of the thigh 2 cun superior to the base of the patella between the vastus lateralis muscle and the rectus femoris tendon(Figure 11-23).

Indications: ①Stomach pain. ②Pain in the knee, atrophy and paralysis of the legs. ③Mastitis.

Manipulation: 1.0-1.5 cun perpendicular insertion.

(12) Zusanli(ST 36) sea point; lower sea point of the stomach

Location: 3 cun inferior to Dubi(ST 35), on the line connecting Dubi(ST 35) and Jiexi(ST 41)(Figure 11-24).

Indications: ①Stomach pain, vomiting, abdominal pain and distension, diarrhea, dysentery, constipation, intestinal abscess. ②Consumptive diseases, palpitation, shortness of breath. ③Atrophy and paralysis of the legs, edema. ④Psychosis and epilepsy. ⑤This point has the function to strengthen the body. It is an important point for health care.

Manipulation：1.0-2.0 cun perpendicular insertion, moxibustion is applicable.

(13) Shangjuxu(ST 37) lower sea point of the large intestine

Location：6 cun inferior to Dubi(ST 35), on the line connecting Dubi(ST 35) and Jiexi(ST 41) (Figure 11-24).

Indications：①Abdominal pain and distension, dysentery, constipation, intestine abscess, stroke, paralysis. ②Atrophy and pain of the legs.

Manipulation：1.0-2.0 cun perpendicular insertion.

(14) Xiajuxu(ST 39) lower sea point of the small intestine

Location：9 cun inferior to Dubi(ST 35), on the line connecting Dubi(ST 35) and Jiexi(ST 41) (Figure 11-24).

Indications：①Lower abdominal pain, borborygmus, diarrhea. ②Atrophy and paralysis of the legs. ③Mastitis.

Manipulation：1.0-1.5 cun perpendicular insertion.

(15) Fenglong(ST 40) connecting point

Location：8 cun superior to the prominence of the lateral malleolus at the lateral border of the tibialis anterior muscle, one finger breadth lateral to Tiaokou(ST 38) (Figure 11-24).

Indications：①Headache, vertigo. ②Psychosis, epilepsy. ③Cough with phlegm. ④Atrophy and paralysis of the legs. ⑤Abdominal distension, constipation.

Manipulation：1.0-1.5 cun perpendicular insertion.

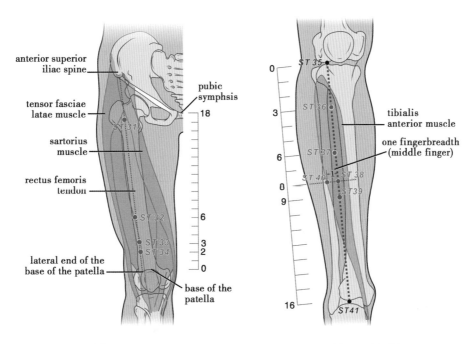

Figure 11-23   Figure 11-24

(16) Jiexi(ST 41) river point

Location：On the anterior aspect of the ankle in the depression between the extensor hallucis longus tendon and the extensor digitorum longus tendon(Figure 11-25).

Indications：①Atrophy and paralysis of the legs, pain in the ankle and wrist. ②Abdominal distension, constipation. ③Headache, vertigo. ④Psychosis, epilepsy.

Manipulation: 0. 5-1. 0 cun perpendicular insertions.

(17) Neiting(ST 44) spring point

Location: On the instep of the foot, at the junction of the red and white skin proximal to the margin of the web between the 2nd and 3rd toes(Figure 11-26).

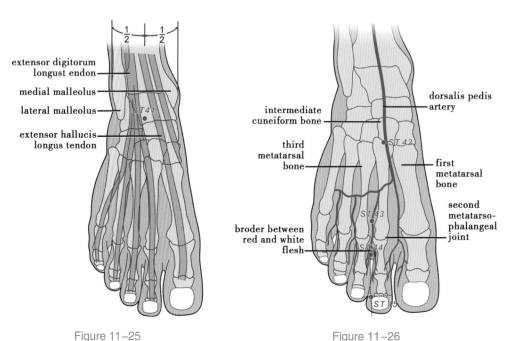

Figure 11-25 Figure 11-26

Indications: ① Toothache, swollen and sore throat, nosebleed, deviated mouth. ② Febrile diseases. ③ Stomach pain with sour regurgitation, diarrhea, dysentery, constipation. ④ Swelling and pain in the dorsum of the foot.

Manipulation: 0. 5-0. 8 cun perpendicular insertion.

(18) Lidui(ST 45) well point

Location: On the lateral side of the distal segment of the 2nd toe, 0. 1 cun from the corner of the toe nail(Figure 11-26).

Indications: ① Toothache, nosebleed, swollen and sore throat. ② Febrile diseases. ③ Profuse dreaming, nightmares, psychosis.

Manipulation: 0. 1 cun superficially insertion.

Other points on stomach meridian of foot yangming see Table 11-13.

Table 11-13 Other points on stomach meridian of foot yangming

Points	Code	Location	Indication
Juliao	ST 3	With the eyes looking straight forward, the point is vertically below the pupil, at the level of the lower border of the ala nasi, on the lateral side of the nasolabial groove	Deviation of the mouth and eye, twitching at the angle of the mouth, nosebleed, toothache
Daying	ST 5	Anterior to the mandibular angle, on the anterior border of the masseter muscle, where the pulsation of the facial artery is palpable	Toothache, deviation of the mouth and eye, swollen cheeks, facial pain, twitching of the facial muscles

Continue to Table 11-13

Points	Code	Location	Indication
Renying	ST 9	In the anterior region of the neck, level with the superior border of the thyroid cartilage, anterior to the sternocleidomastoid and above the common carotid artery	①Swollen and sore throat. ②Scrofula, goiter. ③Hypertension. ④Asthma
Shuitu	ST 10	On the neck, on the anterior border of sternocleidomastoid muscle, at the midpoint of the line linking the Renying (ST 9) and Qishe(ST 11)points	①Sore throat. ②Cough, gasp. ③Scrofula, goiter
Qishe	ST 11	On the neck and on the upper border of the medial end of the clavicle between the sternal and clavicular heads of the stemocleidomastoid muscle	①Swollen and sore throat, scrofula. ②Hiccup. ③Goiter, gasp. ④Pain and rigidity of the neck
Quepen	ST 12	In the midpoint of the supraclavicular fossa, 4 cun lateral to the anterior midline of the chest	①Cough, asthma. ②Swollen and sore throat. ③Pain in the supraclavicular fossa. ④Scrofula
Qihu	ST 13	At the lower border in the center of the clavicle, 4 cun laterals to the anterior midline of the chest	① Cough, asthma, hiccups. ②Pain in the chest
Kufang	ST 14	In the 1st intercostal space, 4 cun lateral to the anterior midline of the chest	①Cough, asthma. ②Distension and pain in the chest
Wuyi	ST 15	In the 2nd intercostal space, 4 cun lateral to the anterior midline of the chest	①Cough, asthma. ②Distension and pain in the chest. ③Mammary abscess
Yingchuang	ST 16	In the 3rd intercostal space, 4 cun lateral to the anterior midline of the chest	①Cough, asthma. ②Distension and pain in the chest. ③Mammary abscess
Ruzhong	ST 17	In the 4th intercostal space, 4 cun lateral to the anterior midline of the chest, at the center of the nipple	This point serves only as a landmark for locating points on the chest and the abdomen
Rugen	ST 18	In the 5th intercostal space, vertically below the nipple, 4 cun lateral to the anterior midline of the chest	①Mastitis, insufficient lactation. ②Cough, asthma, hiccups. ③Chest pain
Burong	ST 19	On the upper abdomen, 6 cun above the center of the umbilicus, 2 cun lateral to the anterior midline of the abdomen	Vomiting, stomachache, abdominal distension, and poor appetite
Chengman	ST 20	On the upper abdomen, 5 cun above the center of the umbilicus, 2 cun lateral to the anterior midline of the abdomen	Stomachache, vomiting, borborygmus, and poor appetite
Guanmen	ST 22	On the upper abdomen, 3 cun above the center of the umbilicus, 2 cun lateral to the anterior midline of the abdomen	Abdominal pain and distension, borborygmus, diarrhea, and poor appetite

Continue to Table 11-13

Points	Code	Location	Indication
Taiyi	ST 23	On the upper abdomen, 2 cun above the center of the umbilicus, 2 cun lateral to the anterior midline of the abdomen	①Abdominal pain and distension. ②Vexation, psychosis
Huaroumen	ST 24	On the upper abdomen, 1 cun above the center of the umbilicus, 2 cun lateral to the anterior midline of the abdomen	①Abdominal pain, vomiting. ②Psychosis
Wailing	ST 26	On the lower abdomen, 1 cun below the center of the umbilicus, 2 cun lateral to the anterior midline of the abdomen	①Abdominal pain, hernia. ②Dysmenorrhea
Daju	ST 27	On the lower abdomen, 2 cun below the center of the umbilicus, 2 cun lateral to the anterior midline of the abdomen	①Lower abdominal distension, difficulty in urination. ②spermatorrhea, premature ejaculation. ③Hernia
Shuidao	ST 28	On the lower abdomen, 3 cun below the center of the umbilicus, 2 cun lateral to the anterior midline of the abdomen	①Lower abdominal distension, difficulty in urination, hernia. ②Dysmenorrhea
Qichong	ST 30	On the lower abdomen, 5 cun below the center of the umbilicus, 2 cun lateral to the anterior midline of the abdomen	①Abdominal pain, hernia. ②Irregular menstruation, infertility, impotence, swelling of the vulva
Biguan	ST 31	On the anterior aspect of the thigh in the depression formed by the sartorius, the tensor fasciae latae, and the proximal portion of the rectus femoris	Weakness, numbness and pain of the lower limbs, pain of the lower back and leg
Yinshi	ST 33	On the anterolateral aspect of the thigh late-ral to the rectus femoris tendon, 3 cun superior to the base of the patella	Pain in the knee, atrophy and paralysis of the legs
Dubi	ST 35	With the knee flexed, on the knee, in the depression lateral to the patella and its liga-ment	Motor impairment of the lower limbs, numbness and pain in the lower limbs, pain in the knees
Tiaokou	ST 38	8 cun inferior to Dubi(ST 35), on the line connecting Dubi(ST 35) and Jiexi(ST 41)	①Atrophy and paralysis of the legs. ②Pain in the abdomen and stomach. ③Pain in the shoulders and arms
Chongyang (source point)	ST 42	At the highest point of the dorsum of the foot, between the tendons of extensor hallucis longus and digitornm longus, where the dorsal artery of the foot pulsates	① Stomach pain, abdominal distension. ②Deviation of the mouth, swollen face, toothache. ③ Swelling and pain in the dorsurm of the foot, weakness and numbness of the foot
Xiangu (stream point)	ST 43	On the dorsum of the foot, between the 2nd and 3rd metatarsal bones in the depression proximal to the 2nd metatarsophalangeal joint	①Facial and general edema. ② Borborygmus, diarrhea. ③ Swelling and pain of the dorsum of the foot

11.3.1.4   Frequently used acupoints on spleen meridian of foot taiyin

This meridian originates from the tip of the big toe, ascends to the front aspect of the medial malleolus, continues going upwards along the posterior side of the lower leg, then it crosses over and goes in front of the liver meridian of foot jueyin, passing through the anterior media aspect of the knee and thigh, it then enters the abdomen and spleen, its pertaining organ, and connects with the stomach. It travels alongside the throat and arrives at the root of the tongue and spreads over the lower surface of the tongue. The abdomen branch of the meridian goes from the stomach through the diaphragm and enters the heart(Figure 11−27).

(1) Yinbai(SP 1) well point

Location: On the medial side of the great toe and about 0. 1 cun lateral to the corner of the toenail (Figure 11−28).

Indications: ①Gynecological diseases like hypermenorrhea, metrorrhagia and metrostaxis. ②Uterine bleeding, menorrhea, blood in the stool and blood in the urine. ③Abdominal distention. ④Psychosis, profuse dreaming and convulsions.

Manipulation: Insert the needle 0. 1 cun into the skin, or insert a three-edged needle to induce bleeding.

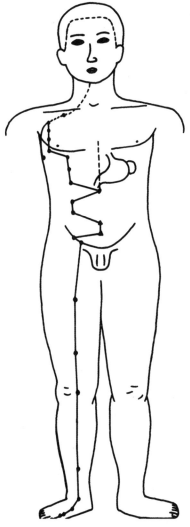

Figure 11 − 27   The course of spleen meridian of foot taiyin

(2)Taibai(SP 3)stream point;source point

Location:On the posterior border of the small head of the 1st metatarsal bone,at the junction of the red and white skin(Figure 11-29).

Indications:①Stomach pain,abdominal distension,abdominal pain,diarrhea,dysentery,anorexia. ②Heaviness of the body,pain in joints.

Manipulation:0.5-0.8 cun perpendicular insertion.

(3)Gongsun(SP 4)connecting point;one of the eight confluent points associating with thoroughfare vessel

Location:On the medial border of the foot,anterior to the proximal end of the first metatarsal,at the junction of the red and white skin(Figure 11-29).

Indications:①Stomach pain,vomiting,abdominal distension,abdominal pain,diarrhea,dysentery. ②Epigastric pain,oppression in the chest. ③Insomnia,irritability,somnolence,beriberi.

Manipulation:0.5-1.0 cun perpendicular insertion.

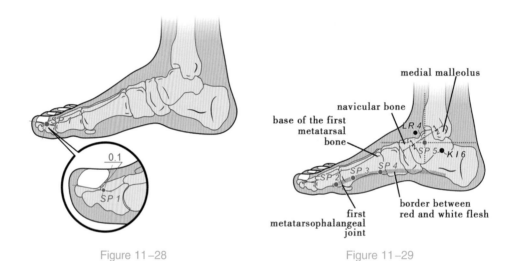

Figure 11-28   Figure 11-29

(4)Sanyinjiao(SP 6)

Location:3 cun above the tip of the medial malleolus and on the posterior border of the medial aspect of the tibia(Figure 11-30).

Indications:①Abdominal pain,abdominal distension,borborygmus,diarrhea. ②Irregular menstruation,dysmenorrheal,menostasis,leucorrhea,prolapse of the uterus,prolonged labor,infertility,impotence, spermatorrhea. ③Difficulty in urination,enuresis,edema. ④Insomnia,dizziness. ⑤Atrophy and paralysis of the legs,beriberi.

Manipulation:1.0-1.5 cun perpendicular insertion. It is contraindicated for pregnant women.

(5)Diji(SP 8)cleft point

Location:On the line connecting the tip of the medial malleolus and 3 cun below Yinlingquan(SP 9) (Figure 11-30).

Indications:①Abdominal distension,abdominal pain,diarrhea. ②Irregular menstruation,dysmenorrheal,uterine bleeding. ③Difficulty in urination,edema. ④Atrophy and paralysis of the legs.

Manipulation:Puncture perpendicularly by 1.0-1.5 cun.

(6)Yinlingquan(SP 9)sea point

Location:In the depression inferior to the medial condyle of the tibia(Figure 11-30).

Indications: ① Abdominal distension, diarrhea, jaundice, abdominal pain. ② Difficulty in urination, edema. ③ Spermatorrhea, pudendal pain. ④ Pain in the knees.

Manipulation: 1.0-2.0 cun perpendicular insertion.

(7) Xuehai(SP 10)

Location: 2 cun superior to the medial end of the base of the patella on the bulge of the vastus medialis muscle(Figure 11-31).

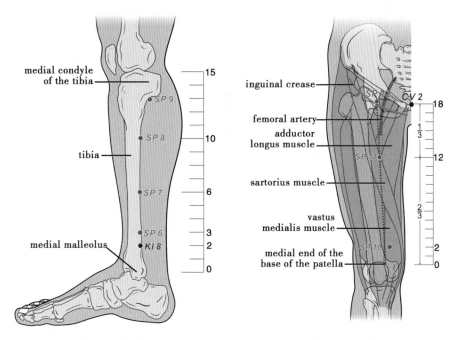

Figure 11-30   Figure 11-31

Indications: ① Irregular menstruation, heavy uterine bleeding, amenorrhea. ② Urticaria, eczema, erysipelas, abdominal distension, diarrhea, jaundice, abdominal pain, difficulty in micturition, edema. ③ Pain and swelling in the knees.

Manipulation: 1.0-1.2 cun perpendicular insertion.

(8) Daheng(SP 15)

Location: 4 cun lateral to the center of the umbilicus(Figure 11-32).

Indications: ① Abdominal pain, diarrhea, and constipation. ② Hernia.

Manipulation: 1.0-2.0 cun perpendicular insertion.

(9) Dabao(SP 21) major collateral of the spleen

Location: On the midaxillary line, in the 6th intercostal space(Figure 11-33).

Indications: ① Cough, dyspnea. ② Chest and hypochondriac regions pain. ③ Pain of the whole body, weariness of the four limbs.

Manipulation: Puncture transversely or obliquely by 0.5-0.8 cun. Deep insertion should be avoided to prevent puncturing the lungs.

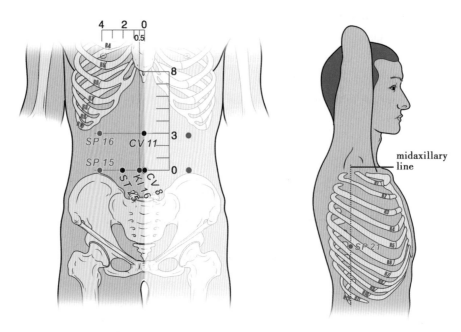

Figure 11-32   Figure 11-33

Other points on spleen meridian of foot taiyin see Table 11-14.

Table 11-14   Other points on spleen meridian of foot taiyin

Points	Code	Location	Indication
Dadu (spring point)	SP 2	In the depression anterior and inferior to the 1st metatarsophalangeal joint of the big toe, at the junction of the red and the white skin	①Abdominal distension, stomach pain, diarrhea, constipation. ②Febrile disease with absence of sweating
Shangqiu (river point)	SP 5	In the depression anterior and inferior to the medial malleolus, at the midpoint of the line connecting the tuberosity of the navicular bone and the tip of the medial malleolus	①Abdominal distension, borborygmus, diarrhea, constipation, jaundice. ② Pain in the foot and ankle
Lougu	SP 7	On the line connecting the tip of the medial malleolus and Yinlingquan (SP 9), 6 cun above the tip of the medial malleolus	①Abdominal distension, borborygmus. ②Seminal emission. ③Weakness and flaccidity of the lower limbs
Jimen	SP 11	On the medial aspect of the thigh between the sartorius and the adductor longus muscle where the femoral artery pulses, at the junction of the upper 1/3 and lower 2/3 of a line connecting the medial end of the base of the patella and Chongmen(SP 12)	Dysuria, enuresis, swelling and pain of the groin
Chongmen	SP 12	At the groin region at the inguinal crease, lateral to the external iliac artery	①Abdominal pain, hernia. ②Uterine bleeding, leukorrhea
Fushe	SP 13	0.7 cun superior and lateral to Chongmen(SP 12), 4 cun lateral to the midline of the abdomen	Abdominal pain, hernia, distension, and masses in the abdomen

Continue to Table 11−14

Points	Code	Location	Indication
Fujie	SP 14	1.3 cun below Daheng(SP 15),4 cun lateral to the midline of the abdomen	Abdominal pain,diarrhea,and constipation
Fuai	SP 16	3 cun above the center of the umbilicus,4 cun lateral to the anterior midline of the abdomen	Abdominal pain, diarrhea, dysentery, constipation,and dyspepsia
Shidou	SP 17	In the 5th intercostal space,6 cun lateral to the anterior midline of the chest	①Belching, abdominal distension. ②Edema. ③Distension and pain in the chest and hypochondrium
Tianxi	SP 18	In the 4th intercostal space,6 cun lateral to the anterior midline of the chest	①Pain in the chest,cough. ②Acute mastitis,insufficient lactation
Xiongxiang	SP 19	In the 3rd intercostal space,6 cun lateral to the anterior midline of the chest	Distension and pain in the chest and hypochondrium
Zhourong	SP 20	In the 2nd intercostal space,6 cun lateral to the anterior midline	①Distension in the chest and hypochondriac regions. ②Cough,asthma

11.3.1.5   Frequently used acupoints on heart meridian of hand shaoyin

It originates from the heart and pertains to the heart system(the tissue where the heart connects other viscera)and connects with the small intestine. The branch that goes upwards through the throat ascends to the head. The straight part of the vessel derived from the heart system runs upwards toward the lungs,runs downwards and emerges from the axilla. It follows along the posterior border of the medial aspect of the forearm and the upper arm and enters the palm. It then travels along the radial side of the little finger and terminates at its tip(Figure 11−34).

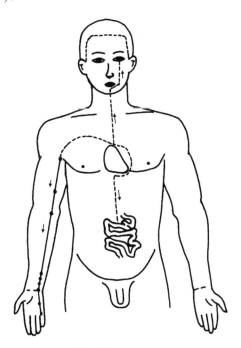

Figure 11−34   The course of heart meridian of hand shaoyin

(1)Jiquan(HT 1)

Location: At the apex of the axilla, on the pulsation point of the axillary artery(Figure 11-35).

Indications: ①Cardiac pain, palpitations. ②Hypochondriac and costal pain. ③Pain in the shoulders and aims, loss of the use of the upper limb. ④Scrofula.

Manipulation: Insert the needle perpendicularly by 0. 3-0. 5 cun deep, avoiding needling the artery.

(2)Shaohai(HT 3)sea point

Location: Anterior to the medial epicondyle of the humerus, level with the cubital crease. With the elbow flexed, at the midpoint of the line connecting the medial end of the cubital crease and the medial epicondyle of the humerus(Figure 11-36).

Indications: ①Cardiac pain. ②Axillary and hypochondriac pain. ③Pain of the arm and elbow, paralysis of the upper limbs. ④Scrofula.

Manipulation: Insert the needle perpendicularly by 0. 5-1. 0 cun deep.

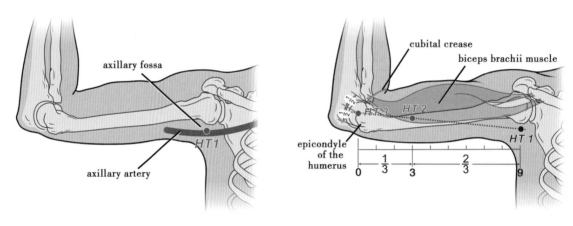

Figure 11-35   Figure 11-36

(3)Tongli(HT 5)connecting point

Location: On the palmar aspect of the forearm, 1 cun above the Shenmen (HT 7) point (Figure 11-37).

Indications: ①Sudden loss of voice, stiffness of the tongue, inability to speak. ②Palpitations. ③Pain in the wrists and arms.

Manipulation: Insert the needle perpendicularly by 0. 3-0. 5 cun deep. It is not advisable to insert deeply to avoid hurting nerves and vessels.

(4)Yinxi(HT 6)cleft point

Location: On the palmar aspect of the forearm, 0. 5 cun above the Shenmen (HT 7) point (Figure 11-37).

Indications: ① Cardiac pain, fright palpitations. ② Hematemesis, epistaxis. ③ Steaming heat, night sweats.

Manipulation: Insert the needle perpendicularly by 0. 2-0. 5 cun deep. It is not advisable to insert deeply to avoid hurting nerves and vessels.

(5)Shenmen(HT 7)stream point; source point

Location: On the palmar ulnar end of the transverse crease of the wrist, in the depression on the radial side of the flexor carpi ulnaris tendon(Figure 11-37).

Indications: ①Insomnia, forgetfulness, dementia, psychosis, epilepsy. ②Cardiac pain, palpitations.

Manipulation: Insert the needle perpendicularly by 0. 2-0. 5 cun deep.

（6）Shaochong（HT 9）well point

Location：On the radial side of the little finger, approximately 0. 1 cun from the corner of the nail（Figure 11–38）.

Indications：①Cardiac pain, palpitations. ②Psychosis, coma. ③Febrile diseases.

Manipulation：Superficially puncture by 0. 1–0. 2 cun, or prick to induce bleeding.

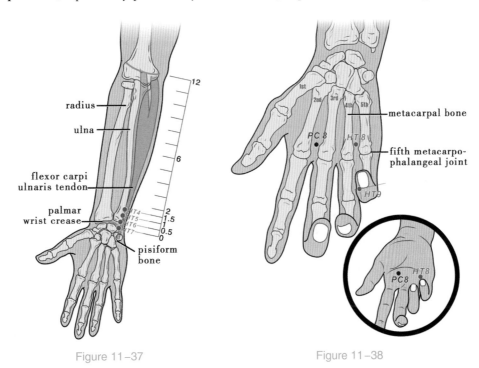

Figure 11–37　　　　　　　　Figure 11–38

Other points onheart meridian of hand shaoyin see Table 11–15.

Table 11–15　Other points onheart meridian of hand shaoyin

Points	Code	Location	Indication
Qingling	HT 2	On the medial side of the arm and on the line connecting Jiquan（HT 1）and Shaohai（HT 3）, 3 cun above the cubital crease, in the groove medial to the biceps muscle of the arm	① Headache, chill. ② Yellowish eyeballs. ③Hypochondriac pain, pain in the shoulders and arms
Lingdao （river point）	HT 4	With the elbow flexed, in the center between the medial end of the transverse cubital crease and the medial epicondyle of the humerus	①Cardiac pain. ② Axillary and hypochondriac pain. ③Pain of the arm and elbow, paralysis of the upper limbs. ④Scrofula
Shaofu （spring point）	HT 8	On the palm, between the 4th and 5th metacarpal bones, where the tip of the little finger rests when a fist is made	①Palpitations, chest pain. ②Itching and pain of the genitals. ③Spasmodic pain of the little finger, heat sensations in the palm.

11.3.1.6　Frequently used acupoints on small intestine meridian of hand taiyang

It originates from the ulnar side of the tip of the little finger, and then runs upwards along the lateral aspect of the forearm. Then it reaches and emerges at the shoulder joint and proceeds in a zigzag course along the scapular region, arriving at Dazhui(GV 14). From here, it descends through the supravicular fossa and connects with the heart, going downwards along the esophagus, passing through the diaphragm to the stomach, and finally ending at the small intestine. A branch from the supraclavicular fossa ascends along the neck to the head.

A branch from the supraclavicular fossa ascends to cross the neck and cheek to the outer canthus of the eye, and finally turns and enters the ear.

Another branch separates from the previous branch on the cheek and ascends to the zygomatic bone, reaching the side of the nose. It finally terminates at the inner canthus to link with the bladder meridian of foot taiyang(Figure 11-39).

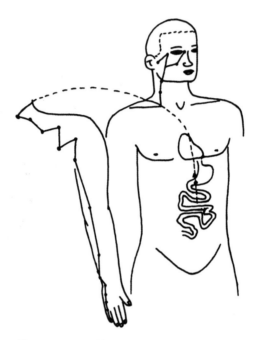

Figure 11-39　The course of small intestine meridian of hand taiyang

(1) Shaoze(SI 1) well point

Location: On the ulnar side of the little finger, approximately 0. 1 cun from the corner of the nail(Figure 11-40).

Indications: ①Headache, superficial visual obstruction, sore and swollen throat. ②Mastitis, insufficient lactation. ③Coma. ④Febrile disease.

Manipulation: Insert the needle superficially by 0. 1 cun deep, or prick to induce bleeding. Contraindicate for pregnant women.

(2) Houxi(SI 3) stream point; one of the eight confluence points associating with the governor vessel

Location: On the ulnar side of the hand, when a loose fist is made, proximal to the 5th metacarpophalangeal joint, at the top of the transverse crease and the junction of the red and white skin(Figure 11-41).

Indications: ①Headache and painful stiff nape of the neck, pain of the lumbar and back region. ②Red eye, deafness, sore and swollen throat. ③Night sweats, malaria. ④Psychosis, epilepsy. ⑤Spasm in the fingers, elbows or arms.

Manipulation: Insert the needle perpendicularly by 0. 5-1. 0 cun deep.

(3) Wangu(SI 4) Source Point

Location: On the ulnar side of the wrist, in the depression between the base of the 5th metacarpal bone and the triquetrum, at the border between the red and white flesh(Figure 11-41).

Indications:①Headache and painful stiff nape of the neck, tinnitus, superficial visual obstruction. ②Jaundice. ③Diabetes, febrile diseases, malaria. ④Pain and spasm in the fingers and wrists.

Manipulation:Insert the needle perpendicularly by 0.3-0.5 cun deep.

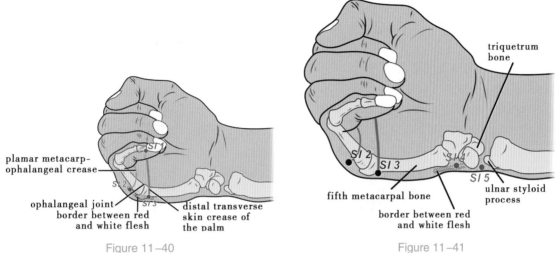

Figure 11-40　　　　　　　　　　Figure 11-41

(4)Yanglao(SI 6)cleft point

Location:On the dorsal ulnar aspect of the forearm, in the depression radial to the head of the ulnar bone,1 cun proximal to the dorsal wrist crease(Figure 11-42).

Indications:①Blurred vision. ②Numbness and pain in the shoulder, back, elbow and arm, stiff neck, acute lumbar pain.

Manipulation:When the palm of the hand is placed on the chest, insert obliquely towards the elbow by 0.5-0.8 cun deep.

(5)Zhizheng(SI 7)connecting point

Location:On the dorsal ulnar aspect of the forearm between the medial border of the ulna and the flexor carpi ulnaris,5 cun proximal to the dorsal wrist crease(Figure 11-43).

Indications:①Headache, stiff neck. ②Febrile diseases. ③Psychosis. ④Aching pain in the elbows and arms.

Manipulation:Insert the needle perpendicularly or obliquely by 0.3-0.8 cun deep.

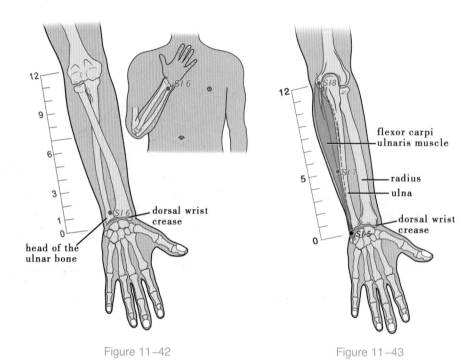

Figure 11-42

Figure 11-43

(6) Tianzong(SI 11)

Location: In the depression of the center of the subscapular fossa, level with the 4th thoracic vertebra (Figure 11-44).

Indications: ①Scapular pain. ②Asthma. ③Mastitis.

Manipulation: Insert the needle perpendicularly or obliquely by 0.5-1.0 cun deep.

(7) Quanliao(SI 18)

Location: On the face, directly below the outer canthus, in the depression below the zygomatic bone (Figure 11-45).

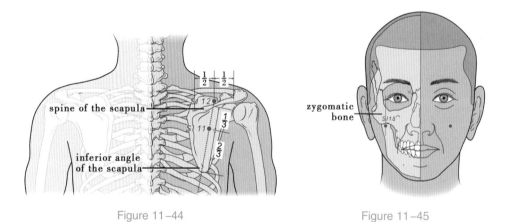

Figure 11-44

Figure 11-45

Indications: Facial paralysis, trembling eyelids, toothache, swollen lips.

Manipulation: 0.3-0.5 cun deep perpendicular insertion or 0.5-1.0 cun deep oblique insertion.

(8) Tinggong(SI 19)

Location: On the face, anterior to the tragus and posterior to the mandibular condyloid process, in the depression found when the mouth is open(Figure 11-46).

Indications:①Tinnitus,deafness,epilepsy. ②Toothache.

Manipulation:1.0-1.5 cun deep perpendicular insertion while opening the mouth.

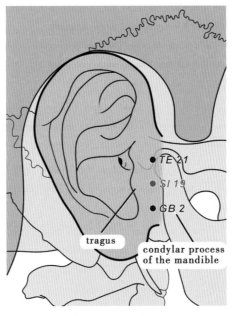

Figure 11-46

Other points onsmall intestine meridian of hand taiyang see Table 11-16.

Table 11-16   Other points onsmall intestine meridian of hand taiyang

Points	Code	Location	Indication
Qiangu(spring point)	SI 2	At the junction of the red and white skin along the ulnar border of the hand, at the ulnar end of the crease of the 5th meta-carpophalangeal joint when a loose fist is made	①Headache, ophthalmalgia, tinnitus, sore throat. ②Febrile disease. ③Acute mastitis
Yanggu(river point)	SI 5	On the ulnar side of the wrist, in the depression between the styloid process of the ulna and the triquetral bone	①Headache, dizziness, tinnitus, deafness. ②Febrile disease. ③Psy-chosis, epilepsy. ④Pain in the wrist
Xiaohai(sea point)	SI 8	With the elbow flexed, in the depression between the olecranon of the ulna and the medial epicondyle of the humerus	①Pain in the elbows and arms. ②Epilepsy
Jianzhen	SI 9	Posterior and inferior to the shoulder joint, 1 cun above the posterior end of the axillary fold with the arm abducted	①Numbness and pain in the shoulder and arm. ②Scrofula
Naoshu	SI 10	On the shoulder, directly above the posterior end of the axillary fold, in the depression inferior to the scapular spine	①Pain in the shoulder and arm. ②Scrofula
Bingfeng	SI 12	At the scapula region, in the supraspinous fossa superior to the midpoint of the scapu-lar spine	Scapular pain and aching numbness of the upper arm

Continue to Table 11-16

Points	Code	Location	Indication
Quyuan	SI 13	At the scapula region, in the depression superior to the medial end of the scapular spine, midpoint of the line connecting Naoshu(SI 10)and the spinous process of the 2nd thoracic vertebra	Pain in the scapula, back and neck
Jianwaishu	SI 14	3 cun lateral to the lower border of the spinous process of the 1st thoracic vertebrae	Stiffness of nape and back, pain in the shoulders and back
Jianzhongshu	SI 15	On the back, 2 cun lateral to the lower border of the spinous process of the 7th cervical vertebrae	①Cough, asthma. ②Pain in the shoulders and upper back
Tianchuang	SI 16	On the lateral aspect of the neck, on the posterior border of the sternocleidomastoideus, posterior to Futu(LI 18), and level with the Adam's apple	①Sore and swollen throat, sudden loss of voice, tinnitus, deafness. ②Pain and stiffness in the nape of the neck
Tianrong	SI 17	Posterior to the mandibular angle in the depression of the anterior border of the sternocleidomastoid muscle	① Tinnitus, deafness, sore and swollen throat. ②Pain and distension in the nape of the neck

11.3.1.7 Frequently used acupoints on bladder meridian of foot taiyang

The bladder meridian of foot taiyang originates from the inner canthus of the eye. It then goes upwards toward the forehead, and connects with the vertex. The straight branch from the vertex enters the brain, and then emerges to descend at the nape of the neck, where the meridian splits into two branches. One of the branches runs downwards along the medial border of the scapular region parallel to the vertebral column, reaching the lumbar region, and then enters the body cavity via the para-vertebral muscle to connect with the kidney and bladder. The branch separates into the lumber region descending via the hip and entering the popliteal fossa of the knee. The branch separates from the nape of the neck and descends along the medial aspect of the scapular region, crosses the hip joint, and then descends along the posterio-lateral aspect of the thigh to meet with the previous branch of the meridian in the popliteal fossa. From here, it descends to emerge at the back of the external malleolus, and ends at the lateral side of the small toe(Figure 11-47).

(1)Jingming(BL 1)

Location: On the face, in the depression between the superomedial parts of the inner canthus and the medial wall of the orbit(Figure 11-47).

Indications: ①Red and swollen eyes, lacrimation upon exposure to wind, unclear vision, myopia, night blindness, color blindness, blurred vision. ②Acute lumbar pain. ③Palpitation and severe palpitation.

Manipulation: Ordering the patient to close the eye, the doctor slightly pushes the eyeball to the lateral side. Insert the point slowly perpendicularly along the orbital wall for 0.3-0.5 cun. Moxibustion is not applicable. For insertion can easily cause bleeding inside, please use a dry cotton ball to press the puncture site for a moment after withdrawing the needle.

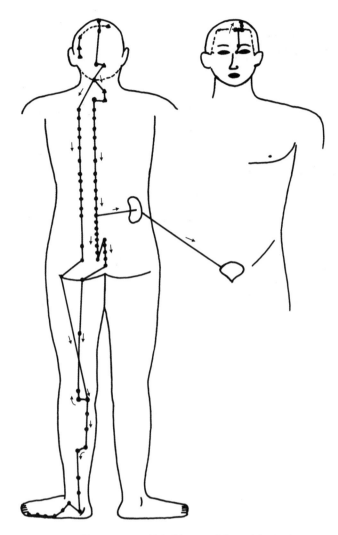

Figure 11–47   **The course of bladder meridian of foot taiyang**

(2)Cuanzu(BL 2)

Location：On the face, in the depression of the medial end of the eyebrow, at the frontal notch(Figure 11–48).

Indications：①Blurred vision, redness, pain and swelling of the eyes, lacrimation, twitching of the eyelid. ②Headache, pain in the supraorbital region, facial paralysis. ③Hiccups.

Manipulation：0. 5–0. 8 cun horizontal insertion. Moxibustion is contraindicated.

(3)Tianzhu(BL 10)

Location：On the nape, in the depression lateral to the trapezius muscle at the level of the superior border of the spinous process of the 2nd cervical vertebra(Figure 11–49).

Indications：①Headache, dizziness. ②Blurred vision, nasal congestion. ③Stiff neck, pain in the upper back and shoulders.

Manipulation：0. 5–0. 8 cun deep perpendicular or oblique insertion. Do not puncture deeply upward or inside so as to avoid damaging the medulla.

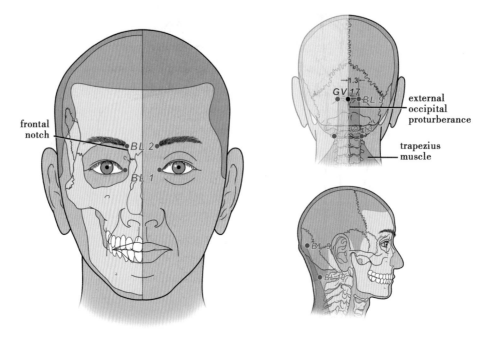

Figure 11-48   Figure 11-49

(4) Fengmen(BL 12)

Location: On the back, below the spinous process of the 2nd thoracic vertebrae, 1. 5 cun lateral to the posterior midline(Figure 11-50).

Indications: ①Cough due to wind invasion, fever and headache, nasal obstruction and nose running. ②Stiffness of nape, pain in the back and shoulders.

Manipulation: 0. 5-0. 8 cun deep oblique insertion. Deep insertion is not advisable.

(5) Feishu(BL 13) back transport point of the lung

Location: On the back, below the spinous process of the 3rd thoracic vertebra, 1. 5 cun lateral to the posterior midline(Figure 11-50).

Indications: ① Cough with asthma, common cold, nasal congestion. ② High fever, night sweating. ③Itching of the skin, urticaria.

Manipulation: 0. 5-0. 8 cun deep oblique insertion.

(6) Xinshu(BL 15) back transport point of the heart

Location: On the back, below the spinous process of the 5th thoracic vertebrae, 1. 5 cun lateral to the posterior midline(Figure 11-50).

Indications: ① Cardiac pain, palpitations, insomnia, forgetfulness, epilepsy. ② Cough, hematemesis. ③Nocturnal emission, night sweats.

Manipulation: 0. 5-0. 8 cun deep oblique insertion.

(7) Geshu(BL 17) one of the eight meeting points(blood convergence)

Location: On the back, below the spinous process of the 7th thoracic vertebrae, 1. 5 cun lateral to the posterior midline(Figure 11-50).

Indications: ①Stomachache, vomiting, hiccups. ②Cough with asthma, hematemesis, high fever, night sweats. ③Urticaria.

Manipulation: 0. 5-0. 8 cun deep oblique insertion.

(8) Ganshu(BL 18) back transport point of the liver

Location: On the back, below the spinous process of the 9th thoracic vertebra, 1. 5 cun lateral to the posterior midline(Figure 11–50).

Indications: ① Jaundice, hypochondriac pain. ② Red eyes, blurred vision, night blindness. ③ Hematemesis, epistaxis. ④Dizziness, depression and psychosis, mania, epilepsy.

Manipulation:0. 5–0. 8 cun deep oblique insertion.

(9) Danshu(BL 19) back transport point of the gallbladder

Location: On the back, below the spinous process of the 10th thoracic vertebrae, 1. 5 cun lateral to the posterior midline(Figure 11–50).

Indications:①Jaundice, bitter taste in mouth, hypochondriac pain. ②Pulmonary phthisis, high fever.

Manipulation:0. 5–0. 8 cun deep oblique insertion.

(10) Pishu(BL 20) back transport point of the spleen

Location: On the back, below the spinous process of the 11th thoracic vertebra, 1. 5 cun lateral to the posterior midline(Figure 11–50).

Indications:①Abdominal distension, diarrhea, dysentery, hematochezia, anorexia. ②Edema, jaundice.

Manipulation:0. 5–0. 8 cun deep oblique insertion.

(11) Weishu(BL 21) back transport point of the stomach

Location: On the back, below the spinous process of the 12th thoracic vertebrae, 1. 5 cun lateral to the posterior midline(Figure 11–50).

Indications:①Epigastric pain, vomiting, abdominal distension, borborygmus. ②Chest and hypochondriac pain.

Manipulation:0. 5–0. 8 cun deep oblique insertion.

(12) Shenshu(BL 23) back transport point of the kidney

Location: On the back, below the spinous process of the 2nd lumbar vertebra, 1. 5 cun lateral to the posterior midline(Figure 11–50).

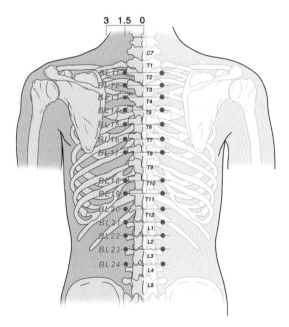

Figure 11–50

Indications:①Tinnitus, deafness. ②Seminal emission, impotence, irregular menstruation, morbid leucorrhea, enuresis, difficulty in urination, edema. ③Lumbar pain. ④Cough, asthma, asthenic breathing.

Manipulation: 0.5-1.0 cun deep oblique insertion.

(13) Dachangshu(BL 25) back transport point of the large intestine

Location: On the back, below the spinous process of the 4th lumbar vertebra, 1.5 cun lateral to the posterior midline(Figure 11-51).

Indications: ①Pain of the lumbar region and lower limbs. ②Abdominal pain, diarrhea, constipation, dysentery, hemorrhoids.

Manipulation: 0.5-1.0 cun deep oblique insertion.

(14) Pangguangshu(BL 28) back transport point of the bladder

Location: On the sacrum, level with the 2nd posterior sacral foramen, and 1.5 cun lateral to the median sacral crest(Figure 11-52).

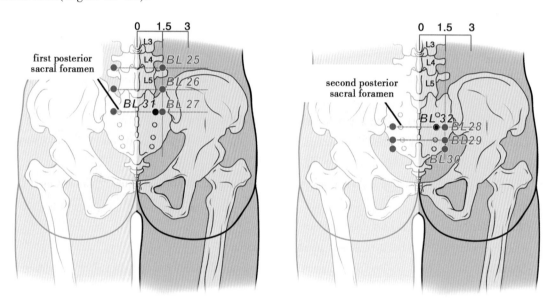

Figure 11-51   Figure 11-52

Indications: ①Difficulty in urination, frequent urination, enuresis. ②Diarrhea, constipation. ③Stiffness and pain in the lower back.

Manipulation: 0.8-1.2 cun deep oblique insertion.

(15) Ciliao(BL 32)

Location: On the sacrum, in the 2nd posterior sacral foramen(Figure 11-53).

Indications: ①Irregular menstruation, dysmenorrhea, morbid leucorrhea. ②Seminal emission. ③Difficulty in urination. ④Hernia. ⑤Low back pain, sacral pain, weakness or paralysis in the lower limbs.

Manipulation: 1.0-1.5 cun deep oblique insertion.

(16) Weiyang(BL 39) lower sea point of the triple energizer

Location: On the lateral end of the transverse crease of the popliteal fossa, on the medial border of the tendon of the biceps femoris(Figure 11-57).

Indications: ①Abdominal distension, edema, difficulty in urination. ②Pain and stiffness in the back, spasm of the lower limbs.

Manipulation: 1.0-1.5 cun deep oblique insertion.

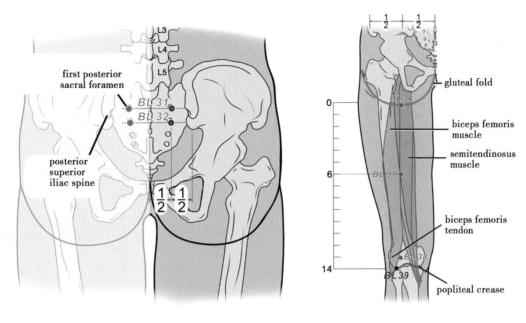

Figure 11-53   Figure 11-54

(17) Weizhong(BL 40) sea point; lower sea point of the bladder

Location: On the midpoint of the transverse crease of the popliteal fossa(Figure 11-57).

Indications: ①Lumbar pain, spasm of the popliteal tendons, weakness or paralysis in the lower limbs. ②Difficulty in urination, enuresis. ③Acute vomiting and diarrhea, abdominal pain. ④Erysipelas, urticaria, furuncles.

Manipulation: 1.0-1.5 cun deep oblique insertion.

(18) Gaohuang(BL 43)

Location: On the back, level with the lower border of the spinous process of the 4th thoracic vertebra, 3 cun lateral to the posterior midline(Figure 11-55).

Indications: ①Cough, asthma, pulmonary phthisis. ②Forgetfulness, seminal, emission, night sweats, consumptive disease. ③Pain of the shoulder and back.

Manipulation: 0.5-0.8 cun deep oblique insertion.

(19) Zhishi(BL 52)

Location: Level with the lower border of the spinous process of the 2nd lumbar vertebra, 3 cun lateral to the posterior midline(Figure 11-55).

Indications: ①Seminal emission, impotence. ②Difficulty in urination, edema. ③Stiffness and pain in the back.

Manipulation: 0.5-0.8 cun deep oblique insertion.

(20) Zhibian(BL 54)

Location: Level with the 4th posterior sacral foramen, 3 cunlateral to the median sacral crest(Figure 11-56).

Indications: ①Pain in the lumbar areas and legs, atrophy or paralysis in the lower limbs. ②Hemorrhoids, constipation, difficulty in urination.

Manipulation: 0.5-0.8 cun deep oblique insertion.

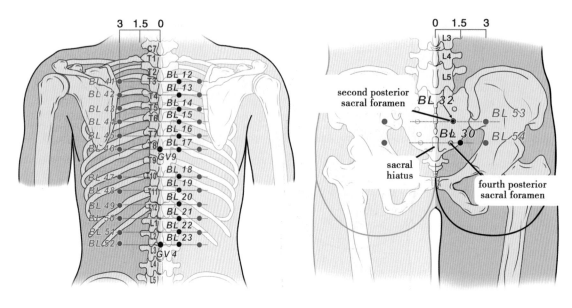

Figure 11-55   Figure 11-56

(21) Chengshan(BL 57)

Location : On the posterior aspect of the leg where the calcaneal tendon connects with the two muscle bellies of the gastrocnemius muscle(Figure 11-57).

Indications : ①Pain in the lumbar and legs. ②Hemorrhoids, constipation. ③Hernia.

Manipulation : 1.0-2.0 cun perpendicular insertion.

(22) Feiyang(BL 58) connecting point

Location : 7 cun directly above Kunlun(BL 60) between the inferior border of the lateral head of the gastrocnemius muscle and the calcaneal tendon(Figure 11-57).

Indications : ①Pain in the low back and legs. ②Headache. ③Dizziness. ④Hemorrhoids.

Manipulation : 1.0-1.5 cun perpendicular insertion.

(23) Kunlun(BL 60) river point

Location : Posterior to the lateral malleolus, in the depression between the tip of the external malleolus and Achilles tendon(Figure 11-58).

Indications : ①Headache, stiffness in the nape, spasm of the back and shoulder, dizziness. ②Low back pain, heel pain. ③Epilepsy. ④Delayed labour.

Manipulation : 0.5-0.8 cun perpendicular insertion. Pregnant woman should not be applied.

(24) Shenmai(BL 62) one of the eight confluence points associating with yang heel vessel

Location : On the lateral side of the foot, in the depression directly below the external malleolus(Figure 11-58).

Indications : ①Headache, dizziness, stiffness in nape. ②Epliepsy, mania, insomnia. ③Pain in the low back and leg.

Manipulation : 0.3-0.5 cun perpendicular insertion.

(25) Shugu(BL 65) stream point

Location : On the lateral side of the foot, posterior to the head of the 5th metatarsal bone, at the border between the red and white flesh(Figure 11-59).

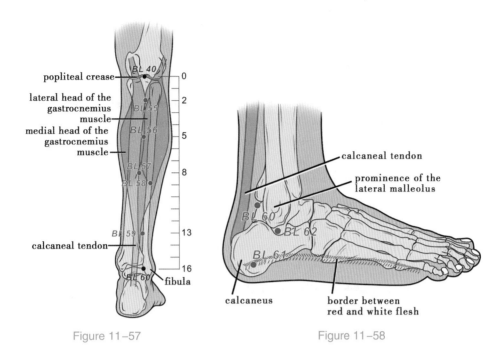

Figure 11–57　　　　　　　　　　　Figure 11–58

Indications:①Headache,stiff neck,dizziness. ②Pain in the lumbar area and lower limbs. ③Psychosis.

Manipulation:0.3–0.5 cun perpendicular insertion.

(26)Zhiyin(BL 67)well point

Location:On the lateral side of the distal segment of the little toe,0.1 cun from the corner of the toenail(Figure 11–60).

Indications:①Malposition of fetus,delayed labour. ②Headache,eyes pain. ③Nasal obstruction,nosebleed.

Manipulation:Insert the needle 0.1 cun into the skin,and moxibustion is applicable for malposition of fetus.

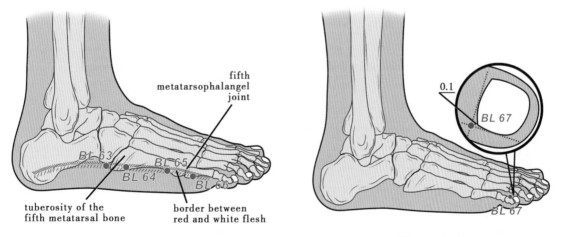

Figure 11–59　　　　　　　　　　　Figure 11–60

Other points on bladder meridian of foot taiyang see Table 11–17.

Table 11-17　Other points on bladder meridian of foot taiyang

Points	Code	Location	Indication
Meichong	BL 3	On the scalp, directly above Cuanzu (BL 2),0.5 cun within the anterior hairline	Headache, dizziness, nasal obstruction, epistaxis
Qucha	BL 4	On the scalp, 0.5 cun within the anterior hairline and 1.5 cun lateral to the midline. At the junction of the medial one-third and lateral 2/3 of the distance from Shenting (GV 24) and Touwei(ST 8)	Headache, dizziness, nasal obstruction, epistaxis
Wuchu	BL 5	On the scalp, 1.0 cun within the anterior hairline and 1.5 cun lateral to the midline	①Headache, dizziness. ②Epilepsy
Chengguang	BL 6	On the scalp, 2.5 cun within the anterior hairline and 1.5 cun lateral to the midline	① Headache, dizziness, nasal obstruction. ②Febrile diseases
Tongtian	BL 7	On the scalp, 4.0 cun within the anterior hairline and 1.5 cun lateral to the midline	①Headache, dizziness, nasal obstruction, epistaxis, nasosinusitis. ②Epilepsy
Luoque	BL 8	On the scalp, 5.5 cun within the anterior hairline and 1.5 cun lateral to the midline	Dizziness, blurred vision, tinnitus
Yuzhen	BL 9	On the posterior aspect of the head, 2.5 cun superior to the posterior hairline, 1.3 cun lateral to the midline and level with the depression on the superior border of the external occipital protuberance	Headache and nape of the neck pain, eye pain, nasal obstruction
Tianzhu	BL 10	On the nape, 1.3 cun lateral to the midpoint of the posterior hairline, and in the depression of the lateral border of the trapezius muscle	Headache, dizziness, stiffness of nape, pain in the back and shoulders, nasal obstruction
Dazhu(one of the eight meeting points-bones convergence)	BL 11	On the back, below the spinous process of the 1st thoracic vertebra and 1.5 cun lateral to the posterior midline	①Stiffness of nape, pain in the back and shoulder. ②Cough
Jueyinshu (back transport point of the pericardium)	BL 14	On the back, level with the lower border of the spinous process of the 4th thoracic vertebra and 1.5 cun lateral to the posterior midline	①Cardiac pain, palpitations. ②Cough, tightness in the chest. ③Vomiting
Dushu	BL 16	On the back, level with the lower border of the spinous process of the 6th thoracic vertebra and 1.5 cun lateral to the posterior midline	①Cardiac pain, tightness in the chest. ②Asthma. ③ Stomachache, abdominal distention, hiccups
Sanjiaoshu (back transport point of the triple energizer)	BL 22	On the back, below the spinous process of the 1st lumbar vertebra and 1.5 cun lateral to the posterior midline	①Edema, difficulty in urination. ②Abdominal distension, borborygmus, diarrhea, dysentery. ③Stiffness and pain in the back and lumbar region

Continue to Table 11-17

Points	Code	Location	Indication
Qihaishu	BL 24	Level with the lower border of the spinous process of the 3rd lumbar vertebra and 1. 5 cun lateral to the posterior midline	①Lumbar pain. ②Dysmenorrhea. ③Abdominal distension, borborygmus, hemorrhoids
Guanyuanshu	BL 26	Level with the lower border of the spinous process of the 5th lumbar vertebra and 1. 5 cun lateral to the posterior midline	① Pain of the lumbar region and lower limbs. ② Abdominal distension, diarrhea. ③Frequent urination or difficulty in urination, enuresis
Xiaochangshu (back transport point of the small Intestine)	BL 27	On the sacrum, level with the 1st posterior sacral foramen, and 1. 5 cun lateral to the median sacral crest	①Lumbar pain, sacral pain. ②Lower abdominal pain and distention, diarrhea, dysentery. ③Seminal emission, morbid leucorrhea. ④Enuresis, hematuria
Zhonglushu	BL 29	Level with the 3rd posterior sacral foramen and 1. 5 cun lateral to the medial sacral crest	①Diarrhea. ②Stiffness and pain in the lower back. ③Hernia
Baihuanshu	BL 30	Level with the 4th posterior sacral foramen and 1. 5 cun lateral to the medial sacral crest	① Seminal emission, enuresis, morbid leucorrhea, irregular menstruation, hernia. ②Pain in the lower back
Shangliao	BL 31	In the region of the sacrum, between the posterior superior iliac spine and the posterior midline, in the 1st posterior sacral foramen	①Irregular menstruation, morbid leucorrhea, prolapsed uterus, seminal emission impotency. ②Difficulty in urination and defecation. ③Pain in the lower back
Zhongliao	BL 33	In the region of the sacrum, medial and inferior to Ciliao(BL 32), in the 3rd posterior sacral foramen	①Irregular menstruation, morbid leucorrhea, difficulty in urination. ② Constipation, diarrhea. ③Lumbosacral pain
Xialiao	BL 34	In the region of the sacrum, medial and inferior to Zhongliao(BL 33), in the 4th posterior sacral foramen	①Lower abdominal pain, lumbosacral pain. ②Difficulty in urination and defecation, morbid leucorrhea
Huiyang	BL 35	In the region of the sacrum, 0. 5 cun lateral to the tip of the coccyx	①Diarrhea, dysentery, hematochezia, hemorrhoids. ②Impotency, morbid leucorrhea
Chengfu	BL 36	At the midpoint of the transverse gluteal crease	①Pain in the lumbar and legs, weakness or paralysis in the lower limbs. ②Hemorrhoids
Yinmen	BL 37	On the line connecting Chengfu(BL 36) and Weizhong(BL 40), 6 cun below Chengfu (BL 36)	Pain in the lumbar and legs, weakness or paralysis in the lower limbs
Fuxi	BL 38	On the lateral end of the transverse crease of the popliteal fossa and 1 cun above Weiyang(BL 39) on the medial side of the tendon of the biceps femoris	①Pain, numbness and spasm in the popliteal fossa and knees. ②Constipation
Fufen	BL 41	On the back, level with the lower border of the spinous process of the 2nd thoracic vertebra and 3 cun lateral to the posterior midline	Stiffness and pain of the neck and back, spasm of the shoulders and back, and numbness of the elbows and arms

Continue to Table 11-17

Points	Code	Location	Indication
Pohu	BL 42	On the back, level with the lower border of the spinous process of the 3rd thoracic vertebra and 3 cun lateral to the posterior midline	①Cough, asthma, pulmonary phthisis. ②Stiff neck, pain of the shoulders and back
Shentang	BL 44	On the back, level with the lower border of the spinous process of the 5th thoracic vertebra and 3 cun lateral to the posterior midline	①Cardiac pain, palpitations. ②Cough, asthma, tightness in the chest. ③Pain in the back
Yixi	BL 45	On the back, level with the lower border of the spinous process of the 6th thoracic vertebra and 3 cun lateral to the posterior midline	①Cough, asthma. ② Malaria, febrile diseases. ③Pain of the shoulders and back
Geguan	BL 46	On the back, level with the lower border of the spinous process of the 7th thoracic vertebra and 3 cun lateral to the posterior midline	① Vomiting, hiccups, belching, dysphagia, tightness in the chest. ②Stiffness and pain of the back
Hunmen	BL 47	On the back, level with the lower border of the spinous process of the 9th thoracic vertebra and 3 cun lateral to the posterior midline	①Distending pain in the chest and hypochondrium, vomiting, diarrhea. ②Pain in the back
Yanggang	BL 48	On the back, level with the lower border of the spinous process of the 10th thoracic vertebra and 3 cun lateral to the posterior midline	①Borborygmus, abdominal pain, diarrhea. ②Jaundice, diabetes
Yishe	BL 49	On the back, level with the lower border of the spinous process of the 11th thoracic vertebra and 3 cun lateral to the posterior midline	Abdominal distension, borborygmus, diarrhea, and vomiting
Weicang	BL 50	On the back, level with the lower border of the spinous process of the 12th thoracic vertebra and 3 cun lateral to the posterior midline	①Epigastric pain, abdominal distension, indigestion. ②Edema
Huangmen	BL 51	Level with the lower border of the spinous process of the 1st lumbar vertebra and 3 cun lateral to the posterior midline	①Abdominal pain, abdominal masses. ②Constipation
Baohuang	BL 53	Level with the 2nd posterior sacral foramen and 3 cun lateral to the median sacral crest	①Difficulty in urination, swollen vulva. ②Abdominal distension, constipation. ③Lumbar vertebral pain
Heyang	BL 55	On the posterior aspect of the lower leg and 2 cun below Weizhong(BL 40)	Stiffness or pain in the low back, atrophy or paralysis in the lower limbs, hernia, uterine bleeding

Points	Code	Location	Indication
Chengjin	BL 56	On the posterior midline of the leg, between Weizhong(BL 40) and Kunlun(BL 60), in the center of the belly of the gastrocnemius muscle and 5 cun below Weizhong(BL 40)	Pain in the low back and legs, hemorrhoids
Fuyang(cleft point of the yang heel vessel)	BL 59	3 cun directly above Kunlun (BL 60) between the fibula and the calcaneal tendon	Pain in the low back and legs, atrophy or paralysis in the lower limbs, headache
Pucan	BL 61	On the lateral side of the foot, posterior and inferior to the external malleolus, directly below Kunlun(BL 60), lateral to the calcaneus at the border between the red and white flesh	①Atrophy or paralysis in the lower limbs, pain in the heel. ②Epilepsy
Jingmen(cleft point)	BL 63	On the dorsum of the foot inferior to the anterior border of the lateral malleolus and posterior to the tuberosity of the 5th metatarsal bone in the depression inferior to the cuboid bone	① Headache. ② Epilepsy, infantile convulsions. ③ Lumbar pain, pain in the lower limbs, pain and swelling in the external malleolus
Jinggu(source point)	BL 64	On the lateral aspect of the foot, distal to the tuberosity of the 5th metatarsal bone at the border between the red and white flesh	①Headache, stiff neck, superficial visual obstruction. ② Pain in the lumbar and lower limbs. ③Epilepsy
Zutonggu(spring point)	BL 66	On the lateral side of the foot, anterior to the 5th metatarsophalangeal join, at the border between the red and white flesh	①Headache, stiff neck, dizziness, epistaxis. ②Psychosis

11.3.1.8　Frequently used acupoints on kidney meridian of foot shaoyin

Kidney meridian of foot shaoyin originates from the inferior aspect of the small toe, and proceeds diagonally to the center of the foot sole emerging from the lower border of the navicular tuberosity. It runs posterior to the inner malleolus and enters the heel. It then ascends along the medial aspect of the lower leg and emerges from the medial aspect of popliteal fossa. From the popliteal fossa, it proceeds upwards along the medial and posterior aspect of the thigh and goes towards the vertebral column. It then pertains to the kidney and connects with the bladder. A straight branch from the kidney ascends to enter the lung, and then travels upwards along the throat to reach the root of the tongue. Another branch emerges from the lung to connect with the heart, and depresses into the chest(Figure 11-61).

(1)Yongquan(KI 1)well point

Location: On the sole, in the depression which appears on the anterior part of the sole when the foot is in the plantar flexion, at the junction of the anterior third and posterior two thirds of the line connecting the base of the 2nd and 3nd toes and the heel approximately(Figure 11-62).

Indications:①Mind diseases like coma, heatstroke, epilepsy, infantile convulsions. ②Headache, vertigo, dizziness, insomnia. ③Lung system diseases like swollen pharynx, aphonia. ④Constipation, dysuria. ⑤Up-rushing gas syndrome. ⑥Feverish sensation in the sole.

Manipulation: 0.5-1.0 cun perpendicular insertion, and to avoid hurting plantar adeep when inserting the needle. Moxibustion is applicable.

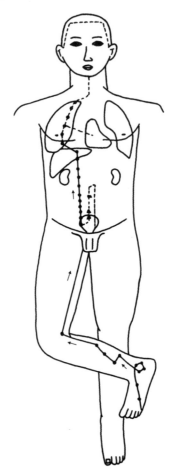

Figure 11–61 **The course of kidney**
meridian of foot shaoyin

(2)Rangu(KI 2)spring point

Location:On the medial border of the foot and in the depression below the tuberosity of the navicular bone, at the border between the red and white flesh(Figure 11–63).

Indications:①Gynecological diseases like irregular menstruation, morbid leucorrhea, prolapsed uterus. ②External genitalia diseases like seminal emission, impotence, and dysuria. ③Sore and swollen throat, hemoptysis. ④Diabetes. ⑤Weakness and flaccidity of the lower limbs, pain instep. ⑥Tetanus, lockjaw. ⑦Diarrhea.

Manipulation:0.5–1.0 cun perpendicular insertion.

(3)Taixi(KI 3)stream point; source point

Location:Posterior to the medial malleolus, in the depression between the tip of the medial malleolus and the calcaneal tendon(Figure 11–63).

Indications:① Headache, dizziness, insomnia, forgetfulness. ② Sore and swollen throat, toothache, tinnitus, deafness. ③Cough, asthma, hemoptysis, pain in the chest. ④Diabetes. ⑤Irregular menstruation, seminal emission, impotence, frequent urination. ⑥Lumbar pain, cold lower limbs, pain and swelling in the medial malleolus.

Manipulation:0.5–1.0 cun perpendicular insertion.

(4)Dazhong(KI 4)connecting point

Location:On the medial side of the foot, posterior and inferior to the medial malleolus, in the depression anterior to the medial side of the attachment of calcaneal tendon(Figure 11-63).

Indications:①Dementia. ②Retention of urine, enuresis, constipation. ③Irregularmenstruation. ④Hemoptysis, asthma. ⑤Lumbago, pain in the heel.

Manipulation:Puncture perpendicularly by 0. 3-0. 5 cun.

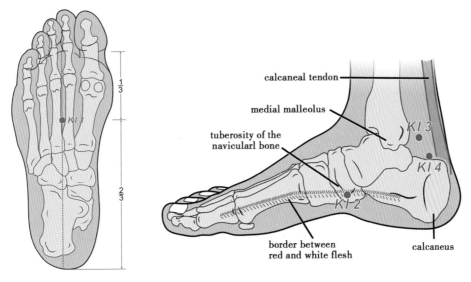

Figure 11-62   Figure 11-63

(5)Zhaohai(KI 6)one of the eight confluence points associated with yin heel vessel

Location:In the depression below the tip of the medial malleolus(Figure 11-64).

Indications:①Insomnia, epilepsy. ②Sore and dry throat, red and swollen eyes. ③Irregular menstruation, dysmenorrheal, morbid leucorrhea, prolapsed uterus. ④Frequent urination, retention of urine, constipation.

Manipulation:0. 5-0. 8 cun perpendicular insertion.

(6)Fuliu(KI 7)river point

Location:2 cun directly above Taixi(KI 3), anterior to the achilles tendon(Figure 11-65).

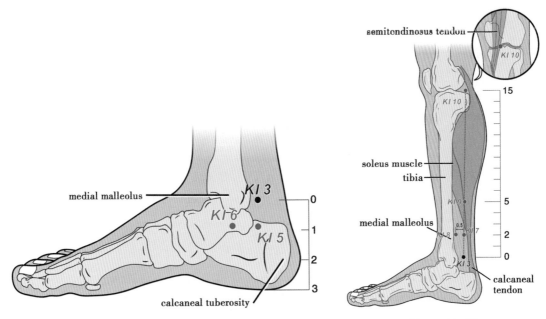

Figure 11-64   Figure 11-65

Indications : ①Edema, night sweat, febrile diseases with anhidrosis or hyperhidrosis. ②Abdominal distension, diarrhea, borborygmus. ③Lumbago, weakness and flaccidity of the lower limbs.

Manipulation : 0. 5–1. 0 cun perpendicular insertion.

Other points on kidney meridian of foot shaoyin see Table 11–18.

Table 11–18　Other points on kidney meridian of foot shaoyin

Points	Code	Location	Indication
Shuiquan	KI 5	1 cun directly below Taixi (KI 3), in the depression of the medial side of the tuberosity of the calcaneus	Irregular menstruation, dysmenorrhea, prolapsed uterus, difficulty in urination
Jiaoxin	KI 8	On the medial aspect of the lower legs, 2 cun above Taixi(KI 3),0. 5 cun anterior to Fuliu(KI 7), posterior to the medial border of the tibia	①Irregular menstruation, uterine bleeding, and prolapsed uterus. ②Diarrhea, constipation
Zhubin	KI 9	On the line connecting Taixi(KI 3) and Yingu(KI 10),5 cun above Taixi (KI 3), medial and inferior to the gastrocnemius muscle belly	①Psychosis. ②Hernia. ③Vomiting. ④Pain on the medial aspect of the lower legs
Yingu (sea point)	KI 10	On the posteromedial aspect of the knee lateral to the semitendinosus tendon in the popliteal crease	①Psychosis. ②Impotence, irregular menstruation, uterine bleeding, difficulty in urination. ③Pain on the medial side of the knees and legs
Henggu	KI 11	On the lower abdomen,5 cun below the umbilicus and 0. 5 cun lateral to the anterior midline	①Pain and distension in the lower abdomen, hernia. ②Seminal emission, impotence, enuresis, difficulty in urination
Dahe	KI 12	4 cun below the center of the umbilicus and 0. 5 cun lateral to the anterior midline	①Seminal emission, impotence. ②Prolapsed uterus, morbid leucorrhea, irregular menstruation. ③Diarrhea and dysentery
Qixue	KI 13	On the lower abdomen,3 cun below the umbilicus and 0. 5 cun lateral to the anterior midline	①Irregular menstruation, morbid leucorrhea, infertility, impotence, difficulty in urination. ②Diarrhea, dysentery
Siman	KI 14	On the lower abdomen,2 cun below the umbilicus and 0. 5 cun lateral to the anterior midline	①Irregular menstruation, morbid leucorrhea, seminal emission, enuresis, edema. ②Abdominal pain, constipation
Zhongzhu	KI 15	In the center of the abdomen,1 cun below the umbilicus and 0. 5 cun lateral to the anterior midline	①Irregular menstruation. ②Abdominal pain, constipation, diarrhea
Huangshu	KI 16	In the center of the abdomen and 0. 5 cun lateral to the anterior midline	①Abdominal pain and distension, vomiting, diarrhea, constipation. ②Hernia. ③Irregular menstruation
Shangqu	KI 17	On the upper abdomen,2 cun above the umbilicus and 0. 5 cun lateral to the anterior midline	Abdominal pain, diarrhea and constipation
Shi guan	KI 18	On the upper abdomen,3 cun above the umbilicus and 0. 5 cun lateral to the anterior midline	①Abdominal pain, vomiting, constipation. ②Infertility

Continue to Table 11-18

Points	Code	Location	Indication
Yindu	KI 19	On the upper abdomen, 4 cun above the umbilicus and 0.5 cun lateral to the anterior midline	① Abdominal pain and distension, borborygmus, constipation. ②Infertility
Futonggu	KI 20	On the upper abdomen, 5 cun above the umbilicus and 0.5 cun lateral to the anterior midline	Abdominal pain and distension, and vomiting
Youmen	KI 21	On the upper abdomen, 6 cun above the umbilicus and 0.5 cun lateral to the anterior midline	Stomachache, vomiting, abdominal distension, and diarrhea
Bulang	KI 22	On the chest in the 5th intercostal space and 2 cun lateral to the anterior midline	①Distension and fullness of the chest and hypochondriac regions, cough, asthma. ②Vomiting. ③Mastiffs
Shenfeng	KI 23	On the chest, in the 4th intercostal space and 2 cun lateral to the anterior midline	① Cough, asthma, distension and fullness of the chest and hypochondriac regions. ②Mastitis. ③Vomiting
Lingxu	KI 24	On the chest, in the 3rd intercostal space and 2 cun lateral to the anterior midline	① Cough, asthma, distension and fullness of the chest and hypochondriac regions. ②Mastitis. ③Vomiting
Shencang	KI 25	On the chest, in the 2nd intercostal space and 2 cun lateral to the anterior midline	①Chest pain, cough, asthma. ②Vomiting
Yuzhong	KI 26	On the chest, in the 1st intercostal space and 2 cun lateral to the anterior midline	Cough, asthma, distending pain in the chest and hypochondriac regions
Shufu	KI 27	On the chest, on the lower border of the clavicle and 2 cun lateral to the anterior midline	①Cough, asthma, chest pain. ②Vomiting

11.3.1.9   Frequently used acupoints on pericardium meridian of hand jueyin

It originates from the center of the chest, and pertains to the pericardium. It descends through the diaphragm, passing through the upper, middle and lower energizer. One branch runs inside the chest to emerge from hypochondrium and runs along the middle of the upper arm, and then it travels along the forearm between the two tendons to enter the palm, passing along the middle finger and ends at its tip. One branch splits from the palm to reach the tip of the ring finger, connecting with the triple energizer meridian of hand shaoyang (Figure 11-66).

(1) Tianchi (PC 1)

Location: On the chest, in the 4th intercostal space, 1 cun lateral to the nipple and 5 cun lateral to the anterior midline (Figure 11-67).

Indications: ①Cough, asthma, pain or distention in the chest. ②Mastitis. ③Scrofula.

Manipulation: Puncture obliquely or transversely by 0.5-0.8 cun. Do not puncture deeply to avoid injuring the lung.

(2) Quze(PC 3)sea point

Location：On the transverse cubital crease and on the ulnar side of the tendon of the biceps muscle of the arm(Figure 11-68).

Indications：①Heart system diseases like cardiodynia,palpitations,etc. ②Stomach diseases like stomachache,haematemesis,vomiting,etc. ③Sunstroke. ④Pain and cramps in the elbows and arms.

Manipulation：1.0-1.5 cun deep perpendicular insertion. Pricking to induce bleeding is applicable.

(3) Jianshi(PC 5)river point

Location：On the palmar side of the forearm,3 cun above the transverse crease of the wrist,and between the tendons of the palmaris longus and flexor carpi radialis(Figure 11-68).

Indications：①Heart system diseases like cardiodynia,palpitations,etc. ②Stomach diseases like stomachache,vomiting,etc. ③Febrile disease, malaria. ④Psychosis, epilepsy. ⑤Brachialgia,cramps in the elbow,axillary swelling.

Manipulation：0.5-1.0 cun deep perpendicular insertion.

(4) Neiguan(PC 6)connecting point；one of the eight confluent points associating with yin link vessel

Location：On the palmar side of the forearm,2 cun above the transverse crease of the wrist,and between the tendons of the palmaris longus and flexor carpi radialis(Figure 11-68).

Indications：① Heart system diseases like cardiodynia, palpitations, chest pain, oppression in the chest,etc. ②Stomach diseases like stomachache,vomiting,hiccups,etc. ③Stroke,dizziness,hemiplegia,migraine. ④Insomnia,depression,epilepsy,febrile disease. ⑤Pain and spasm in the elbows and arms.

Manipulation：0.5-1.0 cun deep perpendicular insertion.

(5) Daling(PC 7)stream point；source point

Location：In the middle of the transverse crease of the wrist,and between the tendons of the palmaris longus and flexor carpi radialis(Figure 11-68).

Indications：①Cardiodynia,palpitations,pain and distension in the chest,hypochondriac pain. ②Stomachache,vomiting,bromopnea. ③Epilepsy,madness. ④Pain and spasm in the elbows and arms.

Manipulation：0.3-0.5 cun deep perpendicular insertion.

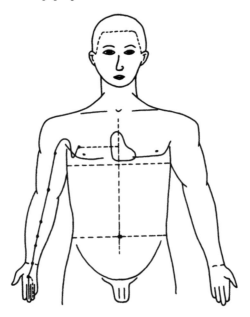

Figure 11-66　The course of pericardium meridian of hand jueyin

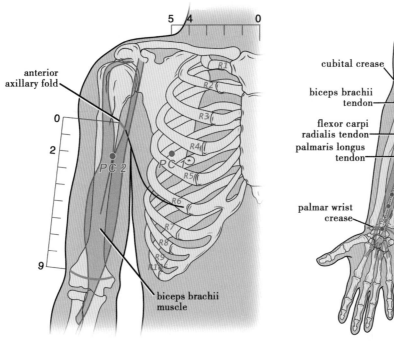

Figure 11-67   Figure 11-68

(6) Laogong(PC 8) spring point

Location: In the middle of the palm, between the 2nd and 3rd metacarpal bones. When the fist is made, the point is just below the tip of the middle finger(Figure 11-69).

Indications: ①Stroke and coma, sunstroke. ②Cardiodynia, restlessness, epilepsy. ③Stomatitis, foul breath. ④Tinea manus.

Manipulation: 0.3-0.5 cun deep perpendicular insertion.

(7) Zhongchong(PC 9) well point

Location: In the center of the tip of the middle finger(Figure 11-69).

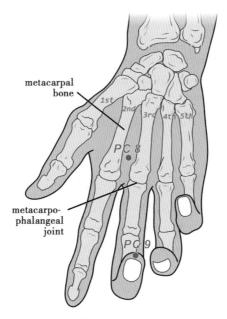

Figure 11-69

Indications : ①Stroke and coma, stiff tongue impeding speech, infantile convulsion, sunstroke, syncope. ②Febrile disease, pain in the hypoglottis

Manipulation : 0. 1 cun shallow insertion or prick with three-edged needle to induce bleeding.

Other points on pericardium meridian of hand jueyin see Table 11-19.

Table 11-19 Other points on pericardium meridian of hand jueyin

Points	Code	Location	Indication
Tianquan	PC 2	On the palmar side of the upper arm, 2 cun below the level of the anterior axillary fold, between the two heads of the biceps brachii muscle	Cardiodynia, cough, distention in the chest, pain in the chest, upper back, and medial side of the upper arms
Ximen(cleft point)	PC 4	On the palmar side of the forearm, 5 cun above the transverse crease of the wrist, and between the tendons of the palmaris longus and flexor carpi radialis	①Cardiodynia, palpitations, restlessness, pain in the chest. ②Hemoptysis, hematemesis, epistaxis. ③Furunculosis. ④Epilepsy

11.3.1.10 Frequently used acupoints on triple energizer meridian of hand shaoyang

It originates from the tips of the ring finger and runs upward between the 4th and 5th metacarpal bones along the dorsum of the hand then continues going upwards between the radius and ulna. It ascends along the lateral aspect of the upper arms to the shoulders and enters the supraclavicular fossa to connect with the pericardium and connects along its pathway with the upper, middle, and lower energizer. One branch separates in the chest region, ascending to emerge from the supraclavicular fossa and rising to the head.

One branch separates in the chest region, ascending to emerge from the supraclavicular fossa and rising along the neck to the posterior border of the ear. It crosses from the superior aspect of the ear to the corner of the forehead, turning downwards the cheek and reaching the inferior aspect of the eye.

Another branch separates behind the ear and enters the ear, and reemerges in front of the ear, crossing the previous branch on the cheek. It then goes to the outer canthus, where it connects with the gallbladder meridian of foot shaoyang(Figure 11-70).

(1)Guauchong(TE 1)well point

Location : On the ulnar side of the distal segment of the 4th finger, 0. 1 cun from the corner of the nail.

Indications : ①Headache, red eyes, deafness, sore throat, stiff tongue. ②Febrile diseases, coma, sunstroke(Figure 11-71).

Manipulation : Insert the needle shallowly by 0. 1 cun deep or prick with three-edged needle to induce bleeding.

(2)Zhongzhu(TE 3)stream point

Location : On the dorsum of the hand proximal to the 4th metacarpophalangeal joint, in the depression between the 4th and 5th metacarpal bones(Figure 11-71).

Indications : ①Headache, red eyes, tinnitus, deafness, sore throat. ②Febrile diseases, sunstroke.

Manipulation : 0. 3-0. 5 cun deep perpendicular insertion.

(3)Yangchi(TE 4)source point

Location : At the midpoint of the dorsal crease of the wrist, in the depression on the ulnar side of the tendon of the extensor muscle of the finger(Figure 11-72).

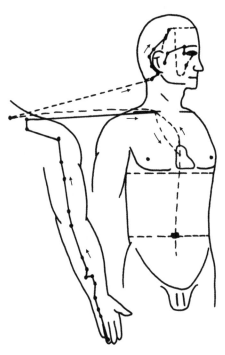

Figure 11-70   **The course of triple energizer meridian of hand shaoyang**

Indications:①Red and swollen eyes,deafness,sore throat. ②Diabetes,febrile diseases. ③Pain in the arms and wrists. ④Malaria.

Manipulation:0.3-0.5 cun deep perpendicularl insertion.

(4)Waiguan(TE 5)connecting point;one of the Eight Confluent Points Associating with Yang Link Vessel.

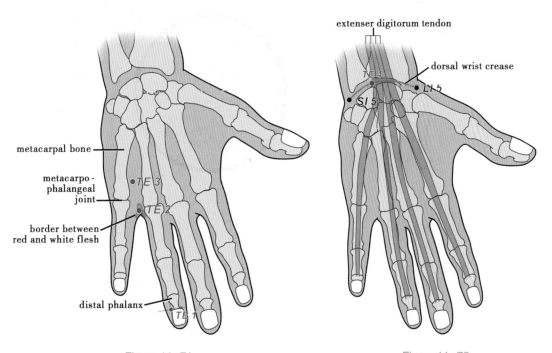

Figure 11-71   Figure 11-72

Location: On the dorsal side of the forearm and on the line connecting Yangchi(TE 4) and the tip of the olecranon, 2 cun proximal to the dorsal crease of the wrist and between the radius and ulna(Figure 11-73).

Indications: ①Febrile disease. ②Headache, cheek pain, red and swollen eyes, tinnitus, deafness. ③Scrofula. ④Hypochondriac pain. ⑤Pain, numbness, flaccidity and muscle atrophy in the upper limbs.

Manipulation: 0.5-1.0 cun deep perpendicular insertion.

(5) Zhigou(TE 6) river point

Location: On the dorsal aspect of the forearm, 3 cun above the transverse crease of the dorsum of the wrist between the ulna and radius(Figure 11-73).

Indications: ① Tinnitus, deafness, sudden loss of voice. ② Hypochondriac pain. ③ Constipation. ④Scrofula. ⑤Febrile disease.

Manipulation: 0.5-1.0 cun deep perpendicular insertion.

(6) Jianliao(TE 14)

Location: On the shoulder girdle in the depression between the acromial angle and the greater tubercle of the humerus(Figure 11-74).

Indications: ①Pain in the shoulders and arms, heaviness of the shoulder with inability to raise the arm. ②Pain in the hypochondriac regions.

Manipulation: 1.0-1.5 cun deep perpendicular insertion.

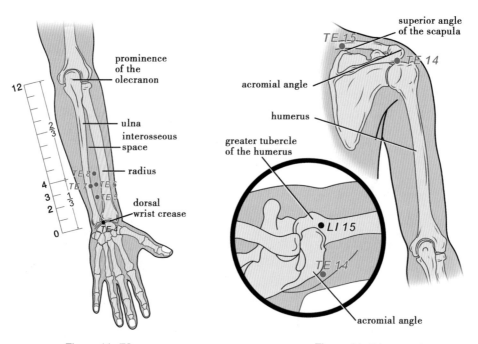

Figure 11-73   Figure 11-74

(7) Yifeng(TE 17)

Location: Posterior to the ear lobe, in the depression between the mastoid process and the angle of the mandible(Figure 11-75).

Indications: ①Tinnitus, deafness. ②Deviation of the mouth and eye, locked jaw, toothache. ③Scrofula.

Manipulation: 0.5-1.0 cun deep perpendicular insertion.

(8) Ermen(TE 21)

Location: In front of the supratragic notch, in the depression of the posterior border of the condylar process of the mandible when the mouth is open(Figure 11-76).

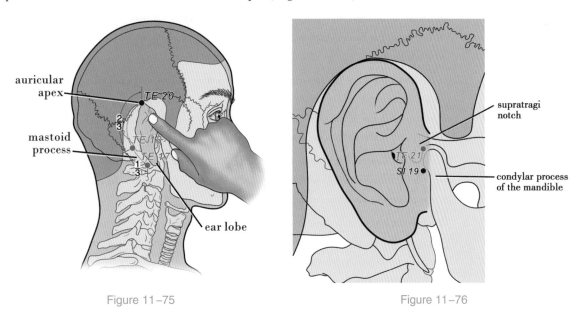

Figure 11-75   Figure 11-76

Indications: ①Tinnitus, deafness. ②Toothache.

Manipulation: 0.5-1.0 cun deep perpendicular insertion.

(9) Sizhukong(TE 23)

Location: On the face and in the depression of the lateral end of the eyebrow(Figure 11-77).

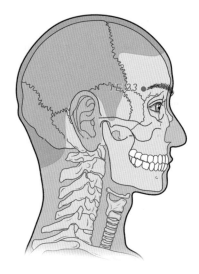

Figure 11-77

Indications: ①Psychosis and epilepsy. ②Redness, swelling and pain of the eyes, twitching of the eyelids, migraine. ③Toothache.

Manipulation: 0.3-0.5 cun deep horizontal insertion.

Other points on triple energizer meridian of hand shaoyang see Table 11-20.

Table 11–20 Other points on triple energizer meridian of hand shaoyang

Points	Code	Location	Indication
Yemen (spring point)	TE 2	On the dorsum of the hand, proximal to the margin of the web between the 4th and 5th fingers, at the border between the red and white flesh	①Headache, red eyes, tinnitus, deafness. ②Malaria. ③Pain in the upper limbs
Huizong (cleft point)	TE 7	On the dorsal aspect of the forearm, 3 cun above the transverse crease of the dorsum of the wrist, on the ulnar side of Zhigou (TE 6), and on the radial side of the ulna	①Tinnitus, deafness. ②Epilepsy
Sanyang luo	TE 8	On the dorsal aspect of the forearm, 4 cun above the transverse crease of dorsum of the wrist, between the ulna and radius	①Deafness, sudden loss of voice, toothache. ②Atrophy or paralysis in the upper limbs
Sidu	TE 9	On the dorsal aspect of the forearm, on the line connecting Yangchi(TE 4) and tip of the elbow, 5 cun below the tip of the elbow between the ulna and radius	①Numbness and pain of the upper limbs. ②Deafness, sudden loss of voice, toothache, headache
Tianjing (sea point)	TE 10	On the lateral aspect of the arm, when the elbow is bent, the point is in the depression about 1 cun above the olecranon of the ulna	①Migraine, deafness, epilepsy. ②Scrofula. ③Pain in the elbows and arms
Qinglengyuan	TE 11	On the lateral aspect of the arm, 2 cun proximal to the prominence of the olecranon on a line connecting the prominence of the olecranon and the acromial angel	①Pain in the shoulders and arms, paralysis of the upper limbs. ②Headache, eye pain
Xiaoluo	TE 12	On the lateral aspect of the arm, 5 cun proximal to the prominence of the olecranon on a line connecting the prominence of the olecranon and the acromial angel	①Numbness and pain of the upper limbs. ②Headache, toothache, stiff neck. ③Epilepsy
Naohui	TE 13	On the lateral aspect of the arm, 3 cun inferior to the acromial angel, on the posterior and inferior border of the deltoid muscle	①Scrofula, goiter. ②Spasm and pain in the upper limbs
Tianliao	TE 15	In the scapula region, in the depression above the superior angle of the scapula, midpoint of a line connecting Jianjing(GB 21) and Quyuan(SI 13)	①Pain in the shoulders and arms. ②Spasm of the nape of the neck
Tianyou	TE 16	On the side of the neck, directly inferior to the posterior aspect of the mastoid process, at the level of the angle of the mandible, on the posterior border of the sternocleidomastoideus	①Headache, stiff neck, dizziness, eye pain, deafness. ②Scrofula

Continue to Table 11-20

Points	Code	Location	Indication
Chimai	TE 18	On the head, posterior to the ear in the center of the mastoid process, at the junction of the middle and lower third of the curved line along the ear helix connecting Jiaosun(TE 20) and Yifeng(TE 17)	①Migraine, tinnitus, deafness. ②Infantile convulsions
Luxi	TE 19	On the head, at the junction of the upper and middle third of the curved line along the ear helix connecting Jiaosun(TE 20) and Yifeng(TE 17)	①Migraine, tinnitus, deafness. ②Infantile convulsions
Jiaosun	TE 20	On the head, on the hairline directly above the ear apex where the ear is folded forward	① Migraine, stiff neck. ② Mumps, toothache. ③Cataracts, red and swollen eyes
Erheliao	TE 22	On the side of the head, on the posterior border of the hairline of the temple, at the level with the root of the ear, posterior to the superficial temporal artery	①Migraine, tinnitus. ②Locked jaw

11.3.1.11　Frequently used acupoints on gallbladder meridian of foot shaoyang

Gallbladder meridian of foot shaoyang originates from the outer canthus, ascends to the corner of the forehead, and then descends to the posterior of the ear. Descending further along the neck to the shoulder, it enters the supraclavicular fossa.

One branch emerges behind the ear and enters the ear, reemerging in front of the ear, and then reaching the posterior aspect of the outer canthus.

Another branch starts from the outer canthus, descends to the Daying(ST 5) and ascends to the infraorbital regions, passing near Jiache(ST 6) and descending along the neck where it joins the previous branch at the supraclavicular fossa.

These meridians descend from head to the supraclavicular fossa, and meet a branch coming from lateral side of eye. Then it descends to enter the chest to connect with the liver and pertains to the gallbladder. It then travels along inside the hypochondriac region to reach qi pathway, curving along the margin of the pubic hair and running transversely into Huantiao(GB 30). The straight branch in pelvis descends from the supraclavicular fossa to Huantiao(GB 30) to meet the previous branch passing through the axillary region, the lateral side of the chest and the free ends of the ribs. It continues going down the lateral side of the thigh and knee to descending along the anterior side of fibula to reach the anterior aspect of the lateral malleolus. It then follows the dorsum of the foot to end on the lateral side of the tip of the 4th toe. One branch splits from Zulinqi(GB 41) and emerges from the tip of the big toe. Then it comes back to enter the nail and go out of the hairy region to connect with the liver meridian of foot jueyin(Figure 11-78).

(1)Tongziliao(GB 1)

Location:In the depression 0.5 cun lateral to the outer canthus and on the lateral side of the orbital margin(Figure 11-79).

Indications:①Pain and red eyes, cataracts. ②Migraine, deviation of the mouth and eye.

Manipulation:0.3-0.5 cun deep horizontal insertion.

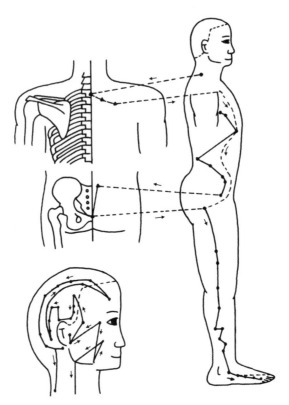

Figure 11 −78　The course of gallbladder meridian of foot shaoyang

（2）Tinghui（GB 2）

Location：Anterior to the intertragic notch, in the depression posterior to the condyloid process of the mandible when the mouth is open（Figure 11−80）.

Indications：①Tinnitus, deafness. ②Toothache, deviation of the mouth and eye.

Manipulation：0.5−0.8 cun perpendicularly insertion.

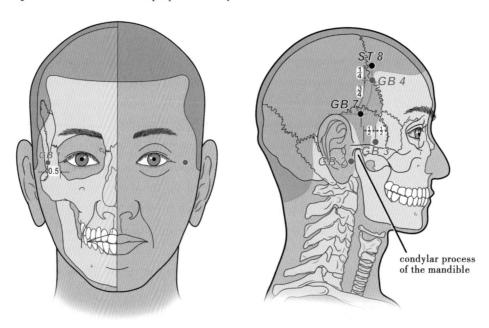

condylar process of the mandible

Figure 11−79　　　　　　　　　　　　　　　　Figure 11−80

(3) Yangbai(GB 14)

Location: On the forehead, directly above the pupil, 1 cun above the eyebrows(Figure 11-81).

Indications: ①Headache, vertigo. ②Deviation of the mouth and eye. ③Pain in the eyes, blurred vision, trembling eyelids.

Manipulation: 0.5-0.8 cun horizontal insertion.

(4) Toulinqi(GB 15)

Location: On the head, directly above the pupil and 0.5 cun above the anterior hairline(Figure 11-81).

Indications: ①Headache. ②Vertigo, lacrimation. ③Nasal obstruction. ④Infantile convulsion.

Manipulation: 0.5-0.8 cun horizontal insertion.

(5) Fengchi(GB 20)

Location: On the nape, below the occipital bone, in the depression between the upper ends of the sternocleidomastoid and trapezius muscles, on the level of Fengfu(GV 16)(Figure 11-82).

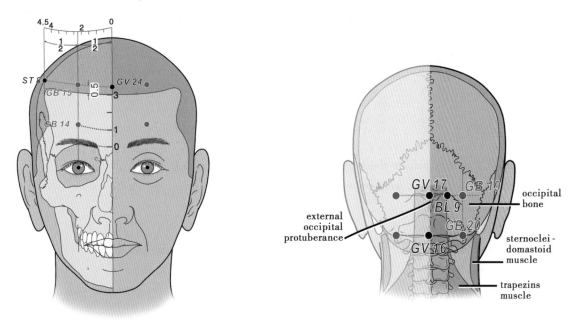

Figure 11-81   Figure 11-82

Indications: ①Headache, vertigo, red and swollen eyes, tinnitus, deafness. ②Common cold, nasal congestion, nasosinusitis, mania and epilepsy, apoplexy, febrile diseases, malaria and goiter. ③Rigidity and pain in the nape and back.

Manipulation: Puncture with the needle tip slightly pointed downwards, or toward the tip of the nose for 0.8-1.2 cun, or puncture horizontally towards Fengfu(GV 16). The medulla is located in the deep part; to insert the needle must strictly grasp the depth and angle.

(6) Jianjing(GB 21)

Location: At the midpoint of a line connecting the spinous process of the 7th cervical vertebra and the lateral end of the acromion(Figure 11-83).

Indications: ①Pain in the shoulders and upper back, stiffness and pain in the neck. ②Mastitis, insufficient lactation. ③Delayed labor. ④Scrofula.

Manipulation: 0.5-0.8 cun deep perpendicular insertion. Do not insert the needle too deep. Acupuncture is contraindicated for pregnant women.

(7) Riyue(GB 24) alarm point of the gallbladder

Location: Directly below the nipple, 4 cun lateral to the anterior midline, in the 7th intercostal space (Figure 11−84).

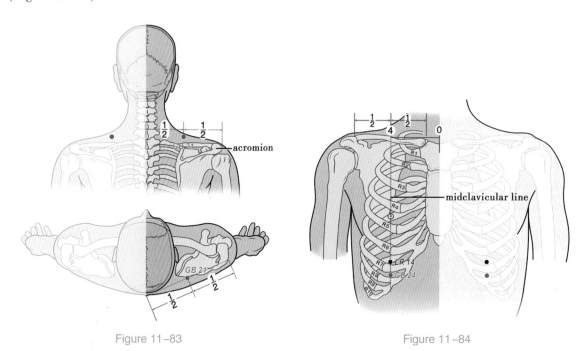

Figure 11−83   Figure 11−84

Indications: ①Jaundice, pain in the hypochondriac regions. ②Epigastric pain, vomiting, hiccups.

Manipulation: 0.5−0.8 cun deep perpendicular insertion. Do not insert the needle too deep so as to avoid hurting the inner viscera.

(8) Daimai(GB 26)

Location: At the junction of the vertical line of the free end of the 11th rib and the horizontal line of the umbilicus(Figure 11−85).

Indications: ①Irregular menstruation, morbid leucorrhea, amenorrhea, lower abdominal pain. ②Lumbar pain. ③Hernia.

Manipulation: 1.0−1.5 cun deep perpendicular insertion.

(9) Huantiao(GB 30)

Location: On the lateral side of the thigh, at the junction of the middle third and lateral third of the line connecting the prominence of the great trochanter and the sacral hiatus when the patient is in a lateral recumbent position with the thigh flexed(Figure 11−86).

Indications: ①Pain in the lumbar areas and legs, hemiplegia, and atrophy or paralysis in the lower limbs. ②Rubella.

Manipulation: 2.0−3.0 cun perpendicular insertion.

(10) Fengshi(GB 31)

Location: On the lateral aspect of the thigh, in the depression posterior to the iliotibial band where the tip of the middle finger touches when one stands with arms extended downward(Figure 11−87).

Indications: ①Hemiplegia, atrophy or paralysis in the lower limbs. ②Itching of the entire body, beri-beri.

Manipulation: 1.0−1.5 cun perpendicular insertion.

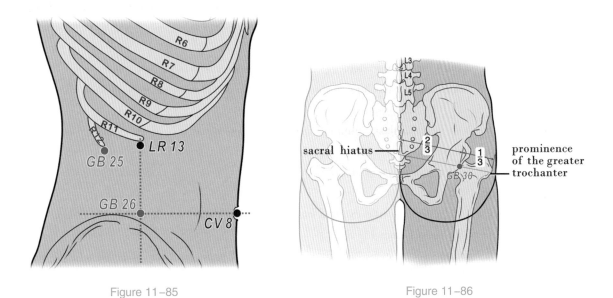

Figure 11-85   Figure 11-86

(11) Yanglingquan (GB 34) sea point; lower sea point of the gallbladder, one of the eight meeting points(sinews convergence)

Location: On the lateral side of the leg, in the depression anterior and inferior to the head of the fibula (Figure 11-88).

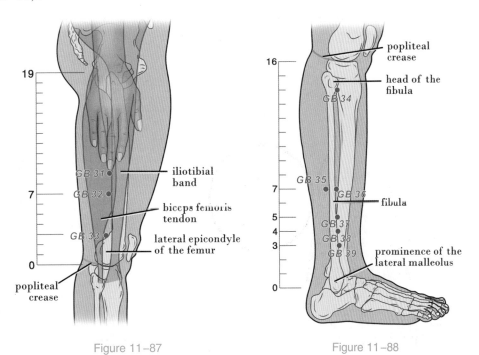

Figure 11-87   Figure 11-88

Indications: ①Jaundice, pain in the hypochondriac region, bitter taste in mouth, vomiting. ②Hemiparalysis, atrophy or paralysis in the lower limbs, beriberi. ③Infantile convulsion.

Manipulation: 1.0-1.5 cun perpendicular insertion.

(12) Guangming(GB 37) connecting point

Location: On the lateral side of the leg, 5 cun above the tip of the external malleolus, on the anterior border of the fibula(Figure 11-88).

Indications : ①Pain in the eyes, night blindness. ②Atrophy or paralysis in the lower limbs. ③Distention in the chest.

Manipulation : 0. 5-0. 8 cun perpendicular insertion.

(13) Xuanzhong(GB 39) one of the eight meeting points(marrow convergence)

Location : On the lateral side of the legs, 3 cun above the tip of the external malleolus, on the anterior border of the fibula(Figure 11-88).

Indications : Dementia, hemiparalysis. Stiffness in the nape, pain and distention in the hypochondriac region, atrophy or paralysis in the lower limbs, sore throat, beriberi, hemorrhoid.

Manipulation : 0. 5-0. 8 cun perpendicular insertion.

(14) Qiuxu(GB 40) Source Point

Location : Anterior and inferior to the external malleolus, in the depression lateral to the tendon of the long extensor muscle of the toes(Figure 11-89).

Indications : ①Red and swollen eyes. ②Stiffness in neck and nape, pain and distention in the hypochondriac region. ③Atrophy or paralysis in the lower limbs.

Manipulation : 0. 5-0. 8 cun perpendicular insertion.

(15) Zulinqi(GB 41) stream point; one of the eight confluence points associated with belt vessel

Location : On the lateral side of the instep of the foot, in the front of the junction of the 4th and 5th metatarsal bones, in the depression lateral to the tendon of the extensor muscle of the small toe (Figure 11-89).

Indications : ①Red and swollen eyes, pain in the hypochondriac region, migraine. ②Irregular menstruation, enuresis, mastitis, malaria, swelling and pain of the dorsum of the feet. ③Scrofula.

Manipulation : 0. 3-0. 5 cun perpendicular insertion.

(16) Zuqiaoyin(GB 44) well point

Location : On the lateral side of the distal segment of the 4th toe, 0. 1 cun from the corner of the toenail (Figure 11-90).

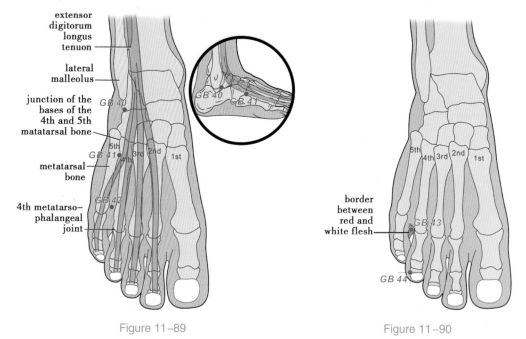

Figure 11-89   Figure 11-90

Indications : ①Headache, red and swollen pain, deafness, sore throat, febriel disease, cough, insomnia, ②Pain in the hypochondriac region. ③Irregular menstruation.

Manipulation: Insert the needle 0. 1–0. 2 cun into the skin, or insert a three-edged needle to induce bleeding.

Other points on gallbladder meridian of foot shaoyang see Table 11–21.

Table 11–21　Other points on gallbladder meridian of foot shaoyang

Points	Code	Location	Indication
Shangguan	GB 3	Directly above Xiaguan(ST 7), in the depression above the upper border of the zygomatic arch	①Tinnitus, deafness, toothache, facial pain, ② Deviation of the mouth and eye, locked jaw
Hanyan	GB 4	In the hair above the temples, at the junction of the upper 1/4 and lower 3/4 of the curved line connectingTouwei(ST 8) and Qubin (GB 7)	①Migraine, vertigo, tinnitus. ②Toothache
Xuanlu	GB 5	In the hair above the temples, at the midpoint of the curved line connecting Touwei(ST 8) and Qubin(GB 7)	①Migraine, red and swollen eyes. ②Toothache
Xuanli	GB 6	In the hair above the temples, at the junction of the upper 3/4 and lower 1/4 of the curved line connecting Touwei(ST 8) and Qubin (GB 7)	①Migraine, red and swollen eyes. ②Toothache
Qubin	GB 7	At a crossing point of the vertical posterior border of the temples and horizontal line through the ear apex	① Headache. ② Toothache, swelling and pain in the cheeks and jaw
Shuaigu	GB 8	1. 5 cun from the apex of the ear straight into the hairline	① Migraine, dizziness, tinnitus, deafness. ② Infantile convulsions
Tianchong	GB 9	2 cun from the posterior border of the ear straight into the hairline and 0. 5 cun posterior to Shuaigu (GB 8)	① Migraine, dizziness, tinnitus, deafness. ② Goiter. ③Fright, epilepsy
Fubai	GB 10	At the junction of the central 1/3 and upper 1/3 of the curved line connecting Tianchong(GB 9) and Wangu(GB 12)	①Migraine, tinnitus, deafness. ②Goiter, scrofula
Touqiaoyin	GB 11	Posterior and superior to the mastoid process, at the junction of the middle third and lower third of the curved line connecting Tianchong (GB 9) and Wangu(GB 12)	①Headache, dizziness, stiffness and pain in the neck. ②Tinnitus, deafness
Wangu	GB 12	In the depression posterior and inferior to the mastoid process	①Migraine, tinnitus, deviation of the mouth and eye. ②Stiffness and pain of the neck. ③Epilepsy

Continue to Table 11-21

Points	Code	Location	Indication
Benshen	GB 13	0. 5 cun above the anterior hairline and 3 cun lateral to Shenting (GV 24)	①Headache, dizziness, insomnia, epilepsy. ②Infantile convulsions, stroke
Muchuang	GB 16	1. 5 cun within the anterior hairline and 2. 25 cun lateral to the midline of the head	Headache, dizziness, redness, swelling and pain of the eyes, infantile convulsions
Zhengying	GB 17	2. 5 cun within the anterior hairline and 2. 25 cun lateral to the midline of the head	Headache, dizziness, and epilepsy
Chengling	GB 18	4 cun within the anterior hairline and 2. 25 cun lateral to the midline of the head	Headache, dizziness, disease of the eyes, nasosinusifis and epistaxis
Naokong	GB 19	On the lateral side of the superior border of the external occipital protuberance and 2. 25 cun lateral to the midline of the head	①Febrile diseases, headache, stiffness and pain around neck, dizziness, red and swollen eyes. ②Palpitations, infantile convulsion, epilepsy
Yuanye	GB 22	On the midaxillary line and in the 4th intercostal space	①Pain in the hypochondriac region, swollen axilla, tightness in the chest. ②Spasm and pain in the upper limbs
Zhejin	GB 23	1 cun anterior to the midaxillary line and in the 4th intercostal space	①Pain in the hypochondriac region. ②Tightness in the chest, asthma. ③Vomiting, acid regurgitation
Jingmen (alarm point of the kidney)	GB 25	On the inferior free end of the 12th rib	①Difficulty in urination, edema. ②Pain in the hypochondriac region, lumbar pain. ③Abdominal distension, diarrhea, borborygmus
Wushu	GB 27	Anterior to the superior iliac spine, level with 3 cun below the umbilicus	①Irregular menstruation, morbid leucorrhea, prolapsed uterus, lower abdominal pain. ②Pain of the lumbar and hip
Weidao	GB 28	Anterior and inferior to the superior iliac spine, 0. 5 cun anterior and inferior to Wushu(GB 27)	①Irregular menstruation, morbid leucorrhea, prolapsed uterus, lower abdominal pain. ②Pain of the lumbar and hip
Juliao	GB 29	On the midpoint of the line linking the anterio superior iliac spine and the prominence of the greater trochanter	①Pain in the lumbar and hip, atrophy or paralysis in the lower limbs. ②Hernia, lower abdominal pain
Zhongdu	GB 32	On the lateral aspect of the thigh, posterior to the iliotibial band and 7 cun superior to the popliteal crease	Atrophy or paralysis of the lower limbs and hemiplegia

Continue to Table 11-21

Points	Code	Location	Indication
Xiyangguan	GB 33	On the lateral aspect of the knee, in the depression between the biceps femoris tendon and the iliotibial band, posterior and proximal to the lateral epicondyle of the femur	Swelling, pain and spasm in the knees, numbness of the lower legs
Yangjiao (cleft point of yang link vessel)	GB 35	7 cun above the tip of the external malleolus and on the posterior border of the fibula	Distending pain in the chest and hypochondriac region, psychosisi, atrophy or paralysis of the lower limbs
Waiqiu (cleft point)	GB 36	7 cun superior to the tip of the external malleolus and on the anterior border of the fibula, level with Yangjiao(GB 35)	①Distending pain in the chest and hypochondriac region. ②Psychosis. ③Stiffness and pain in the neck. ④Atrophy or paralysis in the lower limbs
Yangfu (river point)	GB 38	4 cun superior to the tip of the external malleolus and slightly anterior to the anterior border of the fibula	①Migraine, pain in the outer canthus. ②Pain in the chest and hypochondriac region. ③Scrofula. ④Atrophy or paralysis of the lower limbs
Diwuhui	GB 42	On the dorsum of the foot, between the 4th and 5th metatarsal bones, in the depression proximal to the 4th metatarsophalangeal joint	①Headache, redness, swelling and pain of the eye, tinnitus, deafness. ②Mastiffs. ③Pain in the hypochondriac region, swelling and pain of the dorsum of the feet
Xiaxi (spring point)	GB 43	Between the 4th and 5th toes, at the border between the red and white flesh, proximal to the margin of the web	① Palpitation. ② Headache, dizziness, tinnitus, deafness, red eye pain. ③Distending pain in the chest and hypochondriac region, swelling and pain in the dorsum of the feet. ④Acute mastitis. ⑤Febrile diseases

11.3.1.12   Frequently used acupoints on liver meridian of foot jueyin

The liver meridian of foot jueyin originates from the dorsal hairy region of the big toe that proceeds upwards along the dorsum of the foot anterior to the medial malleolus. It then travels to the place 8 cun above the medial malleolus where it crosses and runs behind the spleen meridian of foot taiyin and ascends along the medial aspect of the knee. It runs further along the medial aspect of the thigh and enters the pubic region, where it curves around the genitalia. From the genitalia, it goes upwards and enters the lower abdomen, then it pertains to the liver and connects with the gallbladder, it ascends to spread over the hypochondriac region. From here it runs upwards along the posterior aspect of the throat and goes upwards to the face. The branch splits from the liver, crosses the diaphragm and proceeds upwards to converge in the chest. It runs upwards along the posterior aspect of the throat, entering the nasopharynx, and connecting with the "eye system". It then proceeds upward and emerges on the forehead and connects with the governor vessel at the vertex(Figure 11-91).

(1)Dadun(LR 1)well point

Location: On the lateral side of the great toe, approximately 0.1 cun lateral to the corner of the toenail (Figure 11-92).

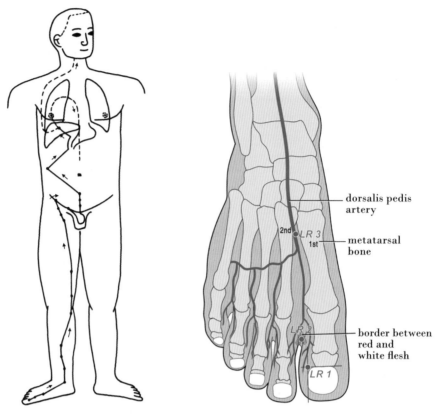

Figure 11-91　The course of
liver meridian of foot jueyin

Figure 11-92

Indications:①Hernia, low abdominal pain. ②Enuresis, dysuria, hematuria. ③Irregular menstruation, metrorrhagia, contraction of scrotum, colpalgia, prolapsed uterus. ④Epilepsy, somnolence.

Manipulation:Insert the needle shallowly by 0.1 cun into the skin, or insert a three-edged needle to induce bleeding.

(2)Xingjian(LR 2)spring point

Location:On the dorsum of the foot, proximal to the web margin between the 1st and 2nd toes, at the border between red and white flesh(Figure 11-92).

Indications:①Dizziness, headache, redness, swelling and pain in the eyes, deviation of the mouth and eyes, epilepsy, stroke, distending pain in the chest and hypochondriac region. ②Irregular menstruation, dysmenorrhea, amenorrhea, metrorrhagia, morbid leucorrhea. ③Colpalgia, hernia, enuresis. ④Difficulty in urination. ⑤Pain in the medial aspect of lower limbs, pain and swelling in the dorsum of foot.

Manipulation:0.5-0.8 cun perpendicular or oblique upward insertion.

(3)Taichong(LR 3)stream point; source point

Location:On the dorsum of the foot, between the 1st and 2nd metatarsal bones in the depression distal to the junction of the bases of the two bones where the dorsalis pedis artery pulses(Figure 11-92).

Indications:①Vertigo, headache, redness, swelling and pain in the eyes, tinnitus, angina, deviation of the mouth and eyes, epilepsy, stroke, infantile convulsions. ②Irregular menstruation, amenorrhea, dysmenorrhea, metrorrhagia, morbid leucorrhea. ③Hernia, distending pain in the chest and hypochondriac region, distention in the abdomen, jaundice, vomiting and hiccup. ④Enuresis, dysuria. ⑤Weakness and flaccidity of the lower limbs, pain and swelling in the dorsum of foot.

Manipulation：0. 5-0. 8 cun perpendicular upwards insertion.

(4)Ququan(LR 8)sea point

Location：When the knee is flexed,at the medial end of the popliteal crease,in the depression medial to the semitendinosus and semimembranosus tendons(Figure 11-93).

Indications：①Dysmenorrhea, irregular menstruation, prolapsed uterus, morbid leucorrhea. ②Seminal emission,impotence,hernia. ③Difficulty in urination. ④Weakness and flaccidity of the lower limbs,pain and swelling in the knees.

Manipulation：1. 0-1. 5 cun perpendicular upwards insertion.

(5)Zhangmen(LR 13)alarm point of the spleen,one of the eight meeting points(zang viscera convergence)

Location：Below the free end of the 11th floating rib(Figure 11-94).

Indications：①Diarrhea, abdominal distention and pain, vomiting, borborygmus. ②Pain in the hypochondriac region,jaundice,abdominal mass.

Manipulation：0. 8-1. 0 cun oblique insertion.

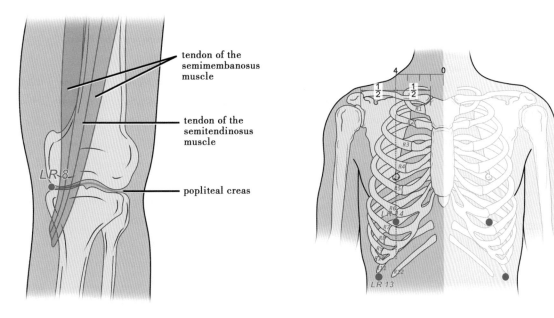

| Figure 11-93 | Figure 11-94 |

(6)Qimen(LR 14)alarm point of the liver

Location：Directly below the nipple,at the 6th intercostal space,4 cun lateral to the anterior midline(Figure 11-94).

Indications：①Distending pain in the chest and hypochondriac region, mastitis, diarrhea, abdominal distention,vomiting,acid regurgitation,hiccup. ②Up-rushing gas syndrome. ③Acute mastitis.

Manipulation：0. 5-0. 8 cun oblique insertion. Do not puncture too deeply in order to prevent hurting the internal viscera.

Other points on liver meridian of foot jueyin see Table 11-22.

Table 11-22 Other points on liver meridian of foot jueyin

Points	Code	Location	Indication
Zhongfeng (river point)	LR 4	On the dorsum of foot, 1 cun anterior to the medial malleolus and in the depression on the medial side of the tendon of the anterior tibial muscle	①Hernia, seminal emission, difficulty in urination. ②Pain in the abdomen, swelling and pain in the feet and ankles
Ligou	LR 5	5 cun above the tip of the medial malleolus and on the midline of the medial surface of the tibia	①Irregular menstruation, morbid leucorrhea, prolapsed uterus. ②Difficulty in urination, enuresis. ③Pain in the lumbosacral region. ④Hernia
Zhongdu (cleft point)	LR 6	7 cun above the tip of the medial malleolus and on the midline of the medial surface of the tibia	①Hernia, lower abdominal pain. ②Uterine bleeding, prolonged uterine discharge
Xiguan	LR 7	Posterior and inferior to the medial condyle of the tibia and 1 cun posterior to Yinlingquan (SP 9)	Swelling and pain of the knees, atrophy or paralysis of the lower limbs
Yinbao	LR 9	On the medial aspect of the thigh between the gracilis and the sartorius, 4 cun proximal to the base of the patella	①Irregular menstruation, difficulty in urination, enuresis. ②Pain in the lumbosacral region
Zuwuli	LR 10	3 cun directly below Qichong (ST 30) and inferior to the pubic tubercle	①Lower abdominal pain and distension, swelling and pain of the testicles, pruritus vulvae, prolapsed uterus, difficulty in urination. ②Scrofula
Yinlian	LR 11	2 cun directly below Qichong (ST 30), inferior to the pubic tubercle	Lower abdominal pain, irregular menstruation and morbid leucorrhea
Jimai	LR 12	Lateral and inferior to Qichong (ST 30), in the crease of the groin where the femoral artery pulsates and 2.5 cun lateral to the anterior midline	①Lower abdominal pain. ②Phallalgia, prolapsed uterus, and hernia

11.3.2 Frequently used acupoints on the eight extra meridians

11.3.2.1 Frequently used acupoints on governor vessel

The governor vessel travels backwards along the interior side of the spinal column, reaching Fengfu (GV 16). From there it enters the brain and ascends towards the vertex. From the vertex, it proceeds downwards along the forehead to the columnella of the nose, ends in the upper lip and connects to Yinjiao (GV 28) (Figure 11-95).

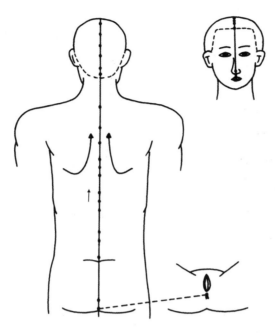

Figure 11-95   The course of governor vessel

(1) Changqiang(GV 1) connecting point

Location: The central point between the tip of the coccyx and the anus below the tip of the coccyx (Figure 11-96).

Indications: ①Hemorrhoids, prolapse of anus, bloody stool, diarrhea, constipation. ②Psychosis, epilepsy. ③Lumbago, lower back and coccyx pain.

Manipulation: Insert the needle obliquely towards the anterior side of the coccyx by 0. 5 – 1. 0 cun deep, deep insertion is not advisable, in order to prevent injuring the rectum.

(2) Yaoyangguan(GV 3)

Location: On the posterior midline, in the depression below the spinous process of the 4th lumbar vertebra(Figure 11-96).

Indications: ①Lower back pain, atrophy or paralysis in the lower extremities. ②Irregular menstruation, morbid leucorrhea. ③Nocturnal emissions, impotence.

Manipulation: Insert the needle perpendicularly by 0.5–1. 0 cun deep, moxibustion is applicable.

(3) Minmen(GV 4)

Location: In the depression below the spinous process of the 2nd lumbar vertebra(Figure 11-97).

Indications: ① Impotence, seminal emission. ② Irregular menstruation, morbid leucorrhea. ③ Lower back pain. ④Diarrhea.

Manipulation: Insert the needle perpendicularly by 0. 5–1. 0 cun deep, moxibustion is applicable.

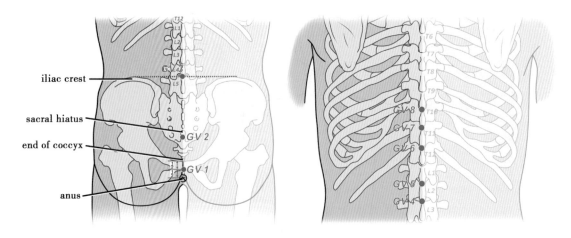

Figure 11-96 Figure 11-97

(4) Zhiyang(GV 9)

Location: In the depression below the spinous process of the 7th thoracic vertebra(Figure 11-98).

Indications: ①Jaundice, distension and fullness in chest and hypochondriac region. ②Cough, asthma. ③Stiffness of the spine, pain in the back.

Manipulation: Insert the needle obliquely upwards by 0.5-1.0 cun deep.

(5) Dazhui(GV 14)

Location: On the posterior midline, in the depression below the 7th cervical vertebra(Figure 11-98).

Indications: ① Febrile diseases, malaria, headache, cough, asthma. ② Epilepsy. ③ Night sweating. ④Pain in the back and shoulder, stiffness of the lumbar spine. ⑤Rubella.

Manipulation: 0.5-1.0 cun perpendicular insertion.

(6) Yamen(GV 15)

Location: On the nape at the posterior midline, in the depression superior to the spinous process of the 2nd cervical vertebra(Figure 11-99).

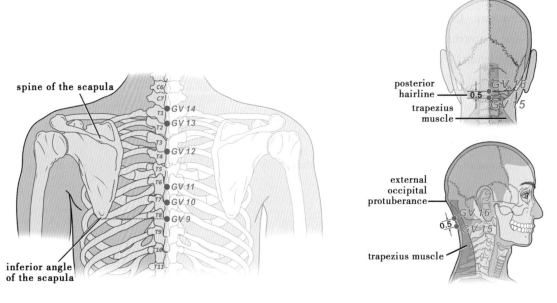

Figure 11-98 Figure 11-99

Indications：①Sudden aphonia, inability to speak due to stiffness of the tongue. ②Mania, epilepsy. ③Headache, stiffness in the neck.

Manipulation：0.5–1.0 cun perpendicular or oblique insertion downwards. Do not insert too deep perpendicularly or obliquely upwards to prevent from pricking the medulla. Pay attention to the angle and depth of insertion.

(7)Fengfu(GV 16)

Location：On the nape directly below the external occipital protuberance in the depression between the trapeziuses(Figure 11-99).

Indications：①Headache, stiffness in the neck, dizziness, swollen and pain throat. ②Apoplexy with aphasia, mania and epilepsy, hemiplegia.

Manipulation：0.5–1.0 cun perpendicular or oblique insertion downwards. Do not insert deeply to prevent from pricking the medulla.

(8)Baihui(GV 20)

Location：On the head, 5 cun directly above the midpoint of the anterior hairline, at the midpoint of the line connecting the apexes of both ears(Figure 11-100).

Indications：①Headache, dizziness, swollen and painful throat. ②Hemiplegia, apoplexy with aphasia, mania and epilepsy, insomnia, forgetfulness. ③Prolapsed anus, prolonged diarrhea, prolapse of uterus.

Manipulation：0.5–0.8 cun horizontal insertion. Moxibustion is applicable.

(9)Shangxing(GV 23)

Location：On the head, 1 cun directly above the midpoint of the anterior hairline(Figure 11-101).

Indications：①Headache, painful eyes, nasosinusitis, nosebleed. ②Malaria, febrile diseases. ③Mania and epilepsy.

Manipulation：0.5–0.8 cun horizontal insertion.

(10)Shenting(GV 24)

Location：0.5 cun directly above the midpoint of the anterior hairline(Figure 11-101).

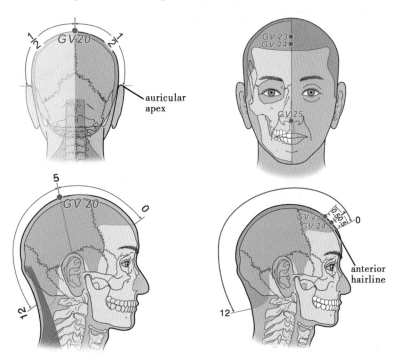

Figure 11-100　　　　　　　　　Figure 11-101

Indications: ①Headache, vertigo, nasosinusitis, nosebleed, conjunctival congestion, corneal opacity. ②Insomnia. ③Psychosis.

Manipulation: 0. 5－0. 8 cun horizontal insertion.

(11)Suliao(GV 25)

Location: At the tip of the nose(Figure 11－101).

Indications: ①Nasosinusitis, nosebleed. ②Unconsciousness, apnea, convulsions.

Manipulation: 0. 5－0. 8 cun horizontal insertion, or pricking to induce bleeding with a three-edged needle.

(12)Shuigou(GV 26)

Location: On the face, at the junction of the upper third and middle third of the philtrum(Figure 11－102).

Indications: ①Coma, syncope. ②Epilepsy, mania and epilepsy, facial paralysis, infantile convulsion. ③Swollen lips and face, rhinobyon, epistaxis, dentalgia, trismus. ④Stiffness of the lumbar spine.

Manipulation: 0. 3－0. 5 cun oblique upwards insertion, or press and knead with fingers.

(13)Yintang(GV 29)

Location: Midway between the medial ends of the two eyebrows(Figure 11－103).

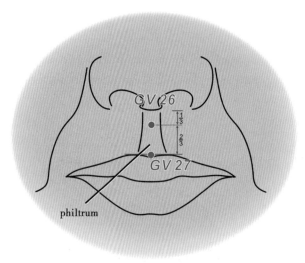

Figure 11－102

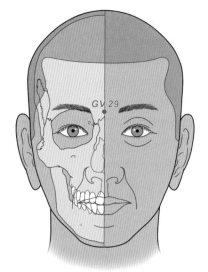

Figure 11－103

Indications: ①Dementia, epilepsy, insomnia, forgelfulness. ②Headache, vertigo. ③Rhinorrhea, epistaxis. ④Infantile convulsions, postpartum anemic fainting, eclampsia.

Manipulation: Pinch the local skin, 0. 3－0. 5 cun horizontal downwards insertion or prick to induce bleeding with three edges needle.

Other points on governor vessel see Table 11－23.

Table 11－23　Other points on governor vessel

Points	Code	Location	Indication
Yaoshu	GV 2	On the posterior midline, in the sacro-coccygeal hiatus	①Dysentery, prolapsed anus, constipation, irregular menstruation. ②Lumbago, atrophy or paralysis in the lower extremities. ③Epilepsy

Continue to Table 11-23

Points	Code	Location	Indication
Xuanshu	GV 5	On the posterior midline, in the depression below the spinous process of the 1st lumbar vertebrae	①Stiffness and pain of the lumbar region. ②Abdominal pain, diarrhea
Jizhong	GV 6	On the posterior midline, in the depression below the spinous process of the 11th thoracic vertebrae	①Diarrhea, jaundice, prolapsed anus, hemorrhoids, infantile malnutritional stagnation. ②Epilepsy. ③Stiffness and pain of the lumbar region
Zhongshu	GV 7	On the posterior midline, in the depression below the spinous process of the 10th thoracic vertebra	①Jaundice. ②Vomiting, distension of the abdomen, stomach pain, poor appetite. ③Lumbar and back pain
Jinsuo	GV 8	On the posterior midline, in the depression below the spinous process of the 9th thoracic vertebra	①Epilepsy. ②Vomiting, flaccidity of limbs, spasms. ③Stomach pain
Lingtai	GV 10	On the posterior midline, in the depression below the spinous process of the 6th thoracic vertebra	①Cough, asthma. ②Furunculosis. ③Stiffness of the spine, pain in the back
Shendao	GV 11	On the posterior midline, in the depression below the spinous process of the 5th thoracic vertebra	①Palpitation, angina, pectoris, amnesia. ②Cough and asthma. ③Stiffness of the spine, pain in the back
Shenzhu	GV 12	On the posterior midline, in the depression below the spinous process of the 3rd thoracic vertebra	①Cough, asthma, fever, headache. ②Stiffness of the spine, pain in the back. ③Back carbuncles. ④Epilepsy, convulsions
Taodao	GV 13	On the posterior midline, in the depression below the spinous process of the 1st thoracic vertebra	①Cough and asthma. ②Headache. ③Fever, tidal fever, malaria. ④Mania. ⑤Stiffness of the spine, pain in the back
Naohu	GV 17	2.5 cun directly above the midpoint of the posterior hairline, 1.5 cun above Fengfu(GV 16), in the depression on the upper border of the external occipital protuberance	① Headache, stiff neck, vertigo. ② Aphonia. ③Epilepsy
Qiangjian	GV 18	4 cun directly above the midpoint of the posterior hairline, 1.5 cun above Naohu(GV 17) and on the midpoint of the line joining Fengfu(GV 16) and Baihui(GV 20)	①Headache, stiff neck, vertigo. ②Psychosis
Houding	GV 19	5.5 cun directly above the midpoint of the posterior hairline, 1.5 cun above Qiangjian(GV 18) or 1.5 cun below Baihui(GV 20)	①Headache, sfiff neck, vertigo. ②Psychosis, epilepsy
Qianding	GV 21	3.5 cun directly above the midpoint of the anterior hairline, 1.5 cun above Baihui(GV 20)	①Headache, vertigo. ②Nasosinusitis. ③Psychosis, epilepsy
Xinhui	GV 22	2 cun directly above the midpoint of the anterior hairline, 1.5 cun above Qianding(GV 21)	①Headache, vertigo. ②Nasosinusitis. ③Psychosis, epilepsy
Duiduan	GV 27	On the midline, at the junction of the margin of the upper lip and the philtrum	①Unconsciousness, syncope, psychosis. ②Facial distortion, swollen, painful gums, nosebleed
Yinjiao	GV 28	In the superior frenulum, at the junction of the upper lip and the gums	①Facial distortion, swelling and pain of the gums, halitosis, nosebleed nasal obstruction. ②Psychosis

11.3.2.2 Frequently used acupoints on conception vessel

The conception vessel arises inside of the lower abdomen, passing through some points such as Guanyuan(CV 4), and reaches the throat. It ascends further to curve around the lips, passing through the maxillary part and entering the infraorbital region(Figure 11-104).

(1)Zhongji(CV 3)alarm point of the bladder

Location: On the anterior midline, 4 cun below the umbilicus(Figure 11-105).

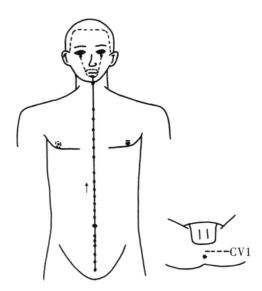

Figure 11-104　The course of conception vessel

Indications: ① Dysuria, enuresis. ② Seminal emission, impotence. ③ Irregular menstruation, morbid leucorrhea, and infertility, metrorrhagia and metrostaxis, prolapse of the uterus, pruritus vulvae.

Manipulation: Insert the needle perpendicularly by 0.5-1.0 cun deep after urination. The point is contraindicated in pregnant women.

(2)Guanyuan(CV 4)alarm point of the small intestine

Location: On the anterior midline, 3 cun below the umbilicus(Figure 11-105).

Indications: ①Asthenic disease, exhaustion syndrome. ②Abdominal pain, hernia. ③Diarrhea, dysentery, rectocele, hemafecia. ④The five kinds of stranguria, dysuria, hematuria, urodialysis. enuresis. ⑤Seminal emission, impotence, premature ejaculation. ⑥ Irregular menstruation, dysmenorrheal, morbid leucorrhea, and infertility. ⑦Commonly used moxibustion point for promoting health.

Manipulation: Insert the needle perpendicularly by 0.5-1.0 cun deep after urination. Moxibustion is applicable. This point is contraindicated in pregnant women.

(3)Qihai(CV 6)

Location: On the anterior midline, 1.5 cun below the umbilicus(Figure 11-105).

Indications: ①Exhaustion syndrome. ②Abdominal pain, diarrhea, constipation, indigestion, dysentery. ③Dysuria, enuresis. ④Irregular menstruation, dysmenorrheal, morbid leucorrhea. ⑤Seminal emission, impotence, premature ejaculation. ⑥Commonly used moxibustion point for promoting health.

Manipulation: Insert the needle perpendicularly by 1.0-1.5 cun deep. Moxibustion is applicable. The point is contraindicated in pregnant women.

(4)Shenque(CV 8)

Location: In the center of the umbilicus(Figure 11-105).

Indications:①Asthenic disease, exhaustion syndrome. ②Abdominal distension, abdominal pain, constipation, diarrhea. ③Edema, dysuria. ④Commonly used moxibustion point for promoting health.

Manipulation:Acupuncture is prohibited and moxibustion is applicable.

(5)Xiawan(CV 10)

Location:On the anterior midline, 2 cun above the umbilicus(Figure 11-106).

Indications:① Abdominal distension, abdominal pain, diarrhea, vomiting, indigestion. ② Abdominal masses.

Manipulation:Insert the needle perpendicularly by 1.0-1.5 cun deep.

(6)Zhongwan(CV 12)alarm point of the stomach;one of the eight meeting points(fu-viscera convergence)

Location:On the anterior midline, 4 cun above the umbilicus, or midway between the umbilicus and the xiphosternal symphysis(Figure 11-106).

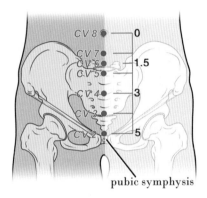

Figure 11-105

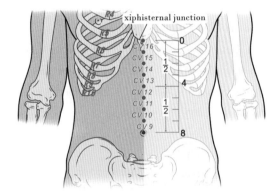

Figure 11-106

Indications:①Stomachache, vomiting, acid regurgitation, hiccup, poor appetite, abdominal distention, diarrhea. ②Jaundice. ③Psychosis, epilepsy.

Manipulation:Insert the needle perpendicularly by 1.0-1.5 cun deep.

(7)Danzhong(CV 17)alarm point of the pericardium;one of the eight meeting points(qi convergence)

Location:On the anterior midline, level with the 4th intercostal space or at the midpoint between the nipples(Figure 11-107).

Indications:①Oppression in the chest, shortness of breath, pain in the chest, palpitations, cough, asthma, vomiting, cardiac spasms. ②Lack of lactation, acute mastitis, nodules of breast.

Manipulation:Insert the needle horizontally by 0.3-0.5 cun deep.

(8)Tiantu(CV 22)

Location:On the anterior midline, at the centre of the suprastemal fossa(Figure 11-108).

Indications:①Cough, asthma, chest pain, swollen and painful throat, apoplexy with aphasia. ②Goiter, globus hystericus, dysphagia.

Manipulation:0.2 cun deep perpendicular insertion at first. Then turn the needle tip downwards and insert it along the posterior side of the sternum closely and slowly by 0.5-1.0 cun deep. Moxibustion is applicable.

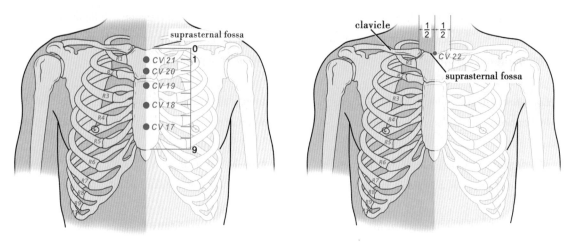

Figure 11-107   Figure 11-108

(9) Lianquan(CV 23)

Location: On the neck and on the anterior midline, above the laryngeal protuberance, on the midpoint above the upper border of the hyoid bone(Figure 11-109).

Indications: Swollen sub-lingual region, increased salivation, aphasia with stiff tongue, sudden loss of voice, dysphagia, difficulty in swallowing.

Manipulation: 0.5-0.8 cun deep oblique insertion towards the root of tongue.

(10) Chengjiang(CV 24)

Location: On the face, in the depression at the midpoint of the mentolabial sulcus(Figure 11-110).

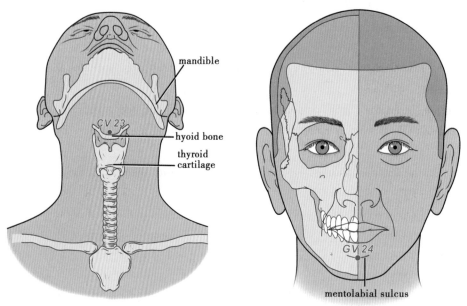

Figure 11-109   Figure 11-110

Indications: ①Facial paralysis, swollen gums, salivation. ②Sudden loss of voice. ③Epilepsy

Manipulation: 0.3-0.5 cun deep oblique insertion.

Other points on conception vessel see Table 11-24.

Table 11-24　Other points on conception vessel

Points	Code	Location	Indication
Huiyin	CV 1	On the perineum, midway between the anus and the scrotum in men, and the anus and the posterior labial commissure in women	①Irregular menstruation, difficulty in urination, nocturnal emissions, vaginal pain, pruritus vulva. ②Asphyxiation from drowning, unconsciousness, psychosis
Qugu	CV 2	On the anterior midline, 5 cun below the umbilicus, in the depression on the midpoint of the upper border of the pubis symphysis	Difficulty in urination, enuresis, irregular menstruation, dysmenorrhea, morbid leucorrhea, nocturnal emissions, impotence, and eczema of the scrotum
Shimen(alarmpoint of the triple energizer)	CV 5	On the anterior midline, 2 cun below the umbilicus	① Abdominal distension, edema, diarrhea. ②Nocturnal emissions, impotence, uterine bleeding, morbid leucorrhea, difficulty in urination
Yinjiao	CV 7	On the anterior midline, 1 cun below the umbilicus	① Abdominal pain. ② Edema. ③ Irregular menstruation, morbid leucorrhea, hernia
Shuifen	CV 9	On the anterior midline, 1 cun above the umbilicus	①Edema, difficulty in urination. ②Abdominal pain, abdominal distension, diarrhea, regurgitation
Jianli	CV 11	On the anterior midline, 3 cun above the umbilicus	① Stomachache, abdominal distention, poor appetite, vomiting. ②Edema
Shangwan	CV 13	On the anterior midline, 5 cun above the umbilicus	①Abdominal distension, stomach pain, vomiting, acid regurgitation, hiccups, poor appetite. ②Epilepsy
Juque(alarm point of the heart)	CV 14	On the anterior midline, 6 cun above the umbilicus, or 2 cun below the xiphosternal symphysis	①Chest pain, palpitation. ②Psychosis, epilepsy. ③Stomach pain, vomiting, acid regurgitation
Jiuwei(connecting point)	CV 15	On the anterior midline, 7 cun above the umbilicus, or 1 cun below the xiphosternal symphysis	①Oppression in the chest, pain in the chest, palpitation. ②Psychosis, epilepsy. ③Abdominal distension, hiccups, vomiting
Zhongting	CV 16	On the anterior midline, level with the 5th intercostal space, on the center of the xiphostemal symphysis	① Oppression in the chest, cardiac pain. ②Vomiting, infantile milk regurgitation
Yutang	CV 18	On the anterior midline, level with the 3rd intercostal space	①Oppression in the chest, pain in the chest. ②Cough, asthma. ③Vomiting
Zigong	CV 19	On the anterior midline, level with the 2nd intercostal space	①Cough, asthma. ②Oppression in the chest, pain in the chest
Huagai	CV 20	On the anterior midline, level with the 1st intercostal space, at the midpoint of the sternal angle	①Cough, asthma. ②Distension and pain in the chest and hypochondriac region
Xuanji	CV 21	On the anterior midline, on the center of the manubrium of the sternum	①Cough, asthma, pain in the chest. ②Swelling and pain in the throat. ③Dyspeptic disease

11.3.2.3　The course of the thoroughfare vessel

It starts inside of the lower abdomen and emerges from the perineum. It runs upwards along the inside part of the spinal column where its superficial branch passes through the region of Qichong(ST 30) and communicates with the kidney meridian, traveling along both sides of the abdomen. It goes up to the throat and curves around the lips.

11.3.2.4　The course of the belt vessel

It starts below the hypochondriac region and runs obliquely downwards Daimai(GB 26), Wushu(GB 27)and Weidao(GB 28). It then runs transversely around the waist like a belt.

11.3.2.5　The course of the yin link vessel

It starts from the medial aspect of the lower leg, ascends along the medial aspect of the thigh to the abdomen to communicate with the spleen meridian. It then runs along the chest, and communicates with the conception vessel at the neck.

11.3.2.6　The course of the yang link vessel

It starts from the lateral aspect of the heel, and runs upwards along the external malleolus, ascending along the gallbladder meridian, passing through the hip region, and running upwards along the posterior aspect of the hypochondriac region and posterior aspect of the axilla to the shoulder, and then to the forehead. It then turns backwards the back of the neck to communicate with the governor vessel.

11.3.2.7　The course of the yin heel vessel

It starts from the posterior aspect of the navicular bone, goes up to the upper portion of the medial malleolus, and runs straight up along the posterior border of the medial aspect of the thigh to the external genitalia. It then travels upwards along the chest to the supraclavicular fossa and runs upwards laterally to the region in front of Renying(ST 9)along the zygomatic arch to reach the inner canthus and communicate with both the bladder meridian and the yang heel vessel.

11.3.2.8　The course of the yang heel vessel

It starts from the lateral side of the heel, runs upwards along the external malleolus and passes the posterior border of the fibula, going up along the lateral side of the thigh and posterior side of the hypochondriac region to the posterior axillary fold. It travels to the shoulder and ascends along the neck to the corner of the mouth, entering the inner canthus to communicate with the yin heel vessel. Finally, it runs up along the bladder meridian to the forehead, where it meets the gallbladder meridian at Fengchi(GB 20).

11.3.3　Extra points

11.3.3.1　Extra points of head and neck(EX-HN)

(1)Sishencong(EX-HN 1)

Location:This name refers to four points located on the vertex,1 cun posterior, anterior and lateral to Baihui(GV 20)(Figure 11-111).

Indications:①Vertigo, headache. ②Forgetfulness, insomnia, epilepsy, mania. ③Paralysis.

Manipulation:0. 5－0. 8 cun horizontal insertion or pricking with a three-edged needle to induce bleeding.

(2)Taiyang(EX-HN 5)

Location:In the position about one finger-breadth posterior to the midpoint between the lateral end of the eyebrow and the outer canthus(Figure 11-112).

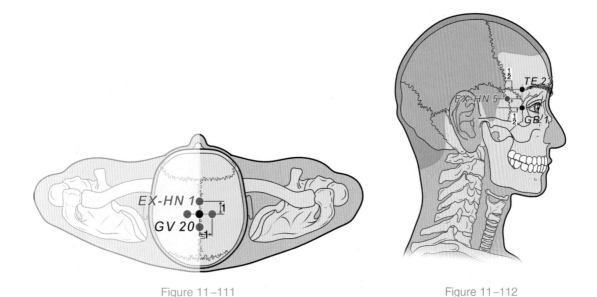

Figure 11-111   Figure 11-112

Indications:①Red and swollen eyes. ②Headache, dizziness. ③Facial paralysis, wry face and eyes, toothache.

Manipulation:0. 3-0. 5 cun perpendicular or oblique insertion or prick to induce bleeding with three edges needle. Moxibustion is applicable.

(3) Qiuhou(EX-HN 7)

Location:In the junction of the lateral 1/4 and medial 3/4 of the infraorbital margin (Figure 11-113).

Indications:Eye diseases.

Manipulation:Gently push the eye ball upward, insert the needle slightly downwards towards the optic foramen along the orbital margin for 0. 5-1. 5 cun without lifting and thrusting.

(4) Jinjin(EX-HN 12), Yuye(EX-HN 13)

Location:In the mouth, on the two veins under the lingual frenum, Jinjin on the left and Yuye on the right(Figure 11-114).

Indications:①Swollen tongue, stiff tongue, ulcers in the mouth, aphasia. ②Vomiting, diarrhea, diabetes.

Manipulation:Prick to induce bleeding.

(5) Qianzheng

Location:0. 5-1. 0 cun anterior to the earlobe(Figure 11-115).

Indications:Facial paralysis, and ulcers in the mouth.

Manipulation:0. 5-0. 8 cun forward oblique insertion.

(6) Yiming(EX-HN 14)

Location:On the neck, 1 cun posterior to Yifeng(TE 17)(Figure 11-116).

Indications:①Vertigo, headache, insomnia. ②Diseases of eyes, tinnitus.

Manipulation:0. 5-1. 0 cun perpendicular insertion, moxibustion is applicable.

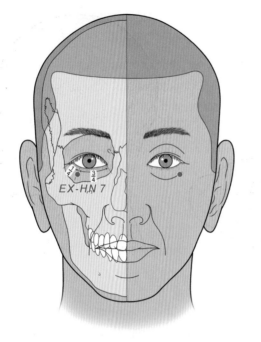

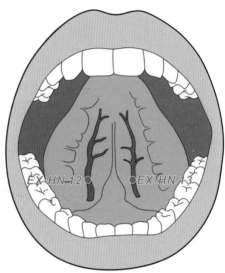

Figure 11-113

Figure 11-114

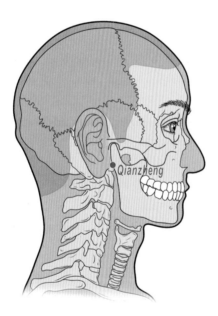

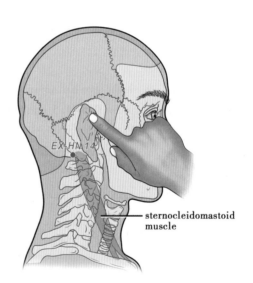

Figure 11-115

Figure 11-116

11.3.3.2　Extra points of chest and abdomen(EX-CA)

(1)Zigong(EX-CA 1)

Location:4 cun below the center of umbilicus,3 cun lateral to Zhongji(CV 3)(Figure 11-117).

Indications:Irregular menstruation,uterine bleeding,dysmenorrheal,prolapsed uterus,infertility,hernia.

Manipulation:0.8-1.2 cun perpendicular insertion.

(2)Sanjiaojiu(EX-CA 2)

Location:On the hypogastric region,making a equilateral triangle with the length of patient's corner of the mouth,the angulus parietalis is on the umbilicus,the bottom margin should be horizontal and the two base angles are the points(Figure 11-117).

Indications：Abdominal pain,hernia.

Manipulation：Moxibustion with 5-7 moxa cone.

11.3.3.3　Extra points of back(EX-B)

(1)Dingchuan(EX-B 1)

Location：Below the spinous process of the 7th cervical vertebra,0.5 cun lateral to the posterior midline(Figure 11-118).

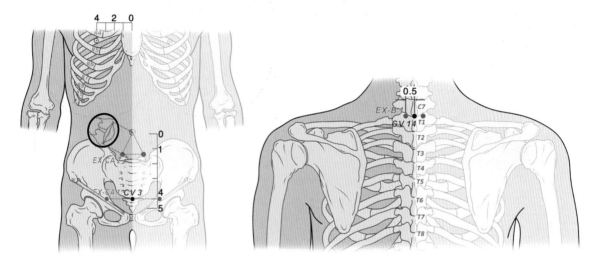

Figure 11-117　　　　　　　　　　　　　Figure 11-118

Indications：①Asthma,cough. ②Rigidity and pain in the shoulder and back,stiff neck.

Manipulation：0.5-0.8 cun perpendicular insertion.

(2)Jiaji(EX-B 2)

Location：0.5 cunlateral to the lower border of each spinous process from the 1st thoracic vertebrae to the 5th lumbar vertebrae. There are 17 points on each side and 34 points in total(Figure 11-119).

Indications：There are many indications. The Jiaji(EX-B 2)points on the upper back are indicated for disorders of the heart,lung and upper limbs,while those on the lower back are indicated for disorders of the spleen and stomach,and those on the lumbar region are indicated for disorders of the lumbar region and lower abdomen,and lower limbs.

Manipulation：0.3-0.5 cun perpendicular or oblique insertion. The plum-blossom needling technique can be utilized.

(3)Yaoyan(EX-B 7)

Location：In the depressed region,3.5 cun lateral to the lower border of the spinous process of the 4th lumbar vertebra(Figure 11-120).

Indications：①Lumbago. ②Morbid leucorrhea,irregular menstruation. ③Consumptive diseases.

Manipulation：1.0-1.5 cun perpendicular insertion.

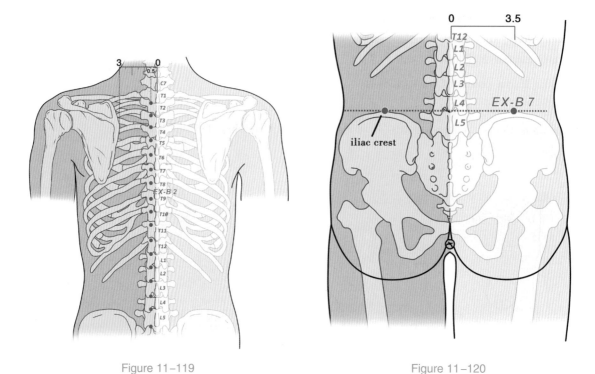

Figure 11-119　　　　　　　　　　　Figure 11-120

11.3.3.4　Extra points of upper extremities(EX-UE)

(1)Jianqian(EX-UE 1)

Location : On the anterior area of the shoulder, the point is on the midpoint between the anterior end of the axillary fold and Jianyu(LI 15)point(Figure 11-121).

Indications : Acute lumbar muscle sprain.

Manipulation : 1.0-1.5 cun perpendicular insertion.

(2)Yaotongdian(EX-UE 7)

Location : On the dorsum of the hand, between the 2nd and 3rd, 4th and 5th metacarpal bones respectively, at the middle points from the line through the metacarpal-phalange-geal joints to the transverse crease of the wrist. There are 2 points on each hand and 4 points in total(Figure 11-122).

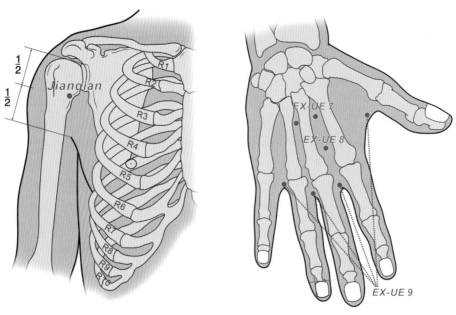

Figure 11-121　　　　　　　　　　　Figure 11-122

Indications：Acute lumbar muscle sprain.

Manipulation：Acupuncture obliquely 0. 5–0. 8 cun towards the center of the palm.

（3）Wailaogong（EX–UE 8）

Location：On the dorsum of the hand, between the 2nd and 3rd metacarpal bones, 0. 5 cun posterior to the metacarpal-phalangeal joint（Figure 11–122）.

Indications：①Stiff neck, swelling and redness in the back of the hands, numbness of the fingers. ②Umbilical tetanus.

Manipulation：0. 5–0. 8 cun perpendicular insertion.

（4）Baxie（EX–UE 9）

Location：Hand slightly flexed, on the dorsum of hands, in the fingerweb between each finger, 8 points on the dorsum of left and right hands（Figure 11–122）.

Indications：①Swelling and pain on the dorsum of the hand, numbness and spasmodic pain in the interphalangeal joints. ②Vexation, fever. ③Eye pain. ④Venomous snake bite.

Manipulation：0. 5–0. 8 cun oblique insertion, or prick to induce bleeding.

（5）Sifeng（EX–UE 10）

Location：On the palmar side of the index, middle, ring and little fingers at the center of the proximal interphalangeal joints（Figure 11–123）.

Indications：①Infantile malnutrition and pertussis, infantile diarrhea. ②Pertussis and asthma.

Manipulation：Prick 0. 1–0. 2 cun deep until yellowish mucus comes out.

（6）Shixuan（EX–UE 11）

Location：At the tips of the ten fingers, about 0. 1 cun distal to the nails, 10 points on left and right fingers in total（Figure 11–124）.

Indications：①Coma, infantile syncope. ②Epilepsy. ③High fever, sore throat, numbness of the fingers.

Manipulation：Insert shallowly about 0. 1 cun into the skin, or insert a three-edged needle to induce bleeding.

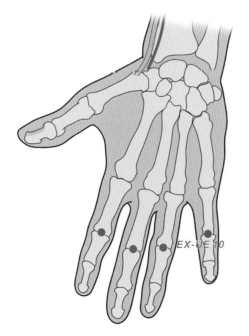

Figure 11–123

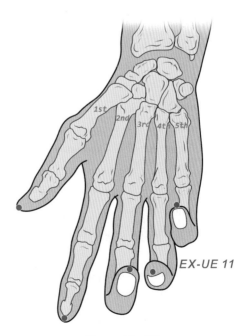

Figure 11–124

11.3.3.5 Extra points of lower extremities(EX–LE)

(1)Heding(EX–LE 2)

Location:On the upper part of the knee,in the depressed region above the midpoint of the base of the patella(Figure 11–125).

Indications:Knee pain,weakness of the leg and foot,paralysis of lower extremities,beriberi.

Manipulation:0.8–1.0 cun perpendicular insertion.

(2)Baichongwo(EX–LE 3)

Location:When the knee is flexed,the point is on the medial side of the thigh,3 cun above the medial side of the patella,1 cun above the point Xuehai(SP 10)(Figure 11–126).

Indications:①Ascariasis.②Itching of the skin,eczema,rubella,skin ulcers on the lower part of the body.

Manipulation:1.5–2.0 cun perpendicular insertion.

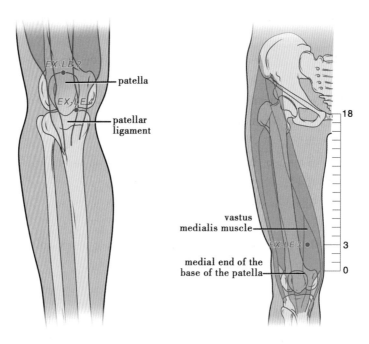

Figure 11–125   Figure 11–126

(3)Neixiyan(EX–LE 4)

Location:In the depressed region,medial side of ligament patellae when the knee is flexed. The medial side is called Neixiyan(EX–LE 4)(Figure 11–125).

Indications:①Pain in the knee and lower limbs. ②Beriberi.

Manipulation:0.5–1.0 cun oblique insertion.

(4)Dannang(EX–LE 6)

Location:On the lateral aspect of the lower leg,2 cun directly below the head of the fibula(Figure 11–127).

Indications:①Pain in the hypochondriac region,cholelithiasis,acute and chronic cholecystitis,biliary ascariasis,jaundice. ②Pain and weakness of the lower limbs.

Manipulation:1.0–2.0 cun perpendicular insertion.

(5)Lanwei(EX–LE 7)

Location:On the superior anterior aspect of the lower leg,5 cun below Dubi(ST35),one-finger breadth from the anterior crest of the tibia(Figure 11-128).

Indications:①Acute or chronic appendicitis,stomachache. ②Poor appetite. ③Weakness and pain of the lower limbs.

Manipulation:1.5-2.0 cun perpendicular insertion.

(6)Bafeng(EX-LE 10)

Location:On the dorsum of the foot,between the web of the toes,proximal to the web margin,4 points on one side and 8 points in total(Figure 11-129).

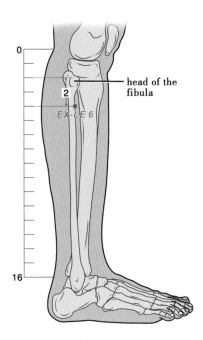

Figure 11-127

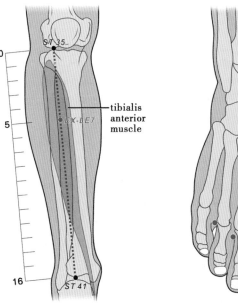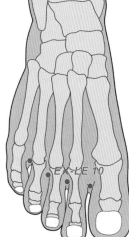

Figure 11-128   Figure 11-129

Indications: ①Pain and swelling on the dorsum of the foot. ②Venomous snake bite. ③Beriberi.

Manipulation: Insert the needle obliquely, 0. 5—0. 8 cun deep, or prick to induce bleeding.
Other Extra point see Table 11—25.

Table 11–25   Other Extra point

Points	Code	Location	Indication
Dangyang	EX–HN 2	On the head directly above the pupil, 1 cun superior to the anterior hairline	Headache, vertigo, insomnia, forgetfulness, epilepsy
Yuyao	EX–HN 4	At the center of the eyebrow in the depression directly above the pupil when the eyes are looking straight ahead	Twiching of the eyelid, deviation of the mouth and eye, ptosis of the eyelid, red and painful eyes, trigeminal neuralgia
Erjian	EX–HN 6	On the top region of the ear. Fold the ear forward and the point is at the apex of the ear	① Swollen and painful eyes, hordeolum. ② Swelling and pain in the throat. ③ Headache, vertigo
Shangyingxiang	EX–HN 8	On the region of the face, at the junction of the cartilage of the ala nasi and the nasal concha, near the upper end of the nasolabial groove	Nasal obstrucfion, sinusitis, soreness and furuncles in the nasal region
Neiyingxiang	EX–HN 9	Inside of the nostrils, on the mucosal membrane at the junction of the cartilage of the ala nasi and the nasal concha	①Diseases of the nose, inflammation of the throat, swelling and pain in the eyes. ②Febrile disease, sunstroke. ③Vertigo
Juquan	EX–HN 10	In the mouth cavity at the midpoint of the center line of the tongue	Cough, asthma, aphasia after cerebrovascular events
Haiquan	EX–HN 11	In the mouth at the midpoint of the lingual frenulum	Aphtha, sore togue, vomiting, diarrhea, hyperpyrexia, unconsciousness, pharyngitis, aphasia after cerebrovascular events, diabetes
Jingbailao	EX–HN 15	On the neck 2 cun directly superior to the 7th cervical spinous process and 1 cun lateral to the posterior midline	Bronchitis, bronchial asthma, phthisis, cervical spondylosis
Anmian	EX–HN 18	On the neck, on the midpoint between Yifeng(TE 17) and Fengchi(GB 20)	①Vertigo, headache, insomnia. ②Madness
Weiwanxiashu	EX–B 3	1. 5 cun lateral to the lower border of the spinous process of the 8th thoracic vertebra	① Stomachache, pain in the chest and hypochondriac region, abdominal pain. ②Diabetes, dry throat
Pigen	EX–B 4	In the lumbar region level with the inferior border of the spinous process of the 1st lumbar vertebra, 3. 5 cun lateral to the posterior midline	Gastrospasm, gastritis, gastrectasia, hepatitis, hepatosplenomegaly, hernia, nephroptosis, lumbar muscle strain

Continue to Table 11–25

Points	Code	Location	Indication
Xiajishu	EX–B 5	In the lumbar region on the posterior midline and below the spinous process of the 3rd lumbar vertebra	Nephritis, enuresis, enteritis, lumbar muscle strain
Yaoyi	EX–B 6	In the lumbar region level with the inferior border of the spinous process of the 4th lumbar vertebra, 3 cun lateral to the posterior midline	Lumbar soft tissue injury, low back pain, profuse uterine bleeding, spinal myospasm
Shiqizhui	EX–B 8	In the lumbosacral region on the posterior midline in the depression below the spinous process of the 5th lumbar vertebra	Irregular menstruation, dysmenorrhea, functional uterine bleeding, hemorrhoids, sciatica, poliomyelitis syndrome, lumbosacral pain
Yaoqi	EX–B 9	In the sacral region 2 cun above the apex of the coccyx in the depression of the sacral horn	Epilepsy, insomnia, headache, constipation
Zhoujian	EX–UE 1	Behind the elbow on the tip of the olecranon process of the ulna	Scrofula, carbuncles, sores
Erbai	EX–UE 2	On the palmar side of the forearm, 4 cun proximal to the transverse crease of the wrist, on both sides of the flexor carpi radialis tendon. Each side has one point; each arm has two points	① Hemorrhoids, Constipation, prolapse of the rectum. ②Pain in the chest and hypochondriac region, pain in the forearm
Zhongquan	EX–UE 3	On the dorsal transverse wrist crease in the depression on the radial side of the extensor digitorum tendon	Bronchitis, bronchial asthma, gastritis, enteritis
Zhongkui	EX–UE 4	The midpoint of the proximal interphalangeal joint of the dorsum of the middle finger	Acute gastritis, cardiac obstruction
Dagukong	EX–UE 5	Midpoint of the interphalangeal joint of the dorsum of the thumb	Conjunctivitis, keratitis, cataract, nasal hemorrhage, acute gastroenteritis
Xiaogukong	EX–UE 6	Midpoint of the proximal interphalangeal joint of the dorsum of the little finger	Eye disorders, pharyngitis, metacarpophalangeal joint pain
Kuangu	EX–LE 1	On the anterior region of the both thighs 1.5 cun lateral to Liangqiu(ST 34); 2 points on each side	Arthritis
Neihuaijian	EX–LE 8	At the prominence of the medial malleolus	Toothache, gastrocnemius spasms
Waihuaijian	EX–LE 9	At the prominence of the lateral malleolus	Toothache, gastrocnemius spasms
Duyin	EX–LE 11	On the sole of the foot, at the midpoint of the plantar surface of the distal interphalangeal joint of the 2nd toe	Angina pectoris, irregular menstruation
Qiduan	EX–LE 12	At the center of the tip of the each of the ten toes 0.1 cun distal to the nails; ten points in total	Cerebrovascular accident, numb toe

11.4　Acupuncture and moxibustion techniques

Acupuncture and moxibustion therapy, which regulate internal functions though outside stimuli, are unique therapy approachs and indispensable components of TCM. The acupuncture treatment is the insertion of different fine needles on the body's surface according to a certain acupoint, to stimulate certain parts of the body and use various methods to evoke the meridians and collaterals as well as the qi of human body, in order to adjust physiological functioning of the body and cure diseases. Moxibustion is the burning of moxa on or near a person's skin as a counterirritant. For a long time, acupuncture and moxibustion treatment are often combined together in clinical practice application, therefore we collectively referred to them as acupuncture-moxibustion therapy.

Acupuncture treatment includes either the administration of manual, mechanical, thermal, electrical stimulation of acupuncture needles, the use of laser acupuncture, and magnetic therapy, etc. Most commonly used acupuncture needles are filiform needle, skin needle, three-edged needle, intradermal needle, fire needle, etc.

11.4.1　Filiform needle therapy

According to ancient Chinese medical records and archaeological findings, the primitive Chinese people used bian stone, the earliest acupuncture instrument, to treat diseases. Afterward, with the further development of the society, bone needles and bamboo needles replaced stone ones. Then the development and improvement of metal casting techniques brought about metal medical needles. Such as bronze, iron, gold and silver ones. Nine types of needles are described in *Miraculous Pivot*, namely, filiform needle, shear needle, round-pointed needle, spoon needle, lance needle, round-sharp needle, stiletto needle, long needle and big needle. At present, filiform needles are widely used.

11.4.1.1　Structure and specification of filiform needles

The filiform needles are usually used in clinical treatment. Most of them are made of stainless steel. The filiform needle may be divided into five parts(Figure 11-130):

- Tail: the part at the end of the handle.
- Handle: the part that the fingers hold. It is wrapped with fine copper or aluminum wire.
- Body: the part between the handle and the tip.
- Root: the connecting section between the body and the handle.
- Tip: the sharp end of the needle.

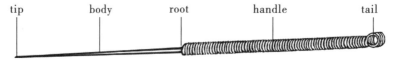

Figure 11-130

As the main tool, the filiform needles should be kept and maintained with great care to avoid damage. The needles should be carefully checked before use. If it is bent, the shaft eroded, or the tip hooked or blunt, the needle is defective and should be discarded.

The length of a filiform needle is also shown as "cun" (Table 11-26). The filiform needles vary in length and diameter(Table 11 – 27). Clinically the needles ranging from gauges 28 – 32 in diameter and 1–3 cun in length are frequently used in clinical treatment.

Points over bony areas, such as the scalp, face, ears and distal limbs require the shortest needles. Those over the thorax, abdomen and lightly muscled areas require medium length needles and those over heavily muscled areas, such as the lumbar area, the hindquarter(buttock and thigh) area and the heavy muscles of the shoulder area require the longest needles.

Table 11–26　Length of different filiform needles

Cun	0.5	1.0	1.5	2.0	2.5	3.0	3.5	4	4.5	5
mm	15	25	40	50	65	75	90	100	115	125

Table 11–27　Diameter of different filiform needles

Gauge	26	28	30	32	34
Dia(mm)	0.45	0.38	0.32	0.28	0.22

11.4.1.2　Practicing needling skills

A filiform needle is slim and soft. Strong and skillful hand manipulation is required to make efficient acupuncture. Beginners must practice the basic manipulation technique. Paper or cotton pads should be used for practice. The method helps to gain personal experience of needling sensation in clinical practice.

Paper pad practice: Fold some soft paper into a pad(8'5'2 cm) and bind it with gauze thread. Hold the pad with left hand. Hold the needle handle with the right thumb, index finger and middle finger similar to holding a brush. Insert needle into packet, rotate in and out clockwise and counter-clockwise (Figure 11–131).

Cotton pad practice: Make cotton ball 5 to 6 cm diameter wrapped in gauze. Hold the ball with left hand and needle handle with right hand. Insert needle into ball and practice rotating, lifting, thrusting procedure. (Figure 11–132).

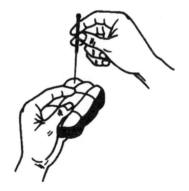

Figure 11–131　**Paper pad practice**

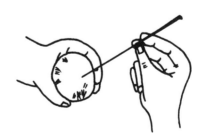

Figure 11–132

11.4.1.3　Preparation prior to treatment

(1)Explanation

In order to get good acupuncture results, the patient cooperation is needed. Some first visiting patients may be afraid of needling. The acupuncturist should explain to the patients in order to make them relax.

(2) Selection and check of the instruments

The suitable needle, long or short, thick or thin, should be selected according to the patien age, sex, body type, constitution, disease diagnosis, the depth and shallowness of the site, and the different acupoints. Generally, for a large or strong male whose disease is deep inside, we choose a large, long filiform needle. We choose slim, short filiform needles for opposite characteristics. Needles should be carefully inspected before use. Prepare needles with different sizes, trays, forceps and some 75% alcohol cotton balls. If the needle body is bent or eroded, or the needle tip is barbed, too sharp or too dull, the needle should be discarded. This will help prevent hurting the patient or breaking the needle.

(3) Sterilization

1) Needle sterilization

Sterilized needles, which should be used only once, are recommended. The needles for repeated use should be sterilized with autoclave; boiling sterilization or medical sterilization with 75% alcohol.

2) Disinfection of the region selected for needling

The area selected for needling must be sterilized with a 75% alcohol cotton ball. The selected area is sterilized from the center to the sides. After sterilization, measures should be taken to avoid recontamination.

3) Disinfection of the acupuncturist fingers

Before needling, the acupuncturist should wash his or her hands with soapsuds or sterilize with 75% alcohol cotton balls.

(4) Selection of the patient postures

Appropriate posture of the patient is important for correct location of acupoints, prolonged retention of the needle and prevention of bending and breaking the needle as well as fainting during acupuncture. Before needling, the patient is advised to relax himself or herself, keep a comfortable and natural posture so as to maintain the position for a longer time.

1) Lying position

It is most frequently used, especially for the aged, the patients with poor constitution or serious diseases or nervousness. Therefore, lying position is significant in preventing fatigue or fainting.

Supine posture: Suitable for needling the acupoints on the head and face, chest and abdominal regions, and the limbs (Figure 11-133).

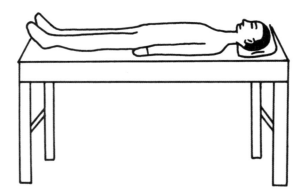

Figure 11-133　**Supine posture**

Lateral recumbent posture: Suitable for needling the acupoints on the posterior region of the head, neck, back, and the lateral side of the limbs (Figure 11-134).

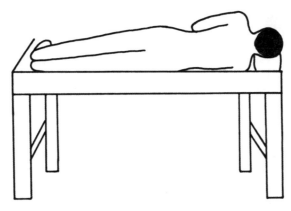

Figure 11-134 Lateral recumbent posture

Pronation posture: Suitable for needling the acupoints located on the posterior region of the head, neck, back, lumbar and buttock regions, and the posterior region of the lower limbs. Sitting position (Figure 11-135).

2) Sitting position

It is suitable for needling the acupoints located on the head, neck, upper extremities or the back of the patient whose illness is mild.

Sitting in pronation posture: Applicable to the acupoints located on the posterior region of the head, neck, and back (Figure 11-136).

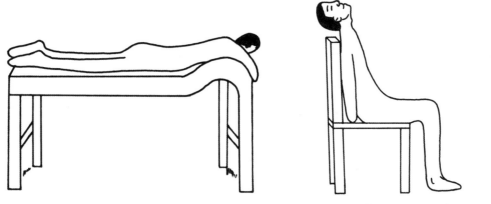

Figure 11-135 Pronation posture   Figure 11-136 Sitting in pronation posture

Sitting in supination posture: Applicable to the acupoints located on the head and face as well as the upper chest region(Figure 11-137).

Sitting in flexion posture: Applicable to the acupoints located on the head, neck and back (Figure 11-138).

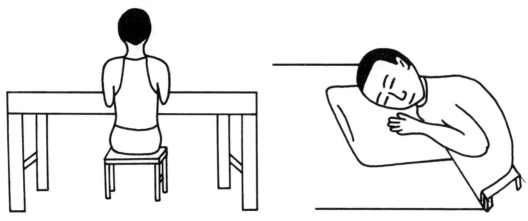

Figure 11-137   Sitting in supination posture   Figure 11-138   Sitting in flexion posture

11.4.1.3   Needle methods

The left hand, known as the pressing hand, presses against the area close to the point to be punctured to fix the skin. The touching and pressing with the pressing hand assist on the accurate location of acupoint. In case of inserting with a long needle, the left hand help to stabilize the body of the needle. The needle usually should be held with the right hand known as the puncturing hand. The thumb and the index finger of the puncturing hand hold the body of the needle, like holding a writing brush (Figure 11-139). The tip of the needle is punctured rapidly into the point with a certain finger force, then the needle is rotated to a deep layer.

Different needle inserting methods are employed according to length of the needle and location of the point. In the clinic, the common methods of insertion are as follows:

(1) Insertion of the needle with single hand

Hold the needle with the thumb and index finger of the right hand, the third finger touching the body of the needle, then insert the needle into the acupoint. This method is suitable for puncturing with short needles.

(2) Insertion of the needle with both hand

1) Fingernail-pressing needle insertion

Press the area close to the acupoint with the nail of the thumb or the index finger of the left hand, then hold the needle with the right hand and keep the needle tip closely against the nail of the left hand, insert the needle into the acupoint. This method is suitable for puncturing with short needles (Figure 11-140).

2) Hand-holding insertion

Hold a sterilized dry cotton ball round the needle tip with the thumb and index fingers of the left hand, leaving 0.2-0.3 cm of its tip exposed, and hold the needle with the thumb and index finger of the right hand. Then insert the needle into the acupoint with the right hand. This method is suitable for puncturing with long needles (Figure 11-141).

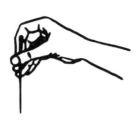

Figure 11-139   Posture of holding the needle

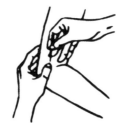

Figure 11 - 140   Fingernail-pressing needle insertion

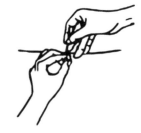

Figure 11 - 141   Hand-holding insertion

3) Skin spreading needle insertion

Stretch the skin where the point is located with the thumb and index finger of the left hand, hold the needle with the right hand and insert it into the acupoint between the two fingers. This method is suitable for the points located on the abdomen where the skin is loose(Figure 11-142).

4) Pinching needle insertion

Lift and pinch the skin up around the acupoint with the thumb and index finger of the left hand, insert the needle into the acupoint with the right hand. This method is suitable for puncturing the points on the face, where muscle and skin are thin(Figure 11-143).

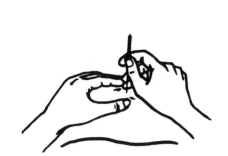
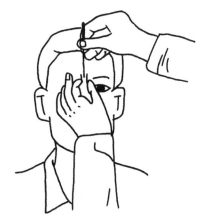

Figure 11-142   **Skin spreading needle insertion**   Figure 11-143   **Pinching needle insertion**

(3) Needle insertion with tube

The guide tube is a hollow tube, made of plastic or stainless steel, about 10-13 mm shorter than the needle. The guide is placed firmly on the point and held with one hand. The needle is inserted into the tube and the needle-handle, protruding from the guide, is tapped firmly with the finger of the free hand to drive the needle 10-13 mm deep. The guide is then removed and the needle is advanced to the correct depth. This method is suitable for beginners.

11.4.1.4   Manipulations

Needle manipulation may induce needling effect, for which several methods can be used. Correct manipulations are prerequisite to better therapeutic effects. Manipulations can be divided into two tapes: primary manipulation techniques and supplementary manipulation techniques

(1) Primary manipulation techniques

1) Lifting and thrusting

Lifting and thrusting manipulation is conducted by lifting perpendicularly from the deep layer to the superficial layer, then thrusting the needle from the superficial layer to the deep layer after the needle is inserted to a certain depth, which is repeatedly performed as required. Generally, lifting and thrusting in a large degree and high frequency may induce a strong stimulation, and in a small degree and low frequency lead to a weak stimulation(Figure 11-144).

2) Twirling or rotating

After the needle is inserted to the desired depth, the needle is twirled and rotated clockwise and counter-clock wise continuously with the thumb, index and middle fingers of the right hand. Generally, the needle is rotated with amplitude from 180° to 360° Rotating clockwise or counter-clockwise alone may twine the muscle fibers and produce pain and difficulty in further manipulation.

Twirling-rotating and lifting-thrusting are the two basic manipulations and can be used individually or in combination. The amplitude of twirling and the scope of lifting-thrusting as well as the frequency and duration of manipulation depend upon the patients constitution, pathological conditions and the acupoints to be needled(Figure 11-145).

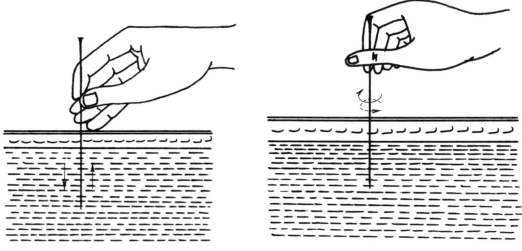

Figure 11-144　Lifting and thrusting　　　　　　Figure 11-145　Twirling or rotating

(2)Supplementary manipulation techniques

During the process of acupuncture, no matter what manipulation it is, the arrival of qi must be achieved. When there is no needling reaction, or the arrival of qi is not apparent after needle is inserted, manipulations for promoting the qi should be conducted. In clinic, following six kinds of Supplementary manipulation techniques are commonly applied.

1)Massage along meridian

Slightly massage the skin along the course of the meridian. The action of this method is to facilitates movement of qi through target meridian and strengthen its sensation at the point. This method is used in patients whose needling sensation is delayed.

2)Flying method

Twirl the needle for several times, and then separate the thumb and the index finger from it(the movement of the fingers looks like the birds wing waving)until the needling sensation is strengthened.

3)Handle-scraping method

The thumb(the index finger or the middle finger)of the right hand is placed on the tail end to keep the needle body steady, then scrape the handle with the nail of the index finger(the middle finger or the thumb)of the right hand upward or downward. The function of this method is to strengthen the needing sensation and promote the dispersion of the sensation(Figure 11-146).

4)Handle-flicking method

Flickthe handle of the needle lightly, causing it to tremble for the enhancement of the stimulation. This is a reinforcing method. This method is used for patients with retarded qi sensation due to qi deficiency(Figure 11-147).

5)Handle-waggling method

Hold the handle of the needle and shake the needle as the movement of a scull. This is an auxiliary method for reducing. "Before withdrawing the needle, shake the needle to drive pathogenic factors out". Shaking is combined with lifting at the withdrawal of the needle in perpendicular insertion. When the needles obliquely or transversely inserted, shake the needle by moving the handle left and right, but the needle body inside the point is kept at the same place. It is used to push the needling sensation in certain direction.

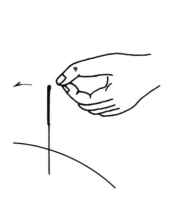
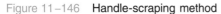
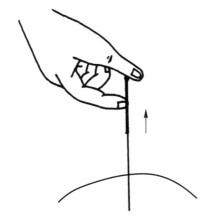

Figure 11-146 **Handle-scraping method**   Figure 11-147 **Handle-flicking method**

6) Trembling method

Hold the needle with the fingers of the right hand and apply lift-thrust or twirl movement in a rapid frequency but small amplitude to cause vibration. It is for promoting the arrival of qi or strengthening the needling sensation.

11.4.1.5   Arrival of qi

After the needle is inserted, physicians will look for the appearance of needling sensation. TCM calls this de qi literally, the "arrival of qi". The sensation of "arrival of qi" is perceived by both patients and practitioners. The patient may feel a dull ache, heaviness, distention, tingling, or electrical sensation either around the needle or traveling up or down the affected meridian. Meanwhile, the practitioner may experience tightness and dragging around the needle similar to a fish taking the bite. This needling sensation varies greatly from person to person.

The needling sensation is influenced by many factors, such as the constitution of a patient, severity of the illness, location of the acupoints and the needling techniques. In general, if the needling sensation occurs easily and the qi can travel to stimulate the lesion, the therapeutic effect will be better; if qi is difficult to secure, then the effect is not so good. For individuals who get this sensation slowly or faintly, the physician will further manipulate to adjust the position, direction and depth of the needle. This includes techniques like lifting and thrusting the needle into place, twirling the needle in a specific manner, plucking or scraping the handle of the needle, and also pressing the skin up and down along the course of the meridian with the fingers.

Techniques are carefully chosen based on the condition of the patient and the location of the acupoints. Common factors to determine the needling techniques include: those with strong bodies or the more muscular regions may be inserted deeper and can accept more vigorous techniques; while the elderly, small children and those with weak bodies, and for those regions with a thinner skin layer should have shallower needle insertions and be stimulated more gently.

11.4.1.6   Reinforcing and reducing manipulations of the filiform needle

Reinforcing manipulation refers to the method which is able to invigorate the body resistance and strengthen the weakened physiological functions. Reducing manipulation refers to the method which is able to eliminate the pathogenic factors and harmonizes the hyperactive physiological functions. Reinforcing manipulation should be selected for deficiency syndrome and reducing manipulation should be selected first for excess syndrome.

(1) Twirling reinforcement and reduction

The reinforcing and reducing of this kind can be differentiated by the amplitude and speed used. Be careful not to rotate and twirl to one direction, otherwise lead to the stuck needle.

1) The reinforcing manipulation

When the needle is inserted to a certain depth and the qi arrives, rotating the needle gently and slowly with small amplitude and lower frequency for relatively a short period using the thumb to twirl the needle forward and the index finger to twirl it backward is called reinforcing.

2) The reducing manipulation

When the needle is inserted to a certain depth and the qi arrives, rotating the needle forcefully with a larger amplitude and higher frequency for relatively a long period using the thumb to twirl the needle backward and the index finger to twirl it forward is called reducing.

(2) Lifting-thrusting reinforcement and reduction

The reinforcing and reducing of this kind can be differentiated by the force and speed used.

1) The reinforcing manipulation

After the needle is inserted to a given depth and the needling sensation appears, the reinforcing method is performed by briefly thrusting the needle forcefully and rapidly and lifting it gently and slowly.

2) The reducing manipulation

After the needle is inserted to a given depth and the needling sensation appears, the reducing method is performed by lifting the needle forcefully and rapidly, thrusting the needle gently and slowly.

(3) Rapid-slow reinforcement and reduction

The reinforcing and reducing of this kind can be differentiated by the speed of insertion and withdrawal of the needle.

1) The reinforcing manipulation

During manipulations, the reinforcing method is performed by inserting the needle to a given depth slowly and lifting it rapidly beneath the skin.

2) The reducing manipulation

During manipulations, the reinforcing method is performed by inserting the needle rapidly to a given depth swiftly and lifting it slowly beneath the skin.

(4) Directional reinforcement and reduction

It is the main leading principles of reinforcing and reducing manipulation in acupuncture.

1) The reinforcing manipulation

During manipulations, the reinforcing method is conducted by guiding the needle tip along the direction of the course of the meridian. The puncture is applied by running along the flowing direction of the meridian qi, to reinforce and benefit the healthy qi, so as to strengthen the hypoactive condition.

2) The reducing manipulation

During manipulations, the reinforcing method is conducted by making the needle tip against the direction of the course of the meridian. The puncture is applied by running against the flowing direction of the meridian qi, to reduce and eliminate the pathogenic qi, so as to weaken the hyperactive condition.

(5) Respiratory reinforcement and reduction

During manipulations, told the patient to breathe deeply and slowly. Respiration can be cooperate by other reinforcing-reducing manipulation for making the blood-qi moving smoothly.

1)The reinforcing manipulation

The reinforcing is achieved by inserting the needle when the patient breathes out and withdraw it when the patient breathes in.

2)The reducing manipulation

The reducing is achieved by inserting the needle when the patient breathes in and withdraw it when the patient breathes out.

(6)Open-close reinforcement and reduction

1)The reinforcing manipulation

When withdrawing of the needle,pressing the needling hole quickly to close it is known as the reinforcing. The purpose of this method is to prevent the health qi from escaping.

2)The reducing manipulation

When withdrawing the needle, shaking the needle to enlarge the needled hole without pressing is known as the reducing. The purpose of this method is to allow the pathogenic factor going out.

(7)Neutral reinforcement and reduction

This method is used to treat diseases atypical to deficiency or excess in nature. Lift,thrust and rotate the needle evenly and gently at moderate speed to cause a mild sensation,withdraw the needle at moderate speed as well.

11.4.1.7 Angle and depth of insertion

The angle and depth of insertion depend on the location of points,the therapeutic purpose,condition, constitution and body type of a patient. Correct angle and depth help to induce the needling sensation,bring about desired therapeutic results and guarantee safety.

(1)Angle

The angle of insertion refers to the angle between the needle and the skin surface when the needle is inserted into the skin. It varies according to the location of the acupoint and the aim of the needling. There are three kinds of angels:perpendicular,oblique and transverse(Figure 11–148).

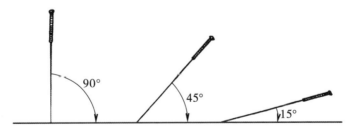

Figure 11–148   Angle of insertion

1)Perpendicular insertion:The needle is inserted perpendicularly,forming an angle of 90° with the skin surface. Most points on the body can be punctured in this way.

2)Oblique insertion

The needle is inserted obliquely,forming an angle of approximately 45° with the skin surface. It is commonly used in areas with few muscles or areas with important viscera underneath. Points on the chest and back are often needled in this way.

3)Transverse insertion

Also known as subcutaneous or transverse insertion,the needle is inserted horizontally,forming an angle of 15° to 25° with the skin. It is commonly used in areas with thin muscle mass,such as the head or sternum.

(2) Depth

The depth is related to the conditions of each acpoint and related to patient's physique, age, state of illness. The principle for depth is to induce better needling sensation but not to hurt any important viscera. Generally, insert shallowly in areas like head, face, chest and back, and deeply in areas like limbs, hips and abdomen. For the elderly often suffering from qi and blood deficiency, infants with delicate constitution, areas such as head and face and certain back region, shallow needle insertions advisable. For the young and middle-aged with musculature or fatty shape, or for the points on the four extremities, buttocks, and abdomen, deep insertion is employed. Oblique and horizontal insertion should be shallow, but perpendicular insertion can be very deep.

11.4.1.8 Retaining and withdrawing the needle

(1) Retaining

Retaining means to hold the needle in place after it is inserted to a given depth below the skin and manipulated. The purpose of it is to prolong the needling sensation and for further manipulation. For common diseases, the needles can be withdrawn or be retained for 10–20 minutes; but for some special diseases, such as chronic, intractable, painful, spastic cases, or for patients with a slow and weak needling sensation, the time for retaining the needle may be prolonged more than 20 minutes. Meanwhile, manipulations may be given at intervals in order to strengthen the therapeutic effects.

(2) Withdrawing

For the withdrawal of the needle, press the skin around the point with the thumb and index finger of the pressing hand, rotate the needle gently and lift it slowly to the subcutaneous level, then withdraw it quickly and press the punctured point with a sterilized dry cotton ball for a while to prevent bleeding. The practitioner should make sure that all the needles are withdrawn. Be sure not to leave any needle on the body.

11.4.1.9 Management and prevention of accident

(1) Fainting in acupuncture

1) Cause of fainting in acupuncture

This is often due to nervous tension, delicate constitution, hunger, fatigue, inappropriate position or fierce needling manipulation.

2) Manifestations of fainting in acupuncture

During acupuncture treatment, there may appear palpitation, dizziness, vertigo, nausea, cold sweating, pallor and weak pulse. In severe cases, there may be cold limbs, drop of blood pressure, incontinence of urine and stool, loss of consciousness, etc.

3) Management of fainting in acupuncture

When fainting appear, stop needling immediately and withdraw all needles. Then make the patient lie flat, offer some warm or sweet water. Symptoms will disappear after a short rest. In severe cases, in addition to above management, press hard with fingernail or needle Shuigou(GV 26), Hegu(LI 4), Neiguan(PC 6) and Zusanli(ST 36), or apply moxibustion to Baihui(GV 20), Qihai(CV 6), Guanyuan(CV 4) and Yongquan(KI 1). The patient will usually respond rapidly to these measures, but if the symptoms persist, emergency medical assistance will be necessary.

4) Prevention of fainting in acupuncture

The needling procedure and the sensations it may cause should be carefully explained before starting. For those about to receive acupuncture for the first time, treatment in a lying position with gentle manipulation is preferred. Needles should not be retained for long time. The complexion should be closely watched and the pulse frequently checked to detect any untoward reactions as early as possible. If there appear some prodromal symptoms such as pallor, sweating or dizziness, management should be taken promptly.

(2)Stuck needle

1)Cause of stuck needle

It may result from nervousness, muscle spasm, rotation of the needle with too wide an amplitude, rotation in only one direction causing muscle fibers to tangle around the needle, or from change of position of the patient after the insertion of the needles.

2)Manifestations of stuck needle

After insertion, one may find it difficult or impossible to rotate, lift and thrust, or even to withdraw the needle.

3)Management of stuck needle

The patient should be asked to relax. If the cause is excessive rotation in one direction, the condition will be relieved when the needle is rotated in the opposite direction. If stuck needle is caused by spasm of muscles temporarily, leave needle in place for a while, then withdraw it by rotating, massaging the muscle near the point, or by inserting another needle nearby to transfer patient's attention and to ease muscle tension. If stuck needle is caused by changed position, resume the original position then withdraw the needle.

4)Prevention of stuck needle

Sensitive and nervous patients should be encouraged to release tensions. Avoid muscle tension during needle insertion. Patient's posture should keep unchanged during the retention of the needles. Fierce needling manipulation should not be applied. Avoid puncturing the muscular tendon during insertion. Do not twirl needle with excessive amplitude or only in one direction.

(3)Bent needle

1)Cause of bent needle

This may arise from unskillful or fierce manipulation, or the needle striking on the hard tissue, a sudden change of the patient's posture, or from an improper management of the stuck needle.

2)Manifestations of bent needle

It is difficult to lift, thrust, rotate and withdraw the needle, and the patient feels painful.

3)Management of bent needle

When the needle is bent, do not lift, thrust or rotate the needle. The needle should be removed slowly and withdrawn by following the course of bending. If bent needle is caused by change of patient's posture, help the patient to resume the original position to relax local muscles and then remove the needle. Never withdraw the needle with force, otherwise, the needle may be broken inside the body.

4)Prevention of bent needle

Perfect insertion and even manipulation should be applied. Prior to treatment, the patient should have a comfortable position and do not change position when needles are retained. The needling place should not be impacted or pressed by an external force.

(4)Broken needle

1)Cause of broken needle

This may result from the poor quality of the needle, erosion between the shaft and the handle, strong muscle spasm or sudden movement of the patient, incorrect withdrawal of a stuck or bent needle, or prolonged use of galvanic current.

2)Manifestations of broken needle

The needle body is broken during manipulation and the broken part is below the skin surface or a little bit out of the skin surface.

3）Management of broken needle

If a needle breaks, the patient should be told to keep calm and not to move, so as to prevent the broken part of the needle from going deeper into the tissues. If a part of the broken needle is still above the skin, remove it with forceps. If it is at the same level as the skin, press around the site gently until the broken end is exposed, and then remove it with forceps. If it is completely under the skin, ask the patient to resume his/her previous position and the end of the needle shaft will often be exposed. If this is unsuccessful, surgical intervention will be needed.

4）Prevention of broken needle

Needles should be of high quality material, preferably stainless steel. All needles should be regularly inspected. Twisted, rusty or imperfect needles should be discarded. During insertion, a needle becomes bent, and it should be withdrawn and replaced by another. Too much force should not be used when manipulating needles, particularly during lifting and thrusting. The junction between the handle and the shaft is the part that is apt to break. Therefore, in inserting the needle, 1/4 to 1/3 of the shaft should always be kept above the skin.

（5）Hematoma

1）Cause of hematoma

This may due to injury of blood vessels during insertion, or from absent pressing of the point after needle withdrawal.

2）Manifestations of hematoma

Local swelling, distension and pain after the withdrawal of the needle. The skin of the local place is blue and purplish.

3）Management of hematoma

Generally, Mild hematoma may disappear by itself. If the local swelling, distension and pain are serious, apply cold compression locally to stop bleeding, hot compression can be applied to promote resolution of the blood stasis, after bleeding completely ceased. Hematoma will disappear by itself. If local swelling and pain are serious, light massage or warming moxibustion to help disperse the hematoma.

4）Prevention of hematoma

Avoid injuring the blood vessels and points are pressed with sterilized cotton ball as soon as the needle is withdrawn.

11.4.1.10　Precautions of acupuncture

It is advisable to delay giving acupuncture treatment to the patient who are very nervous, or over-fatigued. Acupuncture may induce labour and, therefore, unless needed for other therapeutic purposes it should not be performed in pregnancy. Acupunture is contraindicated for puncture points on the lower abdomen and lumbosacral region during women with menstruation. Acupoints on the fontanel is not closed. Acupoints on the areas with infection, ulcer, scar or tumor should not be needled. Needling should be avoided in patients with bleeding and clotting disorders, or who are on anticoagulant therapy or taking drugs with an anticoagulant effect. Acupoints on the ocular area, neck, or close to the vital viscera or large blood vessels should be carefully needled.

11.4.2　Moxibustion therapy

According to *Internal Classic*, "the coldness hidden in the body would bring illness which could be expelled through moxibustion". Moxibustion is a therapy that utilizes cauterization or heating with ignited flammable material(moxa wool or other materials) applied to certain areas on the body.

The material mainly used for moxibustion is moxa. Moxa, the leaf of Aiye, is a perennial, herbaceous plant. Due to its special aroma, bitter and pungent flavor and warm nature, as well as its flammability and moderate heat, moxa is an ideal option of moxibustion. After being dried in the sun, moxa leaves would be pounded and purified. It is thus processed into mugwort wool for clinical application. The reason for using old, dry moxa wool instead of fresh new wool, is that the latter contains so much volatile oil that when burned it releases too much heat.

11.4.2.1　Actions of moxibustion

(1) Warming meridian and dispersing coldness

Moxibustion can warm and dredge the meridians, promote circulation of qi and blood, expel cold and dampness. Clinically, it is applied for all diseases caused by cold obstruction, blood stagnation and blockages of the meridians, such as cold-damp arthralgia, dysmenorrhea, amenorrhea, stomachache, and epigastric pain.

(2) Supporting yang to rescue collapse

Moxibustion can help bring the body into balance and strengthen the original qi. It has active regulating functions of improving and rectifying the disturbance and dysfunction of certain viscera in the body. It has been widely applied to many serious diseases due to insufficiency, sinking or depletion of yang qi, such as enuresis, rectocele, prolapse of the genitalia, menorrhagia, leukorrhea, and chronic diarrhea.

(3) Remove blood stasis and dissipate masses.

Moxibustion can help ensure a consistent flow of qi and blood, remove blood stasis and dissipate pathological accumulation. In the clinical setting, it is commonly used to treat diseases related to qi and blood stagnation, such as the early stages of acute mastitis, scrofula and goiter.

(4) Disease prevention and health maintenance and strengthening the body resistance

Moxibustion on Zusanli(ST 36) or other acupoints, has the function of preventing diseases and maintaining health. It was called healthy moxibustion, which means maintaining the habit by doing moxibustion even though one enjoys good health. This method can invigorate healthy qi and strengthen the immunity to keep one full of vitality and increase longevity.

11.4.2.2　Classifications of moxibustion

There are many kinds of commonly used moxibustion(Figure 11-149).

In the clinic, the common methods of moxibustion with moxa wool are as follows: moxibustion with moxa cone, moxibustion with moxastick and moxibustion with warmed needles.

(1) Moxibustion with moxa cone

To make a moxa cone, roll mugwort fluff into the shape of a cone. The moxa cones vary in size from as small as a grain of wheat to the size of a core of a date. During the treatment with moxibustion, one moxa cone used at one point is called zhuang. Moxibustion with moxa cone is subdivided into direct moxibustion and indirect moxibustion, depending on whether there is something between the moxa cone and the skin.

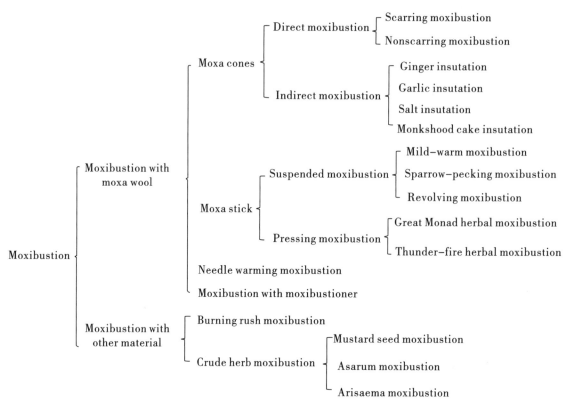

Figure 11-149 The classification of moxibustion

● Direct moxibustion: The ignited moxa is applied to selected acupoints either directly or indirectly. A moxa cone placed directly on the point and ignited is called direct moxibustion. It is subdivided into scarring moxibustion, and no scarring moxibustion. Direct moxibution means that the moxa cone is placed directly on the acupoint and ignited. This type of moxibustion is either scarring or non-scarring according to the degree of burning over the skin(Figure 11-150).

a. Scarring moxibustion: Prior to moxibustion, some garlic juice can be applied to the site in order to increase the adhesion of the moxa cone to the skin, then put the moxa cone on the point and ignite it until it completely burns out and then remove the ash. Repeat the procedure for about 5-10 zhuang. This will cause a local blister, festering and scarring on the skin after healing. It is often used to treat certain chronic diseases, such as asthma and pulmonary tuberculosis.

b. Non-scarring moxibustion: Apply a small amount of Vaseline to the area around the point. Place a moxa cone on the point and ignite. When 2/5 of a moxa cone is burnt, or when the patient feels a burning pain, the cone can be replaced by a new one. The moxibustion continues until the local skin becomes reddish but without blisters. Usually each acupoint can be moxibusted for 3-7 zhuang without suppuration and scar formation. It is often used to treat asthenia-cold syndrome.

● Indirect moxibustion(also known as moxibustion with material insulation) : The ignited moxa cone is insulated from the skin by the materials of ginger, salt, garlic, and monkshood cake, in order not to contact on the skin directly and avoid burning the skin(Figure 11-151). Moxibustion with ginger: Fresh ginger is cut into slices, about 2-3 cm wide and 0.2-0.3 cm thick. Punch several holes on it with needle and place it on the acupoints selected. The moxa cone is then placed on top of the ginger slice where it is ignited and burned. Repeat it for several times until the local skin turns reddish but without blisters formed.

Indications : vomiting, abdominal pain, diarrhea due to cold, and arthralgia syndrome due to wind-cold.

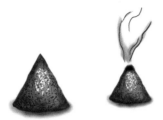

Figure 11-150   **Direct moxibustion**

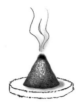

Figure 11-151   **Indirect moxibustion**

Moxibustion with garlic: Garlic cloves are cut into slices, each about 0. 2-0. 3 cm thick, then holes are punched into them. Then place a moxa cone on the garlic and ignite the moxa cone until the patient feels pain. Then remove the cone and place for another one. Repeat it for several times.

Indications: early stage of carbuncle and phlegmon.

Moxibustion with salt: Fill the navel with salt, place a large moxa cone on the top of salt and then ignite it. Replace the burning moxa. This method has the function to restore yang from collapse.

Indications: abdominal pain, diarrhea due to pathogenic cold and flaccid type wind-stroke.

Moxibustion with monkshood cake: Mix monkshood with wine and shape it like a coin, then punch several holes on it with needle for ventilation.

Indications: yang deficiency syndrome like impotence, premature ejaculation, bed-wetting and chronic carbuncle.

(2) Moxibustion with moxa stick

To make a moxa roll, place some mugwort fluff into a sheet of paper and roll it up into a tight stick. Apply a burning moxa stick with a certain distance apart over the selected point. Moxibustion with moxa stick can be performed in two ways: suspended moxibustion and pressing moxibustion

● Suspended moxibustion: This method is done by holding the moxa stick over the acupoint area during the treatment. Note: The end of the moxa stick should not make contact with the skin. It is sub-divided into mild-warming, sparrow-pecking and revolving moxibustion.

Mild moxibustion: Ignite a moxa stick at its one end and place it two to 3 cm away over the site to bring a mild warmth to the local place, but not burning, for some 5 min until the skin becomes slightly red. It is suitable for all the syndromes indicated by moxibustion(Figure 11-152).

Sparrow-pecking moxibustion: In this method, the ignited moxa stick is moved up and down over the point like a bird pecking or moving left and right, or circularly. It is indicated for numbness and pain of the limbs(Figure 11-153).

Circling moxibustion: When using this method, though the end of the moxa stick is kept 2 or 3 cm above the skin. It is moved back and forth or circularly.

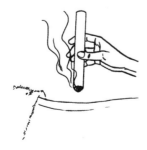

Figure 11-152   **Mild moxibustion**

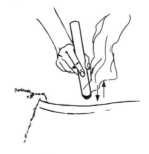

Figure 11-153   **Sparrow-pecking moxibustion**

● Pressing moxibustion: This method of moxibustion is done by pressing the burning end of a moxa stick, partitioned off by several layers of cloth or cotton paper, on the acupoints to allow the heat to penetrate the skin and muscle. After the fire is extinguished, it should be ignited again and repeated. Taiyi miraculous moxa stick and thunder-fire miraculous moxa stick is commonly used.

(3) Warming needle moxibustion

Warming needle moxibustion is a combination of acupuncture and moxibustion, and is used for conditions in which both retaining of the needle and moxibustion are needed. During the manipulation, after the arrival of qi and with the needle retained in the point, affix a small section of moxa stick (about 2cm long) on the needle's handle, ignite the moxa stick from its bottom till it burns out. When the moxa stick burns out, remove the ash and take out the needle. This method has the function of warming the meridians and promoting the flow of qi and blood so as to treat bi syndrome caused by cold-damp and paralysis (Figure 11-154).

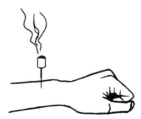

Figure 11-154　Warming needle moxibustion

(4) Moxibustion with moxa burner

The moxa burner is a special instrument used for moxibustion. There are two kinds: the box and the canister. During the manipulation, put some moxa wool, either alone or together with the special ingredients previously mentioned, into the box or canister. Ignite the argyi wool and make sure its lid is properly secured. Then, place it on the acupoints or affected area of the body to be treated. The desired effect is to make the local skin warm and flushed. This method of doing moxibustion is especially useful for children and other individuals who are afraid of being burnt by open flame.

11.4.2.3　Precautions of moxibustion

(1) Order of moxibustion

Generally, it starts from the upper part of the body, then to the low part, first the back, second the abdomen; first the head, then the four limbs. Clinically, it may be applied freely in accordance with the pathological state.

(2) Reinforcement and reduction with moxibustion

For reinforcement do not assist combustion by blowing, let the moxa burn naturally till it burns out; for reduction, while the moxa is burning, blow air to it time after time to make the combustion vigorous. This method is recorded in the book *Miraculous Pivot*.

(3) Moxibustion contraindications

①In principle, excess heat syndrome or the syndrome of yin deficiency with heat signs are contraindicated to moxibustion. ②Direct moxibustion is prohibited to perform on face and head, and the place close to the large blood vessels. ③The abdomen and lumbosacral region are not allowed to use moxibustion in pregnancy. ④Precautions should be taken with patients suffering from skin allergies or ulcers.

11.4.3   Cupping therapy

Cupping is a therapy in which a jar is attached to the skin to induce local congestion and blood stasis through the negative pressure created by consuming the air inside the cup with fire or other methods.

Cupping therapy, also known as "jar suction therapy" or the "horn method" in ancient China, was recorded as early as in *Formulas for Fifty-two Diseases*, a silk book unearthed in Emperor Ma's tomb during the Han Dynasty. Discussions can be found in the TCM literature of other dynasties. Cupping was primarily used to drain stagnant blood and pus from carbuncles and ulcers during surgery. However, with medical progress, not only have the materials and methods of cupping therapy improved, but the scope of its indications has also greatly increased. Clinically, it often employed in conjunction with of acupuncture and moxibustion.

11.4.3.1   Types of cups

Cups are made from a wide variety of materials, among which three types are most common used: bamboo cup, glass cup, pottery cup, and suction cup(Figure 11−155).

(1)Bamboo cup

A section of firm bamboo, 3−6 cm in diameter and 6−9 cm in length, is cut to form a short cylinder. One end is used as the base; the other as the opening at the top. The rim of the cup should be made smooth with a piece of sandpaper. The bamboo jar is light, economical and not easy to break; but it cracks easily from shrinkage if left to dry for long.

(2)Glass cup

The glass cup is transparent, therefore, the skin in the cup can be visualized to help control the appropriate treatment time. However, one disadvantage of glass cups is that they can be easily broken. These cups are shaped like a ball with smooth, open mouth.

(3)Suction cup

Presently, suction cups, for the most part, are made of plastic. Each cup has a fitting on the crown where a suctioning device is attached to remove the air. Through suction, the skin is drawn into the cup by creating a vacuum in the cup placed on the skin over the targeted area. Suction cups are convenient, break-resistant, safe, and the suction force can be easily regulated with very simple adjustments. However, one disadvantage of suction cups is that it cannot provide warm effect.

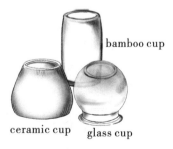

Figure 11−155   Bamboo cup, glass cup and pottery cup

11.4.3.2   Cup-sucking methods

(1)Fire cupping method

A cup is attached to the skin surface through the negative pressure created by an ignited material inside the cup to consume the air. Following are the five methods: fire twinkling method, fire throwing method, alcohol firing method, cotton firing method and firing method for cup laid on treatment location.

1) Flash-fire cupping

Ignite a 95% alcohol soaked cotton ball held with a clamp, put it inside the cup, quickly turn it around in one to three circles and take it out immediately, then press the cup on the selected area; the cup will attached itself to the skin. This is a safe and the most common used method. However, caution should be taken to avoid scalds or burns by over-heating the mouth of the cup.

2) Fire-insertion cupping

A 95% alcohol soaked cotton ball is ignited and placed into the cup. After a short time, the cup is rapidly placed firmly against the skin on the selected area. Since there is burning material inside the cup which is to drop down and burn the skin, it is often applied for the lateral side of the body. The quantity of alcohol should be moderate and avoid of dripping to burn the skin.

3) Alcohol-dropping cupping

Put one to three drops of alcohol into a cup (only a small amount should be used, to prevent it from dripping out of the cup and burning the skin), turn the cup to distribute the alcohol evenly on the surface of the walls. Promptly place the cup on the area to be treated after igniting the alcohol for a few seconds.

4) Cotton-burning cupping

Stick an appropriate-sized alcohol soaked cotton ball on the inner wall of the cup; ignite the cotton ball and quickly place the cup on the area to be treated. With this method, the cotton ball should not be soaked with too much alcohol, otherwise the skin would be burned when the burning alcohol drops down.

(2) Waterboiled cupping

With this method, the negative pressure is created when boiling water draws the air out of the cup so that it can attach to the skin. Generally, a bamboo cup is chosen to put in the boiling water or herbal liquid for several minutes; then the cup is grasped with clamped, with the mouth facing downwards. The cup is immediately placed on the selected location and attached to the body surface.

(3) Suction cupping

A suction cup is placed firmly on the chosen area, where a device is used to withdraw the air. When a sufficient amount of negative pressure is produced, the cup will attach itself to the skin. The negative pressure can be adjusted according to the quantity of air withdrawn, to regulate the suction force.

11.4.3.3　Cupping methods

(1) Retaining cupping

This could also be called the cup-waiting method, as it involves attaching the cup to the skin and retaining it on the selected location for 10−15 minutes before removal. In clinical practice, a single-cup or multi-cup retaining can be used.

(2) Sliding cupping

A lubricant, such as Vaseline or oil, should be applied to the skin over the treatment are, the cup then is sucked to the skin. Hold the cup with hand and slide it across the skin until the skin becomes congested, or even blood stagnation is seen. It is suitable for treatment of a large, thickly-muscled area, such as the back, the lumbus, the buttocks, and the thigh.

(3) Flash cupping

This method is applied by rapidly placing and removing the cup repeatedly over the same place until the skin becomes hyperemic. It is suitable for treating local numbness of the skin or diseases of deficiency with impairment of viscera functions.

（4）Pricking and cupping

After disinfecting the treatment area, prick the points with a three-edged needle to cause bleeding, or tap with plum-blossom needle, then apply cupping. Retain the cup on the area for 10–15 minutes. It enhances blood circulation and relieves swelling and pain by removing the blood stasis. It is indicated for erysipelas, sprains and acute mastitis.

（5）Cupping with retaining of needle

Sometimes referred to as needle cupping for short, this method is done by applying a cup over the center of the site where a needle has been inserted. The cup is removed when the skin turns rosy, congested and blood stagnation appears. This method combines cupping with acupuncture.

（6）Medicated cupping

There are actually two methods involved here. One is to boil a bamboo cup in an herbal decoction for 10 to 15 minutes and place it on the affected area; the other is to put the herbal decoction in the suction cup and apply it to the affected location. The prescription is made according to the illness, for example, herbal medicinal with the properties of dispelling wind and promoting blood circulation, such as Qianghuo, Duhuo, Danggui. Honghua, Mahuang, Aiye, Chuanjiao, Mugua, Chuanwu and Caowu, can be selected for treating wind-cold-dampness syndrome.

11.4.3.4　Effects and indications of cupping

Cupping therapy has the action of warming the meridians, promoting qi and blood circulation, relieving blood stagnation, alleviating pain and swelling, and dispelling dampness and cold. It is commonly applied for wind-cold-dampness impediment disease; acute strains and sprains, soft tissue sprains and contusions, common colds, headaches, facial paralysis, hemiplegia, cough, stomach pains, diarrhea, abdominal pain, the early stages of abscesses, and dysmenorrheal.

11.4.3.5　Removal of cup and precautions

（1）Removal of cup

Generally, the cup is retained in the location for 10 to 15 minutes, then it should be removed. Hold the cup with the one hand and press the skin by the edge of the jar, break the seal created by the suction, let the air come into the cup, and release cup. If the strength of suction is too strong, the cup should not be pulled forcibly, to avoid injuring the skin.

（2）Precautions

①Generally, select areas with abundant muscle mass, and ensure the patients are comfortably positioned. Sites with hair, joints and depressions are not suitable for cupping therapy since it is difficult to achieve a seal and the jar may fall off. Flash cupping should be used on areas that are difficult for cups to stick. ②The size of the cups must be chosen according to the cupping location. The mouth of the jar must be round and smooth, without chips or cracks. Otherwise the skin may be injured. ③Precautions should be taken to avoid scalding the skin. It is normal if small blisters appear on the skin after cupping therapy. It is not necessary to treat them. Prolonged retention and overheating of the mouth of the cup may cause blisters to arise. If the local blood stasis is severe, it is inadvisable to apply more cupping therapy to the same area. In the event that this occurs, small blisters should be covered with sterile gauze to avoid scraping; bigger ones should be punctured with a sterile syringe, followed by the application of a sterile dressing to prevent infection. If there is purple or even black agglomeration left, the warm towel can be used; or we can press the local area, in order to promote the blood circulation, and relieve the symptom. ④It is not advisable to apply cupping therapy to a patient with skin ulcers, skin sensitivity, or edema, as well as on the precordium and places supplied with large blood vessels. It is also contraindicated for those that have high fevers accompanied by convulsions, and on the abdominal and sacral regions of pregnant women.

11.4.4　Other acupuncture related therapies

11.4.4.1　Three-edged needle therapy

The three-edged needle, which is used for bleeding. Presently made of stainless steel, being 2 cun long, is a thick, round-handled needle with a triangular head and a sharp tip(Figure 11-156).

(1)Manipulations

1)Point-pricking method

Hold the handle of the three-edged needle with the right thumb and index finger, prick the selected sterilized acupoint or local reactive spot quickly and induce bleeding, withdraw the needle immediately. Then squeeze and press the area to cause bleeding for several drops. Finally, press the punctured acupoint by a sterilized dry ball to stop bleeding. For instance, pricking Shaoshang(LU 11)to treat sore throat, pricking Taiyang(EX-HN 5)or apex of the auricle to treat acute conjunctivitis, and pricking Weizhong(BL 40)to treat lumbago due to stagnation of blood.

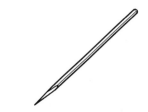

Figure 11-156　**Three-edged needle**

2)Collateral Pricking method

Sterilize the skin, prick the selected superficial vein to let a little blood, then press the punctured hole with a sterilized dry cotton ball to stop bleeding. For instance, pricking the superficial vein at the popliteal space and the medial side of the elbow for sun stoke.

3)Scattered needling method

Prick around a small area or a reddened swelling, then press the skin or apply cupping to let the stagnated blood escape to alleviate swelling and pain. It is indicated for intractable tinea, carbuncles, erysipelas, sprain and contusion, etc.

4)Piercing method

Press and fix the local skin by the left hand, prick the sterilized acupoint or local reactive spot with a three-edged needle to let blood or fluid, or further prick 0.5 cm deep to break the white subcutaneous fibrous tissue and induce bleeding, afterwards, cover the punctured site with a clean dressing. For multiple folliculitis, try to find the red spots at the both sides of the vertebra, and then prick them with a three-edged needle till bleeding.

(2)Effects and indications

The three-edged needling has the function of dispelling blood stasis, eliminating heat, removing toxin, dispersing swelling to alleviate pain and assisting resuscitation. It is advisable to treat syndromes such as acute heat syndromes especially fever, emergency condition of coma, heat-stroke, convulsion and syncope, sore throat, carbuncles, hemorrhoids, intractable Bi syndrome, local hyperemia, swelling, numbness, paralysis, etc.

（3）Precautions

Aseptic operation is applied to avoid infection. The pricking should be slight, superficial, and rapid. The bleeding should not be excessive. Avoid injuring the deep large arteries. It is not advisable to be applied for those who are weak, pregnant, and those susceptible to bleeding.

11.4.4.2　Dermal needle therapy

The dermal needle is also known as the plum-blossom needle, seven-star needle and temple-guard needle, which is made of five, seven and eighteen stainless steel needles inlaid onto the end of a handle. The seven-star needle is composed of seven short stainless steel needles attached vertically to a handle five to six inches long. The plum-blossom needle is composed of five stainless steel needles in a bundle. The temple-guard needle is composed of 18 stainless steel needles in a bundle(Figure 11-157).

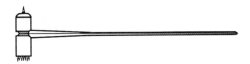

Figure 11-157　**Dermal needle**

（1）Manipulations

After routine sterilization, hold the handle of the needle with the index finger and tap vertically on the skin with a gentle and flexible movement of the wrist. The area to be tapped may be along the course of the meridians, or on the points selected, or on the affected area, or along the both sides of the spinal column. The intensity of tapping may be light, moderate or heavy in accordance with the constitution, the age, the pathological state and the location of the patient.

1）Light tapping

Light tapping is applied with slight force, and shorter time of contact of the needles with the skin until the skin becomes congested without bleeding spots. It is applied for the kids, the women, the weak and the elderly, or for areas on the head and face with thin muscles.

2）Moderate tapping

The force exerted in the moderate tapping is between that of the light and heavy tapings. Moderate tapping is required to cause congestion and with slight pain, but no bleeding, suitable for the majority of the patients, ordinary diseases and general locations.

3）Heavy tapping

Heavy tapping is conducted by exerting a relatively strong force and longer time of contact of the needles with the skin until the skin becomes congested with bloody spots, associated with a little pain. It is applied for patients with the strong, the excess syndrome, or for areas with thick muscles.

（2）Effects and indications

The dermal needling is used to prick the skin superficially by tapping to promote the smooth flow of qi in the meridians and regulate the functions of the zang-fu viscera. It is particularly suitable to treat disorders of the nervous system and skin disease such as headache, dizziness and vertigo, insomnia, hypertension, myopia, alopecia, neurodermatitis, as well as general disorders-painful joints and paralysis, gastrointestinal disease, gynaecological disease, etc.

（3）Precautions

First, check the needles carefully before needling. The tips of the needle should be sharp, smooth and free from any hooks. When tapping, the tips of the needles should strike the skin at a right angle to the surface to reduce pain. Sterilize the needles and the location of treatment should be disinfected. After heavy tapping, the local skin surface should be sterilized to prevent infection. Tapping should be avoided to apply to the location of trauma and ulcers.

11.4.4.3 Intradermal needle therapy

The intradermal needle is a kind of short needle made of stainless steel, used for embedding in the skin or subcutaneously. It can exert the continuous stimulation produced by the implanted needle. There are two types: the thumbtack type and grain-like type, the former is about 0.3 cm long with a head like a thumbtack. Theater is about 1 cm long with a head like a grain of wheat.

(1) Manipulations

The thumbtack-type needle is generally applied to the ear region, while the grain-like needle is applied to points or tender spots on various parts of the body. Embed the sterilized needle into the point, leaving its handle lying flat on the skin surface, and fixing it with a piece of adhesive tape.

(2) Effects and indications

The intradermal needle is mostly used to treat some chronic or painful diseases which need long time retaining of the needle, such as headache, stomachache, asthma, insomnia, enuresis, abnormal menstruation, dysmenorrhea, etc.

(3) Precautions

The points selected for embedding should be located in an area of the body where the needle can be fixed relatively easily. Avoid embedding the intradermal needle around the joints to prevent pain on motion. During the embedding, if pain is experienced, the needle should be removed and embedded again do not select too many points for embedding for each treatment, 2–3 points selection is recommended. The duration of implantation depends on the pathological conditions in different seasons. In summer, the retaining of needle should not be for more than 2 days. In autumn or winter, retain the needles for 2–7 days. During the embedding period, keep the area around the needle clean to prevent infection. The intradermal needle is not suitable for ulcer, inflammation and hard masses with unclear reasons.

11.4.4.4 Skin scraping

Skin scraping, also known as Gua Sha, is based on the skin theory of TCM: by using a smooth edged tools such as jade, ox horn, a ceramic Chinese soup spoon, or a coin, scraping and rubbing repeatedly the relevant parts of the skin, to dredge the meridian, and activate blood circulation to dissipate blood stasis. Gua means to scrape or rub. Sha is the term used to describe blood stasis in the subcutaneous tissue before and after it is raised as petechiae (Figure 11–158).

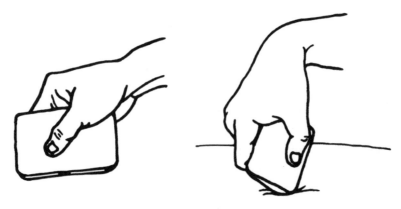

Figure 11–158 **Skin scraping**

(1) Manipulations

Skin is typically lubricated with massage oil. The smooth edge of skin scraping tool is placed against the skin surface, pressed down firmly, and then moved down the muscles or along the pathway of the meridians, with each stroke being about 4-6 inches long. The intensity of scraping may be light, moderate or heavy in accordance with the constitution, the age, the pathological state and the location of the patient. The places to be scraped may be along the course of meridian, or on the points selected, or on the affected locations, especial at the both sides of the vertebra.

(2) Effects and indications

Skin scraping has the function of dredging the meridian, improving the circulation, removing toxin, promoting metabolism, streng thening the body resistance and maintaining healthy. Skin Scraping is mostly used to treat soft tissue pain, stiffness, fever, headache, insomnia, cough, vomiting, diarrhea, heat stroke, and health care, etc.

(3) Precautions

It is not advisable to apply skin scraping therapy to patients with skin ulcers, allergies. It is also contraindicated for those susceptible to bleeding, and on the abdominal and sacral regions of pregnant women. During skin scrapingtherapy, keep the room warm, avoid the wind blowing directly. After the treatment, drink a cup of warm boiling water(preferably add a bit sugar and salt in the water) , and rest for 15-20 minutes. The next scraping therapy should be applied until the bruise(Sha) caused by the scraping has disappeared, so the interval between two treatment should be 3-7 days.

11.4.4.5　Electroacupuncture

Electroacupuncture is a form of acupuncture by which the needle is attached to a trace pulse current after it is inserted to the selected acupoint for the purpose of producing synthetic effect of electric and needling stimulation. It substitutes for prolonged hand maneuvering, otherwise, it is easier to control the frequency of the stimulus and the amount of stimulus than with hand manipulation of the needles.

(1) Electroacupuncture device

Electroacupuncture device is an electric pulse generator and the low frequency impulse current is generated by an oscillator. The device is equipped with host, electrode wire, electrode plates and electrode clip, etc. With special rotary knob to adjust wave form, time, frequency, and output strength, it is easy to be operated.

(2) Manipulation

Insert the needle on the selected acupoints, after the needling sensation is obtained and reinforcing or reducing needling manipulation is conducted, set the output potentionmeter of the electroacupuncture device to "0", connect the two wires of the output respectively to the handles of the two needles switch on the power supply, select the desired wave pattern and frequency, gradually increase the output current until the patient gets a tolerable soreness and numbness sensation. Duration of standard treatment with electroacupuncture is usually 10-20 minutes, usually no more than 30 minutes. When the treatment is over, turn the potential to "0" and switch off the electroacupuncture device, disconnect the wires from the needles and withdraw the needles. The negative electrode is attached to what is considered the main point, while the positive electrode is attached to a secondary point attach to an electroacupuncture device in the case of a direct current. However, in the case of alternating current, the two electrodes in any pair are equivalent, so there is no strict distinction between positive and negative electrode.

Electroacupuncture uses the same points as acupuncture, and operates on a similar principle. In general, 1 to 3 pairs of points are selected from the same side of the body or limbs. Generally, and avoid to apply electro-stimulation at high intensities in the head or across the midline of the body.

(3) Stimulating parameters

1) The actions of electro-pulse

The low frequency pulsation of the stimulator would stimulate the point via the inserted filiform needle so as to affect the physiological function of the body, relieve the muscular spasm and pain, induce sedation and promote the blood circulation. As the pulsation varies in frequency and wave pattern, the actions of the pulses may be different. The high frequency pulse 50−100/sec is known as dense wave, the low frequency pulse 2−5/sec termed as rarefaction wave.

2) Undulate wave forms, amplitude of waves

● Undulate wave forms

Dense wave: High frequency wave (>30Hz, 50−100 pulse). It may reduce the nerve irritability, produce inhibition on sensory never and motor nerve, commonly used for acupuncture analgesia, sedation and pain relief, relaxation of muscles and vessels spasm, etc.

Sparse wave: Low frequency wave (<30Hz, or 2−5 pulse/sec). It is comparatively strong and can cause contraction of the muscles and enhance the tension of muscle and ligaments, commonly used for flaccidity, atrophy and the impairment of muscle, joint, ligament and tendons.

Irregular wave: Alternately dense and sparse wave. This is a kind of wave, which spontaneously alternates appearance of low and high waves within time of 1.5 seconds. It has a better excitation effect during treatment, can promote metabolism and blood circulation, improve tissue nutrition, and eliminate inflammatory edema. It is commonly used for sprain and contusion, periarthritis, facial paralysis, etc.

Intermittent wave: Rhythmically-interrupted electric dense wave for 1.5 second each phase. As a regular intermittent rarefaction wave, it can increase the excitation of muscular tissue and produce good stimulation to the muscle and make it contract perfectly, especially for striated muscle. It is commonly used for muscular weakness and atrophy, paralysis, etc.

Serrated wave (saw-tooth wave): This is an undulated wave in which impulse amplitude undulates automatically in a serrated form 16−20 times or 20−25 times a minute, which is close to human's respiration, therefore also known as respiratory wave. It is used for rescuing a person with respiratory failure by making artificial electro-respiration through stimulation of the phrenic nerve.

● Amplitude of waves: The difference between the maximum and minimum voltage and current, the intensity of electroacupuncture mainly depends on the amplitude of the wave, (0−20 V, or 1−2 mA). In the clinic practice, the intensity can be selected according to the tolerance of the patient.

(4) Effects and indications

The indications of electroacupuncture is quite similar to that of traditional acupuncture, particularly for manic-depressive psychosis, neurasthenia, neuralgia, sequelae of cerebrovascular accident, sequelae of poliomyelitis, muscular flaccidity, gastrointestinal diseases, arthralgia syndrome, painful joints as well as acupuncture analgesia.

(5) Precautions

①Check the electric stimulator to make sure that its output is normal before each treatment. Turn the output to 0 before treatment. ②Adjust the flow of the electric current from small to large gradually, so as not to cause a sudden strong muscular contraction or pain to the patient. ③In treating patient with serious heart disease, take care to prevent the current going through the heart. It is generally recommended to avoid placing electrodes on patient with pacemaker. ④Do not apply electroacupuncture on the lower abdomen or lower back, and sacrum regions of pregnant women. For the elderly, people with weak constitution, drunk, over-hungry, over-eating or overstrain, electroacupuncture should be used with caution. ⑤ A filiform needle, which has been burned during the process of moxibustion and has lost the capability of conduction due to the oxidation of its handle, is not suitable for electric needling use.

11.4.4.6   Scalp acupuncture

Scalp acupuncture refers to the acupuncture technique that targets functional zones on the scalp. The needling points are scalp areas corresponding to the functional areas of the cerebral cortex, the nomenclature of the areas(lines) are in accordance with the functional area of the cerebral cortex.

Scalp acupuncture is based on ancient fundamental theories of Chinese medicine and modern knowledge of western biomedicine. In the 1970's, scalp acupuncture was developed as a complete acupuncture system. Three major contributors to the development of this system, *Jiao Shunfa*, *Fang Yunpeng*, and *Tang Songyan*, each proposed different diagrams and groupings of scalp acupuncture points. A standard of nomenclature for acupuncture points has been published(adopted in 1984 and reconfirmed in 1989), indicating 14 therapeutic lines or zones based on a combination of the thoughts of the different schools of scalp acupuncture. In our book the name and location of scalp therapeutic lines are based on the 1989 edition.

(1)The locations and indications of the stimulating areas

1)MS 1 Middle line of forehead

Location: On the front of the forehead, draw a straight line from Shenting(GV 24), the length of the line will be 1 cun(Figure 11–159).

Application: Headache, dizziness, epilepsy, redness swelling and pain of the eyes.

2)MS 2 Lateral line 1 of forehead(thoracic region)

Location: On the front of the forehead, draw a straight line from Meichong(BL 3), the length of the line will be 1 cun(Figure 11–159).

Application: Allergic asthma, bronchitis, angina, rheumatic heart disease(palpitation, edema, short of breath, oliguria), tachycardia.

3)MS 3 Lateral line 2 of forehead(gastric region, liver and gallbladder region)

Location: on the front of the forehead, draw a straight line from Toulinqi(GB 15), the length of the line will be 1 cun(Figure 11–159).

Application: Acute chronic gastritis, gastric ulcer, duodenal ulcer.

4)MS 4 Lateral line 3 of forehead(reproductive region, intestine region)

Location: On the front of the forehead, draw a straight line from the point[0.75 cun lateral to Touwei (ST 8)], the length of the line will be 1 cun(Figure 11–159).

Application: Dysfunctional uterine bleeding, combine with both foot motor sensory area to treat acute cystitis(frequent urination, urgent urination) or diabetes(thirst, profuse urination, polydipsia, impotence, prolapse of uterus, spermatorrhea), especially relieve the lower abdomen pain.

5)MS 5 Middle line of vertex

Location: on the top of the head, draw a straight line from Baihui(GV 20) to Qianding(GV 21) (Figure 11–160).

Application: headache, vertigo, stroke, aphasia, syncope, mental disorder, epilepsy.

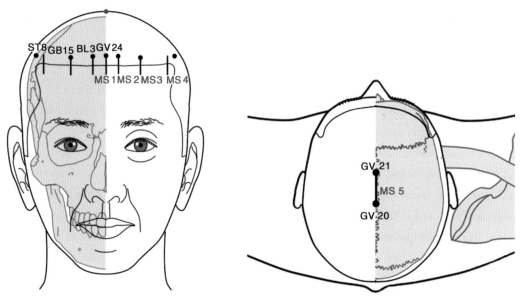

Figure 11–159   Lines of the forehead   Figure 11–160   Middle line of vertex

6)MS 6 Anterior oblique line of vertex-temporal(motor region)

Location: Draw a oblique line from Qianshencong(EX–HN 1) to Xuanli(GB 6), then divided into 5 segments(Figure 11–161).

Application: Superior 1/5 segment will treat the contralateral lower limbs paralysis. Middle 2/5 segment, treat the contralateral upper limbs paralysis, inferior 2/5 segment(the first speech area), for the contralateral facial paralysis, motor aphasia, salivation, dysphonia.

7)MS 7 Posterior oblique line of vertex-temporal(sensory region)

Location: Draw an oblique line from Baihui(GV 20) to Qubin(GB 7), then divided into 5 segments (Figure 11–161).

Application: Superior 1/5 segment will treat the contralateral waist and legs pain, numbness, paresthsia, stiff neck, tinnitus Middle 2/5 segment, treat the contralateral upper limbs pain, numbness, paresthsia, inferior 2/5 segment(the first speech area), for the contralateral facial pain, numbness and so on.

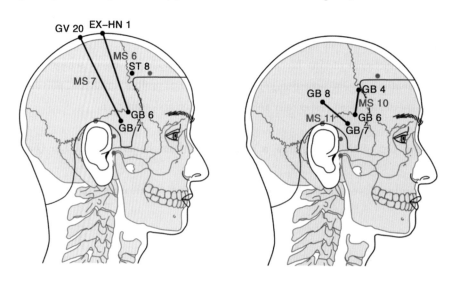

Figure 11–161   Anterior oblique line of vertex-temporal and posterior oblique line of vertex-temporal

8) MS 8 Lateral line 1 of vertex

Location : On the front of the head, draw a straight line from Chengguang(BL 6), the length of the line will be 1. 5 cun(Figure 11–162).

Application : Headache, vertigo, tinnitus, blur vision.

9) MS 9 Lateral line 2 of vertex

Location : On the front of the head, draw a straight line from Zhengying(GB 17), the length of the line will be 1. 5 cun(Figure 11–162).

Application : Headache, vertigo, migraine.

10) MS 10 Anterior temporal line

Location : Draw a straight line from Hanyan(GB 4) to Xuanli(GB 6).

Application : Headache, migraine, tinnitus, epilepsy.

11) MS 11 Posterior temporal line

Location : Draw a straight line from Shuaigu(GB 8) to Qubin(GB 7).

Application : headache, migraine, vertigo, febrile convulsion.

12) MS 12 Upper middle line of occiput

Location : Draw a straight line from Qiangjian(GV 18) to Naohu(GV 17) (Figure 11–163).

Application : headache, dizziness, vertigo, stiff neck, mental disorder, epilepsy.

13) MS 13 Upper lateral line of occiput(optic area)

Location : At the posterior of head, 0. 5 cun lateral beside, draw a straight line parallel to upper middle line of occiput(Figure 11–163).

Application : Cortex vision impairment, cataract.

14) MS 14 Lower lateral line of occiput(balance area)

Location : At the posterior of head, below the external occipital protuberance, draw a straight line from Yuzhen(BL 9), the length of the line will be 2 cun(Figure 11–163).

Application : Headache, stiff neck, vertigo, balance disorder caused by cerebellum impairment.

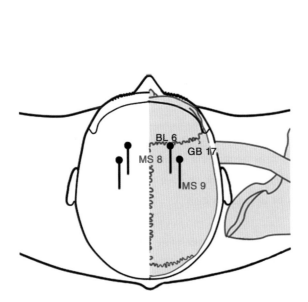

Figure 11–162   **Lines of the temporal**

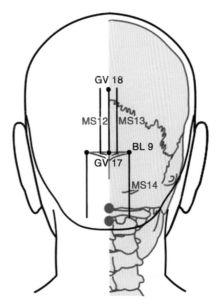

Figure 11–163   **Lines of the occiput**

(2) Manipulation

Patient may be treated with a sitting position or lying position. Disinfect the local place routinely, select a 1.5 cun or 2.0 cun long filiform needle No. 28-30, swiftly insert the needle subcutaneously, in 30 angle to the scalp, when the needle reaches the subgaleal layer and the practitioner feels the insertion resistance becomes weak, further insert the needle by twirling method, which parallels with the scalp until it goes to the periosteum, the depth of insertion varies with the areas, generally 0.5-1.5 cun. After the needle being inserted to the required depth, conduct manipulation.

In scalp acupuncture, the needle is manipulated only by twirling method, no lifting or thrusting of the needle. The depth of insertion keeps constant, and the needle is twirled in a frequency of 130-200 times per minute, it is first manipulated for 2-3 minutes and the needle is retained for 5 to 10 minutes, then the needle is withdrawn. For hemiplegia, during the manipulation and retention of the needle, the patient is encouraged to exercise the affected limbs so as to raise the therapeutic effect. (In severe case, passive movement of the limbs of the patient is conducted).

Electro-stimulation can be connected to the needles in the main areas to replace the hand manipulation. It is in a mode of high frequency and weak stimulation(Figure 11-164).

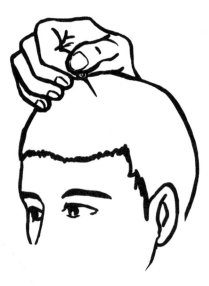

Figure 11-164　Manipulation of the scalp acupuncture

(3) Indications

It is mainly indicated for cerebral disorders, such as hemiplegia, numbness, aphasia, dizziness and vertigo, tinnitus, chorea, etc. It is also applied for headache, low back and leg pain, nocturia, triginimal neuralgia, scapulohumeral periarthritis and other diseases of nervous system.

(4) Precautions

Generally, scalp acupuncture is a strong stimulation, fainting therefore should be avoided. The practitioner should keep a close eye on the complexion of the patient and the intensity of the stimulation should be appropriately controlled. Wind stroke due to cerebral hemorrhage with coma, fever, high blood pressure, etc. In the acute stage, it is not suggested to treat by scalp acupuncture. The treatment may be applied until the pathological state is stable. Patients with acute inflammation, high fever and heart failure should be dealt with great care if scalp acupuncture is used.

11.4.4.7 Auricular acupuncture

Auricular acupuncture is one of the acupuncture therapies used to prevent and treat diseases by stimulating certain points in the auricle with needles or other tools.

(1) The history of auricular acupuncture

Auricular acupuncture has been utilized in the treatment of diseases for thousands of years. In the moxibustion classic of *11 Yin and Yang Meridians for Moxibustion* excavated from Western Han Dynasty mausoleum, it was first recorded as *Ear meridian*, which was connected with upper limbs, eyes, cheeks and laryngopharynx. In the classic TCM literature of *Internal Classic*, which was compiled in around 500 B C, the correlation between the auricle and the body had been described; each of the six yang meridians has a connection to the ear. Yang meridians connect in pairs to yin meridians. Therefore even yin viscera have contact with the ear. In the literature of *Miraculous Pivot*, it described, "for the deaf who can hear, needle the center of the ear. " It is also recorded in *Essential Prescriptions Worth a Thousand Gold for Emergencies* that needling point "center" is an appropriate treatment for jaundice, diseases due to cold, summerheat or epidemic, pathogenic factors. In other classic medical literary texts there are descriptions of stimulating the ears and certain auricular areas with needles, moxibustion, tuina and tuina suppositories to treat and prevent diseases; as well as inspecting and palpating the auricles to assist in disease diagnoses. Modern auriculotherapy got its start in 1957 when a French neurologist named Dr. Paul Nogier In, developed the map of reflex points on the ear, based upon the concept of an inverted fetus arrangement. Since 1982 the World Health Organization (WHO) has worked to try to bring about a standardization of international acupuncture terminology in naming meridians and acupuncture points. In 1992, the Chinese national standard of nomenclature and location of auricular points was published, and it was revised in 2008. In our book, auricular points are based on the 2008 revised edition.

(2) The relationship between the ear, meridians and zang-fu viscera

1) Relationship between the ear and meridians

The meridians of the hand taiyang, hand shaoyang, foot shaoyang and the collateral of the hand yangming enter the ear. The meridians of foot yangming and foot taiyang travel to the front of the ear and above the ear respectively; The divergent meridian of the hand jueyin comes out from the back of the ear. The vessels of the yang heel and yin heel go to the back of the ear. The six yin meridians connect to the ear by means of their divergent meridians that separate, enter, resurface and finally join their interior exterior related yang meridians respectively.

2) Relationship between the ear and zang-fu viscera

The ear has close relation with zang-fu viscera as well. According to records in *Classic of Difficult Issues*, the ear links to the five zang viscera physiologically. In *Lizheng Anmo Yaoshu* (The Extensive Techniques of Massage) the back of the ear is divided into five parts that correspond to the five zang viscera respectively.

(3) The anatomy of the auricle

1) Helix and antihelix (Figure 11–165)

Helix: Curling edge of the lateral border of the auricle.

Helix crus: Transverse edge of the helix reaching backward into the ear cavity.

Antihelix: Medial aspect of the helix, on the elevated edge parallel to the helix. Its upper portion branches out into the superior antihelix crus and the inferior antihelix crus.

2) Earlobe, tragus, and antitragus

Earlobe: Lowest part of the auricle without cartilage.

Tragus:Curved flap in front of the auricle.

Antitragus:Small tubercle opposite to the tragus and superior to the ear lobe.

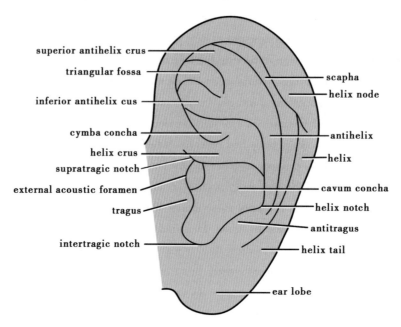

Figure 11-165 The anatomy of the auricle

3)Triangular fossa,cymba concha,cavum concha

Triangular fossa:Triangular depression between the two crura of the antihelix.

Cymba concha:Olive cavum between the helix crus and the inferior antihelix crus.

Cavum concha:Cavum inferior to the helix crus.

4)Scapha,helix tubercle

Scapha:Narrow curved depression between the helix and the antihelix.

Helix tubercle:Small tubercle at the posterior-superior aspect of the helix.

5)Supratragic notch,intertragic notch,helix notch

Supratragic notch:Depression between the upper border of the tragus and the helix crus.

Intertragic notch:Depression between the tragus and antitragus.

Helix notch:Shallow depression between antitragus and antihelix.

(4)The concept and distribution of auricular points

Auricular points are the specific areas distributed over the ear. One of the most popular representations is a picture of a little child huddled up in the foetal position in the form of the external ear. The distribution of auricular points is as follows:Points related to the portion of the head are located on the ear lobe. Points related to the upper limbs are located on the scapha. Points related to the trunk and lower limbs are located on the body of the antihelix and superior and inferior antihelix crus. Points related to the viscera in the abdomen are located on the cymbaconcha. Points related to the viscera in the chest are located on the cavum concha. Points related to the digestive tract are distributed around the helix crus(Figure 11-166).

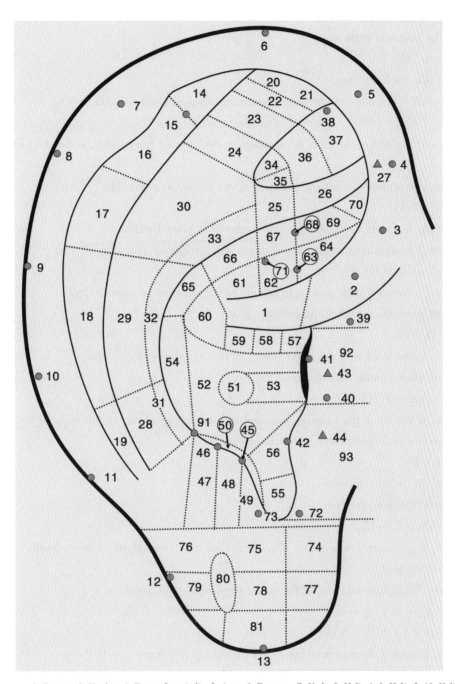

1. Ear center;2. Rectum;3. Urethra;4. External genitalia;5. Anus;6. Ear-apex;7. Node;8. Helix 1;9. Helix 2;10. Helix 3;11. Helix 4;12. Helix 5;13. Helix 6;14. Finger;15. Wind stream;16. Wrist;17. Elbow;18. Shoulder;19. Clavicle;20. Toe;21. Heel;22. Ankle;23. Knee;24. Hip;25. Gluteus;26. Sciatic nerve;27. Sympathetic nerve;28. Cervical vertebrae;29. Thoracic vertebrae;30. Lumbosacral vertebrae;31. Neck;32. Chest;33. Abdomen;34. Shenmen;35. Palvis;36. Middle triangular fossa;37. Internal genitalia;38. Superior triangular fossa;39. External ear;40. External nose;41. Apex of tragus;42. Adrenal gland;43. Pharynx larynx;44. Internal nose;45. Apex of antitragus;46. Central rim;47. Occiput;48. Temple;49. Forehead;50. Subcortex;51. Heart;52. Lung;53. Trachea;54. Spleen;55. Endocrine;56. Triple energizer;57. Mouth;58. Esophagus;59. Cardia;60. Stomach;61. Duodenum;62. Small intestine;63. Appendix;64. Large intestine;65. Liver;66. Pancreas and gallbladder;67. Kidney;68. Ureter;69. Bladder;70. Angle of superior conchae;71. Center of superior concha;72. Anterior intertragal notch;73. Posterior intertragal notch;74. Tooth;75. Tongue;76. Jaw;77. Anterior ear lobe;78. Eye;79. Internal ear;80. Cheek;81. Tonsil;82. Upper ear root;83. Root of ear vagus;84. Lower ear root;85. Groove of posterior surface;86. Heart of posterior surface;87. Spleen of posterior surface;88. Liver of posterior surface;89. Lung of posterior surface;90. Kidney of posterior surface;91. Brain stem;92. Upper tragus;93. Lower tragus.

Figure 11-166　**The distribution of auricular points**

(5) Auricular points

1) Auricular points of helix zone

a. Ear Center(HX 1)

Locations : On the helix crus.

Indications : Hiccup, skin rash, neurodermatitis, enuresis in children, hemoptysis.

b. Rectum(HX 2)

Locations : At the end of the helix approximate to the superior tragicnotch, at the level with point Large Intestine.

Indications : Constipation, diarrhea, prolapse of the rectum, hemorrhoids.

c. Urethra(HX 3)

Locations : At the level with point Bladder, superior to point Urethra.

Indications : Frequent micturition, urgent and painful urination, retention of urine.

d. External genitals(HX 4)

Locations : At the level with point sympathetic nerve, superior to point urethra.

Indications : Orchitis, epididymitis, pruritus vulvae.

e. Anus(HX 5)

Locations : At the level with the lower border of the superior antihelix crus.

Indications : Hemorrhoids, anal fissure.

f. Ear apex(erjian)(HX 6,7i)

Locations : At the tip of the helix, at the level with the upper border of the superior antihelix crus.

Indications : Fever, hypertension, acute conjunctivitis.

g. Node(HX 8)

Locations : On thehelix tubercle.

Indications : Dizziness, headache.

h. Helix 1-6(HX 9-12)

Locations : Region from lower border of auricular tubercle to midpoint of lower border of lobule is divided into five equal parts.

Indications : Tonsillitis, infection of the upper respiratory tract, fever.

2) Auricular points of Scapha

a. Finger(SF 1)

Locations : Scapha is divided into five equal parts, from the upper part to the lower part. The 1st part.

Indications : Finger numbness and pain, paronychia.

b. Wind steam(SF 1,2i)

Locations : The area between point finger and point wrist.

Indications : Urticaria, cutaneous pruritus, allergic rhinitis.

c. Wrist(SF 2)

Locations : The 2nd part.

Indications : Wrist pain.

d. Elbow(SF 3)

Locations : The 3nd part.

Indications : Elbow pain, external humeral epicondylitis.

e. Shoulder(SF 4,5)

Locations : The 4th part.

Indications：Shoulder pain，shoulder peripheral arthritis.

f. Clavicle(SF 6)

Locations：The 5th part.

Indications：Peripheral arthritis of the shoulder.

3)Auricular points of antihelix

a. Heel(AH 1)

Locations：At superior and anterior angle of superior antihelix crus，approximate to the upper part of triangular fossa.

Indications：Heel pain.

b. Toe(AH 2)

Locations：At superior and posterior angle of superior antihelix crus，approximate to ear apex.

Indications：Paronychia，pain of the toe.

c. Ankle(AH 3)

Locations：Midway between point Heel and point Knee.

Indications：Ankle sprain.

d. Knee(AH 4)

Locations：At the middle 1/3 at superior antihelix crus.

Indications：Swelling and pain of the knee joint.

e. Hip(AH 5)

Locations：At the interior 1/3 of the superior antihelix crus.

Indications：Pain of the hip joint，sciatica.

f. Sciatic nerve(AH 6)

Locations：At anterior 2/3 of the inferior antihelix crus.

Indications：Sciatica.

g. Sympathetic(AH 6a)

Locations：At the border between the terminal of the inferior antihelix crus and helix.

Indications：Gastrointestinal colic，biliary colic，angina pectoris，urinary stone，automatic nervous system function disorder.

h. Gluteus(AH 7)

Locations：At the posterior 1/3 of the inferior antihelix crus.

Indications：Pain of the lumbosacral region，sciatica.

i. Abdomen(AH 8)

Locations：On the border of cavum conchae of lumbosacral vertebrae.

Indications：Abdominal pain and distention，diarrhea.

j. Lumbosacral vertebrae(AH 9)

Locations：A curved line from helixtragic notch to the branching area of superior and inferior antihelix crus can be divided into 5 equal parts. The lower 1/5 is cervical vertebrae，the middle 2/5 is thoracic vertebrae，the upper 2/5 is lumbosacral vertebrae.

Indications：Pain in the lumbosacral region.

k. Chest(AH 10)

Locations：On the border of cavum conchae of thoracic vertevrae.

Indications：Pain in the thoracic and hypochondriac regions，fullness sensation in the chest.

l. Thoracic Vertebrae(AH 11)

Locations : Vertebrae, the upper 2/5 is lumbosacral vertebrae.

Indications : Pain in the chest and back.

m. Neck(AH 12)

Locations : On the border of cavum conchae of thoracic vertevrae.

Indications : Stiff neck, swelling and pain of the neck.

n. Cervical vertebrae(AH 13)

Locations : A curved line from helixtragic notch to the branching area of superior and inferior antihelix crus can be divided into 5 equal parts. The lower 1/5 iscervical vertebrae, the middle 2/5 is thoracic vertebrae, and the upper 2/5 is lumbosacral vertebrae.

Indications : Neck pain.

4) Auricular points oftriangular fossa

a. Superior triangular fossa(TF 1)

Locations : Superior to the anterior 1/3 of triangular fossa.

Indications : Hypertension.

b. Internal genitals(TF 2)

Locations : Inferior to anterior 1/3 of triangular fossa.

Indications : Dysmenorrhea, irregular menstruation, dysfunctional uterine bleeding, profuse leukorrhea, nocturnal emission, premature ejaculation.

c. Middle triangular fossa(TF 3)

Locations : Middle 1/3 of the triangular fossa.

Indications : Asthma.

d. Shenmen(TF 4)

Locations : Superior to the posterior 1/3 of triangular fossa.

Indications : Insomnia, dream-disturbed sleep, pain.

e. Pelvis(TF 5)

Locations : Inferior to the posterior 1/3 of triangular fossa.

Indications : Pelvic inflammation.

5) Auricular points of tragus

a. Upper tragus(TG 1)

Locations : Upper half of the external aspect of the tragus.

Indications : Pharyngitis, rhinitis.

b. Lower tragus(TG 2)

Locations : Lower half of the external aspect of the tragus.

Indications : Rhinitis.

c. External ear(TG 1u)

Locations : Supra tragus notch close to the helix.

Indications : Inflammation of the external auditory canal, otitis media, tinnitus.

d. Apex of tragus(TG 1p)

Locations : At the tip of the upper protuberance on the border of the tragus.

Indications : Fever, toothache.

e. External nose(TG 1,2i)

Locations : At the anterior to center of lateral aspect of tragus.

Indications : Nasal obstruction, rhinitis.

f. Adrenal gland (TG 2p)

Locations: At the top of the lower protuberance on the border of the tragus.

Indications: Hypotension, allergic diseases.

g. Pharynxlarynx (TG 3)

Locations: At the upper half of the medial aspect of the tragus.

Indications: Hoarseness, pharyegolaryngitis, tonsillitis.

h. Internal nose (TG 4)

Locations: At the lower half of the medial aspect of the tragus.

Indications: Rhinitis, paranasal sinusitis, epistaxis.

i. Anterior intertragal notch (TG 21)

Locations: Anterior to intertragus, notch, the lowest point of the tragus.

Indications: Stomatitis, pharyngitis.

6) Auricular points of Antitragus

a. Forehead (AT 1)

Locations: At the anterior inferior corner of the lateral aspect of the antitragus.

Indications: Headache, dizziness, insomnia, dream disturbed sleep.

b. Posterior intertragal notch (AT 11)

Locations: Posterior to intertragus notch, anterior and inferior part of antitragus.

Indications: Frontal sinusitis.

c. Temple (AT 2)

Locations: At the midpoint of the lateral aspect of the antitragus.

Indications: Migraine.

d. Occiput (AT 3)

Locations: At the posterior superior corner of the lateral aspect of the antitragus.

Indications: Headache, dizziness, asthma, epilepsy.

e. Subcortex (AT 4)

Locations: On the medial aspect of the antitragus.

Indications: Pain, neurasthenia.

f. Apex of antitragus (AT 1,2,4i)

Locations: At the top of the antitragus.

Indications: Asthma, mumps, cutaneous pruritus.

g. Central rim (brain) (AT 2,3,4i)

Locations: Midway between the antitragic apex and helixtragic notch.

Indications: Enuresis, internal auditory vertigo.

h. Brain stem (AT 3,4i)

Locations: Helix-tragus notch.

Indications: Occipital headache, dizziness, temporary myopia.

7) Auricular points of Conchae

a. Mouth (CO 1)

Locations: Anterior 1/3 of inferior part of helix crus.

Indications: Facial paralysis, stomatitis, gallbladder stone, cholecystitis, withdrawal syndrome.

b. Esophagus (CO 2)

Locations: Middle 1/3 of inferior part of helix crus.

Indications: Esophagitis, esophagus spasm.

c. Cardia(CO 3)

Locations: Posterior 1/3 of inferior part of helix crus.

Indications: Cardio spasm, nervous vomiting.

d. Stomach(CO 4)

Locations: Area where the helix crus terminates.

Indications: Gastro spasm, gastritis, gastric ulcer.

e. Duodenum(CO 5)

Locations: At the posterior part of the superior aspect of the helix crus.

Indications: Duodenal ulcer, pylorospasm.

f. Small intestine(CO 6)

Locations: At the middle part of the superior aspect of the helix crus.

Indications: Indigestion, abdominal pain.

g. Large intestine(CO 7)

Locations: At the posterior part of the superior aspect of the helix crus.

Indications: Diarrhea, constipation, cough, acne.

h. Appendix(CO 6,7i)

Locations: Midway between small intestine and large intestine.

Indications: Simple appendicitis, diarrhea.

i. Angle of superiorconcha(CO 8)

Locations: At the anterior superior angle of cymba conchae.

Indications: Orostatitis, urethritis.

j. Bladder(CO 9)

Locations: Between kidney and angle of superior concha.

Indications: Cystitis, retention of urine, enuresis.

k. Kidney(CO 10)

Locations: On the lower border of the inferior antihelix crus directly above small intestine.

Indications: Lumbago, tinnitus, insomnia, dizziness, enuresis, irregular menses.

l. Ureter(CO 9,10i)

Locations: Between kidney and bladder.

Indications: Colic pain of the ureter calculus.

m. Pancreas and gallbladder(CO 11)

Locations: Between liver and point kidney.

Indications: Pancreasitis, cholecystitis, cholelithiasis.

n. Liver(CO 12)

Location: The posterior and interior border of the cymba conchae.

Indications: Hypochondriac pain, dizziness, irregular menstruation.

o. Center of superior concha(CO 6,10i)

Locations: In the middle of the cymba conchae.

Indications: Abdominal pain, abdominal distention.

p. Spleen(CO 13)

Locations: At the posterior and superior aspect of the cavum conchae.

Indications: Abdominal distention, diarrhea, loss of appetite.

q. Heart(CO 13)

Locations: In the center of the cavum conchae.

Indications: Palpitation, angina pectoris, neurasthenia.

r. Trachea(CO 16)

Locations: Between the orifice of the external auditory meatus and point heart.

Indications: Cough, asthma.

s. Triple energizer(CO 14)

Locations: Posteral-inferior part of the orifice of the external auditory meatus and CO 18.

Indications: Constipation, abdominal distention, stomachache.

t. Lung(CO 17)

Locations: Around the center of the cavum conchae.

Indications: Cough, asthma, skin diseases.

u. Endocrine(CO 18)

Locations: At the base of cavum conchae in the intertragic notch.

Indications: Dysmenorrhea, irregular menstruation, acne.

8) Auricular points of Lobe

On the area from the lower border of the cartilage of the intertragic notch to the lower border of the ear-lobe, draw three horizontal lines by which the area is horizontally and equally divided, then draw two vertical lines by which the area is vertically and equally divided, thus the area is divided into 9 equal sections. These sections are numbered from the anterior section posterior and from the upper section downward.

a. Tooth(LO 1)

Locations: Anterior-superior part of the earlobe.

Indications: Toothache, hypotension, periodontitis.

b. Tongue(LO 2)

Locations: Superomedian part.

Indications: Glossitis, stomatitis.

c. Jaw(LO 3)

Locations: Posterior-superior part of the earlobe.

Indications: Toothache, submandibular arthritis.

d. Anterior earlobe(LO 4)

Locations: Anterior medial part of the earlobe.

Indications: Toothache, neurasthenia.

e. Eye(LO 5)

Locations: Center part of the earlobe.

Indications: Acute conjunctivitis, pseudomyopia.

f. Internal ear(LO 6)

Locations: Posterior medial part of the earlobe.

Indications: Tinnitus, impaired hearing, internal auditory vertigo.

g. Cheek(LO 5,6i)

Locations: Between(LO 5)and LO(6).

Indications: Facial paralysis, trigeminal neuralgia, acne.

h. Tonsil(LO 7,8,9)

Locations: Inferior part of the earlobe.

Indications:Acute tonsillitis,pharyngitis.

9)Auricular points of Posterior Surface

a. Heart of posterior surface(P 1)

Locations:Superior part of the posterior auricle.

Indications:Coronary heart disease,insomnia,dreaminess.

b. Lung of posterior surface(P 2)

Locations:Medial to the central part of the posterior auricle.

Indications:Asthma,neurodermatitis.

c. Spleen of posterior surface(P 3)

Locations:Central part of the posterior auricle.

Indications:Stomachache,indigestion,anorexia.

d. Liver of posterior surface(P 4)

Locations:Lateral to the central part of the posterior auricle.

Indications:Cholelithiasis,cholecystitis,hypochondriac pain.

e. Kidney of posterior surface(P 5)

Locations:Inferior part of the posterior auricle.

Indications:Headache,dizziness,neurosis.

f. Groove of posterior surface(P 6)

Locations:Through the backside of superior antihelix crus and inferior antihelix crus,in the depression as a "Y" form.

Indications:Hypertension,neurodermatitis.

10)Auricular points of Ear Root

a. Upper ear root(R 1)

Locations:At the upper border of the auricular root.

Indications:Hypertension.

b. Root of ear vagus(R 2)

Locations:At the junction of retro auricle and mastoid,level with helix crus.

Indications:Cholecystitis,cholelithiasis,bilaryascariasis.

c. Lower Ear Root(R 3)

Locations:At the lower border of the auricular root.

Indications:Hypotension.

(6)Clinical application of auricular acupuncture

1)Principles for selecting auricular points

①Based on the position of the disease or affected area of the body. The whole body can be mapped on the ear,therefore,every part of an viscera or tissue has a corresponding point on the viscera or tissue's corresponding ear area.

E. g. select the stomach(CO 4)for the treatment of gastritis.

②According to TCM theory

The auricular points corresponding to the five zang and six fu viscera are especially significant in TCM.

E. g. choose the kidney(CO 10)for alopecia. Choose the lung(CO 7)and large intestine(CO 14)for skin diseases

③According to knowledge of modern medicine. E. g. ,Choose Shenmen(TF 4)and Subcortex(AT 4)

for painful conditions and inflammation. Choose the large intestine(CO 7)for toothache.

④According to clinical experience.

E. g. Select external genital(HX 4)for pain in the lower back and legs. Choose Ear apex(HX 6,7i)for bloodletting and for red,swollen and painful eyes.

2)Exploration of auricular points

①Inspection:Auricular inspection is to check for abnormal changes on the ear in order to diagnose diseases or disorders. The most commonly seen positive changes include deformities,discoloration,pimples, desquamation,nodules,congestion,blister and so on. Red color of ear indicates heat. Pale color of ear indicates deficiency. Bluish-black color of ear indicates cold stagnation. Pale purple color of ear indicates qi stagnation. Reddish purple color of ear indicates blood stagnation. Excess moisture on the ear indicates dampness. Pimples on the ear indicates damp heat. Dry flaky skin means blood or yin deficiency.

②Detection of the tender spot:This method searches for the tender spots on the ears with a probe,the head of an acupuncture needle handle,or the end of a matchstick by pressing and moving on the surface of the ear gently and smoothly.

③Measurement of electrical resistance:This technique detects decreased electrical resistance in points with an electrical detector that has an indicator lamp or special sound.

3)Effects and indications of auricular acupuncture

Auricular acupuncture therapy has the action of assistant diagnosis. When there is an illness in the body,especially the organic disease,it may manifest on the ear as positive reactions. There may be tenderness,deformities,discoloration,and disturbance in the skin's electrical properties. We can establish the diagnosis according to these reactions combined with symptoms,signs and medical history. It is commonly applied for acute and chronic pain,addictions,neurological,gynecological,allergic,endocrinal and metabolic disorders,inflammatory conditions,beauty therapy,anti-aging and disease prevention.

4)Manipulation of auricular acupuncture

After diagnosis and point prescription are made,detect the tender spots on the area where the ear points are selected. If marked tenderness is not located,give the treatment with auricular points' therapy. After the selected points are located,strict skin disinfection is necessary. Beside disinfect the needles and fingers of acupuncturist,the auricular points should be swabbed with 2% iodine first and then with 75% alcohol as routine asepsis. If disinfection is not strict,it is easy to lead to auricular perichondritis due to infection. The manipulation techniques are as follows:

①The filiform needle methods:Filiform needles that are 0.5 cun in length or special thumb-tack needle are selected for auricular acupuncture. To begin with the procedure,stabilize the ear with the left hand and insert the needle with right hand,then penetrate the cartilage but do not penetrate through the ear. During the needle retention,the needles should be rotate intermittently. Filiform needles are allow to be retained for 20 to 30 minutes. However,they may be prolonged by 1 to 2 hours or even longer for chronic conditions. After the needle has been removed,press the punctured hole with a dry clean cotton ball for 20 seconds. Once a week treatment,10 times for one course of treatment. For the thumbtack type intradermal needle insertion,the needle should be fastened to the ear with a piece of adhesive tape and kept in place for 2 to 3 days. There will be local pain or heat sensation in most of the patients after the needle insertion.

②Electrotherapy:This method is used to treat diseases of the nervous system,spasm and pain in zang and fu viscera,asthma,etc.

③Needle-embedding therapy:After the thumb-tack needle is embedded,ask the patient to press it 3 times a day by himself;retain the needle on the point for 3-5 days.

④Auricular-seed-pressing therapy: It is a simple stimulating method by tapping small seed-shape herb on the auricular point. This method is safe, painless and fewer side-effects. It will not cause auricular perichondritis. It is suitable for the elderly people and children or the patient who is afraid of acupuncture. The material, such as rape seed, a mung beam, radish seed, a seed of Vaccaria segetalis, or magnetic bead, can be used.

The points may also be treated with the ear-pressing method. Magnetic beads or Vaccaria segetalis are fastened to the ear with a piece of adhesive tape on the auricular points and kept in place for 3 to 5 days. The patient is asked to press the selected points 2 to 4 times a day.

5) Precautions

Filifrom needling on auricular areas may produce strong pain, so explanation is necessary before treatment in order to obtain cooperation from patients. Strict antisepsis to avoid infection. Needling fainting should also be prevented from happening during auricular acupuncture. Prompt intervention is needed if this happens.

For needle-embedding therapy, auricular-seed-pressing therapy, use hypoallergenic adhesive tape for people with adhesive allergies. Do not rub in a sideways or circular motion while pressing the taped auricular points. If it will influence the sleep, only one side points can be used.

6) Contraindications

Auricular acupuncture should be contraindicated for pregnant women or women with a history of abortion. This therapy is not advisable for patients with frostbite, inflammation, or infection of the ear, and patients with severe diseases or bad anemia. In the treatment of severe heart disease or severe hypertension, strong stimulation should be avoided.

11.5　General introduction on acupuncture treatment

11.5.1　The function of acupuncture treatment

The acupuncture treatment has various effectively curing functions to different diseases, such as tranquilizing effect to insomnia, analgesic effect to pain, antitussive effect to cough, etc. But in brief, the functions of acupuncture treatment are worked out by regulating yin and yang, strengthening body resistance and dispelling pathogenic factors, and dredging meridians and collaterals.

11.5.1.1　Regulating yin and yang

As we know, normal physiological states depend on the balance between yin and yang, while diseases mainly result from excess or deficiency of yin or yang. In the fifth chapter of *Miraculous Pivot*, it's said that "how to regulate yin and yang is most important in acupuncture treatment". So that regulation of yin and yang can be recognized as the fundamental effect of clinical acupuncture treatment. Regulation of yin and yang by acupuncture is closely related with point prescription and needling manipulations depending on the different conditions of imbalance of yin and yang. For example, drowsiness due to yin excess and yang deficiency, while insomnia due to yang excess and yin deficiency. Both Zhaohai(KI 6) of yin heel vessel and Shenmai(BL 62) of yang heel vessel could be selected for acupuncture treatment. But different manipulations would be used as for drowsiness reinforcement method is used at Shenmai(BL 62) to strengthen deficient yang and reduction method at Zhaohai(KI 6) to reduce excessive yin, meanwhile for insomnia reinforcement method is used at Zhaohai(KI 6) to tonify deficient yin and reduction method at Shenmai(BL

62) to reduce excessive yang. With these different methods, both drowsiness and insomnia can be treated.

11.5.1.2　Strengthening the body resistance and dispelling pathogenic factors

According to the theories of TCM, the occurrence, development process and outcome of the disease are really the process of struggle between healthy and pathogenic qi in human body. The insufficiency of healthy qi indicates the weakness of body resistance, so the body tends to be attacked by pathogenic qi and cannot dispel the pathogenic factors easily. Another crucial function of acupuncture or moxibustion treatment is strengthening the body resistance and dispelling the pathogenic factors. For example, pricking for bleeding method can be used for dispelling the excessive heat on excessive heat syndrome; reinforcement method like needling and moxibustion can be used for restoring yang qi and helping yang qi warm the body on asthenia cold syndrome; while reinforcement and reduction methods can be used simultaneously on the syndrome complicated with both asthenia and sthenia.

11.5.1.3　Dredging meridians and collaterals

Physiologically speaking, meridians and collaterals can connect exterior and interior, zang-fu viscera and outside limbs; promote qi and blood circulation. If there are some blocks in meridians, the qi and blood circulation will be stagnated and clinically manifested as pain, numbness, nodule, swelling, bruising and other symptoms. However, the appropriate acuppoints and needling methods could solve all problems above easily. The basic and direct function of acupuncture is helping to clear the blocked point in the meridians and collaterals in human body and effectively recover the original functions like connection among viscera and limbs and circulation of qi and blood. Meanwhile, meridians, collaterals and acupoints are also the gateway for exogenous pathogenic qi to infect into and be driven out from the body. So the strengthening the body resistance and dispelling pathogenic factors function of acupuncture treatment is also achieved by dredging meridians and collaterals.

In conclusion, the functions of acupuncture treatment are bidirectional benign effects for human body by dredging qi and blood of meridians and collaterals, and regulating yin and yang. The functions are closely related with the conditions of human body, the methods of acupuncture, and the selection of acupoints.

11.5.2　Principles of acupuncture treatment

11.5.2.1　Tonifying the deficiency and reducing the excess

Tonifying the deficiency and reducing the excess is not only the most important function but also the basic principle of acupuncture.

Deficiency indicates insufficient of healthy qi, including qi or blood deficiency and qi sinking; while excess indicates superabundance of pathogenic factors, including stagnation of qi, blood and phlegm. The deficiency of qi and excess of pathogenic factors results in the entire process of diseases. So the basic principle of acupuncture treatment is tonifying the deficiency and reducing the excess, also referring as strengthening the body resistance and dispelling the pathogenic factors.

According to this principle, to tonify the deficiency, reinforcing methods especially moxibustion can be used at Pishu(BL 20) and Zusanli(ST 36) for spleen qi deficiency, Shenshu(BL 23) and Taixi(KI 3) for Kidney qi deficiency, Qihai(CV 6) and Guanyuan(CV 4) for primordial qi deficiency, and Baihui(GV 20) for qi sinking. To reduce the excess, reducing methods such as needling, pricking for bleeding can be used at Taichong(LR 3) for qi stagnation, Fenglong(ST 40) for phlegm, etc.

11.5.2.2　Clearing the heat and warming the cold

Heat and cold are the key guidelines of the diseases nature and manifested in most process of diseases.

Clearing the heat and warming the cold is the acupuncture treatment principle directing against heat syndromes and cold syndromes.

Many kinds of heat syndromes could be treated by the method of clearing heat. For exterior or interior heat syndromes manifested as sunstroke, sore throat, and fever, needles must be inserted shallowly and pulled out fast, or pricking for bleeding can also be used. For cold syndromes caused by exogenous cold invasion or endogenous yang deficiency, the method of warming cold is applicable. Moxibustion can be used to treat the exogenous cold in meridians; while the excess cold congealing in viscera, needles must be inserted deeply and retained with the manipulation of heat-producing needling.

11.5.2.3 Concentrating on the fundamental contradiction of diseases

The fundamental and incidental contradictions of diseases are relative to each other, but referring to different meanings. The incidental is generally the phenomenon and the secondary aspect, the fundamental causes generally the nature and the primary aspect of a disease. According to different conditions of human body, the genuine qi is fundamental, and the pathogenic factors are incidental; the cause is fundamental, and the symptoms are incidental; the primary disease is fundamental, while the consequent disease is incidental.

Generally speaking, the key principle of acupuncture treatment is concentrating on the fundamental contradiction of diseases. As it is much more effective to solve the fundamental causes than to relieve the symptoms. Mostly when the fundamental contradiction is solved, the incidental contradiction would also be dispelled. Such as for deficiency cold syndromes, nourishing yang will bring out the relieving of cold.

While in emergency, the acute incidental contradiction must be relieved before the fundamental one, so as to save life or relieve emergent condition. For example, severe constipation and dysuria resulted by aeipathias should be treated with the points helping defecation and urinate, to relieve the acute symptoms firstly. After the relief of severe conditions, the points for the primary cause or original disease are selected to treat the disease and prevent the acute constipation and dysuria.

11.5.2.4 Selecting treatment according to the climatic, geographical and individual conditions

This principle is one of the applications of the "holism of human beings and nature". As the continuous changes of the environment, such as season, weather, and living conditions will affect the human body directly or indirectly. While people with different constitutions will have different manifestation to the same pathogenic factors. All above these factors resulting in the corresponding physiological or pathological reaction, should be considered while treating diseases with acupuncture treatment.

(1) Temporal factors

Not only season and climate, day and night, but rhythmic circulation of qi and blood in the meridians, and the regularities of occurrence or aggravation can be considered as temporal factors. For example, midnight-noon ebb-low acupuncture therapy indicating the point selection by midday-midnight flowing of qi-blood, is recognized as one of the Chronomedicine.

(2) Geographical environment

Different areas have different natural conditions, such as climate, cultural customs and habits. For instance, in cold northern China, moxibustion is frequently-used with more moxa cones, but in hot and humid southern China, moxibustion is used fewer.

(3) Individual conditions

The same disease has various syndromes and manifestations in different person according to the age, gender and constitution. For women, acupoints belonging to thoroughfare vessel and conception vessel would be used more frequently, and pregnancy is a very important factors for acupuncture treatment selection. While the manipulations of needling on patients in weak constitution should also be lighter than those with strong constitutions.

11.5.3   Selection of acupoints

Based on the theory of meridians and collaterals, successful acupuncture treatment depends on proper prescription of acupoints. The key principles are selecting according to the symptoms, the causes of the diseases, the functions of the related meridians, and the natures of the points.

11.5.3.1   Principles of acupoints selection

Adjacent or local acupoints are commonly selected to treat the diseases, such as Dicang(ST 4) and Yingxiang(LI 20) for facial paralysis, Zhongwan(CV 12) and Shangwan(CV 13) for stomachache. While distal acuponts especially below the elbows and knees are also selected to treat diseases according to the symptoms or the distributions of the meridians, such as Hegu(LI 4) can be selected for facial paralysis according to the distributions of the meridians, while for ache according to the special analgesia on the symptom.

In addition, the application of the specific acupoints is another important principle of acupoints selection. Such as the eight meeting points are mentioned to the eight specific points where the vital energy of the zang viscera, fu viscera, qi, blood, sinews, pulse, vessels, bones and marrow gather. In clinical application, all diseases of the zang viscera, fu viscera, qi, blood, sinews, pulse, vessels, bones and marrow can be treated by the respective meeting points.

11.5.3.2   Combination of acupoints

(1) Combination of the exterior-interior acupoints

This combining method is based on the exterior-interior relationship of the yin meridians and yang meridians according to the differentiations of zang-fu viscera and meridians. The acupoints of the exterior-interior related meridians can be selected at the same time to strengthen the effect. For example, for lowback pain of kidney deficiency, Taixi(KI 3) of kidney meridian of foot Shaoyin can be selected combining with Kunlun(BL 60) and Weizhong(BL 64) of the bladder meridian of foot taiyang. Additionally, the combination of the source points and the connecting points in specific points is a concrete application of this method in clinic.

(2) Combination of the anterior-posterior acupoints

This combining method is based on the theory the thoracic-abdominal region (anterior) belonging to yin, and the lumbodorsal region(posterior) belonging to yang. Thus, the selection of the points on the anterior and posterior regions makes up a prescription for the diseases of zang-fu viscera and trunk. For example, anterior Zhongwan(CV 12) and posterior Weishu(BL 21) are selected for stomachache.

(3) The Combination of the distal-local acupoints

This combining method is based on the local and distal curative effect of all acupoints. Usually, the adjacent or local acupoints will be selected combining with the distal acuponts especially on the same meridians or the exterior-interior related meridians. For example, Dicang(ST 4) and Yingxiang(LI 20) are selected as the local acupoints combining with Hegu(LI 4) as distal acuponits for facial paralysis.

(4) The combination of the left-right acupoints

The combining method is based on the theory that the symmetrical distribution of the meridians and collaterals, therefore the points on both sides can be selected to strengthen the coordinating effects on the diseases of zang-fu viscera. For example, Hegu(LI 4) on the right side can be selected to treat facial paralysis on the left side according to the distribution of the large intestine meridian of hand yang ming, while Zusanli(ST 36) on both side can be selected to strengthen the effects for stomachache.

11.5.4　Selection of acupuncture and moxibustion technique

Successful acupuncture treatment depends on not only the proper acupoints selections with correct combinations, but also suitable selection of acupuncture and moxibustion manipulations.

11.5.4.1　Selection of methods

The acupuncture and moxibustion therapy includes various methods, as filiform acupuncture, electroacupuncture, moxibustion, cupping, pricking for bleeding, pyropuncture, auricular acupuncture, etc. These methods can be chosen independently or in combination with each other according to the conditions of the diseases. For example, moxibustiuon will also be used based on filiform acupuncture to treat deficiency cold syndrome.

11.5.4.2　Selection of manipulations

After methods are selected, the manipulations must be confirmed. Such as filiform acupuncture, for acute excessive syndrome, reducing manipulation should be used; while for chronic deficient syndrome, reinforcing manipulation is more suitable. The duration and frequency of needling also depend on the conditions and reactions of the patients.

11.5.4.3　Selection of treatment timing

Treatment timing is another influencing factor to the effect of acupuncture. Generally speaking, for the diseases with obvious time regularity of attack or aggravation, acupuncture therapy should be used before the attack or aggravation. For example, acupuncture could be used at 3 to 7 days before menstruation to treating dysmenorrhea. Additionally, midnight-noon ebb-low acupuncture and eight methods of sacred tortoise are specific application of treatment timing selection.

Yang Zhonghua, Zhang Liang, Tang Lilong, Tu Wenzhan, Qu Shanshan

Chapter 12

Other Therapies

The other therapies of TCM are plentiful, which include traditional Chinese tuina, dietary therapy, qigong, Tai Chi, etc. They use different ways to treat and prevent diseases according to different theories and methods. Some therapies such as tuita, dietary therapy, have a full theory to guide the practice. Nowadays, the qigong and Tai Chi are usually taken as physical exercises to prevent diseases. Due to the non-invasive, non-pharmaceutical features, now the other therapies of TCM are getting more and more attention in the world.

12.1 Traditional Chinese tuina

12.1.1 General introduction to tuina

Tuina is based on TCM theory, using body parts to perform manipulations on human in order to take precaution of disease and alleviate pain from illness. The earliest record of tuina dates back to 3 000 years ago and the long history has enriched its connotation which makes it one of the most important medical therapies in TCM. In modern TCM, massage is generally classified into adult tuina and infantile tuina. Adult tuina also includes a unique classification namely Spinal manipulation. With its characteristic theory and special manipulations, tuina is used to treat many kinds of illness in a natural and mostly harmless way. Moreover, basic exercises for tuina practice(tuina gongmethod) is an essential part of tuina practicing which requires long-time hard training for students of tuina and will certainly determine the curative effect. Due to the wide spreading of TCM, tuina is now studied by more and more people all around the world.

12.1.1.1 History of tuina

Tuina was created by ancient Chinese during labor activity and struggles with cruel nature. Human inevitably got injured when fighting with beasts or defending themselves in ancient times. The Chinese ancestors instinctively pressed the injured part of their body and by accident found it relieving pain. After years and years of practice, they summed up the primitive experiences and developed it into a mature medical mode nowadays we called tuina.

Traditional Chinese tuina has a very long history. The earliest reference to massage dates back to the culture of Yin Ruin(about 3 000 years ago) according to the archaeological studies in recent years. Tuina was early recorded in the inscriptions on bones or tortoise shells of the Shang Dynasty. This reveals the fact that tuina had been widely used to treat illness since this period of time.

(1)Qin and Han dynasties

The dynasties of Qin and Han are considered to be an important stage in the history of tuina. According to *Han shu*(History of the Han Dynasty), there was a monograph about massage——*Huangdi Qibo Anmo Shijuan*(*Ten Volumes on Massage Therapies* by *Yellow Emperor* and Qibo)that was the first medical book, not only in Chinese history but also in the history of the world, specially discussed tuina therapy. Unfortunately, this book was lost due to various reasons. *Internal Classic* is the earliest existing medical book of TCM. It was published in the same period with the former book and contained a great amount of ancient literature about tuina. *Internal Classic* pointed out that tuina was originated in the central area of ancient China and the book clearly put forward the positive effects of treating illness with tuina. It also covers a dozen of tuina manipulations such as pushing, pressing, rubbing, nailing, flicking, stretching, searching, stroking, shaking, bending, stepping and pulling. Because the manipulation of pressing(An)and rubbing(Mo)were used together at that time, so tuina was once called Anmo. In Han Dynasty, an extraordinary doctor named Zhang Zhongjing wrote a book——*Synopsis of Prescriptions of the Golden Chamber*. In his work, ointment rubbing manipulation was adopted and suggested as a way for disease prevention for the first time. Also, in his great piece of work he recorded a tuina method used for saving people in danger after trying to commit a suicide by hanging. Another famous doctor named Hua Tuo created a conduction exercise imitating five kinds of animals called five mimic-animal exercise, which is still practiced by people today to improve health. Therefore, *Qin* and *Han* dynasties are the first peak in the development process of massage.

(2)Sui and Tang dynasties

The Sui and Tang dynasties were a flourishing period in massage history. In tuina dynasty, the Imperial Hospital set up a position for specialists of Anmo(At this time massage it was called Anmo). Later, the Emperor Taizong of Tang developed the Imperial Hospital and set up the Anmo department, dividing Anmo manipulators into four levels from high to low, namely Anmo doctor, Anmo technician, Anmo worker and Anmo student. The Anmo doctor will teach Anmo student to practice Anmo with the assistance of Anmo technician and Anmo worker. In addition, self-tuina(one performing tuina to himself/herself)was highly advocated and put into an important position of people's daily life. Self-tuina was both recorded in *Ge Hong's Handbook of Prescriptions for Emergencies* and *Sun simiao's Essential Prescriptions Worth a Thousand Gold for Emergencies*. The widespread use of self-tuina reveals that patients are more self-helping in fighting with illness. Also, the ointments used in rubbing manipulation were improved by Sun Simiao and its application was enlarged, for example, using it to prevent or treat infantile diseases. It was also in this period of time that tuina was introduced to Korea, Japan, India, Arabian and European countries for the first time.

(3)Song Jin and Yuan dynasties

In Song Jin and Yuan Dynasties, tuina was mostly used in orthopedics and infantiles which contributed to the classification between the Spinal manipulation in adult tuina and infantile tuina. With the development of massage in this time, study of manipulation became more valued by the erudite for tuina. The work *Shengji Zonglu*(*General Records of Holy Universal Relief*)devoted a special chapter and gave the summary and induction about tuina. The book turns out to be the earliest and most complete special record of tuina. However, tuina department was canceled in medical organizations of government in this time. But the position of erudite for tuina still exists.

(4)Ming and Qing dynasties

Ming and Qing dynasties were another flourishing period in tuina history. In this time, the number of monographs about infantile tuina sharply increased. In 1601, the first special monograph about infantile tuina was born——*The Canon of Anmo for Children*. Then several monographs were gradually published and until this time infantile tuina formally became an independent system. In addition, tuina department was back in the Imperial Hospital in Ming Dynasty but canceled again later. Although there was no department of tuina in Qing's Imperial Hospital, tuina was still commonly and widely used in official occasion and among the civilians due to its remarkable curative effects. It was in this period of time that the name tuina was first introduced and later replaced Anmo for the name of this subject.

(5) Modern times

Traditional Chinese tuina has come into a brand new stage for integrated development with its golden opportunity, especially since the founding of the People's Republic of China. Firstly, more and more ancient literatures about tuina were unearthed and had been carefully studied and published. Secondly, main schools of tuina began to form and got the chance to be propagated. There are several present main schools of tuina with great influence, namely qi-concentrated single-finger pushing manipulation tuina, *Ding's* rolling manipulation tuina, internal exercise tuina etc. Thirdly, education system and scientific studies about tuina have developed significantly; also there continually occurs spirited innovations which keep enriching the content of this both ancient and dynamic subject.

12.1.1.2　Theory of traditional chinese tuina

Traditional Chinese tuina theory is based on TCM theories. Several important TCM theories that are highly related to tuina will be introduced below.

(1) Defense qi and nourish blood(wei qi ying xue) theory

TCM thinks human's physiological activity is greatly based on qi and blood. Qi and blood are needed to nourish from zang-fu viscera, bones and muscle, collaterals, meridians to fur and skin. So it is very important for tuina to take qi and blood into account when treating diseases. The conception of qi refers to two aspects: one is the refined nutritive substance that builds up human body and maintains human living activities. Another one is the physiological function or power of zang-fu viscera. The most essential qi in human body is the original qi, and its existence relies on innate essence and acquired essence. The function of original qi is to regulate qi movement. There are other two important kinds of qi. One is defense qi and the other is nutrient qi. Defense qi moves outside vessels, protecting human body from pathogenic qi of six climatic influences. Nutrient qi moves inside vessels, nourishing human body. Nutrient qi can also generate blood and flow with blood, so it is also known as nutrient blood. Blood flows in vessels and carries nutrient substance to all parts of human body. Qi and blood are tightly connected. Qi is able to generate blood, impel blood and control blood while blood is the foundation of qi. Blood carries qi all the way through the vessels and blood also nourishes qi. Because of the high-activity of qi, qi must rely on blood to stay regular. Diseases can be divided into four levels(wei, qi, ying and xue) according to the level of illness from mildness to seriousness. Tuina therapy uses this theory to instruct different treatments or manipulations for different level of illness.

(2) Meridian and collateral theory

As we know from the previous chapter that specially discusses meridian and collateral, there are fourteen meridians and lots of branches distributing in human body carrying qi and blood. Meridian and collateral also connect the zang-fu viscera and body extremities to communicate internal parts and external parts of the body. As the ancient literature says about meridian and collateral "No blockage, no pain", only if we keep the meridian and collateral unblocked are we able to do with the pain of our body. Once blockages are in meridian and collateral, qi and blood stop flowing regularly, which leads to the loss of nutrients and weakness of skin, muscles, tendons, vessels and joints. The effect of tuina is to propel the circulation of qi and blood, adjust yin and yang, and nourish tendons and joints. All these effects happen through the meridian and collateral by performing manipulations on the meridian and collateral or on the projected superficial portion of the body corresponding to a certain zang-fu viscera inside. Moreover, tuina manipulations will cause stimulation on an acupoint or even the whole meridian and collateral system which improve physiological functions of viscera, tissues and organs throughout the passing meridian and collateral.

(3) Tendons along twelve meridians

Tendons along twelve meridians are subsidiary part of the twelve meridians. It is the gathering and distributing of qi from twelve meridians to limbs and body. The function of the tendons along twelve meridians is connecting limbs and body, restraining bones, managing joint movements and maintaining natural body position. Tendons along twelve meridians are huge balanced biological structure of soft tissue. The word 'jin' in Chinese means strong fibrous tissue that contains and generates power and force for body movement. Different from the twelve meridians, the twelve musculature start at the tendons along the bladder meridian of foot taiyang. In other words, the twelve musculature start at limbs, gather in joints, distribute in chest and back, finally connect all parts of body. Therefore, tendons along twelve meridians generally run centripetally. Pathological changes of the tendons along twelve meridians system usually appear as spasm, stiffness and convulsion. Tuina can prevent and treat this kind of diseases by acting on the tendons along twelve meridians system.

(4) Muscle and bones theory

A series of diseases will happen due to certain abnormal changes of anatomical position with soft tissues(mostly muscle) and bones. Tuina manipulation is used to correct these abnormal changes and deal with dislocation of joints as well as soft tissues. In TCM, the famous saying "Tendons are out of line, bones are out of place" describes the pathogenesis of this kind of diseases. When a part of soft tissues of our body like muscle or tendon is in injury, a pain will be felt and then act on related body part through reflexion of nerves to alarm us that there is an injury. This kind of injuries can happen due to some anatomical changes such as dislocation and subluxation. However, the pain is a protective action for human body which is to reduce body movements and avoid a second injury. In tuina theory we adopt traction and counter-traction, rotating and pulling or flicking-poking manipulation to repair joint dislocation and joint subluxation, return the sprained soft tissue to normal position and put slipped tendons in order. The effect of this kind of manipulations is instant and remarkable. It can eliminate spasm of muscle, alleviate pain and promote the recovery of the injured soft tissues or joints. Furthermore, diseases that are commonly seen on patients in tuina department such as cervical spondylosis, periarthritis of shoulder and lumbar disc herniation can be well treated with tuina manipulation.

(5) Pediatrics of TCM

In pediatrics of TCM, there are special diagnostics and treatment for children. For example, younger children can easily caught by exogenous contraction and have problem in digesting milk. In TCM, children are considered to be immature in yin yang and zang-fu viscera. Generally, for children heart and liver viscera are in excess while lung, spleen and kidney viscera are in deficiency. This characteristic leads to a high occurrence of lung diseases caused by wind pathogen. Children can also be easily harmed by dryness pathogen and summerheat pathogen which result in lung and stomach yin deficiency. Moreover, children's diseases are likely to become heat diseases due to their constitution of pure yang. Pestilent qi is another common factor that always threatens children's health. It is a kind of strongly infectious pathogenic factor bringing serious and fast-developing syndromes.

There are several things we should pay attention to when treating pediatric diseases with tuina therapy.

First of all, the timing to start treatment should be as early as possible. Because of the pure yin and yang constitution, diseases develop rapidly in pediatrics. The earlier treatment begins, the less possibly illness is going to develop. Therefore, accurate and on time treatment is the guarantee of effect. Secondly, principles of pediatric tuina are gentle, mild and moderate. We should be cautious when choosing treatment in order to protect the young and weak healthy qi of child. Moreover, we should attach importance to taking care of spleen-stomach zang-fu viscera(always in deficiency)while the avoid abuse of treating deficiency with reinforcement. Last but not the least, always remember to treat the earlier coming syndromes first, and then the latter coming ones. Especially when treating exogenous contractions, controlling the former syndrome is important for ceasing the development of illness.

12.1.1.3　Categories

Before we begin, we should understand that there are differences between tuina in traditional Chinese medicine and the commonly seen tuina. Firstly, tuina is instructed by traditional Chinese medicine theory which includes yin-yang theory, meridian and collateral theory, zang-fu viscera theory, five elements theory and so on. General tuina does not have a basic theory instruction. Secondly, the slaying of tuina in western country refers to manipulations with no joint movement and adjustment. A number of manipulations in tuina need to have joint movement and aim at adjusting irregular joint location. Thirdly, tuina is a non-medical behavior for relaxation and leisure. On the opposite, performing tuina is a medical behavior that happens in medical setting like hospital and clinics. Tuina therapy is used to treat certain diseases which have clear and accurate diagnosis. For practitioner, tuina practitioner must have the license of doctor. Tuina is often practiced by people with no practitioner's license. In a word, there are differences between tuina in traditional Chinese medicine and the commonly seen tuina. In ancient times, tuina was not classified into adult tuina and infantile tuina. In modern times, scholars put forward the conception of adult tuina in order to make it different from the well-developed infantile tuina. After a history of more than 3 000 years, tuina is now generally divided into adult tuina, infantile tuina and a special kind named spinal manipulation.

12.1.1.4　Tuina manipulation

Manipulation is an important way to treat disease in traditional tuina. It refers to the standard techniques performed with performer's hand or other part of the body to exert a stimulating effect on the body part to the patient for medical purpose. The promising quality of manipulation with correct clinical differentiation is the key to a good therapeutic effect. The performers are required to perform a manipulation continuously, forcefully, evenly, softly and thoroughly. "Continuously" means performer should keep the manipulation for a certain period of time according to the requirement. "Forcefully" means performers should have a certain force and be able to adapt different patients and different situations. "Evenly" means the force and frequency of the manipulation should be the same during the whole time. "Softly" means the force of manipulation should be well controlled and be gentle but not superficial, and heavy but not retained. The change of movements should be natural and fluent. "Thoroughly" means the manipulation should reach deep down to the affected part of the patient's body on the basis of achieving the four previous key points.

Students can practice tuina manipulations on sand bag or rice bag first, and then on human body. The sand bag or rice bag is squared and about 8 cun(about 3.3 cm)in length and 5 cun in width. The training and practice of fingers, wrist and arms are the key point of practicing tuina manipulations.

Tuina manipulations can be classified by movements into pushing manipulation, pressing manipulation and pulling manipulation, classified by targeted body parts into soft issue manipulation and joint manipulation, classified by schools which we've introduced in the previous paragraph, classified by difficulties and divided into simple manipulation and complex manipulation. In this book, we adopt the first classification to introduce tuina manipulation.

12.1.2　Adult tuina

Adult tuina is used to take precaution of adult diseases as well as treating diseases. Compared with infantile tuina, manipulation in adult tuina has a greater range with heavier strength. Adult tuina manipulation is generally divided into categories of pushing rolling manipulations, scrubbing manipulations, squeezing-pressing manipulations, tapping manipulations, vibrating manipulations, and mobilizing manipulations.

12.1.2.1　Basic exercises for tuina practice

The basic exercises for tuina practice are a series of training designed for erudite for tuina. It is also called tuina gong fa. Gong means function and ability, fa means method of specialized training. Therefore, basic exercises for manipulation practice refer to a process for tuina practitioner to improve their body and adapt the ability of practicing tuina through long-term repeated and diligent practice and training of specific exercises. Traditional tuina attaches great importance to basic exercises and consider it as the guarantee of clinical curative effect. There is also a saying of "the more effort, the more effect" which indicates the great connection between basic exercises and curative effect. To be an erudite for tuina, a basic exercise of the specific training is not only a kind of medical technology that needs to master but also a compulsory training for his professional technique.

Generally, basic exercises for tuina practice include Taijiquan, Shaolin internal cultivation exercise and Sinew-transforming exercises. The functions of basic exercises for tuina practice are as follows: first, enhance the health status of practitioner and fully develop strength, endurance, sensibility and flexibility which give the practitioner the ability in persistent, continuous manipulation of tuina. Second, the structure and function of manipulating part of human body will be improved through basic exercises practice. Third, concentrate on practicing basic exercises can improve the coordination of organisms used in tuina manipulation. Last, practicing basic exercise can cultivate the beneficial qi which makes erudite for tuina stay healthy and have a high efficiency of work. It is the guarantee of manipulation quality and curative effort. Furthermore, practicing basic exercises of tuina can strengthen muscles, bones, ligaments and joint, promote blood circulation, and improve respiratory system, nerve system and digestion system according to recent research.

Some basic exercises for tuina practice are not only for erudite for tuina but also practiced by patients. Patients can practice basic exercises under the instruction of erudite for tuina to improve their health status and accelerate the recovery.

12.1.2.2　Adult tuina manipulations

Adult tuina manipulations mainly include 6 categories: pushing rolling manipulations, scrubbing manipulations, squeezing-pressing manipulations, tapping manipulations, vibrating manipulations and mobilizing manipulations. The five key points of performing adult tuina manipulations especially on soft tissue are "continuously, forcefully, evenly, softly and thoroughly".

(1) Category of pushing rolling manipulations

Continuously and regularly swaying the forearm to exert force on part of body is the basic operation for category of pushing rolling manipulations, including qi-concentrated single-finger pushing manipulation, and rolling manipulation with the ulnar side of the palm and kneading manipulation.

1) Qi-concentrated single-finger pushing manipulation

Pushing with the tip of the thumb or the whorled surface of the thumb on the region to be treated by swaying your forearm to lead your finger is called qi-concentrated single-finger pushing manipulation. It is the typical manipulation of the qi-concentrated single-finger pushing manipulation school.

● Direction for performing manipulations: Clench a hollow fist with suspended and flexed wrist and palm, then stretch the thumb straight naturally to cover your fist hole. Push the targeted region with the tip or the whorl surface of the thumb. Lower the shoulder, drop the elbow and suspend the wrist. Sway the forearm to lead the wrist swing inward and outward while flexing and extending the thumb joint to reach a frequency of 120–160 times per minute. The thumb should go heavily and come lightly continuously and alternately (Figure 12–1).

The key point of performing this manipulation are lowering shoulders, dropping elbow, suspending wrist, exerting force to thumb, emptying palm and pushing forcefully and moving slowly.

● Medical application: The characteristics of this manipulation are that the targeted region is small but the applied force is great and thorough, and the stimulation is regular and mild. This manipulation is commonly used on all the meridians and collaterals and acupoints all over the body. In departments of internal medicine, gynecology, traumatology, five sense organs, and pediatrics, it is used to treat common diseases such as headache, dizziness, insomnia, hypertension, stagnation of the liver qi, arthralgia-syndrome and especially diseases of gastrointestinal alimentary system.

2) Rolling manipulation with the ulnar side of the palm

Rolling manipulation with the ulnar side of the palm refers to using the ulnar side of the palm to press the affected region. Sway the forearm to drive the wrist to extend and flex, and roll on the target region. It is the typical manipulation of the rolling manipulation school (Ding's rolling manipulation).

● Direction for performing manipulations: The performer straightens the thumb naturally and makes a hollow fist. The little finger and the ring finger flex naturally and the flexed angle of the other two fingers reduces gradually to make the palm round along the palm surface. Press the target region with the dorsal palm of the hand near the lateral side of the little finger. Sway the forearm to extend and flex the wrist in a wide range and rotate the forearm as well. Roll the ulnar side of the hand of the target region continuously in a frequency about 120 times per minute (Figure 12–2).

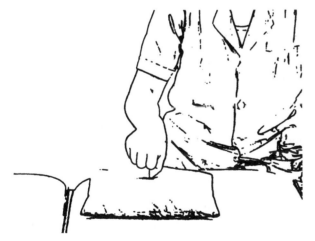

Figure 12 – 1   Qi-concentrated single-finger pushing manipulation

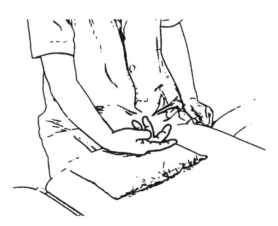

Figure 12–2   Rolling manipulation

The key points of performing this manipulation are lowering shoulders and dropping elbow with the wrist joint flexed naturally. Keep a hollow fist. Fix on the target region with the dorsal part of your palm near the little finger. The stimulation should be done lightly and heavily alternately. Roll forward three times heavier than rolling back.

● Medical application: Rolling manipulation has a large area of stimulation with strong effect, evident deepness and thoroughness. It is one of the most commonly-used manipulations in clinical work, especially suitable for the lunbodorsal region, lunbo-buttock region and thick muscle regions of the limbs. It is good for treating the diseases in motor system and nerve system.

3) Kneading manipulation

Fixing on targeted body surface with certain part of your hand and kneading in circles to rotate slowly and softly the subcutaneous tissues is called kneading manipulation. According to different touching areas, it can be divided into palm-base kneading manipulation, major thenar kneading manipulation, finger kneading manipulation and forearm kneading manipulation.

● Direction for performing manipulations: The key points of kneading manipulation are quite similar. The key points are lowering your shoulders. Fix on the targeted body surface with certain part of your hand. Bring the subcutaneous tissue to move when performing this manipulation. Avoid rubbing or slipping between the treated part and the body surface. The wrist is relaxed in major thenar kneading manipulation but should keep tight in palm-base kneading manipulation and finger kneading manipulation.

● Medical application: The effect of kneading manipulation is light, soft and slow but deep and thorough. Warm effect can be delivered to the deep of tissue by the internal rubbing caused by kneading. Major thenar kneading manipulation is suitable for swelling or aching parts of the limbs caused by acute sprain and contusion. Palm-base kneading manipulation is commonly used on the well-developed muscular regions of the limbs, lumbodorsal region and buttock region. Finger kneading manipulation is used for pointing acupoints or meridians and collateral all over the body. Forearm kneading manipulation is good at treating deep tissue problem.

(2) Category of scrubbing manipulations

Use the tip of finger or palm to touch the targeted region and precede rhythmic and circular movements. This is called scrubbing manipulations.

1) Circular rubbing manipulations

Using the palm or the finger to make a circular rubbing movement on surface of human body is called circular rubbing manipulations. It is mainly divided into finger circular rubbing manipulation(zhi mo method) and palm circular rubbing manipulation(zhang mo method).

● Direction for performing manipulations: Finger circular rubbing manipulation: use your finger tip as the touching area with the fingers juxtaposed. The palm straightened naturally and the wrist joint flexed slightly. Use the elbow joint as a pivot, and move the forearm to rub with the palm side of the fingers circularly on the target region. It can be clockwise or counter-clockwise with a frequency of 100 to 120 times per minute.

Palm circular rubbing manipulation: press on the body surface with the fingers juxtaposed. Straighten your palm naturally and the wrist joint slightly tight. Consider the elbow as a pivot, move the forearm to rub circularly with the palm on the target region. It can be clockwise or counter-clockwise with a frequency of 100 to 120 times per minute.

● Medical application: Rubbing manipulation is mainly applied to treating problems on the chest, hypochondrium and the epigastric region. It has an effect of relieving the depressed liver and regulating the circulation of qi, warming the middle energizer and regulating the stomach. It is also good at treating diseases in digest system.

2) Pushing manipulation

Using the touching part to make a one-way pushing in a straight line is called pushing manipulation. It can be divided into linear-pushing with the finger, linear-pushing with the palm and linear-pushing with the elbow. We take linear-pushing with the palm as an example to introduce. The following direction is for linear-pushing with the palm. Linear-pushing with the palm is the most commonly used pushing manipulation in clinical work.

● Direction for performing manipulations: Use the palm or palm-base as the touching part. Stretch the elbow to make a linear pushing. Use both palms to perform in the same time can also be called separating pushing manipulation.

● Medical application: This manipulation can exert both "warmth and force". Therefore, it has a good effect on warming and dredging the meridians and collaterals, promoting blood circulation and qi, warming the yang, etc. It is suitable for thoracodorsal region and lumbo-abdominal region. It is commonly used to treat oppressed feeling in the chest, diseases in the upper energizer; diseases in digest system for example throw up, nausea and stomachache, depression of the liver qi, lumbago, deficiency of the kidney etc.

3) Scrubbing manipulation

Exert force on the target region with the major thenar to perform straight to-and-fro rubbing movement. Make the warm effect penetrate into the deep layer of tissue. This is called scrubbing manipulation. It can be divided into to-and-fro rubbing manipulation with palm, to-and-fro rubbing manipulation with finger, to-and-fro rubbing manipulation with minor thenar and to-and-fro rubbing manipulation with major thenar.

● Direction for performing manipulations: Keep your wrist in tense. Put the touching part on the body surface and make a little pressing. Use shoulder joint and elbow joint to combine a bend and stretch movement. Make the touching part move evenly to-and-fro in a straight line(Figure 12-3).

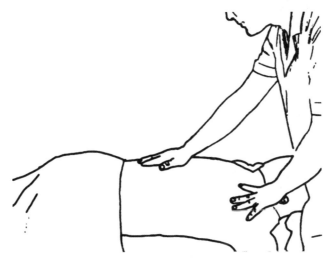

Figure 12-3   Scrubbing manipulation with the palm

● Medical application: This manipulation has a strong rubbing force with a large range of movement. So it has evident warming effect and the function of removing obstruction. It is suitable for all parts of the body. It can warm the body and dispel dampness pathogen. It is good at treating cold manifestation syndrome. Be careful not to rub for a long time in case the surface skin will be injured.

(3) Category of squeezing-pressing manipulations

Using finger, palm or other parts of body to press vertically or squeezing oppositely is called squeezing-pressing manipulations. It can be divided into vertical press and opposite squeeze. Pressing manipulation and grasping manipulation are two typical manipulations for this category.

1) Pressing manipulation

Press a certain acupoint or part of the body surface with finger, palm or elbow. Then exert force gradually is called pressing manipulation.

• Direction for performing manipulations: Vertically press the target region with the touching part, press gradually from lightly to heavily. When using pressing with palm, you should lean your body to strengthen the force on your palm. Performing this manipulation should make patients cooperate with breath like press with exhale and leave with inhale(Figure 12-4).

• Medical application: This manipulation has small and concentrated acting area, and the acting layer is deep with evident stabbing pain effect, and it is applied to indurate tissue of muscles or between bones or tenderness points. It is good for relieving pains.

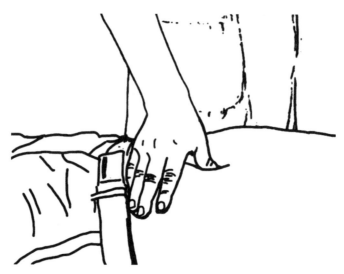

Figure 12-4　Pressing manipulation with the thumb

2) Grasping manipulation

Exert force symmetrically with the thumb and the other four fingers to lift, pinch or clip the extremities or the skin. Such a manipulation is called grasping manipulation. It can be divided into three fingers grasping manipulation and five fingers grasping manipulation.

• Direction for performing manipulations: Relax the wrist joint and clip the operated part tightly with the thumb, index finger and middle finger or with the thumb and the whorl surface of the other four fingers. Lift the skin and repeat the performance of kneading and pinching continuously and alternatively in a form of forceful and gentle way.

• Medical application: This manipulation is deep and heavy but has a mild stimulation. It is commonly suitable for the cord soft tissues such as the muscles and tendons of the neck, shoulder, back, lateral abdomen, upper and lower limbs, etc. It is good at inducing resuscitation and restoring consciousness, expelling pathogenic wind and cold, relaxing muscles and tendons to promote blood circulation, relieving spasm and pain, etc.

(4) Category of tapping manipulations

Using hand or tools to tap the body face in a rhythm is called tapping manipulations. It mainly includes patting manipulation and knocking manipulation. The most commonly used tool in this manipulation is mulberry stick.

1) Patting manipulation(pai method)

Patting on the body surface rhythmically with an empty palm is called patting manipulation.

● Direction for performing manipulations:Coalesce the fingers and slightly flex the metacarpohalangeal joint so as to form an empty palm. Then pat the operated part rhythmically in a frequency of 100 to 120 times per minutes.

● Medical application:This manipulation is mainly used on the shoulder and back,lumbosacral portion and the thigh. Light patting can also be used on thoracic-abdominal region and the head. It is used to treat various kinds of diseases such as arthralgia due to pathogenic wind-dampness,stiffness and pain in the chest and dizziness,etc.

2) Knocking manipulation

Hit the operated part rhythmically with the palm base,the minor thenar,the back of a fist,the finger tip or a mulberry stick. This is called knocking manipulation.

● Direction for performing manipulations:Steadily use finger,palm or mulberry stick to knock on the targeted region. When using hand to perform,relax your wrist and keep a hollow fist or slightly bent fingers. Before performing,the patient should be noticed previously.

● Medical application:Fist-back-knocking manipulation is mainly used on Dazhu(GV 14) and the lumbosacral portion. Palm-knocking manipulation is for the Baihui(GV 20). It is good at activating the flow of blood and qi in the meridians and collateral.

(5)Category of vibrating manipulations

Continuously stimulating the targeted region with a rhythmic high frequency is called vibrating manipulations. It generally includes shaking manipulation and vibrating manipulation.

1) Shaking manipulation

Hold the distal end of the patient's target extremities with one hand or both hands to shake constantly up and down or from the left to the right. This is called shaking manipulation.

● Direction for performing manipulations:Hold the distal end of the patient's targeted extremities. Lift the treated extremity to a certain angle. While pulling with slight force shake constantly in small amplitude to cause the parenchyma of the target region to shake and transmit to the proximal end of the extremity.

● Medical application:This manipulation is mainly applied to extremities and mostly after twisting manipulation with both palms as a combination and reinforcement. It is commonly used in the lumbar area to treat lumbar intervertebral disc protrusion with shaking both two lower limbs simultaneously. It can enlarge the space inside the lumbar vertebrae to help reduce projecting nucleus pulpous,relax adhesion between the projection and nerve roots to remit or release its pressure upon nerve roots. It has a great effect on relieving pain for lumbar intervertebral disc protrusion.

2) Vibrating manipulation

Using finger or palm to make a vertical rapid vibrating movement is called vibrating manipulation. It generally includes vibrating with the palm and vibrating with the finger.

● Direction for performing manipulations:Drop the elbow and put the tip of the middle finger or the palm on the targeted region. Exert force statically with the forearm and hand,and contract the muscle alternatively to direct the vibration produced by arm to the body in a frequency of 300 to 400 times per minute (Figure 12-5).

● Medical application:This manipulation is suitable for all the acupoints on the body,especially to the craniofacial region and the thoracic-abdominal region. It is good far relaxing anxious feeling.

（6）Category of mobilizing manipulations

Make the joint passively move and generate sliding, separation, twisting, bending and stretching. Such manipulation is called mobilizing manipulations. It generally includes rotating manipulation and pulling-stretching manipulation

1）Rotating manipulation

A passive movement performed within the range of joint or semi-joint is called rotating manipulation. It is one of the common manipulations of tuina and performed with different methods when applied to different parts. It generally includes rotating of the neck, rotating of the shoulder, rotating of the elbow, rotating of the wrist, rotating of the lumbar, rotating of the hip, rotating of the knee and rotating of the ankle.

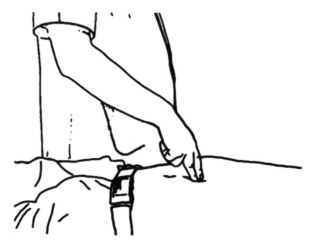

Figure 12-5　Vibrating manipulation with finger

● Direction for performing manipulations: There are many kinds of rotating manipulation based on different parts, but there are still something in common. Movements of rotating manipulation should be moderate and mild with steady force. The frequency of the rotation should be slow and even, especially at the beginning. The amplitude of the rotation should be gradually increased and adjusted according to individual conditions. Generally, the joint should be kept within the limitation of normal physical movement. Rotating manipulation should not be done violently or violate the movement of normal physical activity. Rotating manipulation is forbidden to be used to treat patients with fracture or dislocation of joint.

● Medical application: This manipulation is suitable for joints all over the body. It has the effect of lubricating joints, releasing adhesion, relaxing muscles and tendons, relieving spasm, strengthening and renewing articular moving ability.

2）Pulling-stretching manipulation

Fix one end of a joint or an extremity, pull and extend the other end with constant force to enlarge the joint space. Such a manipulation is called pulling-stretching manipulation. It can be applied to different joints in many regions such as neck, shoulder, elbow, wrist, fingers, waist, hip, knee and ankle.

● Direction for performing manipulation: According to different regions, the patient should take different positions to adjust. This manipulation should make it stable and gentle with the strength intensified gradually. When the traction reaches a certain degree, it should be kept steady for a while. The angle of the traction should be well adjusted and the pulling should be done around the longitudinal axis of the extremity.

● Medical application: This manipulation can be applied to joints of cervical vertebrae, lumbar vertebrae and extremities, with the effect of restoring and treating injured soft tissues, reducing dislocation of joints, enlarging joint spaces, remitting nerve compression, and relaxing adhesion.

(7)Comprehensive manipulations & special manipulations

Comprehensive manipulations are a series of manipulations composed by more than one of the six basic manipulations. Special manipulations are a series of manipulations that cannot be classified into the six basic manipulations but used commonly in clinical work.

1)Grasping-kneading manipulation

Grasping-kneading manipulation is a combination with grasping manipulation and kneading manipulation.

● Direction for performing manipulations：The methods for performing this manipulation are similar to performing grasping manipulation. Grasping-kneading manipulation uses grasp as main manipulation and knead as assistance. Also, the thumb and other fingers need to knead in rotation.

● Medical application：This manipulation has advantages in both grasping manipulation and kneading manipulation. It is mainly applied to extremities and neck region. It is generally used to treat neck pain, cervical spondylosis and periarthritis of shoulder, etc.

2)Thumb-pushing and circular-rubbing manipulation(tui mo method)

The thumb performing qi-concentrated single-finger pushing manipulation while the other four fingers performing finger-rubbing manipulation are called thumb-pushing and circular-rubbing manipulation. It is often applied on the chest, abdomen and back.

● Direction for performing manipulations：Exert force with the side of the thumb；swing the forearm to perform qi-concentrated single-finger pushing manipulation. At the same time, the other four fingers straighten and coalesce to perform rubbing manipulation.

● Medical application：This manipulation is mainly used in chest, abdomen, lumbosacral region and shoulder. It is good for treating distension and pain in abdomen, digestive system problem, genital system problem and periarthritis of shoulder, etc.

3)Sweeping manipulation(sao san method)

Using the radial side of the thumb and other finger tips quickly sweeping from the head of temporal to the back of ear forward and backward is called sweeping manipulation.

● Direction for performing manipulations：The doctor gently supports the patient's head with one hand and touches the patient's temporal region with the radial side of the thumb and the tips of the other fingers of the other hand, then moves the hand along an arc route from the temporal region to the occipital region (along the running route of the gallbladder meridian)from the anterior-superior to the posterior-inferior.

● Medical application：Sweeping manipulation is performed with even force, mainly used for operation on the head. It has the effect of calming the liver to suppress hyperhepatic yang, dispelling wind and dispelling pathogenic cold, tranquilizing and inducing resuscitation, relaxing tendons and relieving pain. Headache, vertigo, hypertension, insomnia, poor memories are often treated with this technique.

4)Pinching of the two sides of spine

Continuously pinching the skin of spine from top to bottom is called the pinching of the two sides of spine. It is a special manipulation first used in adult but lately mainly used in infantiles.

● Direction for performing manipulations：The operator may first push the skin with the tip of thumb, and then use the index finger or other finger to pinch up the skin. Then grasp and lift the skin up with the three fingers simultaneously. Do the lifting and pinching operation with both hands alternately and move forward. Or use the radial aspect of the middle knuckle of the flexed index finger to support the skin, the thumb to press forward. Then grasp and lift the skin forcefully with the two fingers and move forward while both hands are alternately doing the manipulation.

● Medical application: The technique has the effect of promoting digestion to eliminate stagnation, strengthening the spleen-stomach, regulating the spleen-stomach to dissipate dampness, relaxing tendon and removing obstruction and promote qi circulation to activate blood. Epigastria distension and fullness, indigestion, anorexia and chronic diarrhea can be treated with the manipulation.

12.1.2.3 Cautions

Tuina is a safe, effective and generally side-effect free therapy. However, there may have some accidents like dizziness, pain, bruise, and fracture when manipulations are used in a wrong way. In case these situations would happen, we should have emergency response plan and be careful when performing tuina.

Tuina manipulations have several contraindications. First, people should not be treated with tuina after sports or in a condition of tiredness or weakness. Second, people should not be treated with hunger or too fullness and within an hour after a meal. Third, abdomen and lumbosacral region of pregnant women should not be treated while other parts can be treated with light strength, but some acupoints that can possibly cause abortion must be avoided. Fourth, drunk people should not be treated with tuina. Finally, patients with fracture, spinal cord injury, body part with cancer, infectious disease and serious should be forbidden from tuina.

12.1.3   Infantile tuina

Infantile tuina is a series of tuina manipulation designed for infants through the long term practices. It comes from the summary of infantile characteristics, physiological characteristics, pathological characteristics and special acupoints. Also, it is well known for its great curative effect on infantile diseases. In infantile tuina, a number of acupoints are different from adult and some of them are special designed for infantile. In manipulation aspects, infantile tuina manipulation attaches great importance to softness, steadiness, smoothness, correctness and painlessness. Furthermore, many manipulations in infantile tuina require the external use of medical medium. There are eight general manipulations in infantile tuina, namely pressing, rubbing, pinching, circularly pushing, kneading, pushing, nipping and pounding. Although some of those manipulations have the same name as in adult tuina, their performing may be quite different.

12.1.3.1   Acuppoints of infantile tuina

Acupoints of infantile tuina have several characteristics: First, most of acupoints of infantile tuina are not located on the fourteen meridians but located in hand. It is called hundreds of channels and vessels of child gathering in the hand. Secondly, the form of acupoint of infantile tuina is classified into point form, line form and cover form. Thirdly, most of the infantile acupoints are combined with specific manipulation and tend to specific effect.

(1) Erhougaogu (prominent bone behind the ear)

Location: In the depression inferior to the mastoid process behind the eye and superior to the posterior hairline.

Manipulation: kneading the point with the tip of the thumbs or middle fingers. Repeat 30-50 times.

Indication: headache, dysphoria and common cold.

(2) Tianmen

Location: The line from the midpoint between the two eyebrows to the anterior hairline.

Manipulation: Push the point straight upward with the pads of both thumbs alternately, known as opening Tianmen. Repeat 30-50 times.

Indication: Headache, cold, vertigo, night cry and insomnia.

（3）Kangong

Location：The transverse line from the medial end to the lateral end of the eyebrow.

Manipulation：Push the points respectively from the medial ends of the eyebrow to the lateral ends with both thumbs.

Indication：Exogenous fever, redness and pain of eyes, convulsion and myopia.

（4）Tianzhu

Location：The line from the midpoint of the posterior hairline to Dazhui(GV14)

Manipulation：Pushing the point straight downward with the pads of the thumb or the index and middle fingers. Repeat 100-500 times.

Indication：Nausea, vomiting, cold, fever, sore-throat and stiff nape.

（5）Spleen meridian

Location：On the radial border of the thumb and from the tip to the root.

Manipulation：Flex the thumb of the child patient, and then push along the radial border of the thumb towards the wrist. This is called reinforcing spleen meridian. Pushing the opposite direction is called clearing spleen meridian. Repeat 100-500 times.

Indication：Diarrhea, constipation, abdominal distension, dysentery, anorexia and jaundice due to damp heat.

（6）Stomach meridian

Location：At the junction of red and white skin of the greater thenar.

Manipulation：Pushing from the root to the palmar root is considered as a reinforcing method, called reinforcing stomach meridian. Pushing the opposite direction is called clearing stomach meridian. Repeat 100-500 times.

Indication：Nausea, vomiting, belching, no appetite, abdominal distension, halitosis and constipation.

（7）Liver meridian

Location：The whorl surface of the distal interphalangeal joint of the index finger.

Manipulation：Pushing from finger tip to the root is considered as a reinforcing manipulation, called reinforcing liver meridian. Pushing the opposite direction is called clearing liver meridian. Repeat 100-500 times.

Indication：Conjunctive congestion, bitter taste in the mouth, dry throat, convulsion, restlessness and feverish sensation over five centers.

（8）Heart meridian

Location：The whorl surface of the distal interphalangeal joint of the middle finger.

Manipulation：Pushing from finger tip to the root is considered as a reinforcing manipulation, called reinforcing heart meridian. Pushing the opposite direction is called clearing heart meridian. Repeat 100-500 times.

Indication：Orolingual ulceration, short and hot urination, coma due to high fever and feverish sensation over the palms and soles.

（9）Lung meridian

Location：The whorl surface of the distal interphalangeal joint of the ring finger.

Manipulation：Pushing from finger tip to the root is considered as a reinforcing manipulation, called reinforcing lung meridian. Pushing the opposite direction is called clearing lung meridian. Repeat 100-500 times.

Indication：Cold, cough, panting, wheezy phlegm, spontaneous sweating, night sweat, pale face, prolapse of the rectum, enuresis and constipation.

(10) Kidney meridian

Location: The ungual whorl surface of the distal part of the small finger.

Manipulation: Pushing from finger tip to the tip is considered as a reinforcing manipulation, called reinforcing kidney meridian. Pushing the opposite direction is called clearing kidney meridian. Repeat 100 - 500 times.

Indication: Congenital defect, weakness due to lingering illness, diarrhea, enuresis, cough, panting, redness of the eyes and painful urination.

(11) Four transverse creases

Location: On the surface of palm, at the midpoint of the transverse creases of the first interphalangeal joints of the index, middle, ring and little fingers.

Manipulation: Pressing and kneading the point with the nail of the thumb is called nipping Sihengwen. Repeat 100-300 times.

Indication: Indigestion, abdominal distention, abdominal pain, disharmony of qi and blood, panting and fissure on the lip.

(12) Large intestine

Location: On the radial border of the index finger, from the finger tip to the margin between the index finger and the thumb.

Manipulation: Pushing from the finger tip to the wed margin is considered as a reinforcing method, known as reinforcing large intestine. Pushing to the opposite direction is considered as a clearing method, known as clearing large intestine. Repeat the manipulation 100-300 times.

Indication: Diarrhea, dysentery, constipation and abdominal pain.

(13) Small intestine

Location: On the ulnar side of the little finger and the line from the finger tip to the root.

Manipulation: Pushing form the finger tip to its root is considered as a reinforcing method known as reinforcing small intestine. Pushing to the opposite direction is considered as a clearing method, known as clearing small intestine. Repeat the manipulation 100-300 times.

Indication: Hot and difficult urination, watery diarrhea, boils in the mouth and tidal fever in the afternoon.

(14) Shending

Location: On the tip of the small finger.

Manipulation: Pressing and kneading the point with the tip of the thumb or index finger is called kneading Shending. Repeat the manipulation 100-500 times.

Indication: Spontaneous perspiration, night sweating and metopism in child.

(15) Small palmar transverse crease

Location: On the surface of palm, at the root of the little finger, on the ulnar end of transverse crease.

Manipulation: Pressing and kneading the point with the tip of the thumb or middle finger is called kneading small palmar transverse crease. Repeat the manipulation 100-500 times.

Indication: Orolingual ulcer, salivation, pneumonia, phlegm retention and panting.

(16) Small transverse crease

Location: On the surface of palm, the transverse crease of metacarpal interphalangeal joints of the index, middle, ring and little finger.

Manipulation: Nipping the crease with the nail of the thumb is called small intestine; pushing the crease with the side of the thumb is called pushing small transverse crease. Nipping the crease of each finger for five times or pushing 100－300 times.

　　Indication：lip ulcer, boils in the mouth, abdominal distention, fever and restlessness.

　　(17) Major thenar

　　Loction：On the surface of the greater thenar.

　　Manipulation：Kneading the point with the finger tip is called kneading major thenar. Pushing from finger root to the transverse crease of the wrist is called pushing manipulation from Banmen to Hengwen and the opposite direction is called pushing manipulation from Hengwen to Banmen. Repeat the kneading manipulation 30－50 times or pushing manipulation 100－300 times.

　　Indication：Anorexia, indigestion, vomiting, diarrhea, abdominal distension, panting and belching.

　　(18) Small center of sky

　　Location：In the depression of the junction between the major thenar and the minor thenar eminences.

　　Manipulation：Kneading the point with the tip of the middle finger is called kneading small center of sky.

　　Indication：Spasm, night crying, hot and difficult urination, conjunctival congestion with pain, orolingual ulcers and strabismus.

　　(19) Triple pass

　　Location：On the radial aspect of the forearm and the line between Yangchi (TE 4) and Quchi (LI 11).

　　Manipulation：Pushing from the transverse crease of the wrist to that of the elbow with the index finger pulp and middle finger pulp is called pushing Sanguan. Repeat the manipulation 100－300 times.

　　Indication：Abdominal pain, diarrhea, aversion to cold, lassitude of limb, weakness due to illness, wind cold and all other deficiency and cold syndrome.

　　(20) Tianheshui

　　Location：Along the mid-line of forearm from convergent tendon to Hongchi (middle of transverse cubital crease).

　　Manipulation：Pushing from the transverse crease of the wrist to that of the elbow is called clearing Tianheshui. Repeat the manipulation 100－300 times.

　　Indication：All heat symptoms, such as exogenous fever, tidal fever, internal heat, restlessness, thirst, orolingual ulcers, cough, wheezing phlegm and sore throat.

　　(21) Liufu

　　Location：On the ulnar aspect of the forearm and the line between the ulnar side of palmar transverse striation at wrist and the transverse crease of the elbow.

　　Manipulation：Pushing from the transverse crease of the elbow to that of the wrist with the tip of the thumb, or tips of the index and middle fingers is called pushing Liufu. Repeat 100－300 times.

　　Indication：High fever, polydipsia, convulsion, sore throat and constipation.

　　(22) Ershanmen

　　Location：On the dorsum of the hand and in the depression on both sides of the root of the middle finger.

　　Manipulation：Pinching the point with the nail of the thumb is called pinching Ershanmen. Repeat 5 times.

　　Indication：Cold, fever, adiaphoresis and asthmatic breathing.

(23) Shangma

Location: On the dorsum of the hand and in the depressions proximal to the metacarpophalangeal joint of the ring and little fingers.

Manipulation: Kneading the point with the tip of the thumb is called kneading Shangma. Nipping it with the nail of the thumb is called nipping Shangma. Repeat the nipping manipulation 3–5 times or kneading manipulation 100–300 times.

Indication: Hot and difficult urination, abdominal pain, enuresis, indigestion, asthma and toothache.

(24) Yiwofeng

Location: On the dorsum of the hand and on the midpoint of the transverse crease of the wrist.

Manipulation: Kneading the point with the tip of a finger is called kneading Yiwofeng. Repeat the manipulation 100–300 times.

Indication: Abdominal pain, borborygmus, wind cold, acute and chronic convulsion, and difficult joint movement.

(25) Rupang

Location: 0.2 cun lateral to the breast.

Manipulation: Kneading the point with the tip of the middle finger. Repeat the manipulation 20–50 times.

Indication: Chest oppression, wheezing, cough and vomiting.

(26) Dantian

Location: On the lower abdomen, 2 or 3 cun below the umbilicus.

Manipulation: Kneading or rubbing the point respectively is called kneading Dantian or rubbing Dantian. Knead Dantian 50–100 times or rub it for 5minutes.

Indication: Enuresis and abdominal pain.

(27) Dujiao

Location: 2 cun below the umbilicus and 2 cun lateral to Shimen(CV5).

Manipulation: Grasping with the thumb, index and middle finger is called grasping Dujiao and pressing with the tip of the middle finger is called pressing Dujiao. Repeat the manipulation 3–5 times.

Indication: Abdominal pain and diarrhea.

(28) Qijiegu

Location: On the spine, the part from the fourth lumbar vertebra to the end of the coccyx, or Changqiang(GV1).

Manipulation: Pushing the spine upward with the radial side of the thumb or the pads of the index and middle fingers is called pushing Qijiegu upward. Pushing in the opposite direction is called pushing Qijiegu downward. Repeat 100–300 times.

Indication: Diarrhea, constipation and fever.

(29) Guiwei

Location: At the end of the coccyx.

Manipulation: Kneading the point with the tip of the thumb or the middle finger is called kneading Guiwei. Repeat 100–300 times.

Indication: Constipation, diarrhea and enuresis.

12.1.3.2　Basic manipulations of infantile tuina

(1) Pressing manipulation

Pressing a certain part or point with the fingers or palm steadily is called pressing manipulation. It is divided into finger pressing and palm pressing manipulation.

(2) Rubbing manipulation

Fix the palm surface or the pad of the thumb, index or middle figure on a certain part or point, using the wrist together with the forearm to make clockwise or counterclockwise movements.

(3) Pinching manipulation

Holding the limbs or grasping the skin with the pads of the thumb, index and middle finger, squeezing with opposite force, pinching and releasing repeatedly.

(4) Circularly pushing manipulation

Circularly pushing manipulation is performed by pushing on certain points in an arc rotational way with the whorl surface of the thumb or middle finger.

(5) Kneading manipulation

Kneading manipulation is performed by fixing the thenar or whorl surface of the middle finger or thumb on a certain part or point and making circular movements. Kneading manipulation can be further classified according to different operating methods into middle finger kneading manipulation, thumb kneading manipulation and thenar kneading manipulation.

(6) Pushing manipulation

Exert force on the targeted region or certain acupoint by pushing straight forward or making rotational movements on the point with the pad of the thumb or the pads of the index and middle fingers is called pushing manipulation. It can be divided into straight pushing manipulation, rotational pushing manipulation, and separative-pushing manipulation and combined pushing manipulation.

(7) Nipping manipulation

Nipping manipulation is done by hitting a point or area with the nail of the thumb.

(8) Pounding manipulation

Pounding manipulation is performed by striking certain acupoint with the tip of the middle finger or the interphalangeal joints of the flexed index and middle fingers.

12.1.3.3　Indications & contraindications

Infantile tuina is suitable for children under 6 years old, especially suitable for infant under 3 years old. Indications for infantile tuina are quite a lot, and some of them we have mentioned above in acupoints. Infantile tuina is also commonly used for disease prevention and health care for children.

Although infantile tuina is safe and widely used, there are several contraindications should be noticed. Contraindication for infantile tuina is similar to adult tuina. Skin injury, infectious disease, bleeding tendency, cancer and tuberculosis, serious organism disease should be forbidden to treat with infantile tuina.

12.1.3.4　Cautions

Certain perspectives should be noticed when performing infantile tuina:

①The environment of clinic should be quiet, clean and with appropriate temperature. Wind and sharp light should be avoided. Stop unauthorized people from moving around. Keep the children warm after treatment and cold food or drink is forbidden. ②Keep the performer's hand clean and decorations are not allowed. Performers should be kind, patient and careful. The hand should be kept warm when the weather is cold. ③The time of treatment should be considered according to the age, the illness and the manipulation as well. Generally, infantile tuina treatment should be kept within 20 minutes and only once a day. Acute diseases like high fever can be treated twice a day. ④Acupoints in upper limbs are generally treated for only one side. Other parts can be both sides. ⑤Remember to use medical medium while performing infantile tuina. ⑥For convulsions, be careful for the asphyxia and let the child take a side lying position then find related department for help.

⑦Infantile tuina should be performed an hour after the child had meal. ⑧Sterilize before treating every child in case mutual infection.

12.1.4 Spinal manipulations

Spinal manipulations are also known as the pulling manipulation of spine. It can be generally divided into cervical rotational and local manipulation, thoracic resetting manipulation and lumbar resetting manipulation. Spinal manipulations are widely used in all segments of spine. It has the effect of smoothing the joints and resetting subluxation.

12.1.4.1 Manipulations

(1)Cervical rotational and local manipulation

1)Oblique pulling of the cervical vertebra

Manipulation: The patient has a sitting position with the head slight antexion, and the neck should be relaxed. The operator stands behind the patient, holding patient's head at the occiput with one hand, and the chin with the other. Two hands coordinates to rotate patient's head slowly(rotate patient's head to left side if the disorder is on the left side and vice versa). When the head is turned to certain amplitude and the operator feels resistance on hand, stop rotation for a moment, then do a quick and controlled twisting movement (amplitude increased about 3-5 degrees), and cracking sound is often heard at the moment.

2)Positioning rotating-pulling of the cervical vertebra

Manipulation: The patient is to take a sitting position. Operator steps aside and stands behind the patient. Use the inner side of elbow to hang the patient's jaw, and the palm holds the back head. While the other hand's thumb presses against the spinous process of the targeted vertebrae. Use the former arm to lead the neck to make an antexion movement in a certain degree to open the inner space of cervical vertebrae. Slowly rotate the head to the dislocated direction until there is a resistance. Stop rotation for a moment, then do a quick and controlled twisting movement(amplitude increased about 3-5 degrees); cracking sound is often heard at this time.

(2)Thoracic resetting manipulation

1)Positioning rotating-pulling of the thoracic-vertebrae

Manipulation: The patient is to take a sitting position, and the assistant fixes the patient's leg(normal side of the treating part) to make the pelvis stable. The operator stands behind and uses the thumb of one hand to press on the sublxation vertebrae sponous process. The other hand traverses through the patient's axilla and hold on his neck. Ask the patient to lean forward until the space of thoracic vertebrae is open. Coordinate with two hands to twist the spine to the resistant degrees. Stop rotation for a moment, then do a quick and controlled twisting movement(amplitude increased about 3-5 degrees). In the same time use the thumb to push on the spinous process from the injured side to the normal side in order to reset sublxation. Cracking sound is often heard at this time.

2)Antagonistic reduction of thoracic vertebrae

Manipulation: The patient is asked to have a sitting position and put his hands behind the occiput; the body slightly leans forward. The operator stands behind the operator, puts his knee against the diseased area, extends his arms by passing patient's armpits to hold patient's forearms at posterior aspects. Ask patient to have a few bending forward and extending backward movements. Then, the operator pulls patient's arm backward and upward when his knee tries to push the diseased vertebra forward and downward. Hands and knee coordinate to make thoracic vertebrae move.

（3）Lumbar resetting manipulation

1）Positioning rotating-pulling of the lumbar vertebrae in sitting position

Manipulation：The patient is to take a sitting position, and the assistant fixes the patient's leg(normal side of the treating part)to make the pelvis stable or let the patient bestraddle on the treatment desk. The operator sitting behind, use the thumb of one hand to press against on the sponous process of the dislocated vertebrae. The other hand traverses through the patient's axilla and then hold on his neck. Ask the patient to lean forward until the space of lumbar vertebrae is open. Coordinate with two hands to twist the spine to the resistant degree. Stop rotation for a moment, then do a quick and controlled twisting movement(amplitude increased about 3–5 degree). In the same time use the thumb to push on the spinous process from the affected side to the normal side in order to reset sublxation. Cracking sound is often heard at this time.

2）Oblique pulling of the lumbar vertebrae(yao zhui xie ban method)

Manipulation：The patient is to have a lateral recumbent position—lie on one side with hip and knee flexed. The operator stands by facing the patient, puts one hand over the front of patient's shoulder, the other hand or forearm over patient's hip. Two hands push coordinately and slowly to opposite direction. Make a controlled sudden twisting movement with increased amplitude when lumbar vertebrae are rotated to an extremity(when there is resistance). It implies a successful manipulation if cracking sound is heard.

3）Backward stretching and pulling of the lumbar vertebrae(yao zhui hou shen ban method)

Manipulation：The patient is asked to take a prone position. The operator stands beside on the affected side of body. Use the part of pisiform bone on the palm-base to press on the sublxation spinous process of the lumbar vertebrae. Use the other hand to hold the far end of the opposite leg, and then pull upwards until the resistant area. Enlarge the rear protraction amplitude of lumbar vertebrae for 3–5 degrees. At the same time, use the palm-base to press and push on the sponous process.

12.1.4.2　Indications & contraindications

Indications：Cervical spinal manipulations are suitable for sublxation of cervical vertebrae. Antagonistic reduction of thoracic vertebrae is suitable for the sublxation of fourth to tenth thoracic vertebrae and the reset of costovertebral joint. Positioning rotating-pulling of the thoracic-vertebrae is suitable for dislocation reset under eighth thoracic vertebrae. Oblique pulling of the lumbar vertebrae and positioning rotating-pulling of the lumbar vertebrae in sitting position are suitable for all segments of lumbar vertebrae. Backward stretching and pulling of the lumbar vertebrae is suitable for lower lumbar vertebrae reset.

Cervical spinal manipulations are used to treat diverse kind of cervical spondylosis. Thoracic spinal manipulations are used to treat sublxation of thoracic vertebrae and internal problem due to sublxation. Lumbar spinal manipulations are used to treat protrusion of lumbar intervertebral disc and posterior joint derangement of lumbar vertebrae.

Contra indications：First, for spine injures of unknown reason with symptoms of spinal cord injuries, spinal manipulation is not allowed to use. Second, for the aged people with serious hyperostosis or rarefaction of bone, spinal manipulation is not allowed. Third, patients with tuberculosis and tumor of bones are forbidden to receive spinal manipulations. Fourth, be careful with spinal canal stenosis when spinal manipulation is needed.

12.1.4.3　Cautions

①Spinal manipulation performers should know well of anatomy and must master the structure and characteristics of spinal joint as well as the physiological degree of mobility. ②Control your strength when performing spinal manipulation and violent force is not allowed. Pursuit of cracking sound is not suggested in spinal manipulation. Operators should train for a long time before practicing on human body. ③Every single manipulation should be controlled in the physiological degree of mobility, otherwise spinal cord, cauda and nerve root may be injured. Such points should be noticed especially in cervical manipulation and thoracic manipulation. ④Pay attention to the reaction of patient while performing spinal manipulation. Once the patient has very uncomfortable feelings, stop the manipulation immediately and find the reason.

12.2 Dietary therapy

12.2.1 Introduction to dietary therapy

Dietary therapy has long been a common approach to health among Chinese. A number of ancient Chinese medical books displayed an early Chinese interest in healing effect of Food. The earliest extant Chinese dietary text is a chapter of *Sun Simiao*'s *Essential Prescriptions Worth a Thousand Gold for Emergencies*, which was completed in the 650s during the Tang Dynasty. Sun presented current knowledge about food so that people would first turn to food rather than drugs when suffering from an ailment.

Dietary therapy also called food therapy or nutrition therapy is a method of treating diseases with diet. Traditional Chinese dietary therapy is a subject under the guidance of the theory of Traditional Chinese Medicine to study diet treatment of diseases. It is an important part of TCM clinical medicine.

12.2.2 Characteristic of dietary therapy

(1) Holism

Holism is the guiding ideology of the theoretical system of TCM. Holism means unity, integrity and interconnection. As one of the most essential characteristic of TCM, holism is applied throughout the theory system, including physiology, pathology, diagnostics, syndrome differentiation and treatment. It offers important guidance to dietary therapy too.

Diet is an important factor in overall coordination. Diet has an important impact on the integrity of the human body. The nutrients in the diet are absorbed to generate qi, blood and body fluids. A reasonable diet is an important factor in the coordination of the human body and nature. Diet is the most closely related factor in human contact with nature. Phagoiatreusiology presents the time, local diet view, used to adjust the relationship between man and nature. For example, when the weather is cool, we should avoid eating cold food; when the climate is warm, we avoid eating warm food.

(2) Choose diet based on constitution and syndrome differentiation

First, select different foods according to different constitutions. According to the information collected by four ways of looking, listening, questioning and feeling the pulse, yin, yang, qi, blood conditions are analyzed to make judgment of constitution. Choose different foods to keep health according to the constitution.

Second, choose diet based on syndrome differentiation. Syndrome differentiation is the precondition and basis of food therapy. Dietotherapy is one of the means and methods of treating disease. In the diet treatment, first of all pay attention to the syndrome differentiation, and then the right choice of food selection. For example, when people catch a cold, which may be caused by cold wind or heat wind, we need to choose the hot or cold pungent drugs for the treatment depending on syndrome differentiation.

(3) Pay attention to regulating the spleen-stomach function

One of the major features of TCM dietary therapy is to regulate the function of the spleen-stomach. Dietary activity is one of the important manifestations of human life activities, and is the guarantee of healthy and long life. The place of food digestion and absorption is the spleen-stomach. Digestion and absorption depend on the healthy function of the spleen-stomach. Only when the spleen-stomach function is strong, can the food be transformed into nutriment and transported to nourish the whole body and viscera. Improper diet is harmful for the spleen-stomach function, and various kinds of diseases may appear.

12.2.3   Eating with the seasons

Life cultivation in accordance with seasonal conditions refers to regulating one's mind, living conditions, and diet at opportune times throughout the year in order to achieve and maintain good health, prevent diseases and prolong life. These opportune times are determined according to the principles and features of the climatic variations and the waxing and waning of yin and yang during the year. The name 'life cultivation' suggests that life itself is not something to be taken for granted but something like a farmer's crop that needs to be tilled, sowed, nourished and cultivated.

12.2.4   TCM constitution dietary therapy

The constitution of each person is influenced by congenital and acquired factors, and this varies from person to person. In the other words, the body's metabolism, functioning of organs and organ structure all combine to determine the susceptibility to pathogenic factors. Either for health cultivation or disease treatment, Traditional Chinese Medicine must be used in accordance with each individual's body constitution. What are the body constitutions of modern people? Professor *Wang Qi* of Beijing University of Chinese Medicine has led a research group studying Traditional Chinese Constitutional Medicine. Human constitution can be classified into 9 basic constitutional types. Certain constitutional types can lead to certain diseases. Imbalanced constitutions can be regulated and rebalanced to health.

12.3   Qigong

12.3.1   General introduction of qigong

Qigong is one of the essence of Chinese traditional culture, and a treasure of the Chinese nation. In the field of medicine, qigong therapy is an important part of Traditional Chinese Medicine. It has been developed for thousands of years. Qigong is still used in clinical practice, and in recent years, modern medicine and science have paid more and more attention to it.

Traditional Chinese Medicine qigong (TCM qigong) is a discipline that combines TCM with qigong studies. So the concept of qigong includes "traditional Chinese medicine" and "qigong".

Now the most accepted concept of qigong is "qigong is an exercise skill which has function of 'three in one': coordinating body, breath, and mind". This concept includes four levels of meaning. The first level is the content of qigong practice: coordinating body, breath, and mind. Second, the purposes of this three practices are to integrate this three contents together. Third, according to the position of qigong practice in modern disciplinary classification, it is both physical and mental exercise, relating to both physiological and psychological factors. Fourth, the knowledge category of qigong belongs to a kind of skilled knowledge.

12.3.2   Major schools of qigong

In the long history of development, qigong has gradually absorbed the theoretical perspectives and methods which are beneficial to the physical and mental health of human beings in different periods and different disciplines, and gradually formed different academic schools among which Medical, Taoist, Buddhist, Confucian, and Martial Arts qigong are the most major schools.

Medical qigong is one of the fastest growing, popular and the most abundant schools in these five. Originated in the *Internal Classic*, its history is more than 2000 years. *Internal Classic* involves theory, operation, application etc. about qigong, concise and comprehensive, laid the foundation for the development of medical qigong. Medical qigong has three important characteristics. First, it is guided by the TCM theory, including operation, application and research all aspects. Second, the law of medical qigong is clear, the operation is standard, the popularization is widespread, and the influence is great. The most representative medical qigong includes five mimic-animal exercise, six healing sounds, and eight-sectioned exercise. Third, choose the practice method from other schools like Medical, Taoist, Buddhist, Confucian, and Martial Arts according to specific clinical needs.

Taoist qigong can be traced back to the pre-Qin period. Taoist qigong are claimed to provide a way to achieve longevity and spiritual enlightenment as well as a closer connection with the natural world. The main characteristic is the emphasis on both the life and body. The school incorporates various ancient sects, beliefs and philosophies. Its key concept is "Tao", and it emphasizes living and acting naturally, without premeditation. Taoist practice is the art of "inner alchemy", and it trains the body and the mind simultaneously. The mental training includes the "Tao in mind," a method of practice that facilitates stillness of the mind, or the qigong state. The most representative Taoist qigong is Zhoutian Gong(Figure 12-6).

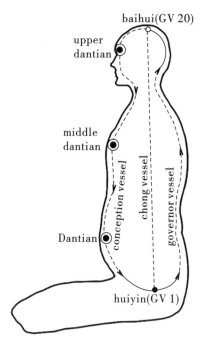

Figure 12-6　Xiao Zhoutian microcosmic orbit

The Buddhist and the Taoist schools of qigong share many elements. In order to adjust heart in Buddhist qigong, breathing exercises are emphasized and keeping static is normal, in which a representative exercise is meditation.

The Confucian branch is based on the ethics-centered philosophy of Confucius. Its goal is to regulate the mind, purge one's emotions, cultivate ethical values, heighten one's creative abilities, and seek perfection for the sake of society. The practitioner seeks peace and tranquility. The name of the Martial Arts(or boxing)school is self-explanatory. Its purpose is to strengthen the body and the spirit so that the practitioner can defeat enemies and defend himself. Martial arts practice enables instant,yet composed reactions in any situation. Self-regulation and healing are also emphasized. After all,a warrior must be in shape and able to recover fast. However,in terms of healing methodology,the Martial Arts school differs significantly from the other schools. It includes a few styles of wushu-qigong. Among them are the well-known hard qigong and the less-known soft qigong.

12.3.3   Different qigong exercises

12.3.3.1   "Yijinjing"(muscle and tendon changing qigong)

The "Yijinjing",muscle and tendon changing qigong is a manual containing a series of exercises,coordinated with breathing,is said to enhance physical health dramatically when practiced consistently. According to legend,the "Yijinjing" was invented by Bodhidharma. In Chinese yi means "change",jin means "tendons and sinews",while jing means "methods". While some consider these exercises as a form of qigong,it is a relatively intense form of exercise that aims at strengthening the muscles and tendons,so promoting strength and flexibility,speed and stamina,balance and coordination of the body.

The basic purpose of "Yijinjing" is to turn flaccid and frail sinews and tendons into strong and sturdy ones. The movements of "Yijinjing" are vigorous and gentle. Their performance calls for a unity of will and strength,using one's will to direct the exertion of muscular strength. It is coordinated with breathing. Better muscles and tendons mean better health and shape,more resistance,flexibility and endurance. It is obtained as follows:①Postures influence the static and nervous structure of the body;②Stretching muscles and sinews affect organs,joints,meridians and qi;③Torsion affects metabolism and jing production;④Breathing produces more and better refined qi;⑤Active working gives back balance and strength to body and mind (brain,nervous system and spirit).

12.3.3.2   Baduanjin(eight-sectioned exercise)

The "Baduanjin" qigong is one of the most common forms of Chinese qigong used as exercise. Variously translated as eight-sectioned exercise,eight-section brocade,eight silken movements or eight silk weaving,the name generally refers to how the eight individual movements of the form characterize and impart a silken quality(like that of a piece of brocade)to the body and its energy. The "Baduanjin" is primarily designated as a form of medical qigong,meant to improve health. This is in contrast to religious or martial forms of qigong. The "Baduanjin" qigong includes standing exercise and sitting exercise.

Standing exercise:

(1)Both hands carry heaven to regulate the triple burner

This move is said to stimulate the triple energizersmeridian. It consists of an upward movement of the hands,which are loosely joined and travel up the center of the body.

(2)Draw the bow left and right as if to shoot a vulture

While in a lower horse stance,the practitioner imitates the action of drawing a bow to either side. It is said to exercise the waist area,focusing on the kidneys and spleen.

(3)Regulate spleen-stomach by lifting one hand

This resembles a version of the first piece with the hands pressing in opposite directions,one up and one down. A smooth motion in which the hands switch positions is the main action,and it is said to especially stimulate the stomach.

(4)Remedy the 5 symptoms and 7 disorders by looking backward

This is a stretch of the neck to the left and the right in an alternating fashion.

(5) Turn the head and swing the tail to eliminate heart fire

This is said to regulate the function of the heart and lungs. Its primary aim is to remove excess fire from the heart. In performing this piece, the practitioner squats in a low horse stance, places the hands on thighs with the elbows facing out and twists to glance backwards on each side.

(6) Two hands grab the feet to strengthen kidneys and waist

This involves a stretch upwards followed by a forward bend and a holding of the toes.

(7) Clench fists and look angry to increase qi and strength

This resembles the second piece, and is largely a punching movement either to the sides or forward while in horse stance. As the most external of the pieces, this is aimed at increasing general vitality and muscular strength.

(8) Jolt the back 7 times and hundred illnesses will disappear

This is a push upward from the toes with a small rocking motion on landing. The gentle shaking vibrations of this piece is said to "smooth out" the qi after practice of the preceding seven pieces or, in some systems, this is more specifically to follow swaying the head and shaking the tail.

12.4 Tai Chi

12.4.1 General introduction of Tai Chi

Tai Chi means "Grand Ultimateness", and in Chinese culture, it represents an expansive philosophical and theoretical notion which describes the natural world(i. e., the universe) in the spontaneous state of dynamic balance between mutually interactive phenomena including the balance of light and dark, movement and stillness, waves and particles. Tai Chi, the exercise, was named after this concept and was originally developed both as a martial art(taijiquan) and as a form of meditative movement. The practice of Tai Chi as meditative movement is expected to elicit functional balance internally for healing, stress neutralization, longevity, and personal tranquility.

The concept of the Tai Chi("supreme ultimateness"), appears in both Taoist and Confucian philosophy, where it represents the fusion or mother of yin and yang into a single ultimateness, represented by the Taijitu symbol.

Tai Chi has become one of the best known forms of exercise or practice for refining qi and is purported to enhance physiological and psychological functions. The traditional Tai Chi is performed as a highly choreographed, lengthy, and complex series of movements. Today, Tai Chi has spread worldwide. Most modern styles of Tai Chi trace their development to at least one of the five traditional schools: Chen, Yang, Wu (wú), Wu(wǔ), and Sun style.

12.4.2 Brief history of Tai Chi

Tai Chi is a gentle and slow boxing, with soft and coherent movements. The word "Tai Chi" is first seen in *Zhouyi*(*The Changes of Zhou*), Tai means supreme, and Chi means the initial beginning or ultimate terminus. Tai Chi is a primitive view of the world of Chinese ancient people. After the combination of boxing and Tai Chi, gradually taijiquan emerged.

There have always been a variety of statements about the origin of Tai Chi. The origin of taijiquan was formed in the late Ming and early Qing Dynasty. There are three main aspects in the origin of taijiquan.

（1）The integrated absorption of the famous Ming Dynasty boxing. The Ming Dynasty martial art was very popular,and there were many famous and new boxing,taijiquan is invented by integrated absorption of the famous Ming Dynasty boxing.

（2）Integrated with ancient skills of breathing and Dao Yin method,Tai Chi is emphasized on both mind and action,so called one of the "Neigong quan"（inner kongfu）.

（3）Tai Chi has adopted Chinese traditional medicine theories of main and collateral meridians and the theories of yin-yang. Tai Chi requires "mind and intention to lead breath,guide the qi to drive body movements."

12.4.3 Main schools of Tai Chi

Chen-style:The most famous forms of taijiquan practiced today are the Chen,Yang,Wu（wú）,Wu（wǔ）and Sun styles. All the five styles can be traced back to Chen style. According to historical records, taijiquan was founded by Chen Wangting（1597-1664）,who lived in Chen Village,in today's Henan Province in China. There are two styles,an old Posture and a New Posture. The characteristics of Chen-style taijiquan include showing hardness and implying softness,coupling hardness with softness,coiling and twisting the movements with changeable,disappearing,and fast-slow techniques. Practicers pay attention to "internal rotation on Dantian" when breathing. The postures are commonly wide and low,containing powerful movements like jumping and foot stamping.

Yang-style:Yang-style taijiquan is one of the important schools of taijiquan with a long history of boxing. The Yang family first became involved in the study of taijiquan in the early 19th century. The founder of the Yang-style was Yang Luchan（1800-1873）,and his grandson Yang Chengfu（1883-1936）created the most popular Yang-style,which spread to the present. The national sports committee has officially publicized the type of Yang-style taijiquan or its evolution,including the 48-style,24-style,and many other styles which are performed popularly in many occasions. The characteristics of Yang-style taijiquan:the movements are stretching,simple and smooth,and the speed is even and continuous. The movements are carefully conceived and practically arranged. It embodies a unique style of beauty and grandeur.

Wu-style（wú）:The Wu-style taijiquan is a traditional boxing,one of the schools of taijiquan,mainly from the boxing development innovation of Yang's taijiquan. Yang-style taijiquan has big and small frames, and Wu-style is gradually revised on the basis of small type Yang-style. Wu-styles is famous for its softness. The movements are easy and continuous with small and nimble fist type. The punches are compact and uninhibited. The hand pushing is tight,delicate,and quiet.

Wu-style（wǔ）:Wu Yuxiang（1813-1880）was the creator of Wu-style. It is a separated family style from the more popular Wu-style. *Wu Yuxiang* was a scholar from a wealthy and influential family who was a friend of *Yang Luchan* and financially supported him in his endeavor to study Tai Chi. Wu-style taijiquan is a distinctive style with small,subtle movements;highly focusing on balance,sensitivity and internal qi development The movements of hands are within the length of toes,and each hand is in charge of the half body.

Sun-style:Sun style taijiquan was developed by *Sun Lutang*,who is considered an expert in two other internal martial arts styles,Xingyiquan and Baguazhang before he came to study taijiquan. Today,Sun-style ranks fourth in popularity and fifth in terms of seniority among the five family styles of taijiquan. The characteristics:linking forwards and back-wards stepping,extending,swift and natural movements,and direction changes with opening and closing movements.

12.4.4　The movement characteristics of Tai Chi

12.4.4.1　Relax body and tranquilize heart

To Relax body and tranquiliz heart are the most important characteristic of Tai Chi. In practice, muscles are in a state of relaxation, naturally stretching, not rigid. "Peaceful heart" means to eliminate all thoughts and concentrate all attentions.

12.4.4.2　Slow and gentle strength

Slow and gentle strength is another important characteristic of Tai Chi. A set of simplified taijiquan, 24 movements, according to the normal speed, should be finished in 5-6 minutes, slow and smooth.

12.4.4.3　Coordination of movements, breath and mind

When practicing Tai Chi, try to cooperate with the breath and the mind. The coordination of movements and mind means that you must remove all the distracting thoughts when practicing, and pay attention to movements. The consciousness should lead the movements, then make the entire body follow the mind.

12.4.5　Health benefits

Before Tai Chi was introduced to western people, the health benefits of taijiquan were largely explained through Traditional Chinese Medicine, based on a view of the body and healing mechanisms which may not always be studied or supported by modern science. Today, Tai Chi is in the process of being subjected to rigorous scientific studies in the west.

Now that the majority of health studies have displayed a tangible benefit in some areas to the practice of Tai Chi, health professionals have called for more in-depth studies to determine mitigating factors such as the most beneficial style, suggested duration of practice to show the best results, and whether Tai Chi is as effective as other forms of exercise.

Li Naiqi, Sui Hua

Chapter 13

Common Diseases

13.1 Wind stroke

The Chinese term "Wind stroke", also known as stroke or apoplexy, refers to an emergency case manifested by sudden loss of consciousness, sensation, accompanied by deviated mouth, slurred speech and hemiplegia. In mild cases, there are just hemiplegia, deviation of mouth, dysphasia or aphasia without sudden coma.

Wind stroke is characterized by symptoms occurring abruptly and pathological changes varying quickly like the wind, from which the Chinese term comes. *Internal Classic* records the symptoms of wind stroke, even if without mentioning the term itself.

This disease corresponds to the western medicine term of cerebrovascular accident(CVA), including cerebral hemorrhage, cerebral thrombosis, cerebral infarction, subarachnoid hemorrhage, cerebral vasospasm, viral encephalitis, etc.

13.1.1 Etiology

The onset of wind stroke is attributed to overworking, emotional stress or irregular diet based on zang-fu viscera deficiency for a long time.

13.1.1.1 Deficiency for a long time

Zang-fu viscera deficiency is caused by yin deficiency constitution or old and feeble for a long time.

13.1.1.2 Overstrain from physical work and sexual activity with inadequate rest

Overstrain from physical work, such as excessive lifting or sport activities and excessive exercise with inadequate rest, weakens the muscles and the meridians and lose too much sweat, causing deficiency of both qi and yin. Overstrain from sexual activity in human combined with inadequate rest consumes essence too much, causing deficiency of kidney yin. The deficient qi and yin lead to the failure in restricting yang. Internal wind is caused by unrestricted yang.

13.1.1.3 Irregular diet

Eating irregularly or eating excessive amounts of fats, sugar, dairy foods, fried foods, barbecueor alcoholic indulgence weakens the spleen and leads to phlegm. Phlegm causes internal fire which brings phlegm into meridians and brain.

13.1.1.4 Emotional disorders

Emotional disorders, such as depression, anxiety, angry and stress, transform heart and liver qi to fire, which makes qi and blood go upward into brain.

13.1.1.5 Exogenous pathogenic factors

External pathogenic qi intrudes into meridians under weakened healthy qi condition when the weather changes.

13.1.2 Pathogenesis

13.1.2.1 Pathogenic site

The pathogenic site of wind stroke is located in brain and heart, involving liver, spleen and kidney.

13.1.2.2 Pathological nature

The pathological nature of wind stroke is deficient in origin and excess in symptom. Deficiency in origin in wind stroke includes liver and kidney yin deficiency and dual deficiency of qi. Excess in symptom in wind stroke consists of pathogenic wind, pathogenic fire, phlegm and blood stasis.

13.1.2.3 Basic pathogenesis

The pathology of wind stroke may be summarized in yin-yang disharmony and qi and blood disorder. Pathogenic wind and fire due to deficient qi and yin of both liver and kidney for long time forces phlegm (caused by spleen yang deficiency) and blood stasis (caused by qi deficiency) to go upward together under emotional fluctuation or weather changing condition. Pathogenic wind, fire, phlegm and blood stasis attacking meridians cause deviated mouth, slurred speech and hemiplegia. If zang-fu viscera and meridians are affected, the diseases will manifest sudden loss of consciousness and sensation in addition to those symptoms.

13.1.2.4 Pathogenesis in different disease stages

During acute stage of wind stroke attack, pathogenic wind, fire, phlegm and blood stasis play the stagnation leading roles. Therefore, wind stroke shows excess in symptom. Liver wind invades meridians with phlegm, blocks qi and blood movement in tendons and muscles, causes losing unilateral limbs activity, facial paralysis and pararthria. If pathogenic wind and fire are so fierce as to ascend to head with the turbid damp phlegm and blood stasis, it will obstruct the clear orifices and brain vessels, make the brain bleeding, and even separate yin and yang and collapse the patient.

During restoration and sequelae stage of wind stroke attack, disordered qi and blood, phlegm and blood stasis staying in meridians and collaterals cause sequelae, including limbs numbness, weakness, less activities, speech and swallowing difficulties.

13.1.3 Diagnosis

Sudden onset, dizziness, unilateral numbness and activity difficulties, deviated mouth and slurred speech, even loss of consciousness.

Occurring in the middle-aged and the aged who are in poor health.

Premonitory symptom, including dizziness, headache, and unilateral limb numbness.

Predisposing factors, including emotional stress, overwork, overdrinking and irregular diet.

13.1.4　Differentiation

13.1.4.1　Differentiation of zang-fu viscera and meridians attacked with wind stroke

Zang-fu viscera being attacked with wind stroke are characterized by loss of consciousness, possible coma, hemiplegia, numbness and aphasia. The loss of consciousness indicates an attack on zang-fu viscera.

Meridians being attacked with wind stroke are characterized by unilateral paralysis, numbness, deviated mouth and slurred speech. There is no loss of consciousness or coma.

13.1.4.2　Differentiation of tense type and flaccid type

There are two types of pattern in wind stroke attacking zang-fu viscera: one called tense type (excessive syndrome corresponding to hard pathogenic qi), and the other called flaccid type (deficient syndrome corresponding to yin and yang separated from each other).

(1) Tense type

Main manifestations are sudden falling down in a fit with loss of consciousness, coma, tightly clinched hands and clenched jaws, closed fists, red face and ears, coarse breathing, rattling in the throat, profuse sputum, constipation, retention of urine, stiff deviated red tongue with thick and yellow or dark and grey fur, wiry slippery and rapid pulse.

(2) Flaccid type

Main manifestations are sudden falling down with loss of consciousness, coma, opening hands and mouth, closed eyes, weak nasal breathing, flaccid tongue, flushed face, oily sweat beads on the forehead, cold limbs, incontinence of urine and stools, weak faint thread pulse.

13.1.4.3　Differentiation of yang tense type and yin tense type

Both yang tense type and yin tense type manifest falling down in a fit and sudden loss of consciousness with closed eyes and mouth.

(1) Yang tense type

Pathogenic factors of yang tense type are phlegm and fire. Main manifestations are red face and ears, coarse breathing, rattling in the throat, profuse sputum, constipation, retention of urine, red tongue with yellow, greasy and thick coating, wiry slippery and rapid pulse.

(2) Yin tense type

Pathogenic factors of yin tense type are cold dampness and phlegm. Main manifestations are white face, purple lips, cold limbs, profuse sputum, and light red tongue with white and greasy coating, deep, slippery and fainting pulse.

13.1.4.4　Differentiation of disease stages

Acute stage: Two weeks.

Restoration stage: From two weeks to six months.

Sequelae stage: More than six months.

13.1.5　Treatment

13.1.5.1　Principles of treatment

①The general principles of treatment for attack on meridians and collaterals are pacifying liver, extinguishing wind, resolving phlegm, dispelling blood stasis and dredging meridians. ②The general principles of treatment for attack of tense type on zang-fu viscera are clearing away fire, extinguishing wind, clearing up phlegm, opening orifices, relaxing bowels and discharging heat. ③The general principles of treatment for attack of flaccid type on zang-fu viscera are restoring yang to stop collapse, activating brain and regaining consciousness. ④The general principles of treatment for restoration and sequelae stage of wind stroke attack are reinforcing healthy qi, clearing pathogenic qi, treating symptoms and root causes, pacifying liver, extinguishing wind, nourishing liver and kidney, resolving phlegm, dispelling blood stasis, reinforcing qi and nourishing blood.

13.1.5.2　Chinese herbal treatment

（1）Attack on meridians and collaterals

1）Syndrome of wind-phlegm attacking collaterals

Characteristic symptoms：Skin numbness, especially one-side of body, sudden deviated mouth and slurred speech, even unilateral paralysis, light red tongue with white and thin coating, floating rapid pulse.

Key pathogenesis：Wind-phlegm attacking collaterals with deficient qi and blood

Therapeutic principle and method：Dispelling wind, resolving phlegm and dredging meridians

Major prescription：Zhenfang Baiwanzi Tang variation

Herbs：Banxia, Tiannanxing, Baifuzi, Tianma, Quanxie, Danggui, Baishao, Jixueteng, Xixiancao

Explanation：

Banxia, Tiannanxing and Baifuzi to dispel wind and resolve phlegm.

Tianma and Quanxie to extinguish wind and dredge collaterals.

Danggui, Baishao, Jixueteng, Xixiancao to nourish blood and dispel wind.

Modification：For cases with slurred speech, add Shichangpu; for cases with purple tongue with blood stasis, add Danshen, Taoren, Honghua, and Chishao.

2）Syndrome of wind and liver yang harassing upper energizer syndrome

Characteristic symptoms：Dizziness, headache and tinnitus as usual, sudden deviated mouth and slurred speech, even unilateral paralysis, red tongue with yellow coating, wiry pulse.

Key pathogenesis：Liver yang transforming into wind which invades into collaterals.

Therapeutic principle and method：pacifying liver and subduing yang, activating blood and dredging meridians.

Major prescription：Tianma Gouteng Yin variation.

Herbs：Tianma, Gouteng, Zhenzhumu, Shijueming, Sangye, Juhua, Huangqin, Zhizi, Niuxi.

Explanation：

Tianma and Quanxie to extinguish wind and dredge collaterals.

Zhenzhumu and Shijueming to settle liver and subdue yang.

Sangye and Juhua to clear the liver and discharge heat.

Huangqin and Zhizi to clear the liver and drain fire.

Niuxi to activate blood, resolve stasis and guide blood to flow downward.

Modification：For cases with chest stuffy, nausea and greasy coating, add Dannanxing, Yujin; for cases with severe headache add, Lingyangjiao, Xiakucao; for cases with heavy legs, add Duzhong, Sangjisheng.

3）Syndrome of stirring wind due to yin deficiency

Characteristic symptoms：Dizziness, tinnitus and soreness of waist as usual, sudden deviated mouth, slurred speech and trembling fingers, even unilateral paralysis, red tongue with greasy coating, wiry thready rapid pulse.

Key pathogenesis：Liver and kidney yin deficiency and wind-phlegm obstructing meridians.

Therapeutic principle and method：Nourishing yin, subduing yang, extinguishing wind and dredging meridians.

Major prescription: Zhenggan Xifeng Tang variation

Herbs: Baishao, Tiandong, Xuanshen, Gouqizi, Longgu, Muli, Guiban, Daizheshi, Niuxi, Danggui, Tianma, Gouteng.

Explanation: Baishao, Tiandong, Xuanshen and Gouqizi to nourish yin, emolliate liver and extinguish wind.

Longgu, Muli, Guiban and Daizheshi to settle liver and subdue yang.

Niuxi and Danggui to activate blood, resolve stasis and guide blood to flow downward.

Tianma and Gouteng to pacify liver and extinguish wind.

Modification: For cases with too much phlegm and fire, nausea and yellow greasy fur, add Dannanxing, Zhuli and Chuanbeimu; for cases with vexing heat in chest, add Zhizi and Huangqin.

（2）Attack on zang-fu viscera

1）Tense type

a. Syndrome of fu-viscera excess caused by phlegm-heat

Characteristic symptoms: Headache, dizziness, dysphoria, testiness, constipation, abdominal distension, sudden loss of consciousness, possibly coma, deviated mouth and slurred speech, muscle rigidity, profuse greasy sputum, dull-red tongue with yellow greasy fur, wiry slippery pulse.

Key pathogenesis: Wind-phlegm attacking upper energizer and phlegm and heat obstructing fu-viscera.

Therapeutic principle and method: Relaxing bowels, discharging heat, extinguishing wind and resolving phlegm.

Major prescription: Taohe Chengqi Tang variation.

Herbs: Taoren, Dahuang, Mangxiao, Zhishi, Dannanxing, Huangqin, Gualou, Taoren, Chishao, Mudanpi, Niuxi.

Explanation:

Taoren, Dahuang, Mangxiao, and Zhishi to relax bowels, discharge heat, cool blood and resolve blood stasis.

Dannanxing, Huangqin, Gualou to clear heat and resolve phlegm.

Taoren, Chishao, Mudanpi to cool blood and resolve blood stasis.

Niuxi to guide blood to flow downward.

Modification: For cases with severe headache and dizziness, add Gouteng, Juhua and Zhenzhumu; for cases with dysphoria, insomnia, dry mouth and red tongue, add Shengdihuang, Shashen and Yejiaoteng.

b. Syndrome of orifices closed by phlegm-fire.

Characteristic symptoms: Sudden loss of consciousness, coma, tightly clinched hands and clenched jaws, closed fists, red face and ears, coarse fetid breathing, rattling in the throat, constipation, retention of urine, red tongue with yellow greasy coating, wiry slippery and rapid pulse.

Key pathogenesis: Phlegm-fire caused by liver yang obstructing orifices.

Therapeutic principle and method: Extinguishing wind, clearing hire, eliminating phlegm and opening orifices

Major prescription: Lingjiao Gouteng Tang variation.

Herbs: Lingyangjiao or Shanyangjiao, Gouteng, Zhenzhumu, Shijueming, Dannanxing, Zhuli, Banxia, Tianzhuhuang, Huanglian, Shichangpu and Yujin.

Explanation:

Lingyangjiao or Shanyangjiao, Gouteng, Zhenzhumu and Shijueming: to pacify liver and extinguish wind.

Dannanxing, Zhuli, Banxia, Tianzhuhuang and Huanglian: to clear heat and resolve phlegm.

Shichangpu and Yujin: to resolve phlegm and open orifices

Modification: For cases with gurgling with sputum in throat, take Zhuli orally; for cases with dry red tongue with yellow rough fur, add Shengdihuang, Shashen, Maidong and Shihu.

c. Syndrome of orifices closed by profuse phlegm

Characteristic symptoms: Sudden loss of consciousness, coma, tightly clinched hands and clenched jaws, red face, lip with dead color, closed fists, profuse sputum, rattling in the throat, lying still, cool limbs, constipation, retention of urine, white greasy coating, slippery deep slow pulse.

Key pathogenesis: Profuse phlegm obstructing orifices.

Therapeutic principle and method: Eliminating phlegm and opening orifices.

Major prescription: Ditan Tang variation.

Herbs: Banxia, Fuling, Hua Juhong, Zhuru, Dannanxing, Shichangpu, Yujin, Tianma, Gouteng, Jiangcan.

Explanation:

Banxia, Fuling, Hua Juhong, Zhuru: to resolve phlegm.

Dannanxing, Shichangpu, Yujin: to eliminate phlegm and open orifices.

Tianma, Gouteng, Jiangcan: to extinguish wind and resolve phlegm.

Modification: For cases with hectic cheek and faint pulse verging on expiry, take Shenfu Tang orally.

2) Flaccid type(Syndrome of collapse of yang and exhaustion of yin)

Characteristic symptoms: Sudden loss of consciousness, coma, opening hands and mouth, closed eyes, weak nasal breathing, flaccid paralysis of limbs, excess sweating, incontinence of urine and stools, weak faint thread pulse.

Key pathogenesis: Pathogenic qi defeating collapsed healthy qi.

Therapeutic principle and method: Restoring yang to save from collapse with replenished qi.

Major prescription: Shenfu Tang plus Shengmai San variation.

Herbs: Renshen, Fuzi, Maidong, Wuweizi, Shanzhuyu.

Explanation:

Renshen and Fuzi: to replenish qi and restore yang.

Maidong, Wuweizi and Shanzhuyu: to nourish yin and astringe yang.

Modification: For cases with excess sweat, add Longgu and Muli.

(3) Restoration and sequelae stage of wind stroke attack

During the acute stage of wind stroke, best results are obtained if treatment is given within 1 month after the attack. However, if treatments are not delivered or good effects are not got, once the occurrence of hemiplegia and facial paralysis is kept more than six months, the sequelae stage comes.

Wind stroke attacking during sequelae stage manifests limb numbness and loss of activities, speech and swallowing difficulties.

The principles of treatment are: reinforcing healthy qi, clearing pathogenic qi, treating both symptoms and causes.

1) Syndrome of wind-phlegm and blood stasis obstructing collaterals

Characteristic symptoms: Limb numbness, hemiplegia, facial paralysis, slurred speech, purple tongue with slippery greasy coating, wiry slippery pulse.

Key pathogenesis: Wind-phlegm and blood stasis obstructing qi and blood in collaterals

Therapeutic principle and method: Dispelling wind, resolving phlegm, activating blood and dredging meridians

Major prescription：Jieyu Dan variation.

Herbs：Tianma, Dannanxing, Tianzhuhuang, Banxia, Chenpi, Dilong, Quanxie, Jiangcan, Yuanzhi, Shichangpu, Jixueteng, Xiqiancao, Sangzhi, Danshen, Honghua.

Explanation：

Tianma, Dannanxing, Tianzhuhuang, Banxia, Chenpi：to extinguish wind and resolve phlegm.

Dilong, Quanxie, Jiangcan：to dispell wind and dredge meridians.

Yuanzhi, Shichangpu：to resolve phlegm and open orifices.

Jixueteng, Xixiancao, Sangzhi, Danshen, and Honghua：to dispel wind, activate blood and dredge meridians.

Modification：For cases with profuse phlegm and heat, add Gualou, Zhuru and Chuanbeimu; for cases with dizziness, headache, red face, red tongue, greasy coating and wiry powerful pulse, add Gouteng, Shijueming and Xiakucao; for cases with dry throat and mouth, add Tianhuafen and Tiandong.

2）Syndrome of qi deficiency and blood stasis in collateral

Characteristic symptoms：Unilateral limbs paralysis, lacking in strength, sallow complexion, purple tongue and weak unsmooth pulse.

Key pathogenesis：Qi deficiency, blood stasis and obstructed collaterals.

Therapeutic principle and method：replenishing qi, nourishing blood, resolving blood stasis and dredging collaterals

Major prescription：Buyang Huanwu Tang variation.

Herbs：Huangqi, Taoren, Honghua, Chishao, Danggui, Chuanxiong, Dilong and Niuxi.

Explanation：

Huangqi：to replenish qi and nourish blood.

Taoren, Honghua, Chishao, Danggui and Chuanxiong：to nourish blood, resolve blood stasis and dredge collaterals.

Dilong and Niuxi：to activate blood, resolve stasis and guide blood to flow downward.

Modification：For cases with blood deficiency, add Gouqizi and Shouwuteng; for cases with cold limbs, add Guizhi; for cases with soreness and weakness of waist and knees, add Xuduan, Duzhong and Sangjisheng.

3）Syndrome of liver and kidney deficiency

Characteristic symptoms：Unilateral paralysis, stiff musculature or amyotrophy limb, slurred speech with tense tongue, deep thready pulse.

Key pathogenesis：Tendon and muscle malnutrition due to liver and kidney deficiency.

Therapeutic principle and method：Nourishing liver and kidney.

Major prescription：Zuogui Wan plus Dihuang Yinzi variation.

Herbs：Shengdihuang, Heshouwu, Gouqizi, Shanzhuyu, Maidong, Shihu, Danggui and Jixueteng.

Explanation：

Shengdihuang, Heshouwu, Gouqizi and Shanzhuyu：to replenish kidney essence.

Maidong and Shihu：To nourish yin and promote fluid production.

Danggui and Jixueteng：To nourish blood and collaterals.

Modification：For cases with soreness lumber and weak legs, add Duzhong, Sangjisheng and Niuxi; for cases with kidney yang deficiency, add Roucongrong, Bajitian, Fuzi and Rougui; for cases with phlegm, add Yuanzhi, Shichangpu and Fuling.

13.1.5.3 Acupuncture and moxibustion treatment

(1)Attack on meridians and collaterals

Acupoints：Shuigou(GV 26),Jiquan(HT 1),Chize(LU 5),Neiguan(PC 6),Weizhong(BL 40),Sanyinjiao(SP 6).

Methods：Reducing manipulation is applied to Shuigou(GV 26),till tears of patients fall out. Apply reducing method with lifting and thrusting to Jiquan(HT 1),Chize(LU 5),Neiguan(PC 6),Weizhong(BL 40)and Sanyinjiao(SP 6)till the patient feel numbness of the diseased limbs.

Explanation：Shuigou(GV 26)for promoting resuscitation and opening orifices;Jiquan(HT 1),Chize(LU 5),Neiguan(PC 6),Weizhong(BL 40)and Sanyinjiao(SP 6)for removing obstruction from the meridians and collaterals.

Modification：For cases with deviation of the mouth：Dicang(ST 4)and Jiache(ST 6);for cases with upper limbs hemiplegia：Jianyu(LI 15),Quchi(LI 11),Shousanli(LI 10),Hegu(LI 4)and Houxi(SI 3);for cases with lower limbs hemiplegia：Huantiao(GB 30),Yanglingquan(GB 34),Zusanli(ST 36)and Taichong(LR 3);for cases with constipation：Tianshu(ST 25),Zhigou(TE 6),Shangjuxu(ST 37);for cases with slurred speech and stiff tongue：Lianquan(CV 23)and Tongli(HT 5).

(2)Attack on zang-fu viscera

Acupoints：Shenque(CV 8),Shuigou(GV 26),twelve Jing(well)points and Yongquan(KI 1).

Methods：Apply indirect moxibustion with salt to Shenque(CV 8). Reducing manipulation is applied to Shuigou(GV 26),till tears of patients fall out. Apply bleeding method to twelve Jing(well)points. Apply reducing method with lifting and thrusting to Yongquan(KI 1).

Explanation：Shuigou(GV 26),twelve Jing(well)points and Yongquan(KI 1)for promoting resuscitation;Shenque(CV 8)for restoring yang from collapse.

Modification：For cases with lockjaw：Jiache(ST 6),Xiaguan(ST 7)and Hegu(LI 4);for cases with profuse sputum：Tiantu(CV22)and Fenglong(ST 40).

(3)Restoration and sequelae stage of wind stroke attack

Acupoints：Baihui(GV 20), Fengfu(GV16), Pishu(BL 20), Zhongwan(CV12), Zusanli(ST 36), Fenglong(ST 40),Guanyuan(CV 4),Sanyinjiao(SP 6)and Taixi(KI 3)

Methods：Apply reducing manipulation to Baihui(GV20)and Fengfu(GV16);reinforcing manipulation is applied to Pishu(BL 20),Zhongwan(CV 12),Zusanli(ST 36),Fenglong(ST 40),Guanyuan(CV4),Sanyinjiao(SP 6)and Taixi(KI 3).

Explanation：Baihui(GV 20)and Fengfu(GV 16)for extinguishing wind;Pishu(BL 20),Zhongwan(CV 12),Zusanli(ST 36)and Fenglong(ST 40)to tonify spleen to resolve phlegm;Guanyuan(CV4),Sanyinjiao(SP 6)and Taixi(KI 3)to nourish kidney and liver yin.

Modification：For cases with deviation of the mouth：Dicang(ST 4)and Jiache(ST 6);for cases with constipation：Tianshu(ST 25),Zhigou(TE 6),Shangjuxu(ST 37);for cases with slurred speech and stiff tongue：Lianquan(CV 23)and Tongli(HT 5).

13.1.6 Prevention

Zhu Danxi considered that people with dizziness were about to get wind stroke. The old people with deficiency of qi,excessive liver yang and phlegm should be cautious about the occurrence of wind stroke,especially those people who feel dizzy and numbness in fingers.

Attention should be paid to diet and life style and overstraining should be avoided. Frequent moxibustion on Zusanli(ST 36)and Xuanzhong(GB 39)is beneficial for high risk group to avoid an attack of wind stroke.

13.2   Arthralgia

Arthralgia(the Chinese term "Bi syndrome") refers to pain, heavy sensation, soreness or numbness of muscles, tendons and joints due to obstructed meridians caused by invasion of pathogenic wind, cold, dampness and heat. The disease is manifested by stiffness, swelling, deformity and limited movement of joints. In mild cases, there are just symptoms are in muscles, tendons and joints; in serious cases, symptoms are in internal organs.

In the book of *Internal Classic*, the Chinese term "Bi syndrome" is proposed and its symptoms, etiology, pathogenesis and prognosis are stated. In Chapter 43 of *Plain Questions*, the invasion of pathogenic wind, cold and dampness causes development of arthralgia. When pathogenic wind predominates, wind arthralgia develops; when pathogenic cold predominates, cold arthralgia develops; when pathogenic dampness predominates, dampness arthralgia develops.

The severity of arthralgia is affected by exposure to climatic factors. The weather of wind and rain tends to cause the occurrence of arthralgia.

In western medicine, arthralgia corresponds to rheumatic arthritis, rheumatoid arthritis, osteoarthritis, tonic rachitis, ankylosing spondylitis, fibrositis, tendinitis, bursitis and gout.

13.2.1   Etiology

The development of arthralgia is related to physical constitution, climate, dwelling environment and diet. The deficient healthy qi and external pathogenic factors cause arthralgia together.

13.2.1.1   Invasion of wind-dampness-cold

Wind-dampness-cold, from damp living environment, cold injury, sleeping in the open, working in the wind and rain and working in water, invades striae, interstice and meridians, stays in muscles, tendons and joints, and causes wind-dampness-cold arthralgia. The excessive yang qi in body or protracted course may give rise to heat syndrome.

13.2.1.2   Invasion of wind-dampness-heat

Unlike wind-dampness-cold, pathogenic heat comes from hot humid living or working environment. Wind-dampness-heat blocks circulation of qi and blood, obstructs meridians and remains in muscles, tendons and joints, and thus arthralgia develops.

13.2.1.3   Overstrain from physical work and sexual activity with inadequate rest

Overstrain from physical work, such as excessive lifting or sport activities and excessive exercise with inadequate rest, injures the muscles and tendons and depletes qi and blood so that human bodies are prone to invasion of external pathogenic factors. Therefore, excessive sport or work activities are likely to develop arthralgia.

Overstrain from sexual activity in human combined with inadequate rest consumes essence too much so as to cause deficiency of qi and blood which decreases the resistance of body, and thus inducing the development of arthralgia too.

13.2.1.4   Weak and aged body with chronic diseases

Losing nourishment of muscles and tendons due to liver and kidney deficiency in aged bodies, or weak bodies caused by chronic disease or childbirth likely lead to the invasion of pathogenic factors. Hence the arthralgia occurs.

13.2.2 Pathogenesis

13.2.2.1 Pathogenic site

The pathogenic site of arthralgia is located in muscles, tendons and joints, even zang-fu viscera.

13.2.2.2 Pathological nature

The pathological nature of arthralgia during beginning course is excess in symptom which manifests obstruction of meridians due to pathogenic factors. Once the healing is delayed, qi and blood are consumed too much, which causes liver and kidney deficiency and phlegm and blood stasis. The pathological nature of arthralgia shows deficiency-excess in complexity under that condition.

13.2.2.3 Basic pathogenesis

The pathology of arthralgia may be summarized that it is the obstruction in the circulation of qi and blood in the meridians that causes the pain, soreness and numbness in muscles, tendons and joints. The obstruction of the meridians is caused by wind, dampness, cold and heat attacking weak body due to oldness, chronic diseases or childbirth.

13.2.3 Diagnosis

Clinic symptoms includes pain, heavy sensation, soreness or numbness of muscles, tendons and joints, even stiffness, swelling, deformity and limited movement of joints.

The exacerbation of arthralgia is related with fatigue, climate, seasonal variation and dwelling environment.

Occurring in any age. Some types of arthralgia are more common in the young and the middle-aged group.

13.2.4 Differentiation

13.2.4.1 Differentiation of predominant pathogenic factors in arthralgia

(1) Wind arthralgia

Wind arthralgia is marked by predominant pathogenic wind which is characterized by constant movement and changes. Therefore, the main manifestations of wind arthralgia are wandering pain moving from joint to joint, especially the elbows, wrists, knees and ankles, leading to limitation of movement.

(2) Cold arthralgia

Cold arthralgia is marked by predominant pathogenic cold which is characterized by property of contraction. The contracted meridians with cold cause qi and blood circulation obstruction. So the main manifestations of cold arthralgia are severe stable pain in the joints with limitation of movement, alleviated by warmth and aggravated by cold, with fixed localization but no local redness and hotness.

(3) Dampness arthralgia

Dampness arthralgia is marked by predominant pathogenic dampness which is characterized by stickiness, heaviness and turbidity. Dampness may impede the qi activity when it attacks the body and impairs yang qi. Therefore, the main manifestations of dampness arthralgia are numbness and heavy sensation of the limbs, fixed pain, soreness and swelling in muscles and joints, aggravated on cloudy and rainy days.

(4) Heat arthralgia

Heat arthralgia is marked by predominant pathogenic heat which is characterized by hotness and consumption of body fluids. The main manifestations of heat arthralgia are local redness, swelling and excruciating pain with limitation of movement involving one or several joints which feel hot when touched, accompanied by fever and thirst. This happens especially with an underlying deficiency of yin.

13.2.4.2 Differentiation of deficiency and excess in arthralgia

During the acute stage of arthralgia, excessive syndrome is composed of severe pathogenic factors, including wind, cold, dampness and heat.

Once symptoms of arthralgia advances to chronic stage, too much essence is consumed and liver and kidney yin become deficient. Blood stasis and phlegm due to qi and yin deficiency obstruct meridians and cause deformity of the joints. Under that condition, arthralgia falls into deficiency and excess in complex.

13.2.5 Treatment

13.2.5.1 Principles of treatment

The general principles of treatment for arthralgia include clearing pathogenic factors and dredging meridians because the pathogenic wind, cold, dampness, heat, phlegm and blood stasis obstruct the meridians and collaterals.

Treatment methods which include expelling wind, dissipating cold, removing dampness, clearing heat, resolving phlegm, activating blood and resolving stasis are chosen based on predominant pathogenic factor.

Moreover, treatment for wind may combine nourishing and activating blood; treatment for cold and warming yang may be applied at the same time; invigorating spleen and replenishing qi may be combined with treatment for dampness; tonifying liver and kidney and replenishing qi and blood are used to patients with chronic arthralgia for long time.

13.2.5.2 Chinese herbal treatment

(1) Invasion of wind-dampness-cold

1) Wind arthralgia

Characteristic symptoms: Wandering pain and soreness in muscles and tendons, involving several joints with limited movements, chill and fever, white and thin coating, floating or slow pulse.

Key pathogenesis: Wind guiding with cold and dampness obstructing qi and blood in meridians.

Therapeutic principle and method: Expelling wind, dissipating cold, removing dampness and dredging variation.

Major prescription: Fangfeng Tang variation.

Herbs: Fangfeng, Mahuang, Guizhi, Gegen, Danggui, Fuling, Shengjiang, Dazao and Gancao.

Explanation:

Fangfeng, Mahuang, Guizhi and Gegen: to expel wind, dissipate cold, release flesh and relieve pain.

Danggui: to nourish and activate blood.

Fuling, Shengjiang, Dazao and Gancao: to invigorate spleen and drain dampness, harmonize nutrient and defensive aspects.

Modification: For cases with soreness and pain in back and lumber, add Duzhong, Sangjisheng, Roucongrong, Bajitian and Xuduan to tonify kidney and liver; for case with swelling heat joints and thin yellow coating, Guizhi Shaoyao Zhimu Tang variation is preferred.

2) Cold arthralgia

Characteristic symptoms: Severe stable pain in the joints with limitation of movement, alleviated by warmth and aggravated by cold, with fixed localization but no local redness and hotness, pale tongue with thin white coating and wiry tight pulse.

Key pathogenesis: Cold guiding with wind and dampness obstructing qi and blood in meridians.

Therapeutic principle and method: Dissipating cold, expelling wind, removing dampness and dredging meridians.

Major prescription: Wutou Tang variation.

Herbs: Zhichuanwu, Mahuang, Baishao, Gancao, Fengmi and Huangqi.

Explanation:

Zhichuanwu and Mahuang: to warm channel, dissipate cold and relieve pain.

Baishao, Gancao and Fengmi: to relieve spasm and pain.

Huangqi: to replenish qi and consolidate exterior.

Modification: For cases with severe pain in joints with cold sense, add Fuzi, Xixin, Guizhi, Ganjiang and Danggui.

3) Dampness Arthralgia

Characteristic symptoms: Heavy sense, fixed pain and soreness in muscles and joints with limited movements, numbness skin, pale tongue with greasy white coating and fainting slow pulse.

Key pathogenesis: Dampness guiding with wind and cold obstructing qi and blood in meridians.

Therapeutic principle and method: Removing dampness, dissipating cold, expelling wind and dredging meridians.

Major prescription: Yiyiren Tang variation.

Herbs: Yiyiren, Cangzhu, Gancao, Qianghuo, Duhuo, Fangfeng, Zhichuanwu, Mahuang, Guizhi, Danggui and Chuanxiong.

Explanation:

Yiyiren, Cangzhu and Gancao: to invigorate spleen, replenish qi, dispersing wind and cold.

Qianghuo, Duhuo and Fangfeng: to expel wind and remove dampness.

Zhichuanwu, Mahuang and Guizhi: to warm channel, dissipate cold and relieve pain.

Danggui and Chuanxiong: to nourish and activate blood.

Modification: For cases with severe swelling joints, add Bixie and Wujiapi; for cases with numbness skin, add Haitongpi and Xixiancao; for cases with edema, add Fuling, Zexie and Cheqianzi; for cases with profuse phlegm, add Dannanxing and Banxia.

(2) Invasion of wind-dampness-heat

Characteristic symptoms: Wandering, redness, swelling and excruciating pain in one or several joints with limited movements, relieved with cool, local subcutaneous nodule or erythema, accompanied by fever, aversion to wind, sweat, thirst and dysphoria, red tongue with yellow greasy coating, slippery rapid pulse.

Key pathogenesis: Pathogenic wind, dampness and heat obstructing qi and blood in meridians.

Therapeutic principle and method: clearing heat, expelling wind, removing dampness and dredging variation.

Major prescription: Baihu Tang, Guizhi Tang plus Xuanbi Tang variation.

Herbs: Shengshigao, Zhimu, Huangbo, Lianqiao, Guizhi, Fangji, Kuxingren, Yiyiren, Huashi, Chixiaodou, Cansha.

Explanation:

Shengshigao, Zhimu, Huangbo, Lianqiao: to clear heat and relieve dysphoria.

Guizhi: to disperse wind and release flesh.

Fangji, Kuxingren, Yiyiren, Huashi, Chixiaodou, and Cansha: to clear heat, drain dampness, diffuse impediment and dredge collaterals.

Modification: For cases with erythema, add Mudanpi, Chishao, Shengdihuang and Zicao; for cases with fever, aversion to wind and throat pain, add Jingjie, Bohe, Niubangzi and Jiegeng; for cases with thirst and dysphria, add Shengdihuang, Maidong and Xuanshen.

(3) Syndrome of phlegm and blood stasis obstructing meridians

Characteristic symptoms: Stabbing pain with fixed localization in the joints, or swelling stiff purple joints, or numbness with heavy sensation limbs, deformity joints with limited movements, local subcutaneous nodule or ecchymosis, darkish complexion, eyelid edema, deep purple tongue with white greasy coating, wiry umsmooth pulse.

Key pathogenesis: Phlegm and blood stasis obstructing meridians.

Therapeutic principle and method: Revolving phlegm, activating blood and dredging meridians.

Major prescription: Shuanghe Tang variation.

Herbs: Taoren, Honghua, Chishao, Danggui, Chuanxiong, Banxia, Fuling, Chenpi, Baijiezi and Zhuli.

Explanation:

Taoren, Honghua, Chishao, Danggui and Chuanxiong: to nourish blood, resolve blood stasis and dredge collaterals.

Banxia, Fuling, Chenpi, Baijiezi and Zhuli: to invigorate spleen and resolve phlegm.

Modification: For cases with subcutaneous nodule, add Dannanxing and Tianzhuhuang; for cases with swelling pain stiff deformity joints, add Ezhu, Sanqi and Tubiechong; for cases with severe continued pain in joints, add Chuanshanjia, Baihuashe, Quanxie, Wugong and Dilong.

(4) Syndrome of liver and kidney deficiency

Characteristic symptoms: Delayed healing of arthralgia, joints with limited movements, becoming thin muscle, soreness and weakness of waist and knees, or aversion cold limbs, impotence and seminal emission, or steaming bone fever, dry mouth and dysphoria, light red tongue with thin white coating, deep thready weak pulse.

Key pathogenesis: Muscles and tendons losing nourishment due to liver and kidney deficiency.

Therapeutic principle and method: Tonifying and replenishing liver and kidney, relaxing sinew, relieving pain and activating collaterals.

Major prescription: Duhuo Jisheng Tang variation.

Herbs: Duhuo, Fangfeng, Qinjiao, Xixin, Rougui, Renshen, Fuling, Gancao, Danggui, Shengdihuang, Baishao, Duzhong, Niuxi and Sangjisheng.

Explanation:

Duhuo, Fangfeng, Qinjiao, Xixin and Rougui: to expel wind, remove dampness and dissipate cold.

Renshen, Fuling, Gancao, Danggui, Shengdihuang and Baishao: to tonify qi and blood.

Duzhong, Niuxi and Sangjisheng: to tonify and replenish liver and kidney.

Modification: For cases with severe soreness and weakness of waist and knees and lacking in strength, add Lujiaoshuang, Xuduan and Gouji; for cases with aversion cold limbs, add Fuzi, Ganjiang and Bajitian; for cases with liver and kidney yin deficiency, pain in lumber and knees, dyphoria, lower fever, or afternoon tidal fever, add Guiban, Shudihuang and Nvzhenzi.

13.2.5.3   Acupuncture and moxibustion treatment

Ashi points located at the diseased areas are selected for the purpose of clearing pathogenic factors. The manipulations of acupuncture and moxibustion should be chosen by symptoms and signs that include the location and the depth of pain. Shallow insertion is for the diseased skin and muscles; while deep insertion is for bones and tendons. The bleeding methods can be used to clear blood stasis and dampness. For eliminating wind and cold,moxibustion can be applied. Prescriptions:

Disease at the shoulder joint:Jianyu(LI 15),Jianliao(TE 14),Jianzhen(TE 19),Naoshu(SI 10).

Disease at the elbow joint:Quchi(LI 11),Chize(LU 5),Tianjing(TE 10).

Disease at the wrist:Yangchi(TE 4),Yangxi(LI 5),Yanggu(SI 5),Waiguan(TE 5).

Disease at the back and lumber:back transport points with pain,points with pain on governor vessel, Jiaji(EX-B 2),Shuigou(GV 26),Shenzhu(GV 12),Yaoyangguan(GV 3).

Disease at the hip joint:Huantiao(GB 30),Juliao(GB 29),Xuanzhong(GB 39).

Disease at the knee joint:Heding(EX-LE 2),Dubi(SI 35),Neixiyan(EX-LE 4),Yanglingquan(GB 34),Yinlingquan(SP 9).

Disease at the ankle joint:Jiexi(SI 41),Shangqiu(SP 5),Qiuxu(GB 40),Kunlun(BL 60),Taixi(KI 3).

Disease at the hands and feet:Yanggu(SI 5),Hegu(LI 4),Houxi(SI 3),Sanjian(LI 3),Baxie(EX-UE 9),Gongsun(SP 4),Shugu(BL 65),Bafeng(EX-LE 10).

13.2.6　Prevention

The patients with arthralgia should keep warm,avoid wind and live in a humid room. The mild exercises are beneficial to the healing. However,people with the sweating body after exercises should not have shower or stay in wind.

13.3　Headache

Headache is a disease which shows the main clinical feature of the head pain. Due to the external and/ or internal injuries,it is resulted in the constraint or loss of the choroid. Headache is not only a common disease,but also a common symptom. It can occur in many kinds of acute and chronic diseases. Sometimes it is also a sign of aggravation or deterioration of some related diseases. There are the records of head illness in Oracle in Shang Dynasty. It is called brain wind or capital wind in the book of *Internal Classic*. In the book of *Treatise on Cold Damage and Miscellaneous Diseases*,there are different treatment methods discussed in detail in the chapter about yangming diseases,shaoyang diseases,jueyin diseases,and so on. *Dong yuan Shi shu(Dongyuan Ten Books)* pointed out that both exogenous and internal injuries were the causes of headache. According to the etiology and symptoms, headache can be recognized as typhoid fever headache, dampness-heat headache,migraine,real headache,qi deficiency headache,blood deficiency headache,taiyin headache,shaoyin headache,and so on. That provides a method for medicine choice according to meridians.

Headache can be induced by various diseases of internal medicine,neurology,surgery,psychiatry,otolaryngology and ophthalmology in western medicine. It involves hypertension,neurosis,intracranial diseases, infectious fever and so on.

13.3.1　Etiology

Headache can be leaded by any of the six external etiological factors,impairment of the function of internal organs,caused by emotional strain,resulting in external pathogens,phlegm and hyperactivity of liver yang. Or it is caused by deficiency of qi,blood,yin and yang,resulting in malnutrition of brain. Trauma, chronic disease and accumulation of stasis also induce headache.

13.3.1.1　The six external etiological factors hurt headache

Wind pathogen may be the main factor. Wind pathogen belongs to yang pathogen. As is known, the head will be hurt first when one is impaired by wind. It is only the wind that can reach the peak. Wind is the chief pathogen of all diseases. When wind pathogen attacks the head, it is usually compounded with coldness, dampness and heat. If wind is compounded with coldness, the coldness will hurt yang, block the qi and blood, and contract the pulse and lead to pain. If wind is compounded with dampness, the sticky qi will make the clear yang turbid, and qi and blood cannot flow smoothly so to lead to pain. If wind is compounded with heat, wind-heat will flow upward to head and make the qi and blood revert upward, leading to headache.

13.3.1.2　Deficiency of qi, blood, yin and yang impair the function of internal organs

The deficiency may be caused by congenital deficiency, aged deficiency, kidney deficiency by sexual strain, being for a long time, after giving birth to a child, losing blood, and etc. The deficient qi, blood, yin and yang cannot nourish head and results in headache.

13.3.1.3　Emotional strain leads to headache

Being in the state of nervousness and melancholy for a long time affects liver qi. Stagnation of liver qi makes the liver meridian loose the stretching, contract together and be painful. An irritable man is easy to be angry. The angry contributes to the production of liver-heat. Liver-heat impairs liver-yin after a long-time damage, goes upward to head, and leads to headache.

13.3.1.4　Irregular diet leads to headache

Just as Zhu Danxi said, most of headache is caused by phlegm. Irregular diet such as excessively having sweet food or meat, eating too much or too little than usual, will damage spleen. Damaged spleen cannot transfer water in body into qi. Stagnant water becomes dampness and phlegm. Dampness and phlegm flow with qi. They stay in head and become pathogenic factors covering the orifices in head. So diet is also one causes of headache.

13.3.2　Pathogenesis

13.3.2.1　Pathogenic site

The pathogenic site of headache is located in head, related to liver, spleen, and kidney closely.

13.3.2.2　Pathological nature

The pathological nature of headache can be related to any of the six external etiological factors, impairment of the function of internal organs, caused by emotional strain, resulting in external pathogens, phlegm and hyperactivity of the liver yang. Deficiency of qi, blood, yin and yang, can result in malnutrition of brain. Trauma, chronic disease and accumulation of stasis also induce headache. The obstruction causes pain.

13.3.2.3　Basic pathogenesis

According to the nature of disease's syndrome, headache can be divided into excess syndrome and deficiency syndrome. Pathogens obstruct qi's flowing in pulses and meridians and cover the clear orifices. Deficiency of essence and blood leads to brain's malnutrition. Both excess and deficiency are the basic pathogen of headache.

13.3.3 Diagnosis

13.3.3.1 The main symptom is headache

It is manifested as forehead pain, frontal and temporal pain, parietal pain, occipital and parietal pain, or even all head pain. It can be jumping pain, stabbing pain, distending pain, vague pain, and empty pain, etc. It will occur suddenly or repeatedly. The duration of pain can vary from several minutes to hours, days, or weeks.

13.3.3.2 About inspection

To do routine blood test and measure blood pressure is regular check. Cerebrospinal fluid test, cerebral blood flow test and EEG are sometimes necessary. Transcranial Doppler check, cranial CT and MRI examination are required. All of these help to make clear diagnosis and exclude organic diseases.

13.3.4 Differentiation

13.3.4.1 Wind-cold type

Wind-cold headache is characterized by acute occurrence, severe headache, being more serious after catching cold, feeling chilly and aversion to wind-cold, nasal congestion, watery nasal discharge, thin white coating of the tongue, floating pulse or tight floating pulse.

13.3.4.2 Wind-heat type

Wind-heat headache is characterized by distending pain and scorching sensation in the head, acute onset, aversion to wind, stuffy nose with turbid discharge, red tongue with yellowish coating, and rapid pulse.

13.3.4.3 Type of hyperactivity of the liver yang

Type of hyperactivity of the liver yang is characterized by distending and radiative pain of the head induced by tension, flushed face and conjunctival congestion, bitter taste, tinnitus, red tongue with thin yellow coating, and tight pulse.

13.3.4.4 Type of accumulation and up-stirring of phlegm

Type of accumulation and up-stirring of phlegm is characterized by heavy feeling in the head, vertigo, oppressed feeling in the chest, nausea, vomiting phlegm, white greasy coating of the tongue, and slippery pulse.

13.3.4.5 Type of stagnation of liver qi in the meridians

Type of stagnation of liver qi in the meridians is characterized by headache with punctured feeling, fixed pain, recurrence due to trauma in the head, purple tongue, and hesitant pulse.

13.3.4.6 Type of deficiency of blood

Type of deficiency of blood is characterized by headache and dizziness worsened by movement, palpitation, insomnia, pale complexion, pale tongue and thready pulse.

13.3.5 Treatment

13.3.5.1 Principles of treatment

The general principles of treatment for headache include strengthening health qi and eliminating pathogens. The pathogens include wind, cold, heat, hyperactivity of the liver yang, phlegm, stagnation of liver qi. The health qi includes qi, blood, yin and yang.

Treatment methods which include expelling wind, dissipating cold, clearing heat, resolving phlegm, activating blood and resolving stasis are applied based on predominant pathogenic factors.

13.3.5.2　Chinese herbal treatment

(1) Wind-cold headache

Characteristic symptoms: Acute occurrence, severe headache, being more serious after catching cold, feeling chill and aversion to wind-cold, nasal congestion, watery nasal discharge, thin white coating of the tongue, floating pulse or tight floating pulse.

Key pathogenesis: Wind-pathogen is one of the main pathogens which hurts the head. If wind is compounded with coldness, the coldness will hurt yang, block the qi and blood, and contract the pulse to lead to pain.

Major prescription: Chuanxiong Chatiao San variation.

Herbs: Chuanxiong, Jingjie, Fangfeng, Baizhi, Qianghuo, Gancao, Xixin, Chaqing.

Explanation:

Chuanxiong, Qianghuo, Baizhi, Xixin: to divergent cold and dredge the meridian.

Jingjie, Bohe: to evacuate the upper wind evil, and to clear the leader.

Fangfeng: to dispel the wind to solve the table, win the wet pain.

Gancao: to supplement qi and harmonize the medicine.

Chaqing: to clear the leader and harmonize the temperature and dryness of wind medicine.

Modification: for cases with colder symptoms, the drugs added are Zhichuanwu, Xixin, Gaoben; for cases with severe headache due to dampness, the drugs added are Cang'erzi, Cangzhu.

(2) Wind-heat headache

Characteristic symptoms: Distending pain and scorching sensation in the head, acute onset, aversion to wind, stuffy nose with turbid discharge, reddened tongue with yellowish coating, and rapid pulse.

Key pathogenesis: When wind is compounded with heat, wind-heat will flow upward to head and make the qi and blood revert to upward, so to lead to headache.

Major Prescprition: Xiongzhi Shigao blood Tang variation.

Herbs: Chuanxiong, Baizhi, Shengshigao (decocted first), Manjingzi, Sangye, Juhua, Qianghuo, Gaoben.

Explanation:

Chuanxiong, Baizhi, Shengshigao, Juhua: to disperse wind and clear heat.

Qianghuo, Gaoben: to dispel rheumatism, and cure headache.

Manjingzi, Sangye, Juhua: to evacuate wind heat and clear head.

Modification: for cases with stuffy with yellow and sticky discharge, add Xinyi, Cang'erzi, Yuxingcao; for cases with severe fever, add Shengdahuang(decocted later); for cases with severe headache, add Xixin.

(3) Type of hyperactivity of the liver yang

Characteristic symptoms: Distending and radiative pain of the head induced by tension, flushed face and conjunctival congestion, bitter taste, tinnitus, red tongue with thin yellow coating, and tight pulse.

Key pathogenesis: The liver loses its characteristic of harmony and accessibility, and the qi is stagnated in body. After a long period of stagnation, the qi is converted into fire, yang qi is type of liver and disturbed the brain.

Major prescription: Tianma Gouteng Yin variation.

Herbs: Gouteng (decocted later), Tianma, Shijueming (decocted first), Niuxi, Huangqin, Zhizi, Duzhong, Sangjisheng, Fuchen, Yejiaoteng.

Explanation:

Gouteng,Tianma: to suppress hyperactive liver and extinguish wind.

Shijueming: to suppress hyperactive liver and subside yang, clear heat and improve eyesight.

Niuxi: to draw blood downward.

Huangqin,Zhizi: to clear heat and purge fire.

Duzhong,Sangjisheng: to nourish liver and kidney.

Fushen,Yejiaoteng: to tranquiliz and sedate the mind.

Modification: For cases with up-stirring of liver and endless radiated pain, add Quanxie,Jiangcan; for cases with deficiency of liver yin and kidney yin, vertigo and tinnitus, add Shengdi,Shudi,Shouwu,Gouqizi

(4)Type of accumulation and up-stirring of phlegm

Characteristic symptoms: Heavy feeling in the head, vertigo, oppressed feeling in the chest, nausea, vomiting phlegm, white greasy coating of the tongue, and slippery pulse.

Key pathogenesis: The function of transport and transformation of spleen is abnormal, which blinds the brain.

Major prescription: Banxia Baizhu Tianma Tang variation.

Herbs: Zhibanxia,Weitianma,Baizhu,Chenpi,Fuling,Gancao

Explanation:

Zhibanxia: to eliminate dampness and phlegm, drop the inverse anti-nausea.

Weitianma: to calm liver and extinguish wind, stop dizziness

Fuling,Chenpi,Baizhu: to invigorate the spleen and infiltrate the dampness, regulate qi and resolve phlegm.

Gancao: to reconcile the medicine.

Modification: For cases with stagnation of phlegm-dampness in the stomach and sticky sputum, add Wuzhuyu,Shengjiang; for cases with accumulation of phlegm forming heat, bitter taste sticky mouth and yellow greasy coating of the tongue, add Zhuru,Chendanxing,Huangqin,Zhishi.

(5)Type of stasis of blood

Characteristic symptoms: Headache with punctured feeling, fixed pain, recurrence due to trauma in the head, purple tongue, and smooth-less pulse.

Key pathogenesis: The congestion blocks the collaterals. Body pain means the balance in body is disrupted.

Major prescription: Tongqiao Huoxue Tang variation.

Herbs: Chishao,Chuanxiong,Taoren,Honghua,Shexiang,Shengjiang,Congbai,Dazao.

Explanation:

Chishao,Chuanxiong,Taoren,Honghua: to promote blood circulation for removing blood stasis and obstruction in collaterals.

Shexiang: Shengjiang,Congbai: to unobstruct the meridians and collaterals.

Modification: For cases with stasis due to cold, headache and aversion to cold, add Xixin,Guizhi; for cases with stagnation of phlegm-dampness, add Baifuzi,Zhinanxing,Jiangcan; for cases with deficiency of qi and blood due to chronic disease, add Huangqi,Dangshen,Gouqizi.

(6)Type of deficiency of blood

Characteristic symptoms: Headache and dizziness worsened by movement, palpitation, insomnia, pale complexion, pale tongue and small pulse.

Key pathogenesis: Insufficient qi and blood on the brain and meridians causes nourishment loss of the brain and headache.

Major prescription：Siwu Tang variation.

Herbs：Shudi, Danggui, Chuanxiong, Baishao.

Explanation：

Shudi：to nourish yin and nourish blood.

Danggui：to nourish the liver and activate blood circulation.

Chuanxiong, Baishao：to nourish blood, invigorate the liver and activate the qi and make the qi and blood harmonious and unobstructed.

Modification：For cases with palpitation and severe insomnia due to blood failure in nourishing heart, add Zaoren, Guiyuanrou, Yuanzhi；for cases with deficiency of qi, add Dangshen, Huangqi.

13.3.5.3 Acupuncture and moxibustion treatment

According to the part of the headache, we should take meridian following acupoint selection and select ashi points as the main. Moxibustion can be added to cold syndrome. Blood stasis headache can use the method of swift pricking blood therapy in ashi points. Patients with severe headache can use strong stimulation and long needle in the ashi points. Prescriptions：

Main acupoint：Baihui(GV 20), Taiyang(EX-HN 4), Fengchi(GB 20), Hegu(LI 4).

Taiyang headache：add Tianzhu(BL 10), Houxi(SL 3), Kunlun(BL 60).

Yangming headache：add Yintang(GV 29), Neiting(SI 44).

Shaoyang headache：add Shuaigu(GB 8), Waiguan(TE 5), Zulinqi(GB 41).

Jueyin headache：add Sishencong(EX-HN 1), Taichong(LR 3), Neiguan(PC 6).

A headache caused by a chill：add Fengmen(BL 12), Lieque(LU 7).

A headache caused by wind heat：add Quchi(LI 11), Dazhui(GV 14).

A headache caused by rheumatism：add Touwei(SI 8), Yinlingquan(SP 9).

A headache caused by upper hyperactivity of liver yang：add Taixi(KI 3), Taichong(LR 3).

A headache caused by phlegm turbid：add Zhongwan(GV 12), Fenglong(SI 40).

A headache caused by congestion：add Xuehai(SP 10), Geshu(BL 17).

A headache caused by blood deficiency：add Pishu(BL 20), Zusanli(SI 36).

13.3.6 Prevention

Appropriate participation in physical exercise, enhance physique, and keep warm, in order to resist the invasion of external evil.

Keep a good mood and avoid bad emotional stimulation.

Do not eat greasy, fast and spicy or fried foods. Stop smoking and drinking.

For severe or gradually worsening headaches accompanied by nausea and vomiting of patients, other lesions and timely examination should be considered.

13.4 Insomnia

Insomnia refers to difficulty in falling asleep, frequent wakening from sleep and sleeplessness by night. It is manifested by dizziness, headache, palpitation and amnesia. In western medicine, it is found in neurosis, anemia and chronic asthenic diseases.

In the book of *Internal Classic* called "must not lie", "eye meditation", that is evil off in the viscera, wei qi through in yang and can not enter the yin. The book *Plain Questions* records "*inverse regulating the stomach and the insomnia*". *Zhang Zhongjing* of the Han Dynasty in *Treatise on Cold Damage and Miscellaneous Diseases* and *Synopsis of prescriptions of Golden Chamber* divided etiology of insomnia into two types: exogenous and internal injuries, and put forward the "dysphoria and consumptive disease leading to insomnia" discussion, which still has application value.

Insomnia can be the main clinical manifestation in various diseases like neurosis, menopausal syndrome, chronic indigestion, anemia and atherosclerosis. These diseases can refer to this section of dialectical treatment.

13.4.1 Etiology

13.4.1.1 Section of the diet

Overeating causes the food retention. Stagnation of food results in spleen and stomach damage, brewing phlegm, and causing the loss of stomach qi. In addition, tea, coffee, wine are also the factors that cause insomnia.

13.4.1.2 Emotional disorders

Emotion failures can lead to dysfunction of zang-fu viscera. For example, rage injures liver and causes stagnation of liver qi. Pathogenic fire derived from stagnation of liver qi disturbs mind, causing lassitude of spirit and insomnia. Joy of laughing, mental excitement, uneasiness can also cause insomnia.

13.4.1.3 Work and rest disorders

Excessive fatigue would hurt the spleen and excessive idleness would weak the spleen qi. Lack of blood and qi due to the dysfunctional transport can not nourish the heart and result in loss of mind and insomnia. Over-thought injures the heart, resulting in consumption of yin blood and failure of the mind to keep to its abode.

13.4.1.4 Deficiency after the illness

Chronic illness causes deficiency including less heart blood, and limited movement of heart qi, leading to insomnia. Some elder patients are physically weak, so the deficiency of yin and yang causes insomnia.

13.4.2 Pathogenesis

13.4.2.1 Pathogenic site

Insomnia is often caused by deficiency of the heart and closely related to the liver, spleen and kidney.

13.4.2.2 Pathological nature

There is difference between deficiency and excess. In clinical practice, type of deficiency of both the heart and spleen, type of hyperactivity of fire due to yin deficiency and type of accumulation of phlegm in the interior are often found.

13.4.2.3 Basic pathogenesis

The basic pathogenesis is the deficiency of the heart, gallbladder, spleen and kidney yin. It leads to pathogenic fire derived from stagnation of liver qi, phlegm-heat attacking internally, deficiency of both heart and spleen, impaired nourishment of heart-mind. Long-term illness can present intermingled deficiency and excess.

13.4.3　Diagnosis

13.4.3.1　Main symptoms

It is difficult to fall asleep and easy to wake up at night for more than 3 weeks, often accompanied with headache, dizziness, palpitation, amnesia, lassitude, hung up, dreaminess and other symptoms. This disease often have improper diet, emotional disorders, fatigue, excessive anxiety, disease, and weakness history.

13.4.3.2　About inspection

Clinically detectable polysomnography:①The duration of the average sleep latency was prolonged(longer than 30 minutes);②The actual sleep time was reduced(less than 6.5 hours per night);③The arousal time increased(more than 30 minutes per night).

13.4.4　Differentiation

13.4.4.1　Liver fire disturbing heart

Insomnia and dreaming a lot, irritability, dizziness with red swollen eyes, tinnitus, dry and bitter taste in mouth, no desire to eat, dark urine, red tongue, wiry and rapid pulse.

13.4.4.2　Phlegm-heat disturbing heart

Upset wakefulness, chest tightness, fullness, belching, nausea, accompanied with pain, headache, dizziness, the yellow coating on the tongue, slippery and rapid pulse.

13.4.4.3　Heart-spleen deficiency

It is not easy to sleep or wake up, accompanied with palpitations, forgetfulness, lassitude, eating less, dizziness, abdominal distension, diarrhea, pale tongue, thready and weak pulse.

13.4.4.4　Disharmony between heart and kidney

Upset wakefulness, sleep difficulties, palpitation and dreaminess, red tongue, little coating, thready pulse.

13.4.4.5　Heart gallbladder deficiency

Virtual trouble insomnia, getting frightened easily, timidness, palpitation, shortness of breath and sweating, fatigue, pale tongue, thready pulse.

13.4.5　Treatment

13.4.5.1　The principle of treatment

The principle of adjusting the yin and yang of viscera should be made in the treatment of deficiency and diarrhea. Treat excess with reinforcement and deficiency with expelling. Tranquillization is necessary on this basis such as nourishing blood, calming the spirit, clearing heart, etc.

13.4.5.2　Chinese herbal treatment

(1) Syndrome of Liver fire disturbing heart

Characteristic symptoms: Wakefulness and excessive dreams, irritability accompanied with dizziness and distention in head, red tongue with thin coating, wiry rapid pulse.

Key pathogenesis: the liver is depressed and the heart is disturbed.

Major prescription: Longdan Xiegan Tang variation.

Herbs: Longdancao, Huangqin, Zhizi, Zexie, Cheqianzi, Danggui, Shengdi, Chaihu, Gancao, Shenglonggu, Shengmuli and Cishi.

Explanation:

Longdancao, Huangqin, and Zhizi: to clear liver fire.

Zexie, Cheqianzi: to clear damp and hot.

Danggui, Shengdi: to nourish yin and yang.

Chaihu: to unblock qi of liver and gallbladder.

Shenglonggu, Shengmuli and Cishi: to clear heart fire, and tranquilize.

Gancao: to supplement qi and harmonize the medicine

Modification: For cases with chest distress, add Xiangfu, Yujin Foshou; *for cases with* dizziness and headache with constipation, use Danggui Longhui Wan.

(2) Syndrome of phlegm-heat attacking heart

Characteristic symptoms: Upset insomnia, chest tightness, fullness, tongue red, yellow greasy coating slippery pulse.

Key pathogenesis: Eating some high-fat food causes phlegm accumulation in the chest, and the phlegm becomes phlegm-fire to affect the consciousness of heart.

Major prescription: Huanglian Wendan Tang variation.

Herbs: Banxia, Chenpi, Fuling, Zhishi, Huanglian, Zhuru, Longchi, Zhenzhumu and Cishi.

Explanation:

Banxia, Chenpi, Fuling and Zhishi: to fortify the spleen, dry dampness, dissolve and remove, phlegm accumulation.

Huanglian and Zhuru: to clear heat, dissolve phlegm, and harmonize the stomach.

Longchi, Zhenzhumu and Cishi: to tranquilize the heart and calm the mind.

Modification: For cases with choking sensation in chest, abdominal fullness and distention, ungratifying defecation, greasy coating and slippery pulse, add Banxia Shumi Tang; if stomach is not comfortable and ache in the belly, add Shenqu, Jiaoshanzha, Laifuzi to promote the digestion.

(3) Syndrome of deficiency of both heart and spleen

Characteristic symptoms: Trouble falling asleep, excessive dream, forgetfulness, pale tongue, thin and weak pulse.

Key pathogenesis: Lack of blood of spleen and heart resulting in failure of nourishment of the heart.

Major prescription: Guipi Tang variation.

Herbs: Renshen, Baizhu, Gancao, Danggui, Huangqi, Yuanzhi, Suanzaoren, Fushen, Longyanrou and Muxiang.

Explanation:

Renshen, Baizhu, Danggui and Huangqi: to boost the qi and fortify the spleen.

Yuanzhi, Suanzaoren, Fushen and Longyanrou: to nourish the heart and clam the mind.

Muxiang: to move qi and relieve the pain.

Gancao: to harmonize nutrient and defensive aspects.

Modification: If blood of heart is not enough, add Shudi, Shaoyao, Ejiao; if insomnia is serious, add Yejiaoteng, Hehuanpi, and Baiziren or Shenglonggu, Shengmuli to tranquilize and allay excitement. If accompanied by food indigestion, greasy coating on the tongue, add Cangzhu, Banxia, Chenpi, Fuling, Houpo to invigorate the spleen and dry the qi and phlegm. If one can not sleep well after giving birth to a baby, or if old people wake up too early, the treatment is the same with that of deficiency of qi and blood.

(4) Syndrome of disharmony between heart and kidney

Characteristic symptoms: Insomnia, palpitation, dreaminess, accompanied with soreness and weakness of waist and knees, red tongue, little coating, thready pulse.

Key pathogenesis: Deficient kidney water fails to nourish the heart and excessive heart fire fails to move down to kidney.

Major prescription: Liuwei Dihuang Wan plus Jiaotai Wan variation.

Herbs: Shudi, Shanzhuyu, Shanyao, Fuling, Zexie, Danpi, Huanglian, Rougui.

Explanation:

Shudi, Shanzhuyu, and Shanyao: to nourish liver and kidney, replenish vital essence and nourish the bone marrow.

Fuling, Zexie, Danpi: to invigorate the spleen to transform dampness and clear ministerial fire.

Huanglian, Rougui: to conduce the fire back to its origin.

Modification: For the shortness of heart yin, use Tianwang Buxin Dan to nourish yin and produce blood, tonify heart and calm the nerves; if insomnia stays all night, add Zhusha, Cishi, Longgu, Longchi to tranquilize and allay excitement.

(5) Syndrome of qi deficiency of heart and gallbladder

Characteristic symptoms: Insomnia, getting frightened easily, with shortness of breath and spontaneaous sweating, pale tongue, thin pulse string.

Key pathogenesis: Heart-gallbladder vacuity timidity, failure of nourishment of the heart, uneasiness.

Major prescription: Anshen Dingzhi Wan plus Suanzaoren Tang

Herbs: Renshen, Fuling, Gancao, Fushen, Yuanzhi, Longchi, Shichangpu, Chuanxiong, Suanzaoren, Zhimu

Explanation:

Renshen, Fuling, and Gancao: to replenish qi of heart and gallbladder.

Fushen, Yuanzhi, Longchi, Shichangpu: to reduce phlegm and calm one's mind, tranquilize and allay excitement.

Chuanxiong, Suanzaoren: to regulate blood and nourish heart.

Zhimu: to clear heat and relieve fidgetiness.

Modification: For cases with shortness of blood of heart and liver, palpitation with fear, reuse Renshen, and add Baishao, Danggui, Huangqi to nourish blood of liver; for cases with heaving deep sighs and eating less food, add Chaihu, Chenpi, Shaoyao, Baizhu to clear the liver and tonify spleen; if one feels more palpitation and restlessness with fear, add Shenglonggu, Shengmuli, Zhusha to tranquilize and allay excitement.

13.4.5.3　Acupuncture and moxibustion treatment

According to the part of the insomnia, we should take meridian-following acupoints selection and select ashi points as the main. Basic moxibustion and acupuncture techniques are very effective in the treatment of insomnia. Different moxibustion and acupuncture selection are for different causes. Prescriptions:

Main acupoints: Shenmen(HT 7), Sanyinjiao(SP 5), Baihui(GV 20), Shenmai(BL 62) and Anmian.

Liver fire disturbing heart: add Xingjian(LR 2).

Phlegm heat disturbing heat: add Fenglong(ST 40), Zhongwan(CV 12) and Neiting(ST 44).

Heart-spleen deficiency: add Xinshu(BL 15), Pishu(BL 20) and Zusanli(ST 36).

Disharmony between heart and kidney: add Taixi(KI 13).

Heart gallbladder deficiency: add Xinshu(BL 15) and Danshu(BL 19).

13.4.6 Prevention

Pay attention to the cultivation of the mind. Pay attention to sleep hygiene. Establish a regular system of interests. Light diet, not overeat, not too much thick tea or coffee.

13.5 Cough

Cough, known as Ke Sou in Chinese, is a common problem that occurs in the lung-viscera system. Ke refers to coughing with sound but without sputum production, while Sou to the presence of sputum without coughing sound. Clinically, the symptoms of Ke and Sou are combined together.

TCM treatment of cough here may be applicable to some respiratory diseases in western medicine in which cough is a major symptom, such as upper respiratory infection, acute and chronic laryngopharyngitis or bronchitis, pneumonia, cough variant asthma and bronchiectasis.

13.5.1 Etiology and pathogenesis

Cough is usually caused by the failure of the lung qi in dispersion and descent or adverse ascent of the lung qi, which results from the attack of six external pathogenic factors or zang-fu viscera dysfunction.

13.5.1.1 Six external pathogenic factors attacking the lung

When the weather changes suddenly or abnormally, the lung is attacked externally from mouth, nose, body hair and skin, by pathogenic wind, cold, summer-heat, dampness, dryness or fire. The lung qi fails in dispersion and descent, which leads to the adverse ascent of the lung qi and causes cough.

13.5.1.2 Deficiency of the lung

Prolonged diseases in the lung-organ system may consume the lung qi and lung yin, which affects function of lung in governing qi and thus causes cough.

13.5.1.3 Dysfunction of other zang-fu viscera

Zang-fu viscera' dysfunction may block the ascent and descent of qi flow and impair the lung's function in governing qi, which also causes cough. The phlegm-dampness due to spleen deficiency, fire transformed from liver qi stagnation or kidney qi deficiency may affect the lung and induce cough.

The following factors like improper diet, excessive drinking or smoking, or excessive intake of spicy, greasy food, may cause the spleen dysfunction of transportation and transformation. Then phlegm-dampness occurs in the body, which affects the lung and causes cough. As the saying goes: "The spleen is the origin of phlegm production and the lung is the place where phlegm stays."

Stress, anger and other emotional upset cause liver qi stagnation, which may transform into liver fire over time. Liver fire flame upwards through the liver channel, which may cause adverse ascent of lung qi and cause cough.

The kidney is the root of qi and takes in qi. Therefore, deficient kidney qi, or yin-yang deficiency may result in the kidney failure in intake of qi and cause the adverse ascent of lung qi, which is followed by cough.

13.5.2 Diagnosis

Cough can be diagnosed by cough with or without sputum. Cough is generally divided into cough due to external attack and cough due to internal injury. The former is characterized by a sudden onset, a short duration and the symptoms of exterior syndrome, while the latter is characterized by recurrent attack, a prolonged duration and the symptoms of other zang-fu viscera' dysfunction.

13.5.3 Differentiation

Cough is mainly caused by the lung and closely related to the liver, spleen, and kidney. As the saying goes, "Dysfunction of all of five zang viscera and six fu viscera can cause cough besides the lung". Cough due to external attack usually manifests excess syndrome and cough due to internal injury manifests deficiency in root but excess in symptoms such as phlegm-dampness, phlegm-heat and liver fire.

13.5.3.1 Cough due to external attack

(1) Wind-cold attacking the lung

Cough with heavy sound, clear thin white sputum, itchy throat, fast breathing, stuffy nose with clear discharge, headache, limbs soreness, aversion to cold, fever, no sweating, thin and white coating and floating and tight pulse.

(2) Wind-heat attacking the lung

Cough with difficult expectoration, fast breathing, dry sore throat, sticky thick yellow sputum, stuffy nose with yellow discharge, thirst, headache, fever, red tongue with thin yellow coating and floating rapid or slippery pulse.

(3) Wind-dryness attacking the lung

Frequent cough with scanty sticky sputum or with no sputum or with blood-streaked sputum, itchy or dry sore throat, dry lips and nose, stuffy nose, headache, aversion to wind or cold, fever, dry red tongue with thin white or yellow coating and floating rapid pulse.

13.5.3.2 Cough due to internal injury

(1) Phlegm-dampness accumulating the lung

Cough with heavy sound, profuse sticky white sputum and easy expectoration, chest tightness, cough relieved after expectoration, lassitude, abdominal distension and fullness, nausea or vomiting, loose stools, greasy white coating, soft moderate pulse.

(2) Phlegm-heat accumulating in the lung

Cough with profuse sticky thick yellow sputum or with foul-smelling or bloody sputum, fast breathing or even wheezing sound in the throat, distension and fullness or even pain in the chest and hypochondriac region, red face, mild fever, dry mouth with a desire to drink water, red tongue with thin greasy yellow coating and slippery rapid pulse.

(3) Liver fire affecting the lung

Paroxysmal cough with scanty sticky sputum, difficult expectoration, flushed face, distending pain in the chest and hypochondriac region, dry throat, bitter taste in the mouth, the symptoms variable with emotional fluctuation, dry red tongue with thin yellow coating and wiry rapid pulse.

(4) Lung yin consumption

Abrupt short cough with scanty sticky white sputum or with blood-streaked sputum or without sputum, tidal fever, flushed cheeks in the afternoon, night sweating, dry mouth and throat, a red tongue with scanty coating, a rapid thready pulse.

13.5.4 Treatment

13.5.4.1 Chinese herbal treatment

（1）Cough due to external attack

To disperse the lung and eliminate external pathogenic factors.

1）Wind-cold attacking the lung

Treatment principle：To eliminate wind，dissipate cold，disperse the lung and stop cough.

Major Prescription：San'ao Tang plus Zhisou San variation.

Herbs：Mahuang，Xingren，Zhigancao，Shengjiang，Jingjie，Jiegeng，Baiqian，Chenpi，Baibu and Ziyuan.

Explanation：

San'ao Tang is applied to disperse the lung and dissipate the cold.

Zhisou San：to slightly disperse the lung，regulate the lung qi and stop cough.

Mahuang：to relieve the exterior and dissipate cold.

Xingren：to descend the lung qi and stop cough.

Zhigancao：to harmonize the actions of other herbs.

Ziyuan and Baibu：to resolve phlegm and stop cough.

Jiegeng and Baiqian：to disperse the lung qi and resolve phlegm.

Jinjie：to eliminate wind and relieve the exterior.

Chenpi：to regulate qi and resolve phlegm.

Modification：For cases with itchy throat，add Niubangzi and Chanyi；for cases with severe stuffy nose，add Cangerzi and Xinyihua；for cases with chest tightness with greasy coating，add Fuling，Banxia and Houpu.

2）Wind-heat attacking the lung

Treatment principle：To eliminate wind，clear heat and stop cough.

Major prescription：Sangju Yin variation.

Herbs：Sangye，Juhua，Lianqiao，Bohe，Jiegeng，Xingren，Lugen and Gancao.

Explanation：

Sangye：to eliminate wind and clear heat.

Juhua，Xingren and Jiegen：to disperse wind-heat and descend the lung qi.

Lianqiao，Bohe and Lugen：to relieve the exterior，clear heat and generate fluid.

Gancao：to coordinate the other herbs and soothe sore throat.

Modification：For cases with severe productive cough，add Chuanbeimu，Qianhu and Pipaye；for cases with fever，add Zhimu，Huangqin，Yuxingcao and Jinyinhua；for cases with sore throat and hoarse voice，add Niubangzi，Shegan and Shandougen；and for cases with thirst，add Tianhuafen and Zhimu.

3）Wind-dryness attacking the lung

Treatment principle：To eliminate wind，moisten dryness and stop cough.

Major Prescription：Sangxing Tang variation.

Herbs：Sangye，Douchi，Xingren，Xiangbeimu，Shashen，Lipi and Zhizi.

Explanation：

Sangye and Xingren：to clear heat，disperse and moisten the lung.

Douchi，Xiangbeimu and Shashen：to clear heat，moisten the throat and relieve cough.

Zhizi and Lipi：to clear the lung-heat，moisten the throat and relieve cough.

Modification：For cases with blood-streaked sputum，add Shengdihuang and Baimaogen；for cases with fluid damage, add Maidong, Shihu and Yuzhu; for cases with the lung-heat, add Shengshigao and Zhimu.

(2) Cough due to internal injury

To eliminate pathogenic factors and supplement anti-pathogenic qi.

1) Phlegm-dampness accumulating the lung

Treatment principle: To dry dampness, resolve phlegm, regulate qi and stop cough.

Major Prescription: Erchen Tang plus Sanzi Yangqin Tang variation.

Herbs: Jiangbanxia, Chenpi, Fuling, Juhong and Zhigancao, Suzi, Baijiezi and Laifuzi.

Explanation:

Erchen Tang: to resolve phlegm-dampness.

Sanzi Yangqin Tang: to warm the lung, resolve phlegm, descend the lung qi and promote digestion.

Jiangbanxia: to dry dampness and resolve phlegm.

Chenpi: to regulate qi and resolve phlegm and dampness combined with Banxia.

Fuling: to strengthen the spleen to resolve phlegm.

Zhigancao: to coordinate other herbs and harmonize the middle energizer.

Modification: For cases with poor appetite due to spleen deficiency, add Dangshen, Baizhu and Fuling; for cases with difficult expectoration, add Gualouren, Zhebeimu and Haifushi; for cases with cold-phlegm with symptoms such as sticky foamy white sputum, aversion to cold and cold sensation in the back, add Xixin and Ganjiang.

2) Phlegm-heat accumulating the lung

Treatment principle: To clear heat, disperse the lung qi, resolve phlegm and stop cough.

Major Prescription: Qingjin Huatan Tang variation.

Herbs: Huangqin, Zhizi, Jiegeng, Maidong, Sangbaipi, Beimu, Zhimu, Gualouren, Juhong, Fuling and Gancao.

Explanation:

Sangbaipi, Huangqin, Zhizi and Zhimu: to clear the lung-heat.

Beimu, Gualouren and Jiegeng: to clear heat and resolve phlegm.

Fuling, Juhong and Gancao: to regulate qi and resolve phlegm.

Modification: For cases with thick yellow sputum or with foul-smelling sputum, add Yuxingcao, Yiyiren and Dongguaren; for cases with profuse sputum, chest fullness and constipation, add Tinglizi and Dahuang; for cases with phlegm-heat impairing the lung fluid with symptoms, add Xianlugen, Tianhuafen and Beisharen; and for cases with fever and restlessness, add Zhimu and Shengshigao.

3) Liver fire affecting the lung

Treatment principle: To soothe the liver, clear the lung, resolve phlegm and stop cough.

Major Prescription: Xiebai San plus Daige San variation.

Herbs: Sangbaipi, Diguapi, Jingmi, Zhigancao, Qingdai and Haigeqiao.

Explanation:

Xiebai San: to clear the lung heat, relieve dyspnea cough.

Daige San: to clear the liver fire, facilitate the function of lung and relieve the restlessness.

Sangbaipi: to clear the lung-heat.

Diguapi: to reduce hidden fire in the lung and nourish the lung yin.

Jingmi and Zhigancao: to nourish the stomach and harmonize the middle energizer.

Qingdai: to clear toxic-heat in the liver channel.

Haigeqiao: to resolve phlegm and relieve cough.

Modification:For cases with pronounced liver fire,add Danpi and Zhizi;for cases with adverse ascent of the lung qi and chest oppression and,add Tinglizi,Zhike,and Gualou;for cases with chest fullness and hypochondriac pain,add Yujin and Sigualuo;for cases with sticky sputum,add Dannanxing,Haifushi and Zhebeimu;and for cases with fire injuring fluid,add Xianlugen,Maidong and Beisharen.

4)Lung yin consumption

Treatment principle:To nourish yin,clear heat,moisten the lung and stop cough.

Major Prescription:Shashen Maidong Tang variation.

Herbs:Shashen,Maidong,Yuzhu,Dong Sangye,Tianhuafen,Shengbiandou and Gancao.

Explanation:

Shashen,Maidong,Yuzhu and Tianhuafen:to nourish yin and moisten the lung.

Dong Sangye:to clear the lung-heat and descend the lung qi.

Shengbiandou and Gancao:to coordinate and harmonize the middle Jiao.

Modification:For cases with prolonged fever and cough due to dryness-heat in the lung,add Sangbaipi and Diguapi;for cases with blood-streaked sputum,add Zhizi,Danpi and Baimaogen;for cases with night sweating,add Shengmuli,Fuxiaomai and Nuodaogen;and for cases with cough with yellow sputum,add Huangqin,Haigefen and Zhimu.

13.5.4.2 Acupuncture & moxibustion treatment

(1)Cough due to external attack

Principal acupoints:Lieque(LU 7),Hegu(LI 4),Feishu(BL 13)and Taiyuan(LU 9)

Modification:For cases with wind-cold attack,add Fengmen(BL 12),for cases with wind-heat attack, add Dazhui(GV 14)and Quchi(LI 11);for cases with sore throat,add Shaoshang(LI 11)with pricking for bloodletting.

Methods:Reducing method is applied to the above points. Moxibustion can also be combined in wind-cold attack.

(2)Cough due to internal injury

Principal acupoints:Feishu(BL 13),Taiyuan(LU 9)and Sanyinjiao(SP 6)

Modification:For cases with phlegm-dampness in the lung,add Fenglong(SI 40),Zusanli(SI 36)and Pishu(BL 20);for cases with liver fire affecting the lung,add Xinjian(LR 2);for cases with lung yin consumption,add Gaohuang(BL 43);for cases with phlegm-heat accumulating the lung,add Chize(LU 5).

Methods:reinforcing manipulation is applied to Pishu(BL 20)and Zusanli(SI 36). Reducing method is applied to the rest points.

13.5.4.3 Tuina treatment

Principal acupoints and locations:Tiantu(CV 22),Danzhong(CV 17),Zhongfu(LU 1),Yunmen (LU 2),Shenzhu(GV 12),Dazhu(BL 11),Fengmen(BL 12),Feishu(BL 13),Dingchuan(EX-B 1), Fengchi(GB 20),Fengfu(GV 16),Jianjing(GB 21),hypochondriac region,chest and upper back.

Manipulations:One-finger pushing,kneading,pushing,rolling,grasping,wiping and scrubbing manipulations.

Basic procedure:

Patient takes a supine position:Apply one-finger pushing or kneading manipulation on the route from Tiantu(CV 22)to Danzhong(CV 17)for 5-10 times;apply pressing-kneading manipulation on Zhongfu(LU 1)and Yunmen(LU 2)for 1 minute each point;apply separate-pushing manipulation on the chest to hypochondriac region for 5-10 times;apply pressing-kneading manipulation on Chize(LU 5),Taiyuan(LU 9), Yuji(LU 10)and Lieque(LU 7)for 1 minute each point;apply grasping-kneading manipulation on Hegu(LI

4) for 1 minute;

Patient takes a prone position: Apply rolling manipulation on upper back along the urinary bladder channel for 3-5 times; apply pressing-kneading manipulation on Dazhu(BL 11), Dingchuan(EX-B 1), Shenzhu(GV 12), Fengmen(BL 12) and Feishu(BL 13) for 1 minute each point; apply grasping manipulation on Jianjing(GB 21).

Modification: For cases with wind-cold attacking the lung, add applying scrubbing manipulation on the upper back along the urinary bladder channel till hot sensation appears; for cases with wind-heat attacking the lung, add applying pressing-kneading Quchi(LI 11) and patting on the upper back till hot sensation appears; for cases with phlegm-dampness accumulating the lung, add pressing-kneading Fenglong(SI 40) and Zusanli(SI 36), wiping on the chest till hot sensation appears; for cases with phlegm-heat or liver fire, add pressing-kneading Taichong(LR 3), palm-twisting hypochondrium.

13.5.5　Prevention

Keep warm. Keep a light diet and avoid sweet, salty, greasy and spicy food. Try to expectorate sputum with the assist of tapping the back or sputum aspirator. Give up cigarette smoking or alcohol drinking, do more outdoor exercises and keep a good ventilation of the room. Keep a peaceful mind.

13.6　Asthma

Asthma is a paroxysmal respiratory disease that occurs when lung qi fails to disperse and descend in the latent phlegm body. It is a joint name for wheezing syndrome and dyspnea syndrome, which is characterized by recurrent attacks of dyspnea with bronchial wheezing. "Wheezing" refers to polypnea with phlegm rale in the throat. "Dyspnea" means hasty panting, with the mouth open and shoulders raised, and inability to lie flat.

According to the *Internal Classic*, which records "The lung may thus be damaged and wheezing will ensue". In the treatise on the differentiation of yin and yang chapter, the clinical feature of wheezing is similar to asthma, though there's not an exact name. In the Han Dynasty, by stating "for coughing with qi ascent and a frog-like rale in the throat, Shegan Mahuang Tang is indicated", Zhang Zhongjing presented the typical symptoms and treatment when asthmatic attack happened. In Yuan Dynasty, Zhu Danxi created the phrases of asthma disease, and pointed out the therapeutic principles. During the Ming Dynasty, Yu Tuan made an explicit differentiation between "wheezing" and "dyspnea". He suggested that wheezing could be confirmed with sound, and panting with breath.

In western medicine the relevant disease includes bronchial asthma, asthmatic bronchitis, allergic asthma and cardiac asthma.

Asthma is a problem worldwide, with an estimated 300 million affected individuals in different countries. The prevalence has been decreasing in Western Europe but increasing in regions such as Africa, Latin America, Eastern Europe and Asia. Annually, asthma causes 346 000 deaths worldwide and 13. 8 million disability adjusted life years(DALYs) each year. Asthma occurs frequently between seasons and is common in child especially under the age of five.

13.6.1　Etiology

13.6.1.1　Exogenous pathogenic factors

Due to the attack of wind-cold, wind-heat or inhalation of extrinsic factors such as smoke, pollen, animals fur and irritant gas, the lung qi may fail to disperse and descend, which causes the disturbance of water metabolism and the stagnation of phlegm-wetness. Thus, asthma happens.

13.6.1.2 Irregular diet

Over-consumption of raw and cold, spicy, sweet and fatty food affects the transportation and transformation of spleen and the digestive function of stomach, leading to phlegm-turbidity or phlegm-heat, and the excessive phlegm could directly flame up along the meridian of lung, block the airway and cause asthma.

13.6.1.3 Deficiency status

The deficiency of lung, spleen or kidney due to the constitutional or post illness may damage body resistance and affect water metabolism. This may cause the susceptibility to allergic factors, such as infant asthma owing to the congenital kidney qi deficiency, and the retention of phlegm-fluid. Also, lung yin deficiency could cause deficient fire which may evaporate body fluids to be the phlegm-turbidity stagnation in the lung, subsequently resulting in asthma.

13.6.2 Pathogenesis

13.6.2.1 Pathogenic site

Asthma is mainly located in lung and closely associated with the spleen and kidney. Besides, because the conditions between each organ are closely related, the heart and liver may also be involved.

Phlegm-dampness, the predominant factor during asthma, may be produced by the dysfunction of spleen due to the improper diet. Phlegm could affect the water metabolism by blocking the normal flow of qi. As the lung dominates qi and is the container of phlegm, and the kidney is responsible for deep breath and is the root of phlegm, the main pathogenic site contains lung, spleen and kidney.

By means of association with the circulation of fluid and qi, liver should also be involved. On one hand, the liver qi stagnation could hinder the fluid movement, On the other hand, such status always transforms into fire conditions and evaporates body fluids. Both of them will lead to phlegm.

Since the blood circulation is closely connected with heart and lung, severe deficiency of lung may damage heart function. Thus, it leads to the deadly wheeling collapse.

13.6.2.2 Pathological nature

Asthma should be divided into acute and relieving stages, which means asthenia in origin and sthenia in superficiality. The sthenia in symptom appears in the acute stage while the asthenia in viscera happens in the relieving stage. The sthenia in symptom exhibits different characteristics for various exogenous pathogenic factors: wind, cold, heat, etc. Besides, the asthenia in zang-fu viscera should distinguish both the main sites and the natures of yin, yang or qi.

13.6.2.3 Basic pathogenesis

The fundamental cause of asthma lies in phlegm-qi binding and obstructing the airway due to the exogenous pathogen induced by the latent phlegm in the body.

13.6.2.4 Pathogenesis in different disease stages

In attack stage, the main pathogenesis is phlegm blocking the airway causing the failure of lung to disperse and descend, which triggers wheezing and panting. The common factors include external pathogen, emotional stress, irregular diet, fatigue, etc. The main factor should be the sudden climate change. Due to the differentiation between constitution and causes, the sthenia in symptom differs in four conditions: cold, heat, deficiency and excess. The categories include:

Cold asthma is due to the exposure to external cold or lack of vital energy.

Pyretic asthma is due to the external heat or the constitutional yang excess.

Frigiopyretic asthma is due to the external cold and the internal pyretic.

Anemophlegmatic asthma is due to the latent phlegm in the lung and the external wind attack.

Deficient asthma is due to the recurrent episode of asthma, manifesting in the insufficient symptoms. The lung, spleen and kidney could be sick concurrently, owing to the interrelationships between viscera.

In the status asthmatics, the sthenia in the root and sthenia in the branch could emerge at the same time, which is characterized with the persistent dyspnea. If the lung qi can't assist the blood circulation and the fire in vital gate is too weak to support the heart yang, the collapse due to dyspnea will happen then.

In the remission stage, the deficiency of qi is the predominate factor to the insufficient symptoms. However, the character is the combination of deficiency and excess. For example, the excess syndrome could transform into the deficient syndrome when yin, yang or qi is damaged by the pathogenic products. Besides, because yin, yang and qi are fundamental materials in metabolism, the deficiency of them create the pathogenic products, which could increase the deficiency symptoms and thus cause the boundless cycle between deficiency and excess.

13.6.3   Diagnosis

13.6.3.1   Disease diagnosis

Because of the factors such as sudden change, unsuitable foods and emotional disorder, it typically has recurrent wheezing, dyspnea, inability to lie flat, even pale complexion, cyanotic lips and nails that could last for minutes or hours. Previous symptoms include rhinocnesmus, sneeze, cough and chest distress.

If the wheezing or panting can't be relieved constantly, it should be treated as the status asthmaticus.

The patient's behavior is usually normal except for a bit fatigue, a poor appetite or abundant phlegm.

A history of other allergic diseases(eczema or allergic rhinitis)or asthma is in first-degree relatives.

The blood tests, the function of lung and the X-ray could be auxiliary examinations.

13.6.3.2   Differential diagnosis

Asthma should be distinguished from dyspnea and pleural fluid retention.

(1)The difference between asthma and dyspnea

Asthma is the combination name of wheezing and dyspnea, which is characterized by paroxysmal whistling sounds in the throat and the breathless while dyspnea involves panting rapidly, not necessarily accompanied by the wheezing sounds.

(2)The difference between asthma and pleural fluid retention

Pleural fluid retention is characterized by coughing, panting, chest fullness or pain after a persistent and forceful coughing, not involving wheezing sounds as asthma.

13.6.4   Pattern identification and treatment

13.6.4.1   Major points

Before the treatment, it is necessary to distinguish a deficiency syndrome from an excess syndrome.

During the acute stage, cold, pyretic, frigiopyretic and anemophlegmatic asthma is included as excessive patterns.

During the remission stage, the deficiency of the lung, spleen, and kidney is often included.

13.6.4.2   Treatment principles

General principles during the acute stage are dispelling phlegm, directing qi and relieving asthma. Specifically, warming the lung, eliminating cold resolving phlegm, regulating the lung qi downward for cold asthma and dissipating heat, dispersing the lung, resolving phlegm, and directing qi downward for pyretic asthma.

General principles during the remission stage are supplying qi, tonifying yang, nourishing yin and also strengthening the lung, spleen or kidney for deficient patterns.

13.6.4.3 Treatment based on pattern identification

(1) Cold asthma

Clinical manifestations: Patients may have wheezing dyspnea, tachypnea, shortness of breath, a sense of fullness and tightness in the chest, mild cough with dilute, whitish and frothy sputum which is difficult to spit out, no thirst or thirst with preference for hot drinks, pale or bluish complexion, cold limbs and coldness intolerance. The typical symptoms could be triggered by cold weather or getting cold.

Tongue: Pale tongue with whitish and greasy coating.

Pulse: Wiry tight pulse or floating tight pulse.

Analysis of clinical manifestations: Wheezing dyspnea and tachypnea may be induced by the latent-cold phlegm in the lung and the narrow airway due to the obstruction of the phlegm-qi conjugate. Cold and phlegm may block the lung and cause an inability of lung qi to disperse, which causes the sensation of fullness or tightness in the chest and mild cough. Lack of heat pathogen or pathogenic products, patients neither bring out thirst nor prefer hot water. Because the esoteric cold could trigger the intent fluid retention, the asthma will attack during the cold weather. As internal yin excess overwhelms yang qi, the bluish complexion, cold limbs and cold intolerance will come together. The features of the tongue and pulse are typical signs for cold excess. Treatment principle: Disseminate the lung, eliminate cold, reduce phlegm and relieve asthma.

1) Chinese herbal treatment

Prescription: Shegan Mahuang Tang or Xiaoqinglong Tang variation.

Herbs: Zhimahuang, Shegan, Ganjiang, Xixin, Zhibanxia, Ziwan, Kuandonghua, Wuweizi, Dazao, Gancao.

Explanation:

Zhimahuang and Shegan: to ventilate lung, relieve dyspnea, resolve phlegm and benefit throat.

Ganjiang, Xixin and Zhibanxia: to warm lung, reduce fluid retention and bring adverse qi downward.

Ziwan and Kuandonghua: to resolve phlegm to stop cough.

Wuweizi: to astringe lung qi.

Dazao and Gancao: to coordinate the drug actions and harmonize the middle energizer.

Modification: For cases with chills, fever and body ache, add Guizhi, Ganjiang to reduce wind and ventilate cold; for cases with excessive phlegm with inability to lie flat, add Tinglizi to purge lung and direct qi downward. It is also necessary to add Xinren, Suzi, Baiqian, and Jupi to resolve phlegm and associate the circulation of qi; for cases with severe cough with breathlessly and profuse sweat, Baishao, should be added to astringe lung qi.

2) Acupuncture & moxibustion

General prescription: Feishu(BL 13), Tiantu(CV 22), Chize(LU 5), Lieque(LU 7), Fengmen(BL 12).

Acupoints & methods: A reduced manipulation should be given to the above points. The needles are retained for 15−30 minutes. Give the treatment qd or qod.

Explanation:

Feishu: to treat cough, asthma, chest pain, spitting of blood, afternoon fever, night sweating, etc.

Tiantu: treat asthma, cough, sore throat, dry throat, hiccup, sudden hoarseness of the voice, difficulty in swallowing.

Chize: treat cough, hemoptysis, afternoon fever, asthma, sore throat, fullness in the chest, infantile convulsions, spasmodic pain of the elbow and arm, mastitis, etc.

Lieque: to treat the headache, migraine, neck rigidity, cough, asthma, sore throat, facial paralysis, toothache, pain and weakness or the wrist, etc.

Fengmen: to treat common cold, cough, fever and headache, neck rigidity, backache, etc.

Modification: For cases of severe asthma add, Dingchuan(EX-B 1); for cases of excessive sputum, add Fenglong(ST 40) to remove the sputum.

(2) Pyretic asthma

Clinical manifestations: The symptoms include ecphysesis with roar like wheezing, breath with gruff voice, fullness in chest and hypochondrium, frequent cough with yellow and thick sputum which is difficult to spit out, a bitter taste in the mouth, fell thirst and prefer to drink water, sweating, red face or general fever. Some cases are triggered in the summer.

Tongue: Red tongue with thin and yellow greasy coating.

Pulse: Slippery rapid pulse or tight slippery pulse.

Analysis of clinical manifestations: Heat and phlegm may block the airway and cause the inability of lung qi to disperse and descend, which causes the ecphysesis with roar like wheezing, breath with gruff voice, fullness in chest and hypochondrium and frequent cough. The combining heat-phlegm evaporates the latent phlegm and causes the yellow and thick sputum which is difficult to spit out. It also evaporates the body fluid and causes the bitter taste in the mouth and thirst fell desire to drink water. Excess of inner heat causes the sweating, red face or general fever. The features of the tongue and pulse are typical signs for heat excess.

Treatment principle: Regulate the lung and clear away heat, resolve phlegm, relieve asthma and sent the adverse qi down.

1) Chinese herbal treatment

Prescription: Dingchuan Tang or Yuebijia Banxia Tang variation.

Herbs: Zhimahuang, Huangqin, Xingren, Banyi, Kuandonghua, Zi Suzi, Baiguo, Gancao.

Explanation:

Zhimahuang: to ventilate lung and relieve dyspnea.

Huangqin and Sangbaipi: to clear heat and regulate the function of lung qi.

Xingren, Banxia, Kuandonghua and Zisuzi: to resolve phlegm and bring adverse qi downward.

Baiguo: to astringe lung qi and restrain the excessive disperse from Mahuang.

Gancao: to coordinate the drug actions.

Modification: For cases with exterior cold binding with internal intense lung-heat, add Shengshigao, Gypsum Fibrosum(initial usage) to clear the internal heat; for cases with inability to lie flat, add Tingliziz and Guangdilong to clear lung and stop panting; for cases with excessive lung heat and spit yellow and thick sputum, add Haigeqiao, Shegan, Zhimu and Yuxingcao to remove heat-phlegm; for cases with constipation, add Dahuang, Gualou, Mangxiao and Zhishi to remove heat by catharsis; for cases with prolonged heat which impairs body fluids and cause the rapid breathing, coughing with a little thick phlegm mixed with blood, dry and sore throat, red and dry tongue and thready rapid pulse, use Maimendong Tang or other drugs such as Shashen, Zhimu, Tianhuafen to nourish yin and clear inner heat.

2) Acupuncture & moxibustion

General prescription: Feishu(BL 13), Tiantu(CV 22), Chize(LU 5), Dazhui(GV 14).

Acupoints & methods: a reduced manipulation should be given to the above points. The needles are retained for 15-30 minutes. Cupping can be applied on the back points too.

Explanation:

Feishu: to treat cough, asthma, chest pain, spitting of blood, afternoon fever, night sweating, etc.

Tiantu: to treat asthma, cough, sore throat, dry throat, hiccup, sudden hoarseness of the voice, difficulty in swallowing.

Chize: to treat cough, hemoptysis, afternoon fever, asthma, sore throat, fullness in the chest, infantile convulsions, spasmodic pain of the elbow and arm, mastitis, etc.

Dazhui could be used in common cold, fever, cough, convulsion, lumbar and back pain.

Modification: The same as type one.

(3) Frigiopyretic asthma

Clinical manifestations: Patients may undergo wheezing dyspnea, tachypnea, shortness of breath, a febrile sensation and fullness in the chest, dysphoria, chills, fever and body ache, absence of sweat, cough with yellow and thick or yellow and white sputum which is difficult to spit out, thirst with desire to drink water and feces lack of fluid.

Tongue: Red tip and margin of tongue with white bias in yellow and greasy coating.

Pulse: wiry tight pulse.

Analysis of clinical manifestations: The airway may be blocked or narrow due to the heat-phlegm binding, thus cause the inability of lung qi to disperse and descend which results in wheezing dyspnea, tachypnea, shortness of breath and febrile sensation and fullness in the chest subsequently. External cold attacking the Taiyang channel and staying in the skin would impair the circulation of defense qi, then causes the chills, absence of sweat, fever and body ache. The combining heat-phlegm evaporates the body fluid and then causes thirst and desire to drink water. The features of the tongue and pulse are typical signs for cold external and heat-phlegm internal excess.

Treatment principle: Relieve superficial pathogenic factors: to dissipate cold, clear away heat and eliminating sputum.

1) Chinese herbal treatment

Prescription: Xiaoqinglong plus Shigao Tang or Houpo Hahuang Tang variation.

Herbs: Mahuang, Shigao, Houpo, Xingren, Shengjiang, Banxia, Dazao, Gancao.

Explanation:

Mahuang: to ventilate lung.

Shigao: to relieve lung-heat, the combination of both two could disseminate exterior cold and remove the interior heat.

Houpo and Xingren: to relieve asthma and stop cough.

Shengjiang and Banxia: to resolve phlegm and bring adverse qi downward.

Dazao and Gancao: to coordinate the drug action.

Modification: For cases with severe outside cold, add Guizhi, Xixin; for cases with excessive phlegm with panting, add Tinglizi, Suzi, Shegan to resolve phlegm and relieve asthma; for cases with yellow and thick sputum which is difficult to spit out, add Huangqin, Qianhu, Gualoupi should to remove the phlegm-heat.

2)Acupuncture & moxibustion

General prescription：Feishu(BL 13),Tiantu(CV 22),Chize(LU 5),Lieque(LU 7),Fengmen(BL 12),Dazhui(GV 14),Hegu(LI 4),Danzhong(CV 17).

Acupoints & methods：A reduced manipulation should be given to the above points. The needles are retained for 15−30 minutes.

Explanation：

Feishu,Tiantu,Chize,Lieque,Fengmen and Dazhui were mentioned above.

Hegu：to treat headache,neck pain,redness,swelling and pain of the eye,epistaxis,toothache,deafness,etc.

Danzhong：to treat asthma,pain in the chest,fullness in the chest,palpitation,insufficient lactation,difficulty in swallowing,etc.

Modification：the same as type one.

(4)Anemophlegmatic asthma

Clinical manifestations：The symptoms include excessive sputum in the throat with the voice similar to sawing wood or whistle,panting and tachypnea,a sense of fullness in the chest,orthopnea and inability to lie flat,frothy sputum or sticky sputum which is hard to spit out,acute break with the sense organs itch,sneeze in the beginning.

Tongue：Thick and greasy coating with normal tongue.

Pulse：Floating pulse.

Analysis of clinical manifestations：Wind could trigger the latent-phlegm in the body,which may affect the function of lung qi and hinder the airway simultaneously. As a result,patients may get the fullness sensation in the chest,wheezing sounds in the throat,typical sputum,panting and hard to lie flat.

Treatment principle：Eliminate wind,resolve phlegm and direct lung qi downward.

1)Chinese herbal treatment

Prescription：Sanzi Yangqin Tang plus Erchen Tang variation.

Herbs：Suzi,Baijiezi,Laifuzi,Jiangbanxia,Chenpi,Xingren,Jiangcan,Houpo,Fuling,Mahuang.

Explanation：

Suzi：to direct lung qi downward and stop asthma.

Baijiezi：to ventilate lung qi and resolve phlegm.

Laifuzi：to assist Suzi to directs lung qi and reduce phlegm.

Mahuang：to ventilate lung and relieve dyspnea.

Xingren and Jiangcan：to eliminate wind,resolve phlegm.

Houpo,Banxia and Chenpi：to resolve phlegm and bring adverse qi downward.

Fuling：to invigorate spleen to dissolve phlegm.

Modification：For cases with severe panting with inability to lie flat, add Tinglizi and Zaojiaoci or Kunxian Dan；for cases with the attack triggered by the exotic wind evil, add Suye, Fangfeng, Caoercao, Chanyi and Dilong.

2)Acupuncture & moxibustion

The same as type one.

(5)Deficient asthma

Clinical manifestations：Patients may have frequent and chronic relapse, wheezing in the throat, low voice,breathlessness which become more serious after exercise,weakness of the lung qi. With the deficiency of yang,dilute and pale sputum,no thirst,wind intolerance,pale or even dark-purple complexion and lips, white coating tongue and thready deep pulse would be exhibited.

As for insufficiency of yang：Stick sputum or lack of sputum，flushed cheeks，fever，red tongue with little far and deep and thready pulse.

Analysis of clinical manifestations：The basic pathogenesis is due to the frequent and chronic relapse，the phlegm and qi binding together，then，cause the blockage of lung qi and also damage the organs such as lung and kidney，and finally create the dysfunction of lung's director of qi and kidney's storage.

Treatment principle：Invigorate the lung，strengthen the kidney，resolve phlegm and bring adverse qi downward.

1）Chinese herbal treatment

Prescription：Pingchuan Guben Tang variation.

Herbs：Dangshen，Huangqi，Chenxiang，Suzi，Qidai，Hutaorou，Banxia，Kuandong，Jupi，Dongchongxiacao，Wuweizi.

Explanation：

Dangshen and Huangqi：to reinforce the lung.

Hutaorou，Chenxiang，Qidai，Dongchongxiacao and Wuweizi：to strengthen the kidney and keep the inspired air going downward.

Suzi，Banxia，Kuandong and Jupi：to keep the inspired air going downward and dispel phlegm.

Modification：For cases with deficiency of kidney yang，add Fuzi，Lujiaopian，Buguzhi and Zhongrushi；for cases with lack of yin，add Shashen，Maidong，Shengdi and Danggui；for cases with excessive panting after moving and direct the qi to be downward，add Zishiyin，Cishi；for cases with dark purple lips and the obstruction of phlegm，add Taoren and Sumu.

2）Acupuncture & moxibustion

General Prescription：Feishu（BL 13），Gaohuang（BL 43），Qihai（CV 6），Danzhong（CV 17），Zhongfu（LU 1）.

Acupoints & methods：A reinforced manipulation should be given to the above points. The needles are retained for 15–30 minutes. Both the moxibustion could be used.

Explanation：

Feishu，Qihai and Danzhong are mentioned above.

Gaohuang：to treat pulmonary tuberculosis，cough，asthma，spitting of blood，night sweating，poor memory，nocturnal emission，etc.

Zhongfu：to treat treating cough，asthma，pain in the chest，shoulder and back，fullness of the chest，etc.

（6）Status asthmatics

Clinical manifestations：Patients may present severe dyspnea with an open mouth，raised shoulders and inability to lie flat，wheezing sound in the throat，restlessness，unconsciousness，cyanotic complexion，peripheral coldness，bead-like sweats.

Tongue：bluish tongue with greasy or floating fur.

Pulse：thready and rapid pulse，large and forceless pulse or fainting pulse.

Analysis of clinical manifestations：The excessive phlegm could not only block the dispersing and descending function of lung qi which cause the severe dyspnea with an open mouth，raised shoulders and inability to lie flat and wheezing sound in the throat，but also block upper orifices which cause the unconsciousness. Due to the blockage of phlegm，the energy can't be transported all over，cyanotic complexion and peripheral coldness happen then. The features of the tongue and pulse are typical signs for deficiency.

Treatment principle: Tonify yang and prevent collapse.

1) Chinese herbal treatment

Prescription: Huiyang Jiuji Tang and Shengmai Yin variation.

Herbs: The ingredients of Huiyang Jiuji Tang: Fuzi, Ganjiang, Rougui, Shengshaishen, Baizhu, Fuling, Ganpi, Zhigancao, Wuweizi, Banxia, and Shexiang.

The ingredients of Shengmai Yin: Renshen, Maidong, Wuweizi.

Explanation:

Huiyang Jiuji Tang: to recuperate depleted yang and rescue the patient from collapse, and supplement qi to activate pulse, to cure syndrome of dominance of internal cold and exhaustion of yang qi.

Shengmai Yin: to strengthen qi and nourish yin, to cure weakness of qi and yin.

Modification: For cases with severe panting, restlessness, bead-like sweat with cold limbs, thick-purple tongue and thready pulse, take Heixi Dan immediately; for cases with serious weakness of yang, breathlessness and sweat with cold limbs, add Rougui and Ganjiang; for cases with rapidly panting, restlessness, bead-like sweat and dry mouth with red tongue, add Shengdi and Yuzhu to nourish yin.

2) Acupuncture & moxibustion

General prescription: Feishu(BL 13), Shenshu(BL 23), Neiguan(PC 6), Shuigou(CV 26), Qihai(CV 6), Guanyuan(CV 3), Shenque(CV 8) and Qishe(ST 11).

Acupoints & methods: A reinforced manipulation should be given to the above points. The needles are retained for 15–30 minutes. Both the moxibustion could be use in Qihai(CV 6), Guanyuan(CV 3), and Shenque(CV 8).

Explanation:

Feishu: same as type one.

Shenshu: to cure nocturnal emission, impotence, enuresis, irregular menstruation, leukorrhea, low back pain, knee weakness, blurring vision, dizziness, tinnitus, deafness, edema, asthma, diarrhea, etc.

Neiguan: to treat cardiac pain, palpitation, stuffy chest, pain in the hypochondriac region, stomachache, nausea, vomiting, hiccup, mental disorders, malaria and pain of the elbow and arm, etc.

Shuigou: to treat mental disorders, epilepsy, hysteria, infantile convulsion, coma, apoplexy-faint, trismus, deviation of the mouth and eye, puffiness of the face, pain and stiffness of the lower back, etc.

Qihai: to cure abdominal pain, diarrhea, enuresis, nocturnal emission, impotence, hernia, edema, dysentery, constipation, asthma, uterine bleeding, irregular menstruation, dysmenorrhea, amenorrhea, morbid leukorrhea, postpartum hemorrhage, etc

Guanyuan: to treat enuresis, nocturnal emission, frequency of urination, retention of urine, hernia, irregular menstruation, morbid leukorrhea, uterine bleeding, postpartum hemorrhage, lower abdominal pain, indigestion, diarrhea, etc.

Shenque: to treat abdominal pain, borborygmus, diarrhea, prolapse of the rectum, etc.

Qishe: to cure treating sore throat, pain and rigidity of the neck, asthma, hiccup, goiter, etc.

(7) The remission stage-the deficiency of lung and spleen

Clinical manifestations: The symptoms include no strength to talk, shortness of breath, slight wheezing occasionally, lot of clear and white sputum, spontaneous sweating, aversion to wind, frequent common cold in changing seasons, sleepy, poor appetite and easy to be diarrhea.

Tongue: pale tongue with thin or white greasy coating.

Pulse: weak and soft pulse.

Analysis of clinical manifestations. Spleen qi deficiency may cause shortness of breath, sleepiness and little strength to talk. Spleen fails to transport and transform leading to poor appetite and easy to have diarrhea. Weakness of wei-defense qi leads to aversion to wind, frequent common cold in season-changing times and spontaneous sweating. Lung fails to handle qi and the dysfunction of lung qi to transform fluid lead to phlegm-fluid stagnation in the lung, causing shortness of breath, lots of clear and white sputum and slight wheezing occasionally.

Treatment principle:

Tonify the lung, invigorating spleen and strengthen the sickness of qi.

1) Chinese herbal treatment

Prescription: Liujunzi Tang variation.

Herbs: Dangshen, Baizhu, Fulin, Zhigancao, Chenpi, Banxia.

Explanation:

Dangshen, Baizhu, Fulin and Zhigancao: to invigorate spleen and replenish qi.

Chenpi and Banxia: to direct qi and dispel phlegm.

Modification: For cases with lack of qi and serious spontaneous sweat, add Huangqi and Fuxiaomai; for cases with lack of resistance of external evils, add Yupinfeng San for usual use; for cases with lack of spleen yang with cold limbs, add Guizhi and Ganjiang to warm yang and resolve fluid retention.

2) Acupuncture & moxibustion

General Prescriptio: Feishu(BL 13), Pishu(BL 13), Gaohuang(BL 43), Qihai(CV 6), Danzhong (CV 17), Zhongfu(LU 1), Zusanli(ST 36), Yinlingquan(SP 9).

Acupoints & methods: A reinforced manipulation should be given to the above points. The needles are retained for 15-30 minutes. Both the moxibustion could be used.

Explanation:

Feishu, Qihai and Danzhong are mentioned above.

Pishu: to treat epigastric pain, abdominal distension, jaundice, vomiting, diarrhea, dysentery, bloody stools, profuse menstruation, edema, anorexia, backache, etc.

Gaohuang: to treat pulmonary tuberculosis, cough, asthma, spitting of blood, night sweating, poor memory, nocturnal emission, etc.

Zhongfu: to treat cough, asthma, pain in the chest, shoulder and back, fullness of the chest, etc.

Zusanli: to treat gastric pain, vomiting, hiccup, abdominal distension, borborygmus, diarrhea, dysentery, constipation, mastitis, aching of the knee joint and leg, beriberi, edema, cough, asthma, dizziness, indigestion, mania, etc.

Yinlingquan: to treat abdominal pain and distension, diarrhea, dysentery, edema, jaundice, dysuria, enuresis, incontinence of urine, pain in the external genitalia, dysmenorrhea, pain in the knee, etc.

(8) The remission stage-the deficiency of lung and kidney

Clinical manifestations: The symptoms include shortness of breath, dyspnea that is triggered by physical exercises, difficulty in inhalation, cough with spicy sputum, tinnitus and rotating dizziness, aching and weakness of waist and knees, fluster and intolerance of work. With the kidney yang deficiency, cold limbs with coldness intolerance and pale complexion will occurr. With the lack of kidney yin, symptoms include feverish sensation of five-palm, hot flush, red cheeks, night sweating and dry mouth.

Tongue: red tongue with lack of liquid and thin coating or pale and plump tongue with white coating.

Pulse: rapid pulse or deep thready pulse.

Analysis of clinical manifestations: Lung fails to handle qi and the dysfunction of lung qi to transform fluid, leading to phlegm-fluid stagnation in the lung, shortness of breath and cough with spicy sputum. Kidney fails to receive qi, leading to shortness of breath, dyspnea and difficult in inhalation that is triggered by physical exercises. Essential deficiency of qi causes tinnitus and rotating dizziness, aching and weakness of waist and knee. The deficiency of kidney yang may cause internal cold with the symptoms such as cold limbs with coldness intolerance and pale complexion. The deficiency of kidney yin may cause internal deficient heat leading to feverish sensation of five-palm, hot flush, red cheeks, night sweating and dry mouth.

Treatment principle: Tonify the lung, strengthen the kidney.

1) Chinese herbal treatment

Prescription: Shengmai Dihuang Tang and Jinshui Liujun Jian variation.

Herbs: Shudihuang, Shanzhuyu, Hutaorou, Renshen, Maidong, Wuweizi, Fulin, Gancao, Banxia, Chenpi.

Explanation:

Shudihuang, Shanzhuyu and Hutaorou: to strengthen the kidney and assist qi to be received.

Renshen, Maidong and Wuweizi: to nourish the kidney yin.

Baizhu, Fulin and Zhigancao: to invigorate spleen and replenish qi.

Chenpi and Banxia: to direct qi and dispel phlegm.

Modification: For cases with tonifying the kidney yang, add Buguzhi, Lujiaopian, Zhifuzi and Rougui; for cases with lack of lung ying and qi, add Huangqi, Shashen, Baihe; for cases with insufficient kidney yin, add Shengdihuang, Dongchongxiacao, also the Heche Dazao Wan could be used to nourish yin; for cases with failing to receive qi, add Dongchongxiacao, Zishiying or Shenge San. In addition, the powder of Ziheche could be used normally.

2) Acupuncture & moxibustion

General prescription: Feishu(BL 13), Shenshu(BL 23), Gaohuang(BL 43), Qihai(CV 6), Danzhong (CV 17), Zhongfu(LU 1), Taixi(KI 3).

Acupoints & methods: A reinforced manipulation should be given to the above points. The needles are retained for 15–30 minutes. Both the moxibustion could be used.

Explanation:

Feishu, Qihai, Gaohuang, Zhongfuand, Danzhong are mentioned above.

Taixi: to treat sore throat, toothache, deafness, tinnitus, dizziness, spitting of blood, asthma, thirst, irregular menstruation, insomnia, nocturnal emission, impotence, frequency of micturition, pain in the lower back, etc.

Notes: In clinical practice, despite the unique features, the deficiency of the lung, spleen or kidney could occur independently or in combination. The symptoms include qi deficiency of the lung and spleen or lung and kidney, lack of yin of the lung and kidney or yang of spleen and kidney. In conclusion, an overall analysis prior to treatment is necessary.

13.6.5 Prognosis

Asthma is a chronic disease which could frequently relapse and hard to be cured. Most teenagers could be cured during the regularly medicine treatment and the resistance will be stronger as times go by. In contrast, as for an elderly or weak person, asthma is hard to be cured. The prolonged asthma and frequent relapse affect the function of spleen, kidney, even heart, which may case the deadly disease named lung distention.

13.6.6 Prevention

Keep warm and avoid being triggered by the sudden change of climate. Take measures to prevent common cold or flu. Try appropriate exercise according to your physical condition. Give up smoking. Be away from inhaling dust or other irritative gas. Avoid excessive intake of cold, greasy, sour, salty, sweet and marine food. Keep off overwork and maintain a peaceful mind. Take patented Chinese medicine such as Yupingfeng San or Shenqi Wan to strengthen body resistance.

13.7 Dysmenorrhea

Dysmenorrhea, also known as painful periods, or menstrual cramps, is characterized by periodic lower abdominal pain or other discomforts before, during or after menstruation. The pain may be even beyond tolerance and cause pale complexion, nausea, vomiting, cold sweating and cold limbs. Clinically, dysmenorrhea can be divided into primary one and secondary one based on the absence or presence of organic problems. Primary dysmenorrhea usually occurs since menarche, while secondary dysmenorrhea occurs after menarche. Dysmenorrhea often occurs among unmarried young women, among whom primary one is more common.

In western medicine, the higher levels of prostaglandins and other inflammatory mediators cause the uterus to contract, which is believed to be a major factor in the occurrence of primary dysmenorrhea. Other developmental problems, such as uterine hypoplasia, cervical stenosis or uterine over-flexion, may cause unsmooth menstrual flow and then cause painful periods. It is the most common gynecologic problem in women of all ages and races. Estimates of the prevalence of dysmenorrhea vary widely (16.8% to 81.3%), and rates as high as 90% have been recorded.

13.7.1 Etiology and pathogenesis

Dysmenorrhea is closely related to thoroughfare vessel, conception vessel and the uterus. Emotional upset, irregular life style or attack by six external pathogenic factors are the common causes of dysmenorrhea.

13.7.1.1 Qi stagnation and blood stasis

Emotional upset or external pathogenic factors may cause the disturbance of qi flow and thus blood stasis in uterus, which causes painful menstruation.

13.7.1.2 Congealed cold and dampness

If being attacked by cold, such as being caught in rain, contracting pathogenic cold, taking in cold drinks, sitting or lying on the cold or damp ground, the uterus may be affected by accumulation of cold and dampness, which leads to the unsmooth flow of qi and blood.

13.7.1.3 Deficiency of qi and blood

Congenital deficiency of qi and blood or consumption of qi and blood due to severe or prolonged diseases can lead to weak blood circulation, which causes pain due to malnutrition.

13.7.1.4 Deficiency of the kidney and liver

Insufficiency of congenital essence, excessive sexual activity or prolonged diseases may injury the liver and kidney, which causes yin-blood deficiency and thus malnutrition of uterus occurs.

13.7.1.5 Down-pouring dampness-heat

Dampness-heat attacks the body and affects thoroughfare and conception vessels or uterus, which leads to the stagnation of qi and blood and thus pain occurs.

13.7.2   Diagnosis and Differential Diagnosis

Periodic lower abdominal pain or painful lumbosacral region during, before or after menstruation. Common among young unmarried women.

Gynecological examination and ultrasound B can be applied to differentiate the primary dysmenorrhea from the secondary one.

Dysmenorrhea should be distinguished from the acute abdominal pain caused by extra-uterine pregnancy or torsion of ovarian cyst and also from the lower abdominal pain caused by acute pelvic inflammation, acute cystitis, urinary lithiasis, appendicitis, colitis or acute gastroenteritis etc.

13.7.3   Syndrome differentiation

13.7.3.1   Qi stagnation and blood stasis

Distending or bearing-down pain in the abdomen during menstruation or one or two days before, abundant amount of or scanty menses or inhibited dripping menses, or dark purple menses with clots or even with big pieces, pain is aggravated by pressing and relieved with clot discharge, distending pain in the breasts and hypochondriac region, dark purple tongue with petechiae on the edges, deep wiry pulse.

13.7.3.2   Congealed cold-dampness

Cold pain in the lower abdomen that occurs before or during menstruation, which may be aggravated by pressing and relieved by warming, scanty dark purple menses with clots, aversion to cold, loose stools, light purple tongue with greasy white coating, wiry deep pulse.

13.7.3.3   Deficiency of qi and blood

Persistent dull pain during or after menstruation, which may be relieved by pressing, bearing-down sensation, abundant amount of menses without any clot or scanty menses, pale complexion, dizziness and palpitation, fatigue, pale tongue with teeth-marked edges, thin coating and thready pulse.

13.7.3.4   Deficiency of the kidney and liver

Dull pain or cold and bearing-down sensation in the lower abdomen with soreness and distension in lumbar region one or two days after menstruation, thin scanty menses dark or light in color, tinnitus, dizziness, blurred vision, or tidal fever, malar flushing, pale tongue with thin white or yellowfur, deep thready pulse.

13.7.3.5   Down-pouring dampness-heat

Pain or burning sensation in the lower abdomen during menstruation, aggravated by pressing, distending pain in the lumbar region, or frequent pain in the lateral lower abdomen which is worsened at the beginning days of menstruation, frequently slight fever, thick darkish red menses with clots, thick yellowish vaginal discharge, scanty dark urine, a red tongue with greasy yellow coating, wiry rapid pulse.

13.7.4   Treatment

13.7.4.1   Chinese herbal treatment

(1) Qi stagnation and blood stasis

Treatment principle: To soothe the liver, regulate qi, remove blood stasis and relieve pain.

Major Prescription: Gexia Zhuyu Tang variation.

Herbs: Danggui, Chuanxiong, Chishao, Taoren, Zhiqiao, Yuanhu, Wulingzhi, Mudanpi, Wuyao, Xiangfu and Gancao.

Explanation:

Zhiqiao, Wuyao and Xiangfu: to regulate qi and harmonize the liver.

Danggui: to nourish and harmonize blood.

Chuanxiong, Chishao, Taoren and Mudanpi: to activate blood circulation and resolve blood stasis.

Yuanhu and Wulingzhi: to resolve blood stasis and relieve pain.

Gancao: to relieve pain and harmonize other herbs.

Modification: For cases with the stomach being attacked by the liver qi, add Wuzhuyu and Banxia; for cases with bearing-down and distending sensation in the lower abdomen, add Chaihu and Shengma.

(2) Congealed cold and dampness

Treatment principle: To warm the meridians to dispel cold, eliminate dampness to remove stasis and relieve pain

Major prescription: Shaofu Zhuyu Tang plus Fuling.

Herbs: Xiaohuixiang, Ganjiang, Yuanhu, Moyao, Danggui, Chuanxiong, Rougui, Chishao, Puhuang and wulingzhi, Fuling.

Explanation:

Rougui, Xiaohuixiang and Ganjiang: to warm the meridians, dispel cold and eliminate dampness.

Danggui, Chuanxiong and Chishao: to nourish blood, activate blood circulation and resolve blood stasis.

Yuanhu, wulingzhi, Puhuang and Moyao: to resolve blood stasis and relieve pain.

Cangzhu: to dry dampness and resolve the turbid.

Fuling: to strengthen the spleen and eliminate dampness by diuresis.

Modification: For cases with pronounced cold pain, add Danggui Jianzhong Tang plus Aiye (Folium Artemisiae Argyi) and Wuzhuyu.

(3) Deficiency of qi and blood

Treatment principle: to strengthen the spleen qi and nourish blood to relieve pain.

Major Prescription: Shengyu Tang variation.

Herbs: Rensheng, Huangqi, Danggui, Chuanxiong, Shudihuang, Baishao, Xiangfu and Yuanhu

Explanation:

Rensheng and Huangqi: to replenish qi.

Danggui, Chuanxiong, Shudihuang and Baishao: to nourish and harmonize blood.

Xiangfu and Yuanhu: to regulate qi and relieve pain.

Modification: For cases with soreness in the lumbar region, add Tusizi and Duzhong.

(4) Depletion of the liver and kidney

Treatment principle: To nourish blood, harmonize the liver, tonify the kidney and supplement the essence.

Major Prescription: Tiaogan Tang variation.

Herbs: Danggui, Baishao, Bajitian, Ejiao, Shanyao and Shanyurou.

Explanation:

Danggui and Baishao: to nourish blood and harmonize the liver.

Shanyurou: to nourish the liver and kidney and supplement the essence-qi.

Bajitian: to warm and tonify the kidney yang.

Ejiao: to nourish blood and yin.

Shanyao: to strengthen the spleen and replenish qi.

Modification：For cases with scanty menses，add Lujiaojiao.

（5）Down-pouring dampness-heat

Treatment principle：to clear heat，remove dampness，resolve blood stasis and relieve pain.

Major prescription：Qingre Tiaoxue Tang plus Yiyiren.

Herbs：Mudanpi，Huanglian，Shengdihuang，Danggui，Baishao，Chuanxiong，Honghua，Taoren，Yuanhu，Ezhu，Xiangfu，Hongteng and Yiyiren.

Explanation：

Mudanpi：to clear heat，cool blood and resolve blood stasis.

Shengdihuang：to clear heat and cool blood.

Huanglian：to clear toxic heat.

Danggui and Baishao：to nourish blood and harmonize the liver.

Chuanxiong，Honghua，Taoren and Ezhu：to activate blood circulation and resolve blood stasis.

Xiangfu and Yuanhu：to regulate qi and relieve pain.

Hongteng and Yiyiren：to remove dampness and resolve blood stasis.

13.7.4.2　Acupuncture & moxibustion

Principal acupoints：Guanyuan（CV 4），Zigong（EX-CA 1），Shiqizhui（EX-B 8），Sanyinjiao（SP 6）and Hegu（LI 4）

Modification：For cases with cold congealing and blood stasis，add Shenque（CV 8）and Guilai（SI 29）；for cases with qi stagnation and blood stasis，add Taichong（LR 3）and Xuehai（SP 10）；for cases with kidney qi deficiency，add Shenshu（BL 23）and Taixi（KI 3）；for cases with qi-blood deficiency，add Qihai（CV 6）and Zusanli（SI 36）.

Methods：Reducing manipulation on Hegu（LI 4）and Sanyinjiao（SP 6）. Reducing manipulation on the rest points for excess syndrome and reinforcing manipulation for deficiency syndrome.

13.7.4.3　Tuina

Principal acupoints and locations：Qihai（CV 6），Guanyuan（CV 4），Baliao（BL 31-34），Zhangmen（LR 13），Ganshu（BL 18），Geshu（BL 17），Pishu（BL 20），Weishu（BL 21），Shenshu（BL 23），Baliao（BL 31-34），Xuehai（SP 10），Sanyinjiao（SP 6），Zusanli（SI 36），Taixi（KI 3）and Yongquan（KI 1），back and lumbar area.

Manipulation：one-finger pushing，rubbing，kneading，pressing，grasping and scrubbing manipulations.

Basic procedure：patient takes a supine position：apply rubbing manipulation clockwise on lower abdomen；apply one-finger pushing or pressing-kneading manipulation on Qihai（CV 6）and Guanyuan（CV 4）for 3-5 minutes each point.

Patient takes a prone position：apply rolling manipulation on bilateral lumbar areas along the urinary bladder channel；apply pressing-kneading manipulations on Shenshu（BL 23），Baliao（BL 31-34）for 2-3 minutes each point；apply scrubbing manipulation on lumbosacral area and Baliao（BL 31-34）until it is warm enough in the local area.

Modification：For cases with qi stagnation and blood stasis，apply pressing and kneading manipulations on Zhangmen（LR 13），Ganshu（BL 18），Geshu（BL 17）and grasp Xuehai（SP 10）and Sanyinjiao（SP 6）until there is local distending feeling；for cases with cold-dampness coagulation，apply scrubbing manipulation first along governor vessel，and then，transversely over lumbosacral region until it is warm enough in the local area and apply pressing-kneading manipulation on Xuehai（SP 10）and Sanyinjiao（SP 6）；for cases with qi and blood deficiency，apply scrubbing manipulation along governor vessel，and then transversely over both sides of the back until it is warm enough in the local area，apply rubbing manipulation clockwise on the lower abdomen, applying pressing-kneading manipulations on Zhongwan(CV 12), apply pressing-kneading manipulations on Pishu(BL 20), Weishu(BL 21) and Zusanli(SI 36); in cases with liver-kidney depletion, apply scrubbing manipulation first along governor vessel, and then transversely over lumbar area until it is warm enough in the local area; apply pressing-kneading manipulations on Taixi(KI 3) and Yongquan(KI 1), Ganshu(BL 18) and Shenshu(BL 23).

13.7.5　Prevention

Keep warm during menstruation. Pay attention to menstrual hygiene. Have a proper rest and avoid over-strain. Avoid irritability and depression. Avoid cold drinks and strenuous exercises before and during menstruation.

13.8　Stomachache

Stomachache may be a paroxysmal, intermittent or seasonal disease which occurs when stomach qi fails to descend, qi stagnation and blood disorder, food retention or stomach qi blockage. The symptom manifests as pain in the stomach and upper abdomen.

Early in *Internal Classic*, there was a record of the stomachache when it still confused with real heart pain yet. Until the Song Jin Yuan Dynasty, "stomach pain" was firstly put forward as an independent disease. The name of "stomach pain" was firstly recorded in *Yixue Qiyuan(Medicine Origin)*. Then *Lanshi Micang(Secret Book of Orchid Chamber)*, for the first time, individually separated "stomach pain" as a disease and elaborated its etiology and pathogenesis, principle and treatment. Since then, "stomach pain" was treated as an independent disease. Also, the etiology and pathogenesis, principle and treatment of stomach pain were relatively and systematically understood. *Treatise on Diseases*, *Patterns*, and *Formulas Related to the Unification of the Three Etiologes* considered that the etiology of stomach pain was resulted from internal cause (damage by excess of seven emotions), external cause(invasion of six climatic exopathogens) and non-endo-non-exogenous cause(diet, overstrain and contacts with foreign substances), and the principle of treatment was to relieve pain by eliminating pathogens and helped the pattern differentiation to be much clear.

In western medicine the relevant disease includes acute and chronic gastritis, peptic ulcer, gastroptosis or prolapsed gastric mucosa, gastroneurosis, functional dyspepsia, gastric cancer and esophagitis.

13.8.1　Etiology

13.8.1.1　Exogenous pathogenic factors

Due to the attack of cold, heat or pathogenic damp especially the cold evil could obstruct the circulation of stomach qi, which caused the dysfunction of stomach qi, leading to pain.

13.8.1.2　Irregular diet

On the one hand, surfeit harms the spleen and stomach, leading to stomach distension and pain, or even abdominal pain and diarrhea. On the other hand, over-consumption of fatty, spicy or sweet food or alcohol will produce inner-heat and impair the descending of stomach qi, subsequently caused the gastric pain.

13.8.1.3　Emotional maladjusted

Emotional disorder such as excessive anger, upset or stress may damage liver and lead to the stagnation of liver qi, which not only hinder the movement of stomach qi, but also restrain the spleen and stomach, resulting in stomachache.

13.8.1.4   Deficiency status of the spleen and stomach

The spleen and stomach are the main organs for digestion. The improper diet or other factors which damage the two organs lead to the deficiency of spleen and stomach. Lack of spleen yang may produce internal deficient cold and neglect the duty to warm the stomach system, which may cause the pain in stomach. Lack of stomach yin may cause malnourishment of the stomach and subsequent pain in stomach.

13.8.1.5   Medicine injury

Over ingestion of cold-natured or hot-natured medications may hurt the stomach qi or stomach yin, which leads to the obstruction of digestion, then, cause the stomachache.

13.8.2   Pathogenesis

13.8.2.1   Pathogenic site

Stomachache is mainly located in the stomach, majorly relates with liver and spleen, and involves gallbladder and kidney.

According to the five elements theory, the liver, known as the resolute viscus, should be ascribed to the character of wood, and stomach, known as the sea of grains and water, should be ascribed to the character of earth. Because of the liver controlling dispersion, the pathogenic products which affect the circulation of qi may cause the stagnation of liver qi. As same as the restriction among wood and earth, the stagnation of liver qi may overact to the stomach and lead to the stomach pain subsequently. In addition, the stagnation of liver qi may transform into inner fire and damage stomach yin, which cause the malnourishment of the stomach.

Lack of spleen yang may produce internal deficient cold and neglect the duty to warm the stomach system, which may cause the pain in stomach.

The kidney is the gate of the stomach. The warm energy from kidney yang is essential to the transportation and transformation of the spleen and stomach. Lack of kidney yang may cause deficient cold in the spleen, leading to stomach pain.

13.8.2.2   Pathological nature

Stomach pain should be divided into cold or heat, excess or deficiency, qi level or blood level patterns. Above all, it should be ascribed to excess patterns and deficiency patterns.

Excess patterns include cold attacking the stomach, food retention, in coordination between liver and stomach, stasis of blood and dampness-heat stagnation of liver and stomach.

Deficiency patterns include deficiency of spleen qi and stomach qi, deficiency cold of spleen and stomach, deficiency of stomach yin.

Between excess syndrome and deficiency syndrome there is complication and transformation.

13.8.2.3   Basic pathogenesis

The fundamental of stomachache lies in disorder of qi and blood, imbalance of cold and heat, accumulation of pathological products such as dampness and stasis, which are consequences of improper diet, emotional disturbance, invasion by six exogenous pathogens or weakness of habitus, resulting in qi disorder, and ascending and descending disorder of spleen and stomach, then the chronic gastritis relative symptoms such as gastric distention and stomach pain are generated. It is usually manifested as asthenia in origin and sthenia in superficiality and deficiency complicated with excess. Asthenia in origin majorly performs as deficiency of spleen qi and stomach yin, while sthenia performs as qi stagnation, dampness-heat and blood stasis. The qi disorder of spleen and stomach is the most direct pathogenic factor.

13.8.3 Diagnosis

13.8.3.1 Disease diagnosis

Because of the external factors such as cold, overeating unsuitable foods, emotional disorder and hurt with medicines with the typical stomachache symptom or other manifestations of pain, with the associated symptoms such as poor palpitation, nausea, vomiting, acid regurgitation and belching with a foul breath.

The young and middle-aged patients are in the majority and the disease may frequently recur from acute or chronic way.

The normal blood tests, bilirubin, diastase tests, ultrasound and the CT scan as well as the X-ray could be the assistants.

13.8.3.2 Differential diagnosis

Before the proper treatment, it is necessary to distinguish stomachache from cardiac pain, hypochondriac pain, intestinal abscesses and abdominal pain.

(1) The difference between stomachache and angina pectoris

The site of the pain for angina pectoris is in the chest while stomachache is in the central of upper abdomen. The symptoms are different in cardiac pain with the severe, persistent stabbing pain, the sense of death, breathless, white complexion with cold limbs and dark purple lips.

(2) The difference between stomachache and hypochondriac pain

The main difference between the two diseases is the site of the pain, in which the hypochondriac pain is left or right flank and stomachache is the central of upper abdomen.

(3) The difference between stomachache and intestinal abscesses

The pain site in intestinal abscesses is epigastric region or the right lower abdomen with the sudden pain in the epigastric region first and then rapidly transfers to the right lower abdomen.

(4) The difference between stomachache and abdominal pain

The site of the pain for abdominal pain is between the stomach and the pubis with the symptoms include distending and dull pain or sever pain with diarrhea or constipation.

13.8.4 Pattern identification and treatment

13.8.4.1 Major points

Firstly, to identify the excess from deficiency: the excess patterns manifest in sudden attack, short duration, and severe pain with tenderness and forceful pulse while the deficient patterns show a chronic episode, long duration, mild pain with preference for pressure and weak pulse.

Secondly, to identify the cold from heat: the cold patterns manifest in the wiry or tight pulse and the pain which could be triggered by cold and removed by warmth while the heat patterns show a sudden, burning pain which could be triggered by the warmth and alleviated by cold, along with yellow coating and wiry-rapid or slippery-rapid pulse.

Thirdly, to identify the conditions between qi level and blood level: the patterns which stay in qi level include qi stagnation with the distending pain associated with emotional fluctuation, qi deficiency with the dull pain, decreased food ingestion, abdominal distension after eating food and weak pulse while that in blood level only include the blood stasis with the symptoms such as stabbing pain with a fixed position, purple tongue and hesitant pulse.

13.8.4.2 Treatment principles

General principles: to direct the movement of qi and harmonize the stomach.

For excess patterns, the principle is to remove the pathogenic factors. Distinguishing the different types from cold accumulation, qi stagnation, blood stasis and stomach heat prior to the proper treatment such as warming the stomach, smoothing the liver, moving the blood and clearing heat is necessary.

For deficient patterns, the main point is to identify the insufficiency in yin or yang, in order to nourish yin or strengthen yang.

13.8.4.3　Treatment based on pattern identification

(1) Accumulation of exotic cold

Clinical manifestations: Patients may present with sudden abrupt of stomachache which could be increased by cold and decreased by warmth, no thirst or preference for hot water.

Tongue: thin and white coating.

Pulse: stringy and tight pulse.

Analysis of clinical manifestations: Cold attacking in the stomach may influence the movement of qi which caused the warming and nourishing dysfunctions beyond the ability of qi, leading to sudden stomachache. Because the heat could warm the body and cold could worsen the stagnation of qi, so the pain could be increased by cold and decreased by warmth. Since cold belongs to the yin pathogen and can't damage the fluid in the body, patients may present with no thirst or preference for hot water. Both the tongue and pulse indicates cold too.

Treatment principle: Dissipate cold and relieve pain

1) Chinese herbal treatment

Prescription: Xiangsu San plus Liangfu Wan variation.

Herbs: Gaoliangjiang, Cuxiangfu, Zisuye, Zisugen, Ganpi, Zhigancao.

Administration: take the herbals decoction for oral use, twice a day.

Explanation:

Liangfu Wan: to warm the stomach and regulate the flow of qi.

Xiangsu San: to dispel cold and relieve the exterior syndrome, regulate qi and the function of the stomach.

Modification: For cases with severe cold, add Wuzhuyu and Chenpi to reduce the effect of cold and associate the circulation of qi; for cases with food intention, add Zhishi, Shenqu, Banxia, Jiaoshanzha to promote digestion.

2) Acupuncture & moxibustion

Prescription: Zusanli(ST 36), Zhongwan(CV 12), Neiguan(CV12), Yinlingquan(SP 9) and Weishu (BL 21).

Acupoints & methods: apply reducing manipulations and combing with moxibustion.

Explanation:

Zusanli: to treat gastric pain, vomiting, hiccup, abdominal dis-tension, borborygmus, diarrhea, dysentery, constipation, mastitis, aching of the knee joint and leg, beriberi, edema, cough, asthma, dizziness, indigestion, mania, etc.

Zhongwan: to treat stomach pain, abdominal distension, borborygmus, nausea, vomiting, acid regurgitation, diarrhea, dysentery, jaundice, indigestion, insomnia.

Neiguan: to treat cardiac pain, palpitation, stuffy chest, pain in the hypochondriac region, stomachache, nausea, vomiting, hiccup, mental disorders, malaria and pain of the elbow and arm, etc.

Yinlingquan: to treat abdominal pain and distension, diarrhea, dysentery, edema, jaundice, dysuria, enuresis, incontinence of urine, pain in the external genitalia, dysmenorrhea, pain in the knee, etc.

Weishu: to treat pain in the chest and hypochondriac and epigastric regions, abdominal distension, borborygmus, diarrhea, vomiting, nausea, etc.

(2) Food retention

Clinical manifestations: The symptoms include: stomach pain, fullness in the gastric, belching, acid regurgitation, vomiting undigested food and fell relief after vomiting.

Tongue: thick and greasy coating.

Pulse: slippery pulse.

Analysis of clinical manifestations: Food retention may block the flow of stomach qi, and cause the stomachache with fullness in the gastric, belching, acid regurgitation, vomiting and fell relief after vomiting. The dysfunction of spleen and stomach may cause inability to digest food.

Treatment principle: Assist digestion and relieve pain.

1) Chinese herbal treatment

Prescription: Baohe Wan Variation.

Herbs: Shanzha, Banxia, Fuling, Shenqu, Chenpi, Lianqiao, Laifuzi.

Explanation:

Shanzha: to digest fatty food.

Shenqu: to promote digestion.

Laifuzi: to assist stomach qi to downward.

Banxia, Chenpi and Fuling: to regulate qi and resolve dampness.

Modification: For cases with severe pain or distention, add Zhishi, Sharen and Binglang to promote digestion and assist the movement of qi; for cases with severe blockage inside the stomach, combine with Zhishi Daozhi Wan or Xiaochengqi Tang; for cases with severe and acute stomachache with yellow and dry add Huangqin and Huanglian; for cases with constipation, combine with Dachengqi Tang.

2) Acupuncture & moxibustion

General Prescription: Zusanli(ST 36), Zhongwan(CV 12), Neiguan(CV12)

Acupoints & methods: apply reducing manipulations

Explanation: same as type one.

(3) Inharmonious between liver and stomach

Clinical manifestations: Distention and ache in gastral cavity or scurrying hypochondrium pain, frequent eructation, exacerbation when emotional discomfort.

Tongue: pink or red tongue with thin white or thin and yello coating.

Pulse: wiry pulse.

Treatment principle: Dispersing stagnated liver qi for regulating stomach qi.

1) Chinese herbal treatment

Prescription: Chaihu Shugan San variation.

Herbs: Chaihu, Baishao, Zhiqiao, Xiangfu, Chuanxiong, Chenpi, Gancao.

Explanation:

Zhiqiao and Chenpi: to regulate qi and coordinate the stomach.

Chuanxiong: to assist the movement of qi and blood.

Baishao and Gancao: to hamonize the stomach and reduce the pain.

Modification: For fullness in the chest, belching and retching, combine with Chenxiang, Xuanfuhua, Sugeng to direct the qi downward; for the transformation trend into fire of stagnation qi, add Huangqin.

2)Acupuncture & moxibustion

General Prescription:Zusanli(ST 36),Zhongwan(CV 12),Neiguan(CV12),Qimen(LR 14),Taichong(LR 3).

Acupoints & methods:A reducing manipulation should be given to the above points. The needles are retained for 15−30 minutes.

Explanation:

Zusanli(ST 36),Zhongwan(CV 12),Neiguan(CV12)were mentioned above.

Qimen:to treat ypochondriac pain, abdominal distension, hiccup, acid regurgitation, mastitis, febrile diseases,etc.

Taichong:to treat headache, dizziness and vertigo, insomnia, congestion, swelling and pain of the eye, infantile convulsion, deviation of the mouth, pain in the hypochondriac region, uterine bleeding, hernia, enuresis, retention of urine, epilepsy, etc.

(4)Heat stagnation of liver and stomach

Clinical manifestations:Urgent burning pain in gastral cavity, dysphoria, gastric discomfort, acid regurgitation, dry mouth, bitter taste in mouth, dry and unsmooth defecation.

Tongue:red tongue with yellow coating.

Pulse:wiry and rapid pulse.

Treatment principle:Dispersing stagnated liver qi and purging heat for regulating stomach.

1)Chinese herbal treatment

Prescription:Danzhi Xiaoyan San or Qingzhong Tang variation.

Herbs:Danggui,Baishao,Baizhu,Chaihu,Fuling,Danpi,Zhizi.

Administration:decoct with water one dose per day, take 2 or 3 times per dose.

Explanation:

Danggui,Baishao and Chaihu:to nourish blood and the liver.

Baizhu and Fuling:to invigorate the splean and dispell dampness.

Zhigancao:to invigorate spleen stomach and replenish qi.

Danpi and Zhizi:to remove heat and soothe liver.

Modification:For disorder of qi and pain or distention in the chest and hypochondrium, add Yujin and Foshou;for cases with fullness in the abdomen and constipation, add Shengdahuang and Binglang;for cases with facilitating the effect of the above formula, add Zuoji Wan to drain the liver fire;for cases with the severe retention of dampness, add Huoxiang, Baidoukou, and Houpo.

2)Acupuncture & moxibustion

General Prescription:Zusanli(ST 36),Zhongwan(CV 12),Neiguan(CV12),Gongsun(SP 4),Taichong(LR 3).

Acupoints & methods:a reducing manipulation should be given to the above points. The needles are retained for 15−30 minutes.

Explanation:

Zusanli,Zhongwan and Neiguan are mentioned above.

Gongsun is used to cure gastric pain, vomiting, abdominal pain and distension, diarrhea, dysentery, borborygmus.

Taichong is used to cure headache, dizziness and vertigo, insomnia, congestion, swelling and pain of the eye, infantile convulsion, deviation of the mouth, pain in the hypochondriac region, uterine bleeding, hernia, enuresis, retention of urine, epilepsy, etc.

(5) Blood stasis

Clinical manifestations : Stomachache with fixed stabbing pain in the epigastrium, tenderness, pain triggered by eating food, hematemesis and black stools.

Tongue : purplish tongue.

Pulse : hesitant pulse.

Treatment principle : Remove blood stasis to reduce the pain.

1) Chinese herbal treatment

Prescription : Shixiao San plus Danshen Yin variation.

Herbs : Puhuang, Wulinzhi, Danshen, Tanxiang, Sharen.

Explanation :

Shixiao San : to promote the flow of blood, remove blood stasis and arrest pain.

Danshen Yin : to promote the flow of blood and remove blood stasis, and promote the flow of qi to arrest pain.

Wulinzhi and Danshen : to move the blood to resolve stasis.

Puhuang and Tanxiang : to promote the movement of qi and blood.

Sharen : to harmonize stomach and resolve dampness.

2) Acupuncture & moxibustion

General prescription : Zusanli(ST 36), Zhongwan(CV 12), Neiguan(CV12), Weishu(BL 21), Geshu (BL 17).

Acupoints & methods : apply reinforce-reducing manipulation should be given to the above points. The needles are retained for 15–30 minutes.

Explanation :

Zusanli(ST 36), Zhongwan(CV 12), Neiguan(CV12), Weishu(BL 21) are mentioned above.

Geshu : to treat vomiting, hiccup, asthma, cough, spitting blood, afternoon fever, night sweating, etc.

(6) Deficiency of stomach yin

Clinical manifestations : Burning pain in gastral cavity, hunger with no appetite, dry mouth, dry and unsmooth defecation, red and dry tongue with scanty fur or without fur or with fissure, thready and rapid pulse or stringy and thready pulse.

Treatment principle : Nourishing yin for benefiting stomach.

1) Chinese herbal treatment

Prescription : Yiguan Jian plus Shaoyao Gancao Tang.

Herbs : Beisharen, Maidong, Danggui, Shengdihuang, Gouqizi, Chuanlianzi, Baishao, Zhigancao.

Explanation :

Yiguan Jian to nourish yin and soothe the liver

Shaoyao Gancao Tang : to harmonize the liver and spleen, and relieve pain.

2) Acupuncture & moxibustion

General Prescription : Zusanli(ST 36), Zhongwan(CV 12), Neiguan(CV12), Weishu(BL 21), Sanyinjiao(SP 6), Taixi(KI 3).

Acupoints & methods : A reinforce manipulation should be given to the above points. The needles are retained for 15–30 minutes.

Explanation :

Zusanli(ST 36), Zhongwan(CV 12), Neiguan(CV12), Weishu(BL 21) are mentioned above.

Sanyinjiao : to treat abdominal pain, borborygmus, abdominal distension, diarrhea, dysmenorrhea, irregular menstruation, uterine bleeding, morbid leukorrhea, prolapse of the uterus, sterility, delayed labour, nocturnal emission, impotence, enuresis, edema, hernia, pain in the external genitalia, etc.

Taixi: to treat sore throat, toothache, deafness, tinnitus, dizziness, spitting of blood, asthma, thirst, irregular menstruation, insomnia, nocturnal emission, impotence, frequency of micturition, pain in the lower back, etc.

(7) Deficient cold of spleen and stomach

Clinical manifestations: Dull ache in gastral cavity, relief with warmness and pressure, relief after diet, cold of limbs, vomitting watery fluid, diarrhea with undigested food, plump and teeth-printed tongue with white and greasy fur, deep and thready pulse or deep and moderate pulse.

Treatment Principle: Warming middle energizer and invigorating spleen

1) Chinese herbal treatment

Prescription: Huangqi Jianzhong Tang variation.

Herbs: Huangqi, Baishao, Guizhi, Gancao, Shengjiang, Dazao, Yitang

Explanation:

Huangqi Dazao and Gancao: to nourish the spleen qi

Guizhi and Shengjiang: to warm the spleen yang and dispel cold

Baishao: to relieve pain

Yitang: to nouish the spleen and relieve pain

2) Acupuncture & moxibustion

General Prescription: Zusanli(ST 36), Zhongwan(CV 12), Neiguan(CV12), Weishu(BL 21), Pishu(BL 20), Shenque(CV 8)

Acupoints & methods: A reinforce manipulation should be given to the above points. The needles are retained for 15–30 minutes.

Explanation:

Zusanli(ST 36), Zhongwan(CV 12), Neiguan(CV12), Weishu(BL 21) were mentioned above.

Pishu: to treat pigastric pain, abdominal distension, jaundice, vomiting, diarrhea, dysentery, bloody stools, profuse menstruation, edema, anorexia, backache, etc.

Shenque: to treat abdominal pain, borborygmus, diarrhea, prolapse of the rectum, etc.

13.8.5   Prognosis

Stomachache often begins with qi level and can resolve with a timely appropriate treatment. However, as time goes by, stomachache can develop into complicated conditions, such as accelerating the circulation of blood which leads to bleeding.

Dysfunctions of spleen and stomach may cause phlegm-dampness, which may block the normal flow of qi and thus cause the pain in stomach.

Chronic stomachache may cause blood obstructing the normal flow of qi, leading to the subsequent vomiting. Long time relapse may affect the blood level in the long run.

13.8.6   Prevention

Patients with stomach pain need to develop good diet habit, and avoid overfeeding of spicy, hot and greasy food. They need to maintain mind at ease, avoid stimulation by unhealthy emotions, and consult psychologist. Enhancing psychological counseling for stomach pain patients has certain help to alleviate disease onset, attenuate symptoms and improve life quality. Also, this kind of patients should avoid long-term overwork, and paid attention to life style regulation especially in winter and spring. Regular physical training is recommended.

13.9 Diarrhea

Diarrhea is a disease referring to frequent defecation with bellyache, the loose stool, even water stool at times ocurring in all seasons but mostly in the summer and autumn.

In traditional Chinese medicine, diarrhea is included in the categories of diarrhea, dysentery and abdominal pain and so forth. The etiology and pathogenesis were detailedly discussed in *Internal Classic*, which laid the foundation for diagnosis and treatment of diarrhea.

In western medicine the relevant disease includes acute and chronic enteritis, gastrointestinal dysfunction, diarrhea-predominant irritable bowel syndrome and intestinal tuberculosis.

13.9.1 Etiology and pathogenesis

It usually results from the influence of cold, heat and dampness attack, improper diet, emotional upsets and a part of which cause weak physique when it takes longer than usual, which leads to functional disorders of the spleen and stomach, accompanied with the dysfunction of the small intestine to digest food and the dysfunction of the large intestine in transportation. In this case, the clear and excreting turbid mix together and transport to the intestines. The main pathogenic factor is dampness and invasion of external pathogenic factors which cause the dysfunction of spleen with the involvement in the spleen, stomach and intestines with relation to the kidney and liver.

13.9.2 Diagnosis

With the pain and hyperactive bowel sounds in the abdomen, diarrhea is mainly marked by mucus, blood, pus present in the stools. By the repeated attacks of damage, long-term diarrhea can cause emaciation and malnutrition. In microscopic stool examination, small amount of leucocytes can be found. Congestion and edema of the intestine mucosa plica and mucous secretion can be seen under colonoscopy. Derangement of the intestinal plica mucosa is examined under X-ray with barium contrast of colon.

13.9.3 Pattern identification and treatment

13.9.3.1 Major points

Excess and deficiency syndromes are usually set apart in this disease. Cold, heat and dampness attack, improper diet damaging the middle energizer and emotional upsets causing the stagnant liver qi and invading the spleen are presented in excess syndromes. A prolonged illness, weak constitution, or an old age will result in deficiency syndromes, including splenic dysfunction of transportation and transformation, declination of kidney yang, qi and yin, which cause the inability to control the defecation.

13.9.3.2 Treatment principles

To clarify the pathogenic factor, the primary treatment is to dispel dampness, strengthen the spleen and adjust the middle energizer, straighten out liver qi and warm kidney yang. Astringents are commonly used in long-term diarrhea also.

13.9.3.3   Treatment based on pattern identification

(1) Cold-dampness attacking the middle energizer

Clinical manifestations : Abdominal pain, loose, watery or even pus and blood stools, gasteremphraxis, borborygmus, anorexia, shiver, and fever, weakness, muscular soreness.

Tongue : thin, white and greasy coating.

Pulse : soft moderate or floating moderate pulse.

Analysis of clinical manifestations : Loose and watery stools are the result of indigestion of water and food as well as mixture of clear and turbid caused by dysfunction of spleen in transportation. Gasteremphraxis, anorexia and shiver are caused by cold-dampness disturbing spleen. Cold-dampness also hampers intestine qi movement, which leads to abdominal pain and borborygmus. If combined with wind-cold attacking exterior, patients can have syndrome like aversion to cold, fever, muscular soreness and *soft-moderate or floating moderate*. Thin, white and greasy are indications of cold-dampness attacking the middle energizer.

Treatment principle : To remove dampness, expel cold and heat with aromatic herbs.

1) Chinese herbal treatment

Prescription : Huoxiang Zhengqi San variation.

Herbs : Huoxiang, Banxiaqu, Chenpi, Baizhu, Fuling, Houpo, Zisuye, Dafupi, Jiegeng, Baizhi.

Explanation :

Huoxiang : to warm cold and resolve dampness.

Banxiaqu, Chenpi, Baizhu and Fuling : to invigorate spleen and resolve phlegm.

Houpo : to invigorate the spleen and drying the qi and phlegm.

Zisuye and Baizhi : to dispel cold to relieve the exterior syndrome.

Dafupi : to refresh the spleen and resolve dampness.

Jiegeng : to disperse the lung qi and resolve phlegm.

Modificaion : If dampness is severely causing abdominal fullness, borborygmus, dripping and lassitude, with white and greasy coating, Weiling Tang should be used to invigorate the spleen to promote dieresis. Besides, add Jingjie and Fangfeng; Baikouren (to be decocted later) ; Sharen (to be decocted later) and Paojiang.

2) Acupuncture & moxibustion

General prescription : Tianshu(ST 25), Yinlingquan(SP 9), Shangjuxu(ST 34), Shenque(CV 8).

Acupoints & methods : Apply indirect moxibustion with Shengjiang to Shenque(CV 8). Needle at Tianshu(ST 25), Yanglingquan (GB34) and Shangjuxu (ST 34) with reducing technique. The acupoints above are respectively needled perpendicularly at a depth of 1–2 cun, bringing about the local soreness and distention sensation. The needles are retained for 20–40 minutes.

Explanation :

Shenque(CV 8) : to restore yang from collapse.

Tianshu(ST 25) and Shangjuxu(ST 34) : to recuperate intestinal function.

Yinlingquan(SP 9) : to treat for abdominal pain and distension, diarrhea, dysentery, edema, jaundice, dysuria, enuresis, incontinence of urine, pain in the external genitalia, dysmenorrhea, pain in the knee, etc.

(2) Dampness-heat attacking the middle energizer

Clinical manifestations : Abdominal pain, urgent watery and yellowish-brown stools with extremely foul smell, difficult defecation, burning pain in anus, fever, thirsty and scanty deep yellow urine.

Tongue : yellow and greasy coating.

Pulse : soft and rapid pulse or slippery and rapid pulse.

Analysis of clinical manifestations: Urgent watery and yellowish-brown stools with extremely foul smell are because of heat in intestine. Difficult defecation is caused by dampness-heat. When dampness-heat flows downward, it leads to burning pain in anus and scanty deep yellow urine. Fever, thirsty, yellow and greasy coating as well as soft and rapid pulse or slippery and rapid pulse are all indications of dampness-heat attacking the middle energizer.

Treatment principle: Clearing heat away to disperse dampness and promote diuresis.

1) Chinese herbal treatment

Prescription: Gegen Qinlian Tang variation.

Herbs: Gegen, Huangqin, Huanglian, Gancao.

Explanation:

Gegen: to clear heat and release flesh.

Huangqin and Huanglian: to clear heat and resolve phlegm.

Gancao: to harmonize nutrient and defensive aspects

Modificaion: For cases with attack of summerheat dampness, which presents fever, headache, thirsty, scanty deep yellow urine and soft-rapid pulse, add Xinjia Xiangru Yin and Liuyi San to clear summerheat dampness; for cases with severe dampness with fullness in the abdomen, add Shichangpu and Fuling.

2) Acupuncture & moxibustion

General prescription: Tianshu(ST 25), Yanglingquan(GB34), Shangjuxu(ST 34), Neiting(ST 44)

Acupoints & methods: The same acupuncture manipulation as type one.

Explanation: Neiting(ST 44) is for reducing heat. The rest are the same as type one.

(3) Food retention

Clinical manifestations: Fullness in the epigastrium and abdomen, foul belching, poor appetite, diarrhea with a foul smell like rotten eggs, abdominal pain alleviated after bowel movements.

Tongue: dirty, thick and greasy fur.

Pulse: slippery pulse.

Analysis of clinical manifestations: Fullness in the epigastrium and abdomen is caused by improper diet, food retention and dysfunction of spleen in transportation. Foul belching is the result of indigestion. Food indigested flowing downward leads to diarrhea with a foul smell like rotten eggs. Abdominal pain alleviates after bowel movements because of excerting indigestion. Dirty, thick and greasy coating and slippery pulse are indications of food retention.

Treatment principle: Promoting digestion to benefit the spleen and relieve stagnation.

1) Chinese herbal treatment

Prescription: Baohe Wan.

Herbs: Shanzha, Shenqu, Banxia, Fuling, Chenpi, Laifuzi, Lianqiao.

Explanation:

Shanzha: to digest fatty food.

Shenqu: to pormote digestion.

Laifuzi: to assist stomach qi to downward.

Banxia, Chenpi and Fuling: to regulate qi and resolve dampness.

Lianqiao: to clear heat and dispersemass.

2) Acupuncture & moxibustion

General prescription: Tianshu (ST 25), Yanglingquan (GB34), Shangjuxu (ST 34), Zhongwan (CV 12).

Acupoints & methods: Apply indirect moxibustion with Shengjiang to Zhongwan(CV 12). The rest acupuncture manipulation is the same as type one.

Explanation:

Zhongwan(CV 12) to treat abdominal pain or distension.

The rest are the same as type one.

(4)Liver qi attacking the spleen

Clinical manifestations: This syndrome includes distending pain, borborygmus, abdominal pain before diarrhea and the pain relieved after diarrhea, which is caused by anger, anxiety, depression, or stress, and the symptoms are belching, stiffness in the chest, anorexia.

Tongue: light red tongue.

Pulse: wiry pulse.

Analysis of clinical manifestations: Distending pain and borborygmus are caused by disorder of qi movement when patients feel anger, anxiety, depression, or stress. These symptoms alleviate after diarrhea. Diarrhea is result of dysfunction of spleen in transportation. Combined with dysfunction of liver in controlling conveyance and dispersion, patients can have belching, stiffness in the chest and anorexia. Light red tongue and wiry pulse are indications of hyperactivity of liver qi.

Treatment principle: To depress the wood(liver) and strengthen the earth(spleen), regulate middle energizer and relieve diarrhea.

1) Chinese herbal treatment

Prescription: Tongxieyao Fang variation.

Herbs: Baizhu, Baishao, Chenpi, Fangfeng.

Explanation:

Baizhu: to invigorate the spleen.

Baishao: to emolliate liver and nourish blood.

Chenpi: to invigorate spleen and regulate qi.

Fangfeng: to ascend clear and relieve diarrhea.

Modificaion: For cases with spleen deficiency with lassitude and loose stools, add Fuling and Shanyao; for cases with recurrent diarrhea, add Mugua and Hezi.

2) Acupuncture & moxibustion

General prescription: Pishu(BL 20), Tianshu(ST 25), Zusanli(ST 36), Sanyinjiao(SP 6), Taichong (LR 3).

Acupoints & methods: The same acupuncture manipulation as type one.

Explanation:

Pishu(BL 20): to treat epigastric pain, abdominal distension, diarrhea, dysentery, bloody stools, etc.

Tianshu(ST 25): to treat recuperat intestinal function.

Zusanli(ST 36): to treat gastric pain, abdominal distension, borborygmus, diarrhea, dysentery, etc.

Sanyinjiao(SP 6): to treat abdominal pain, borborygmus, abdominal distension, diarrhea, etc.

Taichong(LR 3): to treat headache, dizziness and vertigo, insomnia, pain in the hypochondriac region, hernia, enuresis, etc.

(5)Deficiency of the spleen and stomach

Clinical manifestations: Usually the patient of the type diarrhea has distention and stuffiness in the chest and hypochondrium. Loose stools or diarrhea with undigested food, after intaking greasy food bowl movement increases, poor appetite, abdominal flatulence, sallow complexion, tiredness.

Tongue: pale tongue with white coating.

Pulse: thready and weak pulse.

Analysis of clinical manifestations: Loose stools or diarrhea with undigested food are due to deficiency of spleen and stomach deficiency, which cannot digest water and food or separate clear and turbid. Deficiency of spleen yang and dysfunction of spleen in governing movement and transformation leads to poor appetite, abdominal flatulence and increased bowl movement after intaking greasy food. Because of long-time diarrhea and deficiency of spleen and stomach, the source of qi and blood lacks and patients can present with sallow complexion and tiredness. Pale tongue with white coating and thready and weak pulse are indications of deficiency of the spleen and stomach.

Treatment principle: To invigorate the spleen and tonify qi, promote transportation and relieve diarrhea.

1) Chinese herbal treatment

Prescription: Shenling Baizhu San variation.

Herbs: Renshen, Baizhu, Fuling, Shanyao, Lanzirou, Biandou, Yiyiren, Suosharen, Jiegeng, Zhigancao.

Explanation:

Renshen, Baizhu, Fuling and Zhigancao: to nourish spleen qi.

Shanyao, Lanzirou, Biandou, Yiyiren, Suosharen and Jiegeng: to nourish spleen, eliminate dampness and relieve diarrhea.

Modificaion: For cases with declination of spleen yang with cold pain in the abdomen and cold limbs, add Shu Fuzi and Ganjiang; for cases with long-term diarrhea, add Yingsuke and Hezi; for case with indigestion, add Maiya and Jianqu.

2) Acupuncture & moxibustion

General prescription: Pishu(BL 20), Tianshu(ST 25), Zusanli(ST 36), Sanyinjiao(SP 6).

Acupoints & methods: The same acupuncture manipulation as type one.

Explanation:

Pishu(BL 20), Zusanli(ST 36) and Sanyinjiao(SP 6): to treat abdominal distension, diarrhea and indigestion.

Tianshu(ST 25): to recuperate intestinal function.

Modification: For cases with abdominal distention, add Gongsun(SP 4).

(6) Declination of kidney yang

Clinical manifestations: Abdominal pain and borborygmus followed by diarrhea, pain relieved after diarrhea, cold body and limbs, soreness of the waist and knees.

Tongue: pale tongue.

Pulse: deep and thready pulse.

Analysis of clinical manifestations: Kidney yang is too weak to warm spleen and stomach, leading to failure of spleen in governing movement and transformation. Because yang qi hasn't been aroused before dawn and the cold is stronger, patients can have abdominal pain and borborygmus followed by diarrhea, which is also called "morning diarrhea". Pain will relieve after diarrhea. Cold body and limbs, soreness of the waist and knees, pale tongue as well as deep and thready pulse are all indications of declination of kidney yang.

Treatment principle: To warm the kidney, strengthen the spleen, induce astringency and relieve diarrhea.

1) Chinese herbal treatment

Prescription: Sishen Wan variation.

Herbs: Buguzhi, Roudoukou, Wuzhuyu, Wuweizi, Shengjiang, Dazao.

Explanation:

Buguzhi: to warm yang and nourish kidney.

Roudoukou and Wuzhuyu: to warm the interior and disperse cold.

Wuweizi, Shengjiang, Dazao: to relieve diarrhea with astringents

Modificaion: For cases with long-term diarrhea, add Yuyuliang, Yingsuke and Hezi.

2) Acupuncture & moxibustion

General prescription: Pishu(BL 20), Tianshu(ST 25), Zusanli(ST 36), Sanyinjiao(SP 6), Shenshu (BL 23), Mingmen(GV 4).

Acupoints & methods: The same acupuncture manipulation as type one.

Explanation:

Pishu(BL 20): to treat abdominal pain.

Tianshu(ST 25): to recuperate intestinal function.

Zusanli(ST 36): to treat abdominal pain, borborygmus, diarrhea, aching of the knee joint and leg, etc.

Sanyinjiao(SP 6): to treat abdominal pain, borborygmus, abdominal distension, diarrhea, etc.

Shenshu(BL 23): to treat nocturnal emission, impotence, enuresis, irregular menstruation, leukorrhea, low back pain, knee weakness, blurring vision, dizziness, tinnitus, deafness, edema, asthma, diarrhea, etc.

Mingmen(GV 4): to nourish kidney yang.

(7) Deficiency of both qi and yin

Clinical manifestations: Long-term diarrhea with pus and bloody stools, dull pain in the abdomen, low fever in the afternoon, dizziness, insomnia, night sweating, restlessness, irritability, emaciation.

Tongue: red tongue with little fur.

Pulse: thready and rapid pulse.

Analysis of clinical manifestations: This type of diarrhea is usually based on the type of dampness-heat attacking the middle energizer. Because long-term diarrhea, qi, yin and fluid are wasted, leading to dull pain in the abdomen and emaciation. Lack of qi and yin causes low fever in the afternoon, dizziness, insomnia, night sweating, restlessness and irritability. Red tongue with less fur as well as thready and rapid pulse are indications of deficiency of both qi and yin.

Treatment principle: To nourish yin, clear away heat, replenish qi and relieve diarrhea.

Chinese herbal treatment:

Prescription: Shengmai San plus Liujunzi Tang variation

Herbs: Renshen, Maidong, Baizhu, Wuweizi, Fuling, Chenpi, Banxia, Zhigancao

Explanation:

Renshen: to replenish qi to restore yang.

Maidong and Wuweizi: to nourish yin and astringe yang.

Dangshen, Baizhu, Fulin and Zhigancao: to invigorate spleen and replenish qi.

Chenpi and Banxia: to direct qi and dispel phlegm.

Modificaion: For cases with feverish sensation in the chest, palms and soles, add Qinghao and Yinchaihu; for cases with restlessness and insomnia, add Chaosuanzaoren, Huanglian and Danshen; for dizziness, add Tianma and Zhenzhumu; for cases with severe diarrhea, add Chishizhi and Yuyuliang; for red and white mucus in the stools, add Baihuasheshecao and Machixian.

13.9.4   Prevention

During the treatment, patients with diarrhea should pay attention to dietary hygiene and develop a light diet. They should avoid raw, cold, spicy or greasy food.

13.10   Edema

Edema is marked by abnormal fluid retention in body, which affects the head, face, eyelids, limbs, abdomen and back, and even the whole body.

Edema, called "water" in the book of *Internal Classic*, could be divided into three syndromes: the Chinese terms "Fengshui", "Shishui" and "Yongshui". The treatment principles of edema was put forward in *Plain Questions*, "to dislodge blood stasis, open pores and empty bladder". In Song Dynasty, edema was divided into "Yinshui" and "Yangshui" in Chinese terms.

In western medicine the relevant disease includes acute and chronic glomerulonephritis, nephroticsyndrome, secondary glomerulonephropathy.

13.10.1   Etiology and Pathogenesis

Edema is a morbid condition caused by invasion of pathogenic wind, damp toxin, water-dampness, dampness-heat, improper diet which result in dysfunction of lung to regulate the water passage, the spleen to govern the transportion and transformation of body fluids, kidney to regulate water metabolism, and qi transformation in urinary bladder to control urination, thus giving rise to abnormal fluid retention in the body and further involving the muscles and skin.

Invasion of pathogenic wind, noxious dampness, fluid-dampness, improper diet, prolonged illness, stress and anxiety are considered as the main reasons of edema. It usually occurs when the function of qi activity is declined. In the aspect of purtenance, the transportation and transformation of body fluids are related to lung, spleen and kidney, but kidney is more significant to edema. Besides, if there exists blood stasis and the functioning of the triple energizers is impaired, edema will be obstinate and need prolonged treatment. Edema may be seen in acute and chronic glomerulonephritis, nephritic syndrome, congestive heart failure, endocrine disturbance and dystrophy in western medicine.

13.10.2   Diagnosis

Edema usually begins from eyelids or lower limbs, and then spreads to four limbs and entire body. In mild cases, there may be light swelling around the eyelids or in the tibia while in severe cases, generalized swelling, abdominal fullness and enlargement, asthmatic breathing with inability to lie supine may be present. In even more severe cases, retention of urine, nausea, vomiting, foul breath, nasal bleeding, atrophy of the gum or even headache, convulsion, coma and delirium may occur.

The patient may have a history of tonsillitis, palpitation, septicemia or purpura, or invalidism.

Urine routine examination, 24-hour quantitative determination of urinary protein, blood routine examination, determination of blood sedimention rate, plasma albumin, creatinine, urea nitrogen in blood and humoral immunity, as well as electrocardiography, cardiac functional test and B-type ultrasonic examination for the kidneys are the necessary means in the diagnosis of edema.

13.10.3   Pattern identification and treatment

13.10.3.1   Major points and treatment principles

Making the diagnosis of edema, it is essential to clarify whether the complaint is edema of the yang type or edema of the yin type. Usually the yang-type edema is characterized by a short duration, a rapid development, more pronounced edema on the head and face with the skin shiny and thin. However, the yin-type edema is marked by a longer duration, a gradual development, more pronounced pitted edema of lower limbs, sallow and grayish skin. The treatment for the yang-type should aim at eliminating pathogenic factors, with such methods as diaphoresis and diuresis. When necessary, purgation should be used. For the yin-type, it is advisable to support healthy qi to eliminate pathogenic factors, for instance, to promote diuresis by invigorating the spleen and warming kidney. If edema is persistent, promoting diuresis by activating blood circulation and dissipating blood stasis is recommended as the accessory treatment.

13.10.3.2　Treatment based on pattern identification

(1) Invasion by wind and overflow of water

Clinical manifestations: Acute onset, edema starting from the eyelids, followed by four limbs and the whole body, aversion to cold, fever, soreness of the limbs and joints, dysuria, etc.

Tongue: thin white tongue coating.

Pulse: floating, slippery or rapid pulse.

Analysis of clinical manifestations: Edema and dysuria are caused by wind attacking the exterior. Wind evil, mobile and changeable, usually attacks yang portion of body, so edema often starts from the eyelids, followed by four limbs and the whole body. Pathogenic qi stuck on the exterior blocks the movement of wei qi, so patients can have aversion to cold, fever and soreness of the limbs and joints. In case with predominant wind heat, there may also be swelling and pain in the throat, red tougue, floating slippery and rapid pulse. In cases with predominant wind cold, aversion to cold, cough, dyspnea.

Treatment principle: Eliminating wind, dispersing lung qi, circulating water to relieve edema.

1) Chinese herbal treatment

Prescription: Yuebi Jiazhu Tang variation.

Herbs: Mahuang, Shigao(to be decocted first), Xingren, Baizhu, Fuling and Zexie

Explanaion:

Mahuang, Shigao, Xingren, Fuling and Zexie: to induce sweating to release the exterior.

Baizhu: to clear damp and promote diuresis.

Modificaion: For cases with predominance of wind-heat, add Lianqiao, Jiegeng, Banlangen and Xianmaogen; for cases with predominance of wind-cold, remove Shigao and add Zisuye, Guizhi and Fangfeng; for cases with severe cough and dyspnea, add Qianhu and Ziyuan; for cases with sweating with aversion to wind and defensive qi, add Fangji and Huangqi.

2) Acupuncture & moxibustion

General prescription: Sanjiaoshu(BL 22), Shuifen(CV 9), Pishu(BL 20), Zusanli(ST 36), Qihai(CV 6), Feishu(BL 13), Dazhu(BL 11) and Hegu(LI 4).

Acupoints & methods: Reducing excess and reinforcing deficiency. Once a day, and 10 times make up a course of treatment with 2-3 days standby between two courses.

Explanation:

Sanjiaoshu(BL 22) and Shuifen(CV 9): to unclog the water channels of the whole body.

Pishu(BL 20): to treat epigastric pain, abdominal distension, jaundice, vomiting, diarrhea, dysentery, bloody stools, profuse menstruation, edema, anorexia, backache, etc.

Zusanli(SI 36): to treat gastric pain, vomiting, hiccup, abdominal distension, borborygmus, diarrhea, dysentery, constipation, mastitis, aching of the knee joint and leg, beriberi, edema, cough, asthma, dizziness, indigestion, mania, etc.

Qihai(CV 6) : to treat abdominal pain, diarrhea, enuresis, nocturnal emission, impotence, hernia, edema, dysentery, constipation, asthma, uterine bleeding, irregular menstruation, dysmenorrhea, amenorrhea, morbid leukorrhea, postpartum hemorrhage, etc.

Feishu(BL 13) : to treatcough, asthma, chest pain, spitting of blood, afternoon fever, night sweating, etc.

Dazhu(BL 11) : to treat dispel the wind evil.

Hegu(LI 4) : to treat headache, neck pain, redness, swell and pain of the eye, epistaxis, toothache, deafness, etc.

(2)Retention of noxious dampness

Clinical manifestations : Edema of the eyelids followed by generalized edema, dysuria, pyogenic infection, or even ulceration of skin, fever with aversion to wind.

Tongue : red tongue with thin yellow coating.

Pulse : floating, rapid or slippery, rapid pulse.

Analysis of clinical manifestations : Being the primary pathogen, wind evil is often combined with other diseases, so edema often starts from the eyelids, followed by four limbs and the whole body, and patients can have fever with aversion to wind. Noxious dampness flows into lung and spleen, damaging the function of lung in governing regulation of water passages and spleen in governing water and dampness, which leads to dysuria, pyogenic infection, or even ulceration of skin. Red tongue with thin yellow coating as well as floating, rapid or slippery, rapid pulse are indications of retention of noxious dampness.

Treatment principle : To disperse lung qi, remove toxic substance, and promote diuresis to relieve edema.

1)Chinese herbal treatment

Prescription : Mahuang Lianqiao Chixiaodou Tang and Wuwei Xiaodu Yin variation.

Herbs : Mahuang, Xingren, Sangbaipi, Chixiaodou, Jinyinhua, Lianqiao, Yejuhua, Pugongying, Zihuadiding and Zibeitiankui

Explanaion :

Mahuang and Xingren : to release the exterior with acrid-warm

Sangbaipi, Chixiaodou, Lianqiao, Jinyinhua, Yejuhua, Pugongying, Zihuadiding and Zibeitiankui : to clear away heat and toxic material

Modificaion : For cases with predominant dampness with skin ulceration, add Kushen and Tufuling; for cases with predominant wind with itching, add Baixianpi and Difuzi; for cases with blood heat with red and swollen skin, add Mudanpi; for cases with constipation, add Shengdahuang(to be decorated later)and Mangxiao(to be infused separately).

2)Acupuncture & moxibustion

General prescription : Sanjiaoshu(BL 22), Shuifen(CV 9), Pishu(BL 20), Zusanli(SI 36), Qihai(CV 6)

Acupoints & methods : The same as type one.

Explanation : The same as type one.

(3)Water-dampness retentin

Clinical manifestations : Pitted edema of the whole body, scanty urine, heaviness of the body, feeling of oppression in the chest, poor appetite, nausea.

Tongue : greasy white coating.

Pulse : deep, moderate pulse.

Analysis of clinical manifestations：Water and dampness stagnate on skin and the interior, damaging the function of triple energizers and bladder in transformation, which causes pitted edema of the whole body and scanty urine. The pathogen also disturbs spleen yang and spleen qi, resulting in heaviness of the body, feeling of oppression in the chest, poor appetite and nausea. Greasy white fur and deep, moderate pulse are indications of retention of water and dampness.

Treatment principle：To invigorate the spleen, eliminate dampness, activate yang and promote diuresis.

1) Chinese herbal treatment

Prescription：Wupi Yin and Weiling Tang variation.

Herbs：Cangzhu, Houpo, Chenpi, Guizhi, Fuling, Zexie, Shengjiangpi and Dafupi.

Explanaion：

Cangzhu, Houpo, Chenpi and Shengjiangpi：to clear dampness and harmonize the stomach.

Fuling, Zexie, Dafupi and Guizhi：to induce diuresis and alleviate edema.

Modificaion：For cases with severe edema with asthma, add Mahuang, Xingren

2) Acupuncture & moxibustion

General prescription：Sanjiaoshu (BL 22) , Shuifen (CV 9) , Pishu (BL 20) , Zusanli (SI 36) , Qihai (CV 6).

Acupoints & methods：The same as type one.

Explanation：The same as type one.

(4) Excess of dampness-heat

Clinical manifestations：General edema with the skin shiny and taut, fullness in the chest and abdomen, restless fever, thirst, scanty deep yellow urine, or dry stools.

Tongue：red tongue with yellow greasy coating.

Pulse：deep, rapid or soft pulse.

Analysis of clinical manifestations：General edema with the skin shiny and taut is due to long-term dampness-water turning into heat or dampness-heat stagnation on skin or in meridians. Fullness in the chest and abdomen may be caused by dampness-heat stagnation in triple energizers which disturbs the movement of qi. If heat predominates, fluid could be wasted and patients may have restless fever, thirst, scanty deep yellow urine, or dry stools. Red tongue with yellow greasy coating as well as deep, rapid or soft pulse are indications of excess of dampness-heat.

Treatment principle：To clear away heat, promote dieresis and regulate qi circulation.

1) Chinese herbal treatment

Prescription：Shuzao Yinzi variation.

Herbs：Mutong, Zexie, Fulingpi, Chixiaodou, Huangbai, Zhuling, Shanglu, Binglang, Cangzhu and Shengyiren.

Administration：Take the herbals decoction for oral use, twice a day.

Explanaion：

Mutong, Zexie, Fulingpi, Zhuling, Shanglu, Binglang and Chixiaodou：to induce diuresis to alleviate edema.

Huangbai, Cangzhu and Shengyiren：to dry dampness and strengthen the spleen.

Modificaion：For cases with abdominal flatulence and constipation, add Shengdahuang and Tinglizi; for cases with retention of dampness-heat in the urinary bladder damaging the blood vessels, manifested as painful urination and hematuria, add Daji, Xiaoji and Baimaogen; for cases with severe edema accompanied by chest oppression, asthmatic breathing, inability to lie supine, and wiry, forceful pulse, add Tinglizi, Xingren and Fangji; for cases with long-standing rentention of dampness-heat transforming into dryness which further damages yin, manifested as dry mouth and throat and dry stools, add Zhuling, Huashi, Maimendong and Ejiao.

2) Acupuncture & moxibustion

General prescription: Sanjiaoshu (BL 22), Shuifen (CV 9), Pishu (BL 20), Zusanli (SI 36), Qihai (CV 6).

Acupoints & methods: The same as type one.

Explanation: The same as type one.

(5) Deficiency of spleen yang

Clinical Manifestations: Genearal pitted edema which is more pronounced below the loins, abdominal flatulence, impaired appetite, loose stools, lusterless complexion, lassitude, cold limbs, small amout of urine.

Tongue: pale tongue with greasy white coating.

Pulse: deep, moderate or deep, weak pulse.

Analysis of clinical manifestations: Genearal pitted edema which is more pronounced below the loins, abdominal flatulence, impaired appetite and loose stools may be caused by dysfunction of spleen in governing water due to deficiency of spleen yang. Lusterless complexion, lassitude and cold limbs are results of lack of qi and blood generated by spleen due to deficiency of spleen yang, too. Spleen yang cannot transform to spleen qi, so patients have little urine. Pale tongue with greasy white coating or as well as deep, moderate or deep, weak pulse are indications of deficiency of spleen yang.

Treatment principle: To warm and invigorate spleen yang so as to promote diuresis.

1) Chinese herbal treatment

Prescription: Shipi Yin variation.

Herbs: Ganjiang, Caoguo, Baizhu, Fuling, Jiaomu, Houpo, Muxiang and Dafupi

Explanaion:

Zhifuzi and Ganjiang: to warm and nourish spleen and kidney

Baizhu and Fuling: to dry dampness and strengthen the spleen

Caoguo, Jiaomu, Houpo, Muxiang and Dafupi: to refresh the spleen and resolve dampness

Modificaion: For cases with short breath and weak voice, add Danshen and Huangqi; for cases with small amount of urine, add Guizhi and Zexie.

2) Acupuncture & moxibustion

General prescription: Sanjiaoshu (BL 22), Shuifen (CV 9), Pishu (BL 20), Zusanli (SI 36), Qihai (CV 6), Sanjinjiao (SP 6), Yinlingquan (SP 9).

Acupoints & methods: The acupuncture manipulation is the same as type one. Add moxibustion.

Explanation:

Sanyinjiao (SP 6): to treat abdominal pain, borborygmus, abdominal distension, diarrhea, dysmenorrhea, irregular menstruation, uterine bleeding, morbid leukorrhea, prolapse of the uterus, sterility, nocturnal emission, impotence, enuresis, edema, hernia, pain in the external genitalia, etc.

Yinlingquan (SP 9): to treat abdominal pain and distension, diarrhea, dysentery, edema, jaundice, dysuria, enuresis, incontinence of urine, pain in the external genitalia, dysmenorrhea, pain in the knee, etc.

The rest are the same as type one.

(6) Deficiency of kidney yang

Clinical manifestations: General pitted edema which is more pronounced below the loins, palpitation, short breath, soreness and heaviness in the loins, decreased quantity of urine, cold limbs, aversion to cold, lassitude, pale or grayish dim complexion.

Tongue : pale and swollen tongue with white coating.

Pulse : deep and thready or deep, slow and forceless pulse.

Analysis of clinical manifestations : Deficiency of kidney yang leads to deficiency of kidney qi, so water and dampness flows downward and edema is general pitted and more pronounced below the loins. Water pathogen insults heart, so patients may have palpitation short breath. Waist, the house of kidney, could feel soreness and heaviness because of deficiency of kidney yang. Kidney and bladder share the relationship of exterior and interior, so deficiency of kidney yang may cause dysfunction of bladder in qi transformation and decreased quantity of urine. Lack of kidney yang can also cause cold limbs, aversion to cold, lassitude, pale or grayish dim complexion. Pale and swollen tongue with white tongue coating as well as deep and thready or deep, slow and forceless pulse are indications of deficiency of kidney yang.

Treatment principle : To warm the kidney, assist yang, activate qi and promote diuresis.

1) Chinese herbal treatment

Prescription : Jisheng Shenqi Wan and Zhenwu Tang variation.

Herbs : Zhifuzi, Rougui, Bajitian, Yinyanghuo, Baizhu, Fuling, Zexie, Cheqianzi, Niuxi and Shanyao.

Administration : Take the herbals decoction for oral use, twice a day.

Explanaion :

Zhifuzi, Rougui, Bajitian and Yinyanghuo : to warm yang for resolving fluid retention.

Baizhu, Fuling and Zexie : to clear dampness and promote diuresis.

Cheqianzi : to clear away heat and promote diuresis.

Niuxi : to nourish yin and nourish kidney.

Shanyao : to invigorate the liver and benefit the spleen.

Modificaion : For cases with palpitation, cyanotic lips, feeble pulse, or slow-irregular and intermittent pulse, increase Zhifuzi and add Guizhi, Zhigancao and Danshen ; for cases with asthmatic breathing, sweating, and floating, feeble and rapid pulse, add Hongshen (to be decocted separately) , Gejiefen (to be infused separately) , Wuweizi, Shanzhuyu, Muli (to be decocted first) and Longgu (to be decocted first) ; for cases with deficiency of kidney yang is persistent, it impairs yin, giving rise to deficiency of kidney yin. In this case, there appear such manifestations as recurrence of edema, lassitude, soreness in the loins, nocturnal emission, drymouth and throat, feverish sensation in the palms, soles and chest, red tongue and thready, rapid pulse, The treatment should aim at nourishing kidney yin and promoting diuresis concurrently. The alternative prescription is : Shanyao, Shanzhuyu, Gouqizi, Mudanpi, Zexie and Fuling.

2) Acupuncture & moxibustion

General prescription : Sanjiaoshu (BL 22) , Shuifen (CV 9) , Pishu (BL 20) , Zusanli (ST 36) , Qihai (CV 6) , Shenshu (BL 23) , Guanyuan (CV 4) and Mingmen (GV 4) .

Acupoints & methods : The acupuncture manipulation is the same as type one. Add moxibustion.

Explanation :

Shenshu (BL 23) : to treat nocturnal emission, impotence, enuresis, irregular menstruation, leukorrhea, low back pain, knee weakness, blurring vision, dizziness, tinnitus, deafness, edema, asthma, diarrhea, etc.

Guanyuan (CV 4) : to treat enuresis, nocturnal emission, frequency of urination, retention of urine, hernia, irregular menstruation, morbid leukorrhea, uterine bleeding, postpartum hemorrhage, lower abdominal pain, indigestion, diarrhea, etc.

The rest are the same as type one.

13.10.4   Prevention

Patients with edema should develop a regular life style and try to avoid getting cold or tired. During treatment, sexual activity should be abstinent.

Wang Xinjun , Yang Yang , Xiong Ying , Cui Ruiqin , Wang Rui , Cai Xiaowen

Appendix

(1) Basic classics

(*Huangdi's*) *Internal Classic*: Written in the Spring and Autumn states by numerous experts, it is China's earliest comprehensive traditional medical work including two parts, *Plain Questions* and *Miraculous Pivot*.

Classic of Difficult Issues: Written in the Western Han Dynasty by Qin Yueren (Bian Que), it is also known as Classic on 81 Medical, Problems which includes a total of eighty-one difficult issues and covers the basic theory of Chinese traditional medicine through questions and answers.

Treatise on Cold Damage Diseases: Written in the Eastern Han Dynasty by Zhang Zhongjing, it is a monograph on the treatment of exogenous disease.

Synopsis of Golden Chamber: Written in the Eastern Han Dynasty by Zhang Zhongjing, it is the earliest extant monograph on diagnosing and treating diseases.

Treatise on the Pathogenesis and Manifestations of All Diseases: Written in the Sui Dynasty by Cao Yuanfang, it is a monograph on the origins and manifestations of diseases.

(2) Chinese medicinal classics

Shennong's Classic of Materia Medica: Written in the Eastern Han Dynasty by numerous experts, it is the earliest extant monograph on science of Chinese materia medica.

Variorum of the Classic of Materia Medica: Written in the Liang Dynasty by Tao Hongjing, it is written on the basis of *Shennong's Classic of Materia Medica*, adding 365 kinds of medicine.

Newly Revised Materia Medica: Written in the Tang Dynasty by Li Ji, Su Jing and other 23 people following the Emperor's order, it is China's first pharmacopoeia promulgated by the government.

Classified Emergency Materia Medica: Written in the Northern Song Dynasty by Tang Shenwei, it is a brilliant monograph on collective materia medica.

Compendium of Materia Medica: Written in the Ming Dynasty by Li Shizhen, it includes 1,892 kinds of medicine.

Prescription Classics Lei's Treatise on Processing of Drugs: Written in the Northern and Southern dynasties by Lei Xiao, it is China's earliest science of Chinese medicine processing.

Prescriptions for Fifty-two Diseases: Written in the Warrior States period, it is China's earliest extant medical classics.

Handbook of Prescriptions for Emergencies: Written in the Eastern Jin Dynasty by Ge Hong, it is China's first monograph on the clinical emergency treatment.

Essential Prescriptions worth a Thousand Gold for Emergencies: Written in the Tang Dynasty by Sun Simiao, it is the first medical encyclopedia in China.

Supplement to the Essential Prescriptions worth a Thousand Gold: Arcane Essentials from the Imperial Library: Written in the Tang Dynasty by Wang Tao, it is a compilation on medical works in the Tang Dynasty.

Prescriptions from the Great Peace Imperial Grace Pharmacy: Written in the Song Dynasty by Taiping People's Welfare Bureau, it is the first official medicine standard.

Effective Formulas Handed Down for Generations: Written in the Yuan Dynasty by Wei Yilin, it contains a total of more than 3 300 prescriptions, including internal medicine, surgery, gynecology, pediatrics, orthopedics, otolaryngology and other diseases in TCM.

(3) Diagnostic classics

Pulse Classic: Written in the Jin Dynasty by Wang Shuhe, it is a brilliant monograph on sphygmology before the Han Dynasty.

Essentials for Diagnosticians: Written in the Yuan Dynasty by Hua Shou, the book was written by combining pulse theory before Yuan Dynasty and private insight.

Binhu's Sphygmology: Written in the Ming Dynasty by Li Shizhen, this book discusses 27 kinds of pulse conditions.

Pulse Diagnosticians: Written in Ming Dynasty by Li Zhongzi, it is a work on the basic theory and clinical application of the pulse.

Obey the Rules of Inspection: Written in the Qing Dynasty by Wang Hong, it is an all-around monograph on inspection.

(4) Internal medicine classics

Confucian's Duties to Their Parents: Written in the Jin Dynasty by Zhang Congzheng, it charts Zhang Congzheng's academic thinking and clinical experience.

The Origin of Medicine: Written in the Jin Dynasty by Zhang Yuansu, it expounds zang-fu viscrea, meridians, pathogeny and the law of the treatment.

Treatise on the Spleen and Stomach: Written in the Jin Dynasty by Li Dongyuan, it is his representative work of his theory on spleen-stomach.

Treatise on Inquiring the Properties of Things: Written in the Yuan Dynasty by Zhu Zhenheng, it is a collection of medical journals by Zhu and puts forward the famous academic viewpoints such as the theory of ministerial fire, the theory of yang in excess and yin in asthenia and so on.

Complete Works of Jingyue: Written in the Ming Dynasty by Zhang Jiebin, it is a famous book, combining ancient medical experts' and his own experience.

Systematized Identification of Warm Diseases: Written in the Qing Dynasty by Wu Tang in 1798, it is a work on warm diseases.

Treatise on Warm-Heat Diseases: Transcribed in the Qing Dynasty from Ye Gui's dictation, it is a foundational work on warm diseases.

Classified Patterns Clear-Cut Treatments: Written in the Qing Dynasty by Lin Peiqin, it is a work on practice in internal medicine.

Correction of Errors in Medical classics: Written in the Qing Dynasty by Wang Qingren, it corrects some thinking of the ancients on anatomy and physiology.

Secret Formulary Bestowed by Immortals for Treating Injuries and Mending Fractures: Written in the Tang Dynasty by Lin Daoren, it is a monograph on orthopedics and traumatology during the early period in

China.

Orthodox Manual of External Medicine : Written in the Ming Dynasty by Chen Shigong, it is a monograph on orthopedics and traumatology.

Essence on the Silvery Sea : Written in the Ming Dynasty, it is a monograph on ophthalmology.

Longmu's Secret Treatiseon Ophthalmology : Written in the Song and Yuan Dynasty, it concludes the general theory of ophthalmology and the treatment and prescription of 72 kinds of eye diseases.

(5) Gynaecology and pediatrics classics

Tested Treasures in Obstetrics : Written in the Tang Dynasty by Zan Yin, it is the earliest extant monograph on obstetrics and covers the treatment of various diseases for women during the period from pregnancy to puerperium.

Compendium of Effective Prescriptions for Women : Written in the Song Dynasty by Chen Ziming, it is the first all-round monograph on gynecology and obstetrics.

Fu Qingzhu's Obstetrics and Gynecology : Written in the Qing Dynasty by Fu Shan, it is a famous work on gynecology.

Synopsis of Treating Women's Diseases : Written in the Ming Dynasty by Wu Zhiwang, it is a monograph on gynecology.

Standards of Syndrome Identification and Treatment : Written in the Ming Dynasty by Wang Kentang, it is a monograph on gynecology.

Key to Therapeutics of Children's Diseases : Written in the Song Dynasty by Qian Yi, it is a monograph on pediatrics.

(6) Acupuncture classics

Huangdi's Bright Hall Moxibustion Classic : Written in the Tang Dynasty, it covers the acupuncture methods of the general points for adults and children.

Systematic Classic of Acupuncture and Moxibustion : Written in the Western Jin Dynasty by Huangfu Mi, it sums up science of acupuncture and moxibustion again after Internal Classic.

Treatise on the Eight Extra Meridians : Written in the Ming Dynasty by Li Shizhen, it is a monograph on eight extra meridians.

Elucidation of the Fourteen Meridians : Written in the Yuan Dynasty by Hua Shou, it is a monograph on meridians.

Complete Compendium of Acupuncture and Moxibustion : Written in the Ming Dynasty by Yang Jizhou, it compiles the ancients' academic viewpoints and experience on acupuncture and moxibustion.

Liu Yanling, Yao Zengyu

References

［1］王新华. 中医学＝TEXEBOOK OF TRADITOONAL CHINESE MEDICINE［M］. 北京：科学出版社，2016.

［2］高思华，王键. 中医基础理论［M］. 北京：人民卫生出版社，2016.

［3］王天芳. 中医诊断学［M］. 北京：人民卫生出版社，2007.

［4］李飞. 方剂学：上、下册［M］. 2 版. 北京：人民卫生出版社，2011.

［5］孙慧，曹玉麟. 基础中医英语［M］. 青岛：中国海洋大学出版社，2016.

［6］国家药典委员会. 中华人民共和国药典：2017 年版［M］. 北京：中国医药科技出版社，2017.

［7］南京中医药大学. 中药大辞典［M］. 上海：上海科学技术出版社，2006.

［8］宁娜，韩建军. 实用中药英语［M］. 哈尔滨：哈尔滨工业大学出版社，2015.

［9］常章富，贾德贤，JAMES BARE. Chinese Materia Medica（International Standard Library of Chinese Medicine）［M］. 北京：人民卫生出版社，2014.

［10］沈雪勇，王华. 针灸学［M］. 2 版. 北京：人民卫生出版社，2012.

［11］张吉，赵百孝，劳力行. Acupuncture and Moxibustion［M］. 北京：人民卫生出版社，2014.

［12］李义凯，翟伟. 推拿学［M］. 北京：科学出版社，2012.

［13］刘明军，王金贵. 小儿推拿学［M］. 2 版. 北京：中国中医药出版社，2016.

［14］冯天有. 中西医结合治疗软组织损伤的临床研究［M］. 北京：中国科学技术出版社，2002.

［15］施洪飞，方泓. 中医食疗学［M］. 北京：中国中医药出版社，2016.

［16］刘天群，章文春. 中医气功学［M］. 北京：中国中医药出版社，2016.

［17］温搏. 太极拳中英双语初级教程［M］. 北京：北京师范大学出版社，2014.

［18］周仲瑛. 中医内科学［M］. 北京：人民卫生出版社，2007.

［19］李振吉. 中医基本名词术语中英对照国际标准［M］. 北京：人民卫生出版社，2008.

［20］GIOVANNI M. The practice of Chinese medicine：the treatment of diseases with acupuncture and Chinese herbs［M］. New York：Churchill Livingstone/Elsevier，2008.

［21］贾春生，黄泳. 针灸学［M］. 北京：科学出版社，2013.

［22］谈勇. 中医妇科学［M］. 北京：人民卫生出版社，2007.

［23］JAMIESON D J，STEEGE J F. The prevalence of dysmenorrhea，dyspareunia，pelvic pain，and irritable bowel syndrome in primary care practices［J］. Obstet Gynecol，1996，87（1）：55-58.

［24］PROCTOR M，FARQUHAR C. Diagnosis and management of dysmenorrhea［J］. BMJ，2006，332（7550）：1134-1138.

［25］NASIR L，BOPE E T. Management of pelvic pain from dysmenorrhea or endometriosis［J］. J Am Board Fam Pract，2004，17（Suppl）：S43-S47.